Motor Learning and Control

From Theory to Practice

William H. Edwards
California State University, Sacramento

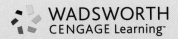

WADSWORTH
CENGAGE Learning™

Australia • Brazil • Japan • Korea • Mexico • Singapore • Spain • United Kingdom • United States

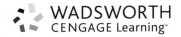

Motor Learning and Control: From Theory to Practice, 1e
William H. Edwards

Publisher: Yolanda Cossio

Acquisitions Editor: Laura Pople

Developmental Editor: Nedah Rose

Assistant Editor: Samantha Arvin

Editorial Assistant: Kristina Chiapella

Media Editor: Miriam Myers

Marketing Manager: Laura McGinn

Marketing Assistant: Elizabeth Wong

Marketing Communications Manager: Linda Yip

Senior Content Project Manager: Carol Samet

Creative Director: Rob Hugel

Art Director: John Walker

Print Buyer: Paula Vang

Rights Acquisitions Specialist, Text: Roberta Broyer

Rights Acquisitions Specialist, Image: Dean Dauphinais

Production Service: MPS Limited, A Macmillan Company

Text Designer: Diane Beasley

Photo Researcher: Raquel Sousa/Pre-PressPMG

Text Permissions Researcher: Isabel Saraiva

Copy Editor: Jill Pellarin

Illustrator: MPS Limited, A Macmillan Company

Cover Designer: Jeanne Calabrese

Cover Images: Moment/cultura/Corbis (left); Andy Sacks/Getty Images (top right); Tommy Olofsson/Getty Images (top middle); Seth Joel/Getty Images (bottom middle); Steve Hix/Somos Images/Corbis (bottom right)

Compositor: MPS Limited, A Macmillan Company

For product information and technology assistance, contact us at **Cengage Learning Customer & Sales Support, 1-800-354-9706**
For permission to use material from this text or product, submit all requests online at **www.cengage.com/permissions**
Further permissions questions can be e-mailed to **permissionrequest@cengage.com**

Library of Congress Control Number: 2010922549

ISBN-13: 978-0-495-01080-7

ISBN-10: 0-495-01080-4

Wadsworth
20 Davis Drive
Belmont, CA 94002-3098
USA

Cengage Learning is a leading provider of customized learning solutions with office locations around the globe, including Singapore, the United Kingdom, Australia, Mexico, Brazil, and Japan. Locate your local office at **www.cengage.com/global**.

Cengage Learning products are represented in Canada by Nelson Education, Ltd.

To learn more about Wadsworth, visit **www.cengage.com/**Wadsworth.

Purchase any of our products at your local college store or at our preferred online store **www.CengageBrain.com**.

Printed in the United States of America
1 2 3 4 5 6 7 14 13 12 11 10

DEDICATION

For Barbara

BRIEF CONTENTS

CONTENTS

PREFACE

The scholarly study of motor learning and control is one of the most fascinating as well as practical of academic disciplines. The fabric of our daily activities is stitched together by thousands of individual motor acts every day. Being able to move—and beyond that, to move skillfully—not only makes life possible but shapes and gives purpose to our lives. The first objective in writing this book was to convey something of the excitement and essential character of this important area of inquiry and scholarship to students studying for careers in movement-related fields. I know from experience that unless students are initially engaged by and interested in a subject, no amount of academic planning and rigor, no manner how well-conceived, will prove favorable in gaining their best efforts and in optimizing their learning potential. In writing this book, I have made every attempt to present information in ways that are meaningful, accessible, and thought provoking to its readers.

A second primary purpose of this book was to offer a comprehensive and contemporary overview of the major areas of study in motor learning and control. Moreover, a major purpose was to present these from the several different perspectives applied to scholarly study and research in the field today. Until fairly recently, the scholarly study of motor skills has been the purview of one dominating theoretical perspective or another, with the particular perspective in vogue at any time shifting with the winds of the favored psychological theories of the day. Today that has changed. Motor learning and control have become major areas of study within a wide variety of disciplines, including neural science, cognitive psychology, computer science, engineering, robotics, developmental studies, philosophy, and kinesiology. The careers in which skill development plays an essential role have also expanded from traditional fields of athletics and physical education, and now include physical and occupational therapy, performing arts, occupational and industrial training, the design of medical assistive devices, and human factors. Courses in motor learning and control, which were historically and are still housed almost exclusively in departments of kinesiology, must serve the needs and goals of a diverse student body. Indeed, kinesiology has become, in the twenty-first century, a major of choice as a gateway field for students preparing in widely diverse career fields.

This wide diversity of scholarly perspectives and career options related to the study of skilled human movement means that a textbook must cover a broad terrain of both theory and application. Traversing that broad terrain is another major goal of the current text. After introducing the basic perceptual and neurological foundations necessary for studying motor learning and control intelligently, the two major contemporary theories applied to the study and understanding of motor skills, cognitively based information processing theories and dynamical systems theories, are presented. Throughout the book, the attempt has been to show how each theory offers advantages and insights into our knowledge of how people control and learn movement skills. Indeed, this book takes the position that both theoretical approaches have much to offer and that in matters of discerning good instructional applications we can learn much from both. In terms of theoretical accuracy, I have constantly attempted to provide a fair presentation and evaluation of both theories, pointing to the values inherent in each, as well as the areas of possible inadequacies needing further development in each.

Beyond the specifics of neurological findings or theoretical assumptions, chapters present examples of research investigations related to the topics presented. The intent here is to demonstrate that much, if not most, of what we do know about effective principles and techniques for instructing motor skills is based upon sound empirical research, even when disagreements may exist over the underlying mechanisms and theoretical assumptions supporting those practical findings.

This book, then, is aimed at providing a comprehensive, authoritative, and engaging overview of the major areas of study in motor learning and control from a broadly encompassing theoretical and scholarly perspective. Its intended audience includes students preparing in any of the diverse career fields in which skillful human movement is an essential component. The text is specifically designed for use in an upper-division undergraduate or beginning graduate course in motor learning and control, and assumes some basic college-level background in human anatomy and physiology.

Finally, it is hoped that this book also serves a more general purpose in highlighting the significance of movement skills in every facet of human life, and helps initiate readers into a lifelong appreciation for the importance and wonder of skillful human actions.

ORGANIZATION OF THE TEXT

This book is organized into 12 chapters. The first two chapters are designed to introduce the field of study covered in the text. Chapter 1 introduces and defines the two disciplines motor learning and motor control, and discusses why it is essential they be studied together when application is a major interest. The chapter also presents a brief history of these two disciplines, identifies their relevance and applicability in a number of career fields, and finishes with a section concerning why the study of motor learning and control is important for students in these movement-related career fields. Chapter 2 introduces the subject matter of the text: human motor skills. The essential characteristics of motor skills are identified and thoroughly discussed, and the major problems confronting researchers and theorists studying motor skills are presented. Methods for classifying motor skills are also presented in this chapter. Together, these two chapters circumscribe the area of study for the text, establish the problems and areas of concern for movement scientists in the area, and relate the field of study to areas of personal and career interests among readers.

After introducing the field of study, the remainder of the book is organized around three groupings of chapters that, if viewed as a progressive series of topics, represent the book's subtitle: "From Theory to Practice." Chapters 3 and 4 present the neurological and theoretical underpinnings of contemporary motor learning and control. Chapter 3 is concerned with relating information on the perceptual and neurological activities and structures of the central nervous system. It conveys a solid understanding of the workings of the motor system in controlling human movement, as well as the changes that occur over the course of learning. Chapter 4 follows with a thorough presentation of the two major contemporary theories of motor learning and control, namely cognitive-based theories focusing on information processing approaches such as schema theory, and dynamical systems approaches focusing on the constructs of constraints, attraction, self-organization, and emergence. Also presented in this chapter is a discussion of the work of Nikolia Bernstein, whose ideas of synergies and learning progressions in many ways form an intellectual bridge between cognitively based information processing and dynamical systems approaches.

Chapters 5 through 8 are aimed at providing a comprehensive introduction to the foundations of learning. Chapter 5 discusses the basic laws and fundamental principles of learning, such as performance curves, the Law of Practice, the asymptotic nature of learning, and the transfer of learning. The chapter also presents a discussion and example of how learning is assessed using acquisition, retention, and transfer measures, and explicitly presents and discusses the distinction between performance and learning, which is carried forward as a major theme throughout the remainder of the text. Chapter 6 presents a discussion of the role of memory in learning. Although most of the work in memory research has been conducted from cognitive-based theoretical models and is covered as such, the chapter also gives due consideration to the concepts of affordances and attunement as prescribed by ecological psychological approaches within dynamical systems models. Chapter 7 discusses the stages of learning. Presented here are the three-stage models of Fitts and Posner representing cognitive-based information processing models, and the more recent model by Vereijken et al., developed from dynamical systems theory. The concept of expertise and high-level performance is also presented and discussed in this chapter. Chapter 8 is concerned with individual differences in motor skill capabilities and discusses the factors responsible for differences in how people acquire and perform motor skills.

The final four chapters of the book complete the progression from theory to practice by focusing on the practice experience. By this time students should possess a solid basis for understanding the implications of theory for practice design. A premise of this book is that practice understood in the context of theory and fundamental principles of learning is a prerequisite to both comprehensive understanding and effective application of practice strategies and techniques. Chapter 9 presents pre-practice considerations concerning motivation and attention, providing techniques for optimizing both among learners. Chapter 10 presents an overview of contemporary findings and thinking related to the provision of verbal instructions and visual demonstrations, both practical areas having undergone considerable rethinking in light of contemporary research findings. Chapter 11 then discusses a number of factors involved in the design of practice experiences, including the scheduling of practice when teaching both a single skill and several skills within a practice session, the distribution or spacing of practice both within and between practice sessions, and part-practice techniques and their appropriate uses. Chapter 12 concludes the chapters on practice with a presentation of the important topic of feedback, including the uses, roles, and strategies for providing effective feedback.

Finally, an appendix is provided covering aspects of laboratory research and the preparation of written laboratory or research reports. This information is provided in appendixes for classes in which laboratory experiences are included, or in which instructors wish to include additional information concerning research techniques and practices.

PEDAGOGICAL FEATURES

A number of features have been added to chapters to aid student learning. A pedagogical approach, based on considerable research support, that students learn best when a text requires constant self-examination and application of content material, was a guiding principle in the preparation and writing of this book. By engaging student interest, critical reflection, and thoughtful application of the materials presented, the text aims to deepen both content knowledge and the students' critical thinking and decision-making abilities related to the control and learning of motor skills.

Figures and tables illustrating textual content have been included wherever necessary and helpful in clarifying chapter topics.

As a special feature of the text, boxes within chapters have been provided to add additional information expanding upon that in the text. These are often in the form of real-life examples in which textual content is applied in actual situations. Other boxes present exercises for students to test their understanding of topics, as well as to develop skills in applying chapter content in movement-related contexts. Boxes help carry students through the chapters by providing constant reinforcement of main topical ideas through real-life examples, professional applications, and personal applications designed to enhance both student interest and learning of the chapter content.

At the conclusion of each chapter are several pedagogical features designed to help students evaluate their grasp of chapter content, provide additional learning experiences, and serve as resources for further study and preparation for course evaluations.

Immediately following the chapter summaries are several Learning Exercises. These exercises include critical analyses and application exercises in which chapter topics must be used to solve professional and movement-skill problems, as well as field observations. The field observations include both interview and observational analyses. In these later examples, students are asked to observe various skill performance situations, collect data, perform critical analyses and draw conclusions, and summarize their findings in written reports. Several exercises covering various areas of concern with varying degrees of complexity, as well as both critical thinking and field analysis exercises, are included for each chapter. These Learning Exercises may be used in a variety of different ways, including as individual assignments, group assignments, class projects, formal laboratory exercises, and additional evaluative tools. Instructors may also find many of the Learning Exercises suited for class assignment and discussion, and might well build some lectures around these projects. As with many of the previous aspects of the text, these exercises are designed expressly to involve students more completely in their own learning.

The For Further Study section begins with a short multiple-choice and completion quiz, testing students' knowledge of the chapter and helping them identify possible areas in need of reevaluation or additional study.

The section Study Questions, as the name implies, lists a number of questions around which students might organize their review and study of the chapter; taken as a whole, the Study Questions offer a thorough overview of the major areas covered within a chapter.

The For Further Study section ends with suggestions for further reading relative to the topics presented within the chapter. All of the suggested readings are from readily available sources, so course instructors can make them available though their respective college and university libraries if desired.

INSTRUCTOR RESOURCES

PowerLecture DVD-ROM: This one-stop course preparation and presentation resource makes it easy for instructors to assemble, edit, publish, and present custom lectures for your course, using PowerPoint. The PowerLecture DVD-ROM includes PowerPoint slides with all art and tables from the book, the Instructor's Manual, the test bank, and videos.

Test Bank: The test bank features an assortment of over 400 multiple-choice, completion, and short answer essay questions. The Test Bank is included on the PowerLecture DVD.

Instructor's Manual: Authored by William Edwards, this comprehensive manual includes chapter objectives, annotated lecture presentation outlines, and classroom activity suggestions. The Instructor's Manual is found on the PowerLecture DVD.

STUDENT RESOURCES

CourseMate: The CourseMate brings course concepts to life with interactive learning, study, and exam preparation tools that support the printed textbook. The CourseMate includes an interactive eBook, interactive teaching and learning tools including quizzes, flashcards, videos, and more. It also contains the Engagement Tracker, a first-of-its-kind tool that monitors student engagement in the course.

ACKNOWLEDGMENTS

Although many people have contributed to this text in ways probably both they and I do not realize or have long forgotten—including my fourth-grade teacher Mrs. LaDue, who made me write essays even when I complained that I was incapable of it and had no reason for learning to do so at any rate, and then both ruthlessly corrected and profusely praised my efforts when I did produce the required paper—there are still a few people that I must identify for special acknowledgment.

No academic should forget those special men and women who taught him and whose teachings, belief in his abilities, and encouragement initiated him into the world of scholarship and academe. I was fortunate to have had several such mentors. These include Art Ridgeway and Lynn Emery at California State Polytechnic University, and Roger Burke, J. Tillman Hall, Earl Pullias, and Ruth Sparhawk at the University of Southern California. Each, in his or her own way, encouraged, inspired, and shaped my academic and professional interests and development. This book hopefully reflects some of the many lessons that they passed on to me.

Rob Carlson, who was my department chair at San Diego State University (now Dean at California State University, San Bernardino), was instrumental in his support at a critical time in my early professional years. Without his professional support and generosity, this book, and possibly the career that spawned it, may never have taken form.

My colleagues and students at California State University, Sacramento, have provided many opportunities for both reflection and development of the ideas in this book. From my students, I have learned that teaching most profitably moves in two directions, from teacher to students and from students to teacher, if an instructor allows. Especially for my motor learning students who used earlier drafts of this book as their class text, and whose interest and many suggestions contributed to its development (and the idea for the cover), I am appreciative.

The good folks at Cengage Learning and their publishing auxiliaries have been a joy to work with and have always displayed high professional expertise in rendering this text in its final form. I must mention especially Nedah Rose, senior development editor at Cengage Learning, who has been the best, and certainly most patient, editor for whom any writer could ask. This book would not have taken initial shape, nor have come to ultimate fruition, without her belief in it.

Finally, I am most grateful for the opportunity to acknowledge the significant contributions of my wife, Barbara Edwards, to the development of this work. She read, reread, edited, and reread again every word in these chapters many times over. Her suggestions for changes in wording and content have significantly contributed to the clarity and usefulness of the text. Her many late nights editing my latest draft before I sent it off to the publisher the following morning deserve an A+ in spousal support. Of course, my greatest support has come, as always, from her love, encouragement, and constant faith shared in our "cord of three." It is to her that this book is dedicated.

Before closing these acknowledgments, I would be remiss not to recall that throughout the preparation of this book I have also been helped by comments from a variety of reviewers. The book is stronger for their comments and suggestions.

Laura Abbott	*Georgia State University*
Harold Barkhoff	*University of Hawaii–Hilo*
Eric Berglund	*Miami University of Ohio*
John Buchanan	*Texas A&M University*
Michael Butler	*Emporia State University*
Brian Church	*Arkansas State University*
Rebecca Crowley	*University of Texas–Arlington*
Daniel Czech	*Georgia Southern University*
Doug Dickin	*University of Idaho*
Mark Fischman	*Auburn University*
Noreen Goggin	*University of North Texas*
Florian Kagerer	*University of Maryland*
Susan Kasser	*University of Vermont*
Chris Kovacs	*Western Illinois University*
Rick Lambson	*Southern Utah University*
Russell Lord	*Montana State University*
Jonathan Metzler	*Georgia Southern University*
Virginia Overdorf	*William Paterson University*
Julie Partridge	*Southern Illinois University*
Monica Pazmino-Cevallos	*Radford University*
Steven Radlo	*Western Illinois University*
Barry Schulz	*University of Utah*
Judy Schulz	*Washington State University*
David Sherwood	*University of Colorado*
Ann Smiley-Owen	*Iowa State University*
Phillip Tomporowski	*University of Georgia*
Howard Zelaznik	*Purdue University*

William H. Edwards,
California State University, Sacramento

Introduction

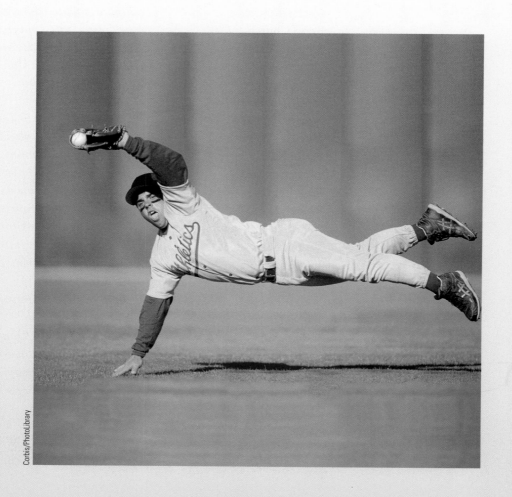

"There is no such thing on earth as an uninteresting subject; the only thing that can exist is an uninterested person."
G.K. Chesterton (1874–1936)

KEY QUESTIONS

- What role do movement skills play in human life?
- What is motor learning?
- What is motor control?
- How are motor learning and motor control studied?
- In what professional fields does knowledge in motor learning and control play a critical role?
- Why should you study motor learning and motor control?

CHAPTER OVERVIEW

Two fundamental questions lie at the heart of human movement. The first asks how humans acquire movement skills. How do we learn the thousands of skills we use every day and which make life possible? How do we learn to walk and to climb stairs, to write our names and to use a keyboard, drive an automobile or fly an airplane, hit a golf ball or perform a triple axel; how do we learn to dance and to use complicated machinery and to hit home runs and to play the violin? How do we learn all of the skills that stitch together the fabric on which the pattern of our life is given expression and meaning?

The second question asks how movement skills are controlled. How do we interpret information within the environment, decide upon movement responses, organize muscular commands to carry out those responses, and adapt our movements to changing conditions? How do we coordinate the movements of a muscular-skeletal architecture capable of assuming an almost infinite variety of movement patterns, harnessing them into the precise skills required by athletes, professional dancers, or surgeons—or even everyday skills like putting on eyeliner, playing a video game, or driving an automobile on a busy street.

Movement scientists who search for answers concerning these two questions organize their inquiries into two separate, yet jointly pursued, scholarly disciples. Motor learning is the discipline concerned with answering the first question: How do people acquire movement skills? How can those skills best be taught? Motor control, the other of these two disciplines, seeks to answer the question: How are movement skills controlled? How are the actions of limbs and bodily segments coordinated in order to achieve a movement goal? Although there are distinct differences between these two disciplines, they also form a unified study of significant importance to professionals in many fields, and for that reason are studied together when our interests are in professional application.

In this chapter, we will introduce these two scholarly disciplines—motor learning and motor control. Together, they form the foundational knowledge concerned with the analysis, instruction, and rehabilitation of movement skills.

———————

Human life is shaped by the capacity for skilled movement. Some movement skills make life possible. Without essential movement skills, we could not protect ourselves from the dangers of our environment, construct shelter, provide food, move from one place to another, or reproduce.

Beyond making survival possible, movement skills underlie virtually every aspect of human existence. The average person completes thousands of voluntary, skilled movement acts every day. Many of these are accomplished with little or no conscious awareness, whereas others may take considerable thought and effort. One thing that they all have in common, though, is that at some point each was learned. People are not born possessing such movement skills, but acquire them in order to adapt to the demands of the environment. These learned capacities are called *motor skills*, and they underlie the many diverse activities comprising human life. (We will define motor skills more completely in Chapter 2.)

What a piece of work is man... in form, in moving, how express and admirable!

—Shakespeare, *Hamlet*

Motor skills are ubiquitous. They form the backdrop against which human life is acted out. Many of our basic motor skills are acquired as we grow and mature. During the first year or two of life, we first learn to crawl and then to walk, to reach for objects, grasp things, and to avoid bumping into obstacles in our environment. As we grow, we learn other skills—how to use eating utensils, dress ourselves, open doors, run, jump, climb, and perhaps ride a bicycle. Many other movement experiences are learned during school years and add to our growing repertoire of motor skills. We learn to write, draw, paint, use musical instruments, play games, dance, and use new kinds of tools and equipment. As we mature into adults, we continually learn new motor skills to meet our growing needs and interests. Many of these skills, especially those that are complex or specialized, we acquire in formal instructional settings. These may include skills learned in school as well as in occupational settings, sports and recreational programs, dance studios, fitness centers, rehabilitation clinics, and the many other places where people acquire the large variety of motor skills making up daily life.

Therefore, the provision of effective instruction in a wide and diverse variety of motor skills is a significant societal need, and one having widespread ramifications for the quality of individual lives as well as the life of the culture as a whole. Meeting these important individual and societal needs requires the preparation of instructional professionals who possess a sound knowledge of the factors underlying the learning or rehabilitation of motor skills. Such knowledge comprises the disciplines of motor learning and motor control.

ACQUIRING KNOWLEDGE CONCERNING MOTOR SKILLS

How is knowledge in the disciplines of motor learning and control acquired? What kind of knowledge about motor skills is important for instructional professionals to possess? That is, how do people best learn motor skills? What are the most effective ways to instruct such skills? How are motor skills controlled, and how does understanding how they are controlled translate into more effective training and rehabilitation programs?

To answer these questions, let us start by first addressing one of the primary ways in which people, including many professionals involved in the instruction of motor skills, gain knowledge about the learning and instruction of skills. For many people, their first and sometimes only way of acquiring knowledge about motor skills is through experience and tradition. Such knowledge is based on the way things have always been done, on the way that one does it oneself, or on the way that experts do it.

Such an appeal to experience and tradition does have much to recommend it, and it would be foolish to neglect experience altogether. Experience is often a good teacher, and the test of time is an important guard against untested fads and the fleeting novelties that often comprise the "latest and best" new methods. The appeal to experience can also be an appeal to authority. Experience tells us that things should be done in a certain way because that is the way that experts do them. The experts in question may include successful athletic coaches, champion athletes, professional dance instructors, experienced therapists, and others having authority that comes with success. Certainly, there is much to be learned from the knowledge possessed by experts and the wisdom gained through experience. But is this the best way to acquire valid knowledge? Should we base our understanding and practice concerning motor skills on experience alone?

Let us answer this question with a thought experiment. Consider where such an appeal to knowledge built only on experience and authority may lead us. Suppose, for the purposes of our experiment, that we were able to sample a large number of experts in various fields involving the instruction of motor skills. These would include individuals such as physical education teachers, athletic coaches, physical and occupational therapists, recreation specialists, and occupational trainers. What could we learn from this sampling of experts? What knowledge would they convey to us?

Let us pretend that we carried out this plan for acquiring information on effective instructional practices for motor skills. What would we discover? Based upon experience and tradition, what is known about the most effective principles for instructing motor skills? Carrying out our experiment, we would arrive at agreement concerning many principles and guidelines for the effective instruction of motor skills. (For the questioning reader, there is a vast literature written by experts in various motor skills from which such principles can be drawn.) Let us offer 15 such guidelines, which you will find listed in Box 1.1. These 15 are all widely held, and supported by considerable experience as well by the weight of authority. Even so, there is nothing particularly special about these specific 15 guidelines in our list. Many more could be added. The list can be considered representative, however, of the many traditionally accepted principles and guidelines for the instruction of motor skills based upon common and widely accepted practice. Before proceeding further, read through the list in Box 1.1. As you do, see how many of the guidelines you are familiar with and how many you accept as good instructional principles.

After reading though the guidelines in Box 1.1, how many of them did you recognize? Based upon your experiences, how many do you accept as valid guidelines about how people learn motor skills and about the best methods for

---

BOX **1.1**   Some Principles Concerning Motor Skills Derived Through Appeals to Tradition and Authority

1. The best measure of how well a person is learning a new skill is how well he or she can perform the skill in practice.

2. Generally, how well a person performs a skill when first learning it is the best indication of his or her potential for learning the skill.

3. Except for strength and running speed, men and women possess the same capabilities for learning movement skills.

4. Some people possess a genetically endowed, generalized motor capacity predisposing them to be good at virtually all movement skills.

5. Skills should never be practiced when a person is so fatigued that his or her performance of the skill suffers, because doing so may lead to the learning of bad habits that can later prove hard to break.

6. When learning complex motor skills having many parts, breaking the skill into smaller component parts and practicing each until it can be performed well before reassembling the parts and performing the skill as a whole is typically an effective practice method.

7. An important goal of practice is the development of muscle memory.

8. When instructing someone in a new skill, an effective teacher should provide corrective feedback as frequently as practically possible.

9. When having learners practice several different new skills during a practice session, instructors should avoid mixing the skills, but instead have learners repeat each skill separately for a number of practice attempts so that they can get the idea of the different skills and be able to more easily perform and learn them.

10. Unless limited by equipment design or game rules, on average, left-handed individuals learn movement skills as easily as do right-handed individuals.

11. A skill that will be performed in one specific way only should be practiced only in that specific way.

12. When learning a new skill, observing a model performing the skill correctly is more beneficial than watching a model who is committing errors while performing the skill.

13. When tracking a moving object such as a pitched ball, it is important to keep the head still so that the eyes can most effectively focus on the object.

14. Beginners should be encouraged to relax and not to overthink how they are performing new skills, but instead to allow nonconscious and automatic processes to operate and aid learning.

15. As a practice goal, instructors should have learners practice new skills in ways that promote the best performance of those skills.

teaching people motor skills? More generally, how many of these 15 principles should a knowledgeable motor skills instructor employ?

If you want to carry this experiment one step further, you could take the list of principles and observe one or more professionals during an instructional session. It would come as no surprise to you, most likely, if you observed many of these suggested guides to good instruction being put into action. It should not come as a surprise, either, if you observed learners improve their levels of skill as a result of instructions based upon these guidelines. After all, they are each the result of observing what has worked in the past, of what experience teaches us. That is, individuals following these guidelines do learn motor skills.

Your next question might be, "If experience is an effective teacher when learning about motor skills and how to instruct them, why a text (or class) on the subject? In fact, why not just learn from experience or, at least, rely upon the authority of professionals and other experts?" Especially for those who have been involved in learning and performing skills at high levels, such as competitive athletes or professional performers, this conclusion can be a tempting one, indeed. Such a question is appropriate and wise to ask at this point. The conclusion that it might be best to skip the formal learning experiences of class and text and instead just rely on the experiences and tradition of those who participate in the teaching and learning of motor skills might be a valid conclusion. That is, it might be valid except for one thing. That one thing is that all 15 principles we have presented, and a good many more we could have likewise convincingly stated, are false!

At this point, the reader may be saying, "Wait a minute, was it not just stated that all 15 principles work, that they do result in the learning of motor skills just as experience shows?" The answer is both yes and no! We did say that individuals following these guidelines improve their motor skills. What we did not say, however, was that the 15 guidelines represent the best and most effective knowledge on which to base instruction. Of the guidelines listed here, some are partially effective, whereas others are almost totally ineffective. None, however, represents the most effective instructional guideline for the particular aspect of practice it addresses (we will see the particular problem with each of theses 15 guidelines in the chapters ahead). The reason that these 15 guidelines appear to work is because practice, even relatively ineffective practice, almost always results in learning. Practice is the single most important variable in learning, and even when it is less than optimally structured, considerable likelihood remains that it will promote improvement in the skills practiced.

The next question an attentive reader might ask is, "Why, if these are not the most effective principles on which to base learning experiences, have they come to be held in such high status by experts?" The answer to that question is something we will be developing throughout this book (but which we can now say is something referred to as a *learning–performance distinction*). The real question is, What kind of knowledge is best, and on what kinds of knowledge should professionals base their practice and methods? The answer advanced in this book is that such knowledge should be arrived at scientifically, through experimentation and critical analyses of experimental findings, rather than by

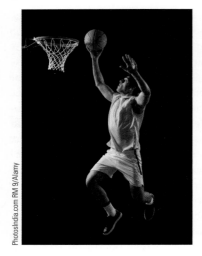

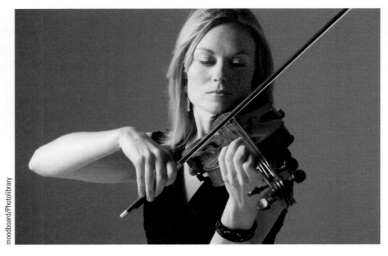

Motor learning entails the study of how individuals acquire and improve the wide variety of human movement skills possible.

appeal to experience and authority. A major premise throughout this book is that the best knowledge for guiding effective practice is gained through scientific inquiry. Although experience can provide many insights, and should not be discounted, we have just seen that experience alone can lead to false conclusions and relatively ineffectual practices. The scientific approach, on the other hand, offers the most valid and reliable method for discovering objective, factual knowledge upon which to base instructional programs and the promise that such programs hold for learners. The two scholarly disciplines of motor learning and motor control are both grounded in the scientific method. A scholarly discipline encompasses accepted methodological approaches, theoretical assumptions, and a body of knowledge addressing some phenomena of interest and study. Motor learning and control are those disciplines in which the phenomena of interest are the acquisition and control of human motor skills, both based upon scientific methods and theoretical constructs resulting in scientifically validated knowledge. We will look more closely at each of these scientific disciplines next.

MOTOR LEARNING AND MOTOR CONTROL

Although the study of motor skills is encompassed by many fields of study, the specific study of how skills are acquired and controlled comprises the scholarly disciplines of motor learning and motor control, respectively. These two closely related disciplines have as their central focus of inquiry the scientific study of the factors responsible for the development of skilled physical behaviors in humans, as well as the factors underlying the execution of those behaviors. These two disciplines are closely intertwined, and indeed their distinction might best be thought of as a useful way of organizing clusters of similar questions for study, rather than marking a strict demarcation among motor skill phenomena. In practice, the processes of motor learning and motor control comprise a symbiotic blending of factors underlying the acquisition and production of motor skills (see Figure 1.1). Factors responsible for the control of motor skills also influence the learning of those skills, and the learning of skills influences the development of those factors responsible for their control and production. Moreover, the processes and conditions subserving motor learning and control constantly change and interact in subtle ways. Like the two sides of a coin, motor learning and motor control differ and may each be inspected for their specific details, but they each remain metal of a single coin.

Motor Learning

motor learning: The discipline concerned with the processes underlying the acquisition and performance of motor skills.

Motor learning is the study of the processes involved in acquiring motor skills and of the variables that promote or inhibit such acquisition. In defining motor skills, we said that they are movement capacities that are learned rather than gained through normal growth and development. Those factors influencing the learning of motor skills, whether through normal daily experiences or within formal instructional settings, entail the study of motor learning. How do people learn skills? Why are some skills more difficult to learn than others? Why do people differ in their capacity for skill learning? What are the best ways to teach somebody a new skill? What is the best way to rehabilitate a skill lost due to injury or disease?

Many factors influence the learning of motor skills, but it is common to classify them into three distinct categories. These categories include the study of (1) the learner, (2) the skill to be learned, and (3) the conditions under which

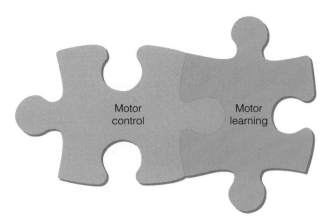

FIGURE **1.1** The Interconnected Relationship of Motor Control and Motor Learning

Source: Created by the author.

the skill is learned. All three factors play a significant role in the acquisition of motor skills. Any complete analysis of the learning of motor skills, therefore, requires the consideration of each of these aspects of learning. Considerations pertaining to the learner include factors such as age, sex, physical condition, intelligence, psychological characteristics, and existing skill levels and previous experiences. Individuals learn at different rates and benefit differently from various kinds of instructions. An understanding of instructional processes must take such differences into account. The nature of a skill being learned also plays a significant role in learning. Different skills benefit from instructional and practice designs differently. The identification of these differences and the classification of skills into categories relative to such differences are important prerequisites to the study of effective instructional design. Motor skill instructors need to know that what works when teaching one skill may not work well when instructing another skill, not because of any differences in learners but because the skills are different. Finally, the environment in which a skill is acquired impacts the effectiveness of learning. This includes both the social and physical environments. Socially, whether a skill is practiced alone or in the company of others, the nature of the instructor–learner relationship, and the emotional experience of the learning environment all influence learning. Aspects of the physical environment that influence learning are many and include the availability and use of equipment, physical features of the environment, time of day, lighting conditions, and environmental distractions. A special class of environmental influences entails the biomechanical aspects of a learner's bodily interaction with the physical environment, and the ways in which both static and dynamic forces impact performance and learning. These three factors influencing the learning of motor skills are illustrated in Figure 1.2.

Though the study of motor learning entails a broad analysis of many features, we can offer as a working definition that motor learning is the process by which the capacity to produce motor skills is changed as a result of instruction, practice, or experience, and of the influences that the learner, task, and environment play in those processes. A consideration of some questions typical to motor learning may provide a good beginning to understanding and appreciating this area of inquiry concerning motor skills. A list of such questions is presented in Table 1.1 (after reading the table, also consider the exercise in Box 1.2).

Motor Control

motor control: The discipline concerned with the underlying mechanisms responsible for human movement and stability.

Motor control involves the study of the neural, behavioral, environmental, and synergistic mechanisms responsible for human movement and stability. All motor skills, regardless of the level of skill with which they are executed, are expressions of the motor control system. The final target of this system is the muscles and joints responsible for executing action. Two outcomes of muscular control are paramount to motor control—the control of movements and the control of stability or posture.

When moving the body from one location to another, or moving the limbs to produce desired skills, the motor control system is responsible for coordinating the activity of over 600 muscles in the body. How are the muscular

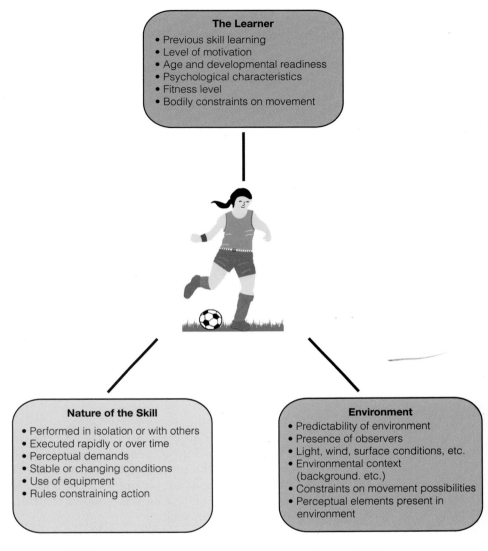

The Learner
- Previous skill learning
- Level of motivation
- Age and developmental readiness
- Psychological characteristics
- Fitness level
- Bodily constraints on movement

Nature of the Skill
- Performed in isolation or with others
- Executed rapidly or over time
- Perceptual demands
- Stable or changing conditions
- Use of equipment
- Rules constraining action

Environment
- Predictability of environment
- Presence of observers
- Light, wind, surface conditions, etc.
- Environmental context (background. etc.)
- Constraints on movement possibilities
- Perceptual elements present in environment

FIGURE **1.2** Factors Influencing the Learning of Motor Skills

Source: Created by the author.

commands to carry out these movements planned, organized, and executed? Certainly, the answer involves an integration of various bodily systems, including the brain and central nervous system, the muscular system, and perceptual systems. But motor control also occurs within a particular context including the physical environment, which both contributes to and constrains movement activities. Additionally, the requirements and nature of the skill executed further influence the way in which movements must be controlled. So

TABLE **1.1**

Examples of Questions Studied by Motor Learning Theorists

- Should instructors demonstrate only how to perform skills correctly, or should errors also be demonstrated?
- Should beginners be taught how to analyze their movement errors?
- Should a performer focus attention on his or her bodily movements?
- How can a coach or instructor estimate an individual's potential for learning a particular skill?
- When should part practice be used in teaching skills?
- Are there recognizable stages in the process of skill learning?
- Should skills which are intended to be performed in only one way, be practiced in only that way?
- How frequently should learners be provided with corrective feedback?
- What information should feedback convey?
- How can bulletin boards and visual displays best be used as teaching aids?
- Is the use of mirrors in teaching skills such as dance effective for learning?
- Can skills be taught in ways to enhance long-term memory and limit forgetting?
- Is slow-motion practice beneficial?
- How much rest should be provided during individual practice sessions?
- How much time should elapse between practice sessions?
- Are there differences in the ways that individuals learn?
- Should practice emphasize consistency, or variability?
- What are the major problems learners face when first practicing a new skill?

both the nature of the skill being performed and the context in which it is performed must be taken into account when explaining the underlying mechanisms responsible for the control of movement skills. There is considerable theoretical debate among motor control scholars today about the relative contributions made by each of these aspects of motor control, and the role and relative importance played by each.

Motor control is also the study of stability or postures. How does a person maintain his or her stability and equilibrium in a changing environment? How does the person remain upright when walking or sitting, for example, or maintain a supportive posture when running or reaching for an object? Motor control theorists seek to understand the mechanisms underlying stability and the

BOX **1.2**   **Asking Motor Learning Questions**

Select a motor skill in which you are interested and possess at least a moderate degree of proficiency. Think about the factors that might affect somebody initially learning this skill. Prepare a list of ten questions, specific to the skill you selected, concerning factors influencing the learning of the skill that would be studied in the discipline of motor learning.

maintenance of various postures, events often taken for granted but essential in virtually every activity in which humans engage.

As a working definition, we can define motor control as the study of the mechanisms that underlie and are responsible for human movement and stability. While the study of motor control is diverse and covers many topics, as was the case with motor learning a good way to begin developing an appreciation for this field of study is to consider some typical questions addressed by motor control theorists. Again, as we did for motor learning, a sampling of such questions is presented in Table 1.2, with a further exercise for consideration presented in Box 1.3.

A BRIEF HISTORY OF MOTOR LEARNING AND MOTOR CONTROL

It is difficult to identify an exact beginning date for motor learning and control as fields of scientific inquiry. The major problem in determining a beginning date is that two different disciplines can equally claim ancestry in the fields of studying motor learning and motor control. The disciplines of

TABLE **1.2**
Examples of Questions Studied by Motor Control Theorists

- How is muscular activity organized and controlled?
- How do the many different systems contributing to movement collectively organize to accomplish a single goal?
- What aspects of a movement are stored in memory?
- How are reflexes involved in the control of movement?
- What is the best way to recover the use of an injured joint?
- Do experts use vision differently than do beginners when performing motor skills?
- How do people maintain their balance when spinning around?
- Why do most people find it difficult, if not impossible, to pat their head while rubbing their stomach?
- Why do some skills become automatic?
- How can people drive their cars for many miles without being conscious of thinking about driving?
- Why do stroke patients have difficulty with speech and gait?
- Why do people find it impossible to stop some movements once they have begun?
- How do humans match perceptual information to appropriate motor commands?
- What are the neurological bases for diseases of the motor control system such as Parkinson's disease and myasthenia Gravis?
- Are people born possessing innate capacities limiting them in certain skills, or is their potential always unlimited given sufficient practice?
- How and why does alcohol affect movement control?
- What changes occur in the brain as a result of learning a new motor skill?
- Why are people good at some skills, but not at others?

neurophysiology and psychology both produced important early work relative to motor skills, setting the stage for what came later. Although both disciplines have origins in the 19th century, they pursued different areas of inquiry. A number of good reviews of the history of motor learning and motor control are available, and the interested reader is directed to them (Adams, 1987; Meijer, 2001; Summers, 2004). We will offer only a brief sketch of this history here, formed around broad periods we will label, somewhat arbitrarily, early, middle, and modern.

Early Period

By the 1870s, a number of physiologists had begun investigating the links between the central nervous system and muscular activity. These inquiries came to represent a specialized area of physiology called *neurophysiology*. A number of early neurophysiologists significantly advanced knowledge concerning how muscles functioned and were innovated by nerve impulses. These studies represent the earliest forays into questions of motor control.

The most important contributions concerning motor control during this period were those associated with the work of the English physiologist Sir Charles Sherrington (1857–1952). Sherrington discovered many of the basic mechanisms underlying the neural control of movement on which contemporary motor control theories are still grounded, He developed, for instance, the concepts of reciprocal innervation and the final common pathway. *Reciprocal innervation* refers to the complementary relaxation of one muscle when its antagonist is contracted. The *final common pathway* was Sherrington's term for his discovery that nerve impulses from many sources, including various areas of the brain, sensory receptors, and reflexes, converged in the spinal column to form a single unified signal to muscles. Sherrington also made important discoveries adding to our knowledge of reflexes and their role in motor control.

The other important physiologist from this period is the Russian Nikolai Bernstein (1897–1966). The addition of Bernstein to the early period is interesting; although he dominated Russian physiology during the 1920s and '30s, his work was not known in the West until the 1970s. Since then, it has experienced somewhat of a rebirth, coming to play a dominant role in contemporary theories of both motor control and motor learning (see Box 1.4).

This period also saw the emergence of psychology as a specialized field of scholarship. The German Wilhelm Wundt (1832–1920) is credited as the

---

BOX **1.3**   *Asking Motor Control Questions*

Select a motor skill in which you are interested and possess at least a moderate degree of proficiency (it can be the same skill used for the exercise in Box 1.2, or an entirely new skill). Think about factors influencing the coordination and control of the skill. Prepare a list of ten questions, specific to the skill you selected, concerning how the skill is controlled and coordination achieved.

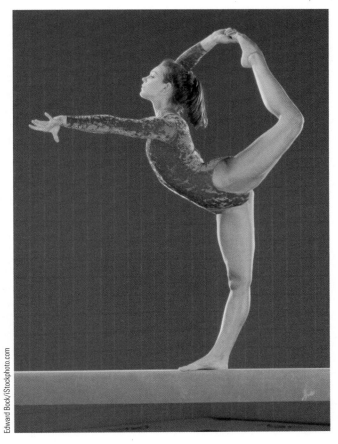

Edward Bock/iStockphoto.com

Motor control entails the study of those factors responsible for the control and coordination of movement, and of the stability of postures.

founder of psychology, having written the first book in the field in 1862. He began the first experimental laboratory devoted to psychological areas of investigation in 1879 and studied variables related to perception, sensation, and attention through the measurement of reaction time, a method of studying motor learning variables extending to the present day.

An early psychological study of learning involving motor skills was reported by Bryan and Harter in 1897, a date some modern-day scholars point to as that of the first true experiment in motor learning. Bryan and Harter investigated the learning rates and patterns of individuals learning to send and receive telegraph messages. Others trace the beginnings to the work of American psychologist Robert Woodworth (1869–1962), who in an 1899 paper reported on his investigations concerning the accuracy with which people are capable of producing voluntary movements.

The most influential psychological developments impinging on the learning of motor skills coming from this period were the learning theories of the American psychologist Edward Thorndike (1874–1949). His major contribution to skill learning is his development of the Law of Effect. This well-known concept, which continues to influence the instruction of motor skills today, is that behaviors that are rewarded are repeated, whereas those that are punished are not, a process gradually reinforcing desired behaviors and promoting learning. Thorndike also developed ideas concerning the transfer of learning and individual differences in learning capabilities that still enjoy contemporary application.

Although both physiologists and psychologists continued to produce work of value in the study of motor skills, work in both fields tended to become more specialized and the direct study of motor skills waned throughout the 1920s and '30s. That was to change with the coming of a world war.

BOX **1.4** Nikolai Bernstein—Movement Scientist Ahead of His Time

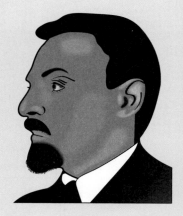

Trained in physiology, Nikolai Bernstein was a dedicated scientist who spent his professional career studying and conducting research concerning how the human brain controls movement. For Bernstein, an overriding problem with the science of his day was that the coordination of movement was not viewed in its true complexity. One of the major concepts he developed is called the *degrees of freedom problem*. This refers to the number of ways that various components of the motor system are free to vary, a number Bernstein showed reached well into the millions at the level of individual cells and neural connections. For Bernstein, the human brain was simply not capable of controlling all of these degrees of freedom involved in complex motor skills. An important part of his answer to this problem was to identify how learning resulted in the development of neurological structures called *synergies*, which greatly reduced the number of degrees of freedom that have to be controlled. He also contributed to learning theory with his concept concerning how learners, in the early stages of learning, "freeze the degrees of freedom" and then gradually release them as they acquire greater skill proficiency (we shall describe these processes in much more detail in Chapters 4 and 7).

Because of the closed nature of Russian society during most of Bernstein's working life, his writings and ideas remained obscure outside of Russia. His major work, a book of his collected papers written in the 1920s and '30s titled *The Co-ordination and Regulation of Movement*, was first published in English in 1967. It is not an exaggeration to say that much of modern thinking in motor learning and control owes a large debt to the rediscovery of Bernstein. Perhaps his greatest achievement, viewed in hindsight, is that he conceived of a new way of viewing and studying human movement nearly a half-century before his more modern peers, who are still discovering the full potential of Bernstein's ideas.

Middle Period

World War II (1939–1945) marked a dramatic shift in research focus among many psychologists. Because of their need to select and train personnel for military service, both England and America quickly enlisted the efforts of many scientists in the war effort. In the United States, programs for testing and selecting personnel, especially pilots and gunnery aircrews, led to development of tests of the motor and perceptual abilities required for these skills. The need to train military personnel, often for very physical tasks, also led to military support for research concerning effective training methods, a research agenda the military still supports in a number of ways today.

An important development in psychology occurring during the same period was a renewed interest in learning theory and in the factors responsible for learning. Clark Hull (1884–1952), in particular, advanced an influential theory of learning and motivation. What was particularly important to motor skill theorists, was that Hull's theory was a "general" theory of learning, meaning that it addressed cognitive, perceptual, and motor skills. Hull's (1943) theory helped initiate new areas of inquiry into the learning of motor skills and was important in much of the research on skill learning conducted during the 1940s and '50s.

Two other important things happened during the postwar period: first, the work of Franklin Henry (1904–1993), who is probably more responsible than any other single person for the evolution of motor learning as an academic field of study (see Box 1.5); and second, the large expansion of physical education programs in the 1950s and '60s as college enrollments swelled with returning GIs, many of whom chose physical education as a career. The growth in these departments led to the development of many new doctoral programs, including ones specializing in motor learning. Much of the research in motor learning and control came from faculty members within these programs, and many new academic journals and textbooks were produced to disseminate their findings.

By the 1950s and '60s, a new emphasis on cognition was beginning to take hold of research agendas in motor learning and control. Ideas first advanced in England that the brain could be conceived of as a computer, as well as ideas borrowed from engineering that the brain used feedback loops like servo-mechanisms used to control mechanical devices, led to a focus on how the brain used and processed information. These ideas would be expanded into the information processing perspective, the dominant theoretical approach to the study of motor learning from the 1950s well into the 1980s, and still viable today (see Chapter 4). The information processing model is the basic idea that distinct cognitive processes are responsible for the learning and control of motor skills, and that their specific functions can be identified and studied. Two important theories coming from this model are the closed-loop theory proposed by Jack Adams (1971) and Schema Theory developed by Richard Schmidt (1975). Both of these theories, particularly Schema Theory, remain viable expressions of the information processing model.

BOX 1.5   Franklin Henry—The Father of Motor Skills Research

In 1919, at the age of 14, young Franklin Henry ran away from the poverty of his family's Colorado farm and joined the Navy. Eager to obtain an education after his discharge, he entered the University of California at Berkeley as a special student (because he had not graduated from high school). Eventually, he earned a Ph.D. in psychology. During his studies, Henry managed to eke out a living and pay his tuition by working in the Physical Education Department, where he maintained and repaired exercise testing equipment. As a psychology student, he began using spare parts from the exercise testing devices to build equipment of his own conception and design for the testing of psychological variables related to motor skill learning. Members of the physical education faculty were impressed with Henry's ideas, and when he received his doctorate, they offered him a faculty position in their department with responsibilities for developing an entirely new discipline devoted to the psychological study of motor skill learning. In 1939 then, the first professor specializing in motor learning developed and taught the first class in motor learning at the University of California at Berkeley.

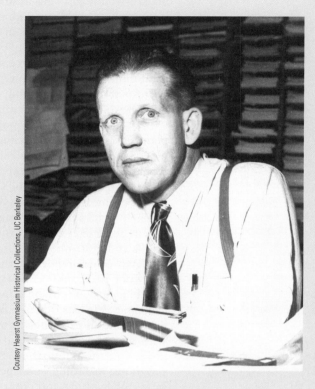

Courtesy Hearst Gymnasium Historical Collections, UC Berkeley

Over a career that spanned the next half-century, Henry developed many of methods and experimental procedures used for investigating the learning of motor skills, as well as conducted a number of important research studies that advanced the new field and helped secure its academic acceptance. For this reason, Henry is known today as "The Father of Motor Skills Research."

Henry's contributions were not limited to research alone. He chaired the graduate committees of many students who went on to become leaders who advanced research and knowledge in motor skill learning. He is responsible for beginning the North American Society for the Psychology of Sport and Physical Activity (NASPSPA), the primary professional organization for those in fields related to behavioral and psychological aspects of sports and motor skills. Perhaps his most significant influence, however, was in the broader professional arena. Henry wrote and argued, long before others in the field, that the study of human movement sciences entailed an academic discipline, and he offered convincing reasons for reorganizing traditional physical education departments into broader-based programs relevant to many professions and scholarly areas of study involving human movement. Today's academic programs in kinesiology are an ongoing testimony to the ideas and accomplishments of Franklin Henry.

Modern Period

Well into the 1980s, information processing approaches, especially Schema Theory, continued to dominate the motor learning and control landscape. But by the end of the decade, new paradigms had emerged to challenge this model of skill learning. The 1990s have been called the "Decade of the Brain," and new techniques for studying brain activities have led to a renewed interest on the part of neuroscientists to investigate the neural mechanisms underlying motor control. There has been a dramatic shift away from focusing on cognition alone when studying brain functions, and a recognition that motor control and learning are intertwined with both cognitive and perceptual processes and must be studied as a unity. This has led to significant research and many new findings on ways in which the brain controls and learns motor skills. Research in the area of brain studies remains promising, particularly in the areas of rehabilitation and treatment of motor-related diseases.

Traditional scientific approaches in many areas have been challenged by a new scientific paradigm in the past two decades or so. This approach which has many descriptors—complexity science, ecological theory, dynamical systems theory, coordination dynamics, chaos theory—focused study on how interacting systems adapt and organize into new patterns of behavior. Inspired by the work of Nikolai Bernstein, a number of movement scientists including Scott Kelso, Karl Newell, and Michael Turvey began applying this perspective to the study of motor skills in the 1980s. We will leave further discussion of this approach until later, because it makes up a major part of Chapter 4.

We can conclude this brief review by noting that although psychology remains the primary parent discipline of motor learning and control studies today, new approaches to the study of skilled movements have increasingly also come from other disciplines, including neuroscience, physiology, genetics, biochemistry, engineering, robotics, physics, computer science, and education. Indeed, the scientific study of motor learning and control seems poised for explorations into many previously uncharted waters of scientific discovery.

OCCUPATIONAL USES OF KNOWLEDGE IN MOTOR LEARNING AND CONTROL

By this point, it has no doubt become obvious to the reader that motor learning and control are comprised of knowledge essential in many professional and occupational fields. In fact, for any career field concerned with how people acquire movement skills, knowledge of motor learning and control is prerequisite to effective practice. As we have seen, many misconceptions and myths surround instruction in motor skills. Those professionals responsible for such instruction need to be especially well-informed concerning knowledge in this important area of human activity.

The goals of many occupations include providing people with effective instructions concerning the performance or learning of movement skills. These include skills underlying recreational and leisure activities, sports participation, artistic and musical expression, and many work and job skills. Other occupations are directly concerned with rehabilitating skills lost or compromised due to injury or disease, often including the skills that make daily life functionally possible.

Skilled movement, as we have seen, touches almost every aspect of human activity. Thus, it is not surprising that specialized knowledge concerning these skills is essential in a broad diversity of career fields. Regardless of the aspect of human movement that may be its primary focus, however, the various occupations and professions concerned with promoting the quality of people's movement skills do share an essential humanistic quality in common. All are concerned, most fundamentally, with the goal of helping people realize better, happier, and more productive lives.

A brief listing of occupations in which the knowledge of motor learning and control plays an especially central and critical role include the following:

Athletic Coach

Motor learning not only helps the coach determine the best methods of structuring practice and teaching sport-specific skills but also is important in understanding performance variables such as fatigue, arousal, motivation, environmental conditions, and travel that can have a significant impact on athletic performance. Because practice activities are necessarily different in many respects from those conditions experienced during a game or contest, an understanding of motor learning helps the athletic coach design practices that will have the greatest transfer from practice to competitive situations. Motor learning knowledge also provides a basis for understanding and accommodating individual differences among athletes during practice experiences, providing the best opportunity for each athlete under the coach's instruction to attain his or her best performance levels. As we have seen, many "traditional" approaches to providing instruction in sports skills are less than optimal; a solid foundation in the science of motor learning provides the athletic coach with the knowledge needed to provide the most successful practice experiences for those athletes under the coach's care.

Athletic Trainer

Returning injured athletes to competition as quickly (and well) as possible requires the ability to properly prescribe effective exercise and rehabilitation training activities, a role in which an understanding of motor control and learning is essential. An understanding of motor learning can also help the athletic trainer to appreciate the limits of skill training and to identify potentially dangerous training situations that can be corrected before injuries occur. Additionally, an appreciation for the factors involved in motor control can help the athletic trainer diagnose the underlying causes of motor impairments and prescribe effective protocols for treating injuries and returning athletes to participation within proper timeframes.

Dance Instructor

Teachers and choreographers constantly attempt to enable their dance students to reach goals of artistic expression. To develop a dancer's artistry, dance teachers must possess the knowledge and skills necessary to instruct the varied and complex motor skills involved in dance. Because dance performers frequently must acquire new and complex performance routines, motor learning principles involving the memory of long sequences of motor skills often play an especially importance role in effective dance instruction. Successful dance instructors must be able to break dance skills down into meaningful elements for practice, identify individual needs of dancers, provide effective instructions and demonstrations, structure the learning experience, provide corrective feedback, and establish realistic goals that motivate performers (Overby, 1993).

Ergonomics Designer

The interface between humans and equipment is an area of professional application called *human factors engineering* or *ergonomic design*. This area is concerned with understanding how human performance and the effective use of various types of equipment are affected by design considerations. Human factors engineers ask the question, "How can equipment be designed for the safest, easiest, most dependable use?" Some examples of concerns in this area: How can an assembly line be designed to optimize both productivity and safety? How can the design of seating, steering, instruments, and acceleration and braking pedals in an automobile be coordinated for optimal use and safety? How can simulators used to teach skills in flying a plane (or driving a car or using complex machinery, etc.) be designed for maximum learning and transfer in actual practice?

Such questions as these are evaluated and answered through application of motor control and learning principles.

Fitness Consultant

Fitness consultants use exercise, sports and games, and other movement skill activities to promote levels of fitness in individuals and groups. It can be easy to focus on the fitness benefits of these activities and forget two important facts. The first is that activities used primarily to promote fitness levels also exhibit a component of skill. Even weight training exercises require a considerable degree of coordination and timing when one is first learning to execute them. The second important fact to remember is that the activities used for fitness promotion must be taught; that is, the fitness specialist or consultant schedules practice and provides instruction about performing skills. Fitness activities are still skills, and they can be instructed in more or less effective ways. The instruction of fitness skills using effective practice methods can significantly impact the quality of the training effect, promoting the attainment and benefits of fitness acquisition.

Movement Scientist

Movement scientists in areas of motor learning and motor control are those having received specialized training, usually at the Ph.D. level, in motor learning and control. Movement scientists are typically employed in universities, although some also find employment as research specialists in government programs or private corporations. The majority employed as university professors generally teach undergraduate and graduate courses in motor learning and motor control, as well as closely related areas involving skill acquisition. They maintain currency with developments in the field through reading current research journals and attending professional meetings where other scholars share their ideas and current research findings. Many movement scientists also maintain robust research agendas, conducting and publishing the results of their investigations.

Depending upon the type of university in which the movement scientist chooses to work, his or her work responsibilities can be balanced more toward teaching or research, though both will typically be required to some degree.

Occupational Therapist

Occupational therapists help people improve their ability to perform functions associated with daily living and work. They work with individuals suffering from mentally, physically, developmentally, and emotionally disabling conditions. Occupational therapists teach their patients how to develop, recover, or maintain daily living and work skills. These can include all types of skills, from using a computer, to dressing, to performing specific work tasks on an assembly line. Almost always these skills are motor skills or include some motor component. The design and delivery of patient services by occupational therapists includes significant instruction of both daily and specialized motor skills.

Physical Educator

The goal of the physical education teacher is to provide effective instruction for sport and movement skills, and knowledge of motor learning can make this goal more easily attainable (Collier and Hebert, 2004; Wiegand, Bulger, and Mohr, 2004). Indeed, a good foundation in motor learning is paramount to effective instruction in physical education settings, especially because research in motor learning has clearly revealed that many traditional and widely used methods of teaching movement skills are often not the most effective methods of instruction. The teaching of sports and movement skills is an important educational objective in most school curricula. Many recreational, community, and private organizations are also devoted to the teaching of sports and other movement skills. The professional physical educator will teach many different skills to a wide variety of students possessing different interests and abilities, and a strong foundation in motor control and learning theory is essential to providing safe and effective instruction in all of these situations.

Physical Therapist

Physical therapists must design effective training programs that address concerns for both physiological improvement and regaining movement skills (Higgins, 1991). An understanding of the mechanisms of motor control can assist the therapist in evaluating the underlying causes of movement impairment, as well as in assessing movement abilities. Once an evaluation is made, motor learning principles then inform the best methods of rehabilitating impaired skills. Providing effective instruction to patients, who may have little experience in skills training as well as apprehension concerning their training, can be challenging and requires a comprehensive understanding of diverse instructional methods and practice scheduling techniques for meeting the individual needs of patients.

Sport Psychologist

Sport psychologists apply psychological principles and techniques to help athletes achieve optimal sport and exercise performance and health. They work with individual athletes or groups to enhance motivation, attentional focus, goal

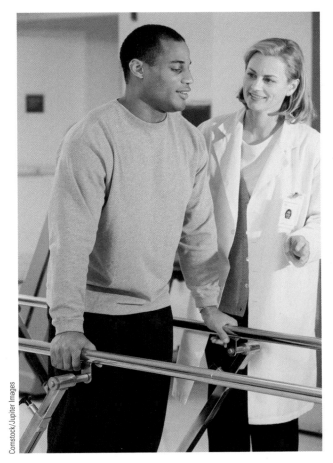

Comstock/Jupiter Images

Motor learning and control are an essential component of the knowledge required of physical and occupational therapists.

achievement, and adherence to training, as well as to overcome inappropriate thoughts, anxiety, and poor practice habits. Although the sport psychologist possesses a powerful array of psychological tools for enhancing mental effort and functioning, ineffective practice methods can hamper even the best psychological performance techniques, causing them to become ineffective. The sport psychologist must assure that his or her therapeutic interventions are supported and enhanced by proper instructional and practice approaches. Improper skills training methods can destroy otherwise significant benefits from psychological performance enhancing techniques. The sport psychologist must be able to blend appropriate instructional and practice designs with his or her performance enhancing methods, as well as to work with coaches and exercise leaders in assuring that their skill training methods are also appropriate. Optimal performance and skill improvement will only result when sound psychological training practices are coupled with effective methods of skills instruction and practice.

Training Specialist

The time needed to acquire occupational skills can be shortened, and the quality of learning skills improved, through the application of motor learning principles. Experts in how people acquire skills comprise an important part of the training professionals in many corporate and industrial work settings where employees must be taught on-the-job motor skills ranging from typing to using machinery or heavy equipment. Also, the identification and selection of those employees most capable of performing necessary job tasks can be made more efficient through testing individuals' motor abilities and then matching those abilities to required job skills. In addition to corporate and industrial career settings, many professional trainers play a critical role in the training of personnel for military, firefighting, and law enforcement service.

Youth Sports Leader

Youth sports leaders find employment in city recreation departments; boys' and girls' clubs; YMCA, YWCA, YMHA, and YWHA agencies; youth camps; and other public and private organizations devoted to activities for children and teenagers. A significant part of the activities in many of these organizations involves the teaching of sports, games, and fitness activities. Instructors working with young children need to be especially well educated and knowledgeable concerning effective instructional and scheduling methods that are age-appropriate, maintain enthusiasm and motivation in these age groupings, and follow careful protocols designed to optimize safety during participation in active movement skills.

REASONS TO STUDY MOTOR LEARNING AND MOTOR CONTROL

Before beginning the study of motor learning and control, each student should come to some understanding concerning both the importance and reasons for such a study. The preceding discussion has attempted to provide some rationale for the importance of motor learning and control as an area of scholarly study; it is left to discuss some of the reasons concerning why students should feel such a study is important to them. Although students are encouraged to think about their reasons for pursuing a study of the topics presented in this text, and to come to answers of their own, the three following reasons are offered for special consideration:

BOX **1.6**   Choosing a Career

Spend some time thinking about how your most basic values and beliefs are reflected in your choice of a career path. Is the career for which you are preparing compatible with your values? How does your choice of a college major reflect and promote your values?

Professional Application

Students taking motor learning and control are typically preparing for professions involving the teaching of motor skills. Physical education teachers, athletic coaches, physical and occupational therapists, dance instructors, industrial trainers, and military trainers, to name perhaps the most obvious examples, all have as a substantive part of their professional work the teaching of motor skills. Motor learning is the science that underlies the teaching of those skills. Without an adequate understanding of motor learning principles, instruction of motor skills can become ineffectual. Many practitioners, as we have unfortunately seen in this chapter, employ relatively ineffective instructional practices. Traditional practices of instruction are frequently wrong—or at least not as effective as they might be. Numerous investigations have observed that even long-time professionals in teaching, coaching, therapy, and training employ outdated and relatively ineffective instructional designs and methods—and this often includes successful professionals (Wiegand, Bulger, and Mohr, 2004). A working knowledge of motor learning and its principles is paramount in the design and teaching of the most effective and beneficial instructional programs for motor skill learning. Experience is a valuable teacher, but incomplete without an adequate base of knowledge to support it.

Intrinsic Interest

Motor learning and control can be studied for its intrinsic value and interest. Indeed, the study of how humans control their movements and acquire new ones is a fascinating subject. Everyone performs thousands of skilled movements every day. Motor learning is really a study of oneself—or at least of a significant area of daily activity in which everyone participates. The complexity of human movement and skill acquisition is an exciting story, filled with surprises and unexpected turns. Much of how humans control movement is still a mystery, perhaps even one that will never fully be explained. A famous scientist once remarked that if we compare the processing capabilities of the human motor system to the most powerful computer in the world, we get a good idea of the challenge in understanding how movement is controlled. Assuming that computers double their calculating capability every year because of rapid advances in computer science, this scientist determined that computers would eventually be capable of the same feats in directing movement skills as is the human brain—in about 200 years! We can add that this scientist probably represents the most optimistic view.

Learning to appreciate the vast resources of the motor system, and something of the story of how we ourselves move and learn, is a branch of learning well worth pursuing for its own intrinsic value. Particularly for students in disciplines involving motor skills, the story of how movements are controlled and learned should be an especially interesting one.

Ethical Considerations

In the near future, most students will probably be professionally employed and teaching people motor skills in one of a variety of settings. Some will be helping students in schools to acquire basic movement skills that will initiate them into lifelong activities promoting health and enjoyment; others will be design-ing instructional programs to help people rehabilitate from injuries and return to normal daily functioning in jobs and recreational pursuits. Still other students will help athletes or dancers reach higher levels of skill in sports or artistic expres-sion. Some students may find themselves helping to train police officers, firefight-ers, military personnel; or perhaps designing programs to help workers learn job skills more effectively. Other students may design equipment to make people safer in their jobs and homes or to assist them in overcoming physical limitations.

Regardless of the professional field in which you may find yourself, as a stu-dent today the choices you make about the seriousness of your study (in this as well as other subjects) will have a direct bearing on your ability to help people tomorrow in your chosen field of professional work. There is no higher call that any of us have than to use our talents to help others achieve worthwhile goals that promote the quality and meaning of life. As a student today, your serious-ness of purpose in this subject (as in others) is really an ethical decision—an indi-cation of your commitment to your chosen profession—to be of help to those who can most benefit from your talents and professional expertise. Failure to acquire requisite skills and knowledge today will mean that you will be less pre-pared to serve others in your professional work tomorrow. It is this writer's sin-cere hope that each student will view his or her efforts in the study of motor control and learning in terms of an ethical decision concerning how best to pre-pare for a satisfying career well selected and of the greatest service to others.

SUMMARY

- Skilled movements encompass a wide range of behaviors making human life possible.
- Humans develop and acquire new motor skills throughout their lifetimes in order to adapt to their surroundings and meet both their needs and interests.
- The study of how people learn motor skills to meet their many needs and interests is an important area for scholarly study.
- Two scholarly disciplines focusing scholarly inquiry on motor skills are the disciplines of motor control and motor learning.
  - Motor learning is the study of those factors responsible for the acquisition of motor skills, including the study of how people learn as well as the instructional methods promoting that learning.
  - Motor control is the study of the underlying processes responsible for the organization, coordination, and execution of motor skills.
  - Although motor control and motor learning represent separate areas for scholarly inquiry, they are highly intertwined in their focus on motor skills and should be studied together by movement skill practitioners.
- The study of motor learning and motor control entails the application of scientific inquiry to questions of motor skill acquisition and control.
- The study of motor learning and control has evolved from early studies conducted in physiology and psychology during the later part of the eighteenth century, with distinct stages in its development over the

years marked by varying theoretical approaches and changing focus of scholarly interests and societal needs.

- Knowledge based upon scientific study is essential to professional practice in many fields concerned with the performance of motor skills, including the coaching of athletic teams, athletic training, dance instruction, human factors and ergonomic design, occupational training, the teaching of physical education, and physical and occupational therapy.
- In approaching the study of motor learning and control, students can benefit from considering the professional application, intrinsic interest, and ethical implications inherent in such study.

LEARNING EXERCISES

1. For this exercise, you will identify and interview a professional in a field related to the instruction of motor skills (most likely one of the 12 discussed in this chapter in the section on occupations). Select an occupation of interest to you, and contact and arrange a meeting time with the professional you have selected (remember that he or she is freely giving time for this interview, so be accommodating, courteous, and professional).

   At the time of the interview, ask the following questions:

   - Please describe a typical day's activities in your job.
   - What do you find most rewarding and enjoyable about your job?
   - What do you find the least enjoyable part of your job?
   - What knowledge do you think is most essential to possess in your job?
   - How much of a role does the teaching of motor skills play in your job?

   - What knowledge concerning the teaching of skills do you think it is most important for someone in your position to have?
   - For a current student of motor learning, what do you think is the most important information for me to acquire? (Be sure that you take good notes, or that you record the interview, obtaining the interviewee's permission first if you record the interview.)

   Prepare a written report of your interview, including what you learned from the exercise. Mention anything that particularly surprised you.

2. Prepare a list of the 10 questions for which you would most like to learn the answers as you study motor learning and control. Keep the list and be aware whenever opportunities to learn more about one of your questions arises. Strive to answer all 10 questions fully and to your satisfaction during your course of study. (You may also want to share this list with your instructor.)

FOR FURTHER STUDY

HOW MUCH DO YOU KNOW?

For each of the following, select the letter that best answers the question.

1. Motor skills are
   a. inherited at birth.
   b. limited to a few well-learned skills.
   c. defined as requiring significant amounts of muscular effort.
   d. diverse and underlie most daily activities.

2. Which of the following topics would be included as an area of study within the discipline of motor control?
   a. Motivation
   b. Visual perception
   c. Practice scheduling
   d. The stages of learning

3. During the 1950s and '60s, research in motor learning and motor control experienced a sharp increase from previous levels due to—
   a. the growth of graduate programs in physical education.
   b. the development of the computer.
   c. new techniques for studying the brain.
   d. increased funding for military research.

4. Nikolai Bernstein focused much of his research attention on solving the _____ problem.
   a. perceptual-motor integration
   b. degrees of freedom
   c. cognitive overload
   d. field-dependency

5. Which of the following is *not* a reason for studying motor learning and motor control recommended specifically for consideration in this chapter?
   a. Professional application
   b. Intrinsic interest

   c. Certification requirement
   d. Ethical considerations

Answer the following with the word or words that best complete each sentence.

6. The scholarly discipline from which motor learning originally emerged and took shape, and which continues to be the dominant disciplinary perspective today, is _____.

7. The scholarly discipline concerned with how motor skills are acquired, and with the variables that influence that acquisition, is _____.

8. Motor learning encompasses the study of three factors influencing the learning of motor skills. These three factors are _____.

9. _____ is known as the "The Father of Research in Motor Skills."

10. Emerging during the middle period in the history of motor learning, the _____ model became the dominant approach to the study of motor skills learning well into the 1980s, and continues to exert considerable influence today.

Answers are provided at the end of this review section.

STUDY QUESTIONS

1. To what extent do motor skills play a role in people's daily activities?
2. Define motor learning and be able to list several examples of questions motor learning theorists study.
3. Define motor control and be able to list several examples of questions motor control theorists study.
4. Why is it important that practitioners study motor learning and motor control together?
5. Describe the origins of motor learning and control as fields of study during the period

from the middle of the nineteenth century to World War II.
6. Who was Nikolai Bernstein, and what were his major contributions?
7. What were the major influences on the growth of motor learning and motor control during the middle period from World War II to roughly the end of the 1980s.
8. Who was Franklin Henry, and what were his major contributions?
9. What major changes from the past are influencing the study of motor learning and motor control today?

10. List the 12 professional occupations discussed in this chapter for which a knowledge of motor learning and control plays an especially critical role, and provide a brief explanation for the importance of these two disciplines in each of these occupations.

ADDITIONAL READING

Adams, JA. (1987). "Historical review and appraisal of research on the learning, retention, and transfer of human motor skills." *Psychological Bulletin, 101*(1), 41–74.

Higgins, S. (1991). "Motor skill acquisition." *Physical Therapy, 71*(2), 123.

Rink, JE. (2003). "Motor learning." In BS Mohnsen (ed.), *Concepts and principles of physical education: What every student needs to know* (pp. 15–37). Reston, VA: NASPE.

Summers, JJ. (2004). "A historical perspective on skill acquisition." In AM Williams and NJ Hodges (eds.), *Skill acquisition in sport: Research, theory and practice*, London: Routledge.

Thomas, JR, and Thomas, KT. (2009). "Motor behavior." In SL Hoffman (ed.), *Introduction to kinesiology: Studying physical activity*, 2nd ed., Champaign, IL: Human Kinetics.

REFERENCES

Adams, JA. (1971). "A closed-loop theory of motor learning." *Journal of Motor Behavior, 3,* 111–150.

Adams, JA. (1987). "Historical review and appraisal of research on the learning, retention, and transfer of human motor skills." *Psychological Bulletin, 101*(1), 41–74.

Bernstein, N. (1967). *The co-ordination and regulation of movements*. London: Pergamon Press.

Collier, D, and Hebert, F. (2004). "Undergraduate physical education teacher preparation: What practitioners tell us." *Physical Educator, 61*(2), 102.

Higgins, S. (1991). "Motor skill acquisition." *Physical Therapy, 71*(2), 123.

Hull, CL. (1943). *Principles of behavior*. New York: Appleton-Century-Crofts.

Meijer, OG. (2001). "Making things happen: An introduction to the history of movement science." In ML Latash and VM Zatsiorsky (eds.), *Classics in movement science*, Champaign, IL: Human Kinetics.

Overby, LY. (1993). "Motor learning in the dance education curriculum." *Journal of Physical Education, Recreation and Dance, 64*(9), 42.

Schmidt, RA, and Lee, TD. (2005). *Motor control and learning: A behavioral emphasis*, 4th ed. Champaign, IL: Human Kinetics.

Shumway-Cook, A, and Woollacott, MH. (2007). *Motor control: Translating research into clinical practice*, 3rd ed. New York: Lippincott, Williams and Wilkins.

Summers, JJ. (2004). "A historical perspective on skill acquisition." In AM Williams and NJ Hodges (eds.), *Skill acquisition in sport: Research, theory and practice*, London: Routledge.

Ulrich, BD, and Reeve, TG (2005). "Studies in motor behavior: 75 years of research in motor development, learning, and control." *Research Quarterly for Exercise and Sport, 76* (Supplement to No. 2), S62–S70.

Wiegand, L, Bulger, SM, and Mohr, DJ. (2004). "Curricular issues in physical education teacher education: Which foundational courses do PETE students really need?" *Journal of Physical Education, Recreation and Dance, 75*(8), 47.

Answers to How Much Do You Know questions: (1) D, (2) B, (3) A, (4) B, (5) C, (6) psychology, (7) motor learning, (8) the learner, the nature of the skill, and the environment, (9) Franklin Henry, (10) information processing.

CHAPTER 2

What Is a Skill?

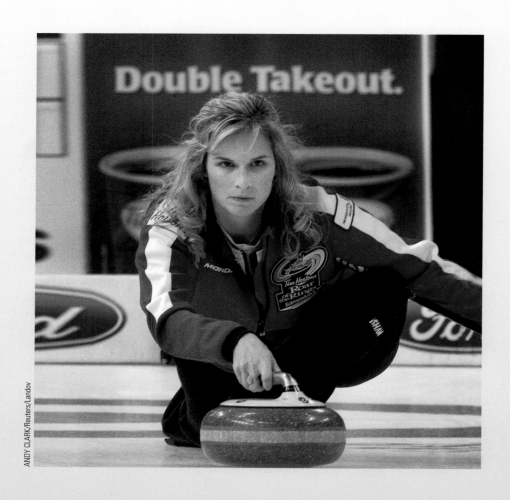

ANDY CLARK/Reuters/Landov

"I was not successful as a ball player, as it was a game of skill."
Casey Stengel (1890–1975), professional baseball manager

KEY QUESTIONS

- What is a skill? How are skills defined?
- How do motor skills differ from other types of skills?
- Are there characteristics common to all motor skills?
- What factors influence the performance of motor skills?
- What problems do researchers confront when studying motor skills?
- How can motor skills be meaningfully classified?

CHAPTER OVERVIEW

If you were presented a list of motor skills including the shot-put, completing a maximal weight bench press, and casting in fly fishing, which two would you select as having the most in common? Most people would probably select the shot-put and bench press as being the most similar. And if you focus only on the muscular effort required to accomplish both of these skills, your choice would be the most logical one. But if you consider all of the essential characteristics of these three skills—the perceptual requirements for each, the patterns of muscular coordination and timing involved in each, the demands imposed on each by the environment, the basic movement goals for each—then fly fishing and the shot-put actually have much more in common with one another than either has with the skill of bench pressing.

Analyzing skills for common features is more than a mere exercise in identifying similarities, however. For one thing, such analysis forms the basis for determining the most effective methods for instructing motor skills. In our example, many of the instructional methods best suited to teaching someone to put the shot are the same as those that should be used when teaching someone to cast a fly line to the spot where the biggest trout hide out, but these same instructions would prove less effective when teaching someone the proper mechanics for performing the bench press.

In this chapter, we will consider questions concerning the nature of skills, including what all skills have in common as well as those features differentiating various types of skill. As we begin our journey of discovery in this book, we will examine the ways in which movement scientists conceptualize skills, the theoretical problems confronted in studying skilled behaviors, and the vocabulary used to communicate effectively about motor skills. This chapter forms an essential component of the foundation upon which our subsequent explorations into motor learning and control are built.

The word *skill* is easily and, for the most part, meaningfully understood by almost everyone. When we say that someone is a skilled typist, or a skilled tennis player, or an unskilled driver, everyone understands what we mean. We can also refer to particular kinds of behaviors as skills. We say that writing is a skill, as are playing the piano, using tools, solving mathematical problems, square dancing, and hitting fastballs. Again, our meaning is clear to everyone.

When we begin to study skills scientifically, however, our everyday use of the term soon leads to disagreement and uncertainty. It does so because our everyday usage of the word *skill* is too vague, lacking the necessary precision to sufficiently illuminate the similarities and differences among skills in which researchers and practitioners alike are interested. What is common to all activities defined as skills? To be a skill, must an activity be performed at some minimum level of proficiency? Are all skills learned, or can some be inherited? What do movement skills have in common, if anything, with other types of skills? What is the best way to study and learn about skills? Addressing such questions requires that our definition of skill be embedded within a theoretical framework that provides consistency and meaningfulness in usage. Defining *skill* scientifically is the first step in developing a theory about how people acquire skillful behaviors, and how practitioners can design more effective evaluation and training programs.

THE DOMAINS OF SKILL

Do we use the word *skill* to mean the same thing when we say that Mary is a skilled mathematician and John is a skilled first baseman? Certainly something about our meaning is the same; in both cases we mean to indicate that our subjects perform their respective skills at a high level of proficiency—Mary gets straight A's in math and John is on the varsity baseball team. What about Hector, a connoisseur of fine wines, who is so skilled that he can tell the vintage, year, and bottler of any wine just by tasting it. Is he skilled in the same way as are Mary and John?

Mary, John, and Hector are each skilled at their respective area of interest. But it is also clear that what each is skilled at doing is very different. Mary's skill comes from her capacity to think about abstract symbols and to manipulate them in her head. Hector's ability to discern various wines indicates a highly developed sense of taste discrimination. Of course, Hector's ability to discern various wines comes from a great deal of experience and knowledge about different vintners. So, in his use of knowledge concerning wines, his skill has some things in common with Mary's (although, if he acquires too much experience at wine sampling, he may not pass many math tests!).

John's ability, compared to Mary's and Hector's, is expressed primarily through bodily movements. He is quick off the ball, can coordinate his limbs to perform complex and exacting movements, and possesses good catching and throwing abilities. But are John's skills merely physical? To be a skilled baseball player, he must also act out of considerable knowledge concerning game situations. Often he must make split-second decisions about a situation and how best to respond—something requiring considerable knowledge on his part. John has also developed keen capabilities at watching a ball fly off of a hitter's bat, and can quickly and accurately perceive how he must move to catch it.

There are similar elements of skill in each of the examples above, as well as elements of each that are different. Mary, John, and Hector are all highly skilled, but they are skilled at different things. Mary is skilled primarily because of her cognitive abilities; Hector, because of his perceptual awareness; and John, because of his movement capabilities. In the study of skilled behavior, these specific capacities are called cognitive, perceptual, and motor skills.

Skill Domains

skill domain:
A categorical classification of skills possessing similarities specific to cognitive, perceptual, and motor characteristics.

A skill is initially defined as belonging to one of three domains. A domain is simply a category into which similar things can be grouped. A **skill domain** is the grouping of skills based upon the underlying capacities most essential for accomplishing them. When defining a skill, our first decision entails deciding whether cognitive, perceptual, or motor capabilities are most necessary to the successful completion of the skill.

Cognitive Skills

cognitive skill: A skill for which success is primarily determined by an individual's knowledge and cognitive capabilities.

A **cognitive skill** is one in which knowing what to do or how to do it is the most important aspect in accomplishing the skill. Although perceptual and motor elements may make up part of a cognitive skill, understanding and knowing are the most essential capabilities for doing the skill well, and are usually the most difficult to master. We can define a cognitive skill as one in which success in accomplishing the goals of the skill is primarily determined by an individual's knowledge and cognitive abilities. Examples of cognitive skills include reading, writing, solving mathematical problems, doing crossword puzzles, memorizing a list of names, constructing a reasoned and persuasive argument, diagnosing an athlete's injury, computer programming, and calling plays in a football game.

Perceptual Skills

perceptual skill: A skill for which the ability to discern and discriminate among sensory stimuli is of primary concern in successfully accomplishing the skill.

A **perceptual skill** is one in which the ability to discern, or to discriminate among, sensory stimuli is of primary importance in accomplishing the skill successfully. More simply stated, it is the ability to recognize important things in the environment—that is, to detect information. In accomplishing a perceptual skill, the primary goal of the performer is not in possessing the movement capabilities necessary for acting, but in sensing when and how to act.

Perceptual skills are intricately intertwined with movement skills, such as those found in sports, so that it can sometimes be difficult to separate the contributions of each type of skill to successful performance. Is the sensory acuity necessary to discern where and when a pitched baseball will cross home plate more or less important than the actual movement patterns required for hitting the ball, for example? So essential are perceptual abilities in accomplishing most motor skills, in fact, that motor skills are often referred to as *perceptual-motor skills.* Still, many skills rely primarily upon an individual's awareness of sensory stimuli and are therefore grouped under the perceptual domain.

A perceptual skill can be defined as one in which successfully accomplishing the goal of a skill is primarily determined by an individual's ability to recognize and discriminate among various sources of perceivable stimuli. Examples of perceptual skills include selecting good melons at the grocery store, adjusting the color on a television set, sorting eggs by size, "reading" a defense in football, identifying the ingredients in food by taste, maintaining balance when walking on an icy path, and spotting a camouflaged enemy in a woody thicket.

Motor Skills

As we have seen, motor skills are not performed in isolation from perceptual and cognitive components necessary for task completion. In many of the skills of interest to the movement specialist, however, it is the quality of the movement itself that is of paramount importance. A motor skill is one in which the primary determinant of success is the quality of movement. For example, a bowler may have no trouble knowing what to do (knock down the pins with the ball) or in perceiving how to do it (the length and width of the bowling lane, the location of pins, and the weight of the bowling ball are constant and easily discernable from trial to trial), but producing the correct movements to accomplish the goal of knocking all 10 pins over with one ball is still a challenge in each frame. Where cognitive skills emphasize knowing what to do, and perceptual skills getting the information to do it, motor skills are concerned with doing it, and doing it correctly.

There is a tendency to think of motor skills only in terms of sports skills or other specialized activities. Catching a football, serving a tennis ball, performing a somersault, skate boarding, and square dancing are certainly all motor skills. But we perform motor skills in most of our daily activities—thousands of them forming the essential and routine, meaningful and pedestrian, events that make daily life possible. Motor skills include washing dishes, brushing your teeth, turning on a lamp, shaking someone's hand, putting on your clothes in the morning, taking a shower, sitting down and standing up, driving to school, dancing for joy when you get an "A" in organic chemistry, and climbing into bed at night (or for a well-deserved nap after your organic chemistry test). Many occupations consist of learning to perform specialized motor skills—using machinery, repairing computers or car engines, sorting and stacking items on shelves, playing the piano professionally, wrapping an injured athlete's ankle, performing surgery, or flying the space shuttle. Even skills that we might first be inclined to consider purely cognitive, like talking and writing, have significant motor elements underlying their successful production (you can think about what you want to say, but speaking requires the sophisticated and finely tuned coordination of muscles within the vocal tract in order to produce words).

As these activities classified as motor skills indicate, many different types of activity rely primarily upon movement for their success. We should again emphasize that motor skills, as with cognitive and perceptual skills, are so labeled because of the degree to which cognitive, perceptual, or motor elements contribute to the successful accomplishment of task goals. Few real-world skills do not contain elements of all three domains; it is convenient both theoretically

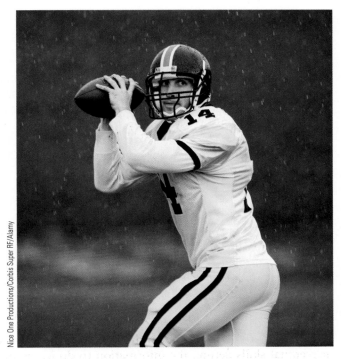

Nice One Productions/Corbis Super RF/Alamy

Many skills include significant components of all three skill domains: cognitive, perceptual, and motor.

and practically, however, to label skills relative to the major domain responsible for successful goal achievement. Any skill, and perhaps especially a motor skill, is a mosaic of cognitive, perceptual, and motor strands woven and blended together into the rich tapestry of skilled human behavior (see Figure 2.1).

Is Skill Learning Domain Specific?

Given both the differences and similarities of the three domains into which skills can be classified, it is reasonable to ask if cognitive, perceptual, and motor skills are acquired in fundamentally different ways. That is, are there three separate and distinct sets of skill-learning principles, a different set for each domain? At first it might seem that differences in the primary modality of success in each domain of skill would naturally lead to differences in methods of acquiring each, and in turn differences in the best ways of instructing each. As we have seen, however, skills are always, at least to some degree, composites of all three domains, so that questions of differences in how each type of skill is acquired are not as clear-cut and easily differentiated as they might on initial reflection seem.

Although there remains some debate on this issue, there is a growing body of evidence that cognitive, perceptual, and motor skills are acquired in essentially the same way (Allman, 1999; Gardner, 1983; Heathcote, Brown, and Mewhort, 2000; Rosenbaum, Carlson, and Gilmore, 2001). Similarities among skills in all three domains include the following:

1. **Transfer specificity**—Practicing a particular skill generally has little if any influence on other skills (Kramer, Strayer, and Buckley, 1990; Singley and Anderson, 1989)
2. **Learning rates**—Charting the rate of learning in all three domains results in similar patterns which can all be described by the same mathematical power function rules (i.e., learning in all three domains follows the same mathematical regularities) (Neves and Anderson, 1981; Singley and Anderson, 1989)
3. **Learning stages**—Learners appear to progress through the same stages of learning regardless of the skill domain (Anderson, 1982; Fitts and Posner, 1967)

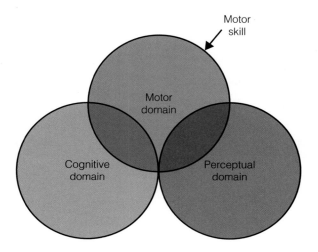

FIGURE **2.1** Motor Skills Include Aspects of the Cognitive and Perceptual Domains of Skill

Source: Created by author.

BOX **2.1**   Into Which Skill Domain Should Driving Be Classified?

All skills are composed of aspects from each of the three skill domains. The contributions of each domain may be so significant, in fact, that it can sometimes be difficult to decide into which domain a particular skill should be classified. How should driving an automobile be classified, for example? Certainly there are essential cognitive demands when driving. A driver must know the rules of the road, as well as understand operating procedures such as shifting gears and steering around corners. Perception is also essential to driving. Detecting changes in road conditions, other traffic, and one's own car speed and direction require constant monitoring of an ever-changing array of sensory information. Finally, a driver must coordinate both the knowledge of driving and the perception of the driving environment with correct motor responses involved in steering, accelerating, braking, and shifting gears in order to accomplish driving skills efficiently and safely. Given the essential contributions of each skill domain when a person is operating an automobile, would you classify driving as a cognitive, perceptual, or motor skill?

4. **Individual differences in skill performance**—The general correlation between how well individuals perform any two dissimilar skills is highly consistent across all three skill domains (Gardner, 1983)
5. **Importance of imagery**—Once thought to play a role only in cognitive learning, recent research has revealed the important role imagery plays in the learning of perceptual and motor skills, as well (Billard, 2001; Crammond, 1997; Jeannerod, 1994)
6. **Involvement of neural substrates**—Recent research has revealed that there is significantly less differentiation than once thought between areas of the brain involved in generating the three types of skills, especially a more important role of the cerebellum in cognitive as well as perceptual and motor skills than was previously believed (Courchesne and Allen, 1997; Fiez, 1996)
7. **Similar training effects**—Many similarities exist in the effects of various training regimens on the learning of skills in all three domains, including practice distribution effects, effectiveness of varied practice scheduling, and the roles of instruction and feedback (Schmidt and Bjork, 1992).

The final point just made, that similarities exist in the training effects of various practice arrangements and methods among all three skill domains, should be especially noted. We will see throughout our study that problems arise, and relatively ineffective instructional methods frequently follow, when we forget that all three skill domains share more commonalities than differences. Indeed, advances in neuroscience have led experts from across the spectrum of skill domains to conclude that common neural mechanisms underlie the acquisition of all skills, and even that all skills are performatory in nature. In this view, all skills are related to an action system. Cognition and perception exist fundamentally to subserve action, and are intrinsically linked to the motor system and to the acquisition of motor skills (Smyth and Haggard, 1999; Rosenbaum, Carlson, and Gilmore, 2001).

BUT WHAT, EXACTLY, IS A SKILL?

Having distinguished among the three domains into which skills are grouped, the reader might still be left with the question, What, exactly, is a skill? Or, to be more precise, What is a motor skill?

BOX **2.2**

Is There a Correlation between Intelligence and Motor Skills?

There is growing evidence that intelligence and proficiency at motor skills, especially motor coordination, are significantly correlated. Large studies of school-age children in both Europe and the United States have reported links between measures of intelligence and levels of motor coordination. In one study, children with higher cognitive status were found more capable of carrying out complex motor tasks than were children of lower cognitive status. Findings like these support the growing conclusion among scientists in several fields of study that a common neurological mechanism or factor supports cognitive, perceptual, and motor activities. Although debate still exists over what this factor might be, scientists studying human intelligence have begun to include motor intelligence as an important field of study.

Defining Skills Generally

Jack Adams, one of the founding fathers of modern motor learning research, in an important review of the history of motor skill research concluded that the term "skill is not favored with a clear outline" and that "analysts have been struggling with its definition for decades" (Adams, 1987, p. 41). Although there are points of contention among researchers and motor learning theorists relative to what should be emphasized given different theoretical perspectives, a workable definition of skill (and motor skill) useful to the student interested in the domain of motor skill learning can still be offered.

Our discussion thus far has resulted in the classification of a diverse array of activities as skills. This leads to the first of three important elements in defining skill: (1) Skills entail a broad range of human behaviors. As we have seen, those behaviors classified as skill range from activities emphasizing cognitive elements to those in which perceptual and motor elements dominate, as well as varying combinations of all three. Thus, the many types of activity classified as skills are broad and diverse, making up a large part of people's daily activities.

Though skills represent a wide range of human behavior, they all have one important feature in common. This leads to the second element in defining skill: (2) Skills are goal-oriented; they are directed toward the attainment of a specific goal. Skills are purpose driven and, therefore, voluntary. A performer purposefully initiates action to achieve a specific goal.

Finally, (3) skills are learned. Individuals acquire an improved capacity to achieve desired goals through experience or, frequently, intentional practice. It is in this sense that we can say that a person is unskilled or highly skilled at an activity, depending on his or her degree of learning rather than on some underlying capacity or ability that is genetically acquired. Some skills, like walking, are learned through developmental processes involving interaction with the environment. Others, like turning a light switch on and off, are learned through often repeated (but not intentionally practiced) experiences. Yet other skills, including most everyday and virtually all specialized skills, are learned through intentional practice.

We can offer the following working definition of a **skill**:

> A skill is a learned, goal-directed activity entailing a wide range of human behaviors.

skill: A learned, goal-directed activity entailing a broad range of human behaviors.

Defining Motor Skills Specifically

Our proceeding discussion resulted in a general definition of skill, regardless of the specific domain of skill addressed. What about motor skills specifically, though? Defining motor skills entails the same three components used with the more general definition of skill but also addresses the contributions of the motor system and movement in accomplishing skill goals. Narrowing our definition of skill to motor skills, we can say that (1) motor skills cover a broad range of behaviors accomplished primarily through the coordination of limbs and body segments brought about through involvement of the musculature. (2) Motor skills are directed toward the accomplishment of specific environmental goals, and goal attainment is importantly dependent on movement. Although any skilled behavior involves combinations of cognitive, perceptual, and motor processes in varying degrees of importance, motor skills refer to performance that is "muscular," that is, where muscular activity is the primary determinant in goal attainment. (3) Motor skills are learned. Motor skills do not result from the activity of reflexes or inherent natural abilities—they must be learned. Motor skills range from simple actions easily learned, such as depressing a telegraph key on signal, to complex sports skills requiring lengthy periods of practice to master.

Folding these features into definitional form, we can offer the following expanded definition of a **motor skill:**

> A motor skill is a learned, goal-directed activity accomplished primarily through muscular contributions to action and entailing a broad range of human behaviors.

This definition, referred to as the classic definition of motor skill, represents a categorical definition. This means that any activity or behavior so described is, by definition, a motor skill. That is, it is a definition that circumscribes all behaviors considered motor skills, regardless of the quality of those behaviors. In this sense, it is a definition of motor skill as a "thing." This is a widely accepted definition pervasive in the literature and echoed by many authors over the years, so that we might label it as the classic definition of motor skills.

motor skill: A learned, goal-directed activity accomplished primarily through muscular contributions to action.

Defining Motor Skills by the Characteristics of Skilled Performance

The classic definition of motor skills just presented highlights an important characteristic of skills—they can be improved! This has led many skill analysts to include in their definition of motor skill those features distinguishing relatively poor, or unskilled, performers from highly skilled performers. That is, the extent and quality of learning becomes an important aspect of how motor skill is defined.

A definition of motor skill in terms of the characteristics separating performers of various skill levels was offered in 1952 by Guthrie and has continued to influence the definition of motor skills to the present. Guthrie posited that all motor skills consist of the ability to bring about some end result with maximum certainty and a minimum outlay of energy, or of energy and time.

There is intuitive appeal in Guthrie's definition. In particular, it highlights the qualitative aspect of motor skills. That is, different individuals performing the *same* skill can exhibit varying quality of performance. Specific in Guthrie's definition are three features separating unskilled from skilled performers. (A comparison of Guthrie's definition of skill with that of the classic definition is shown in Table 2.1.)

1. **Maximum certainty of goal achievement.** An important quality of skill proficiency is the ability to achieve the task goal with a maximum of certainty. In laboratory research concerned with motor skill learning, certainty is measured by the reduction (change) in error measures over acquisition. In sports settings, certainty is the primary determinant of skill. A kicker in football who misses all of his team's attempted field goals, even if his kicking form is perfect, would not be considered skilled.

2. **Minimum energy expenditure.** For many motor skills, proficiency is achieved through the minimization of energy required for performance. The conservation of energy is essential to high-level performance in energy-demanding skills such as wrestling or cross-country running. In these activities, the skilled performer learns to reduce or eliminate unnecessary movement or physical exertion. In addition to reductions in muscular forces through efficient regulation of the body's energy producing systems, individuals also learn to minimize the mental demands required for task attainment. Performers come to produce skills in more automatic fashion, with less conscious attention directed toward movement organization, and are then more able to direct mental resources to other features of the performance or the environment (a topic explored more fully in Chapter 6).

3. **Minimum movement time.** In many motor skills, the quality of performance increases with reduced time (or increased speed) of movement. Skillful performers of such motor skills as volleyball, soccer, baseball, running, and swimming all benefit from increasing the speed of their movements. Success in some sport skills, such as sprinting, is almost entirely determined by the speed of motor actions.

It should be noted, however, that some motor performances are not improved as movement speed continues to increase. In skills requiring considerable movement accuracy, such as hammering a nail or hitting a baseball, too much speed can result in decreased performance success. Attempting to hammer a nail too rapidly will result in misses (and perhaps a smashed finger or two), just as attempting to swing at a pitched baseball with maximum speed can result in a strike rather than a hit. These examples demonstrate one of the oldest principles in skill performance: the speed–accuracy trade-off, which we discuss in Chapter 4.

Limitations to Definitional Use

An important caution must be mentioned in applying Guthrie's definition distinguishing among individuals on the basis of varying skill levels. There is a tendency, when focusing attention too closely on aspects of performance quality, to limit the definition, and therefore the term *skill*, to only those performances of high quality or expertise. Only those skills carried out by highly

TABLE **2.1**
Comparing Two Definitions of Motor Skill

	Classic Definition	Guthrie's Definition
Defining Characteristics	Goal-directed, learned behaviors accomplished primarily through contributions of the muscular system	Maximizes certainty of goal attainment while minimizing energy expenditure and movement time
Defining Perspective	Nature of the task	Quality of performance
Primary Question Addressed	What behaviors constitute motor skills?	What makes a person skillful?

skilled individuals may come to be seen as warranting research and scholarly attention. Too much focus on those qualities indicating high-level performance of motor skills may, as a result, lead us to neglect aspects of skill displayed by beginning or relatively ineffective performers, who may represent those individuals most in need of the movement specialist's attention.

Skills, Movements, and Abilities

Before concluding our consideration of the definition of motor skill, we need to clarify a few other terms that are either frequently used in its place or are incorrectly identified with it. Two terms are especially used in the literature when referring to motor skills; these are the terms *response* and *action*. Both of these terms can be used interchangeably with that of the term *motor skill* though each carries a slightly different theoretical connotation. The term **response** has the longest history of the two, and is rooted in psychological approaches to the study of human behavior going as far back as the early 1900s. The term is particularly favored by theorists emphasizing the behavioral or cognitive aspects of skill acquisition. (It should be noted that some theorists discourage use of the term *response*, feeling it indicates that skills are initiated exclusively by environmental stimuli rather than being voluntary behaviors. This being a valid caution, when using the term *response* in this text it is with the connotation that skills may be initiated both as responses to environmental stimuli, as well as to voluntary decisions). In recent years, the term **action** has emerged in common usage much more recently, especially by those theorists interested in the contributions of the environment and of the interaction of numerous systems in the control and acquisition of motor skills. Thus, *motor skill*, *response*, and *action* may be considered synonymous terms.

The term *movement* is frequently also used as a synonym for motor skill, as in "She has mastered the various movements required to be good at basketball." Movements are not the same thing as motor skills, however, and the two terms should not be confused and used interchangeably. Movements refer to the behavioral characteristics of bodily elements. The change in position of an individual limb or body segment is a **movement**. Movements are the constituent parts of a skill. Motor skills are assembled through a collection of movements organized together to manifest a complex action directed toward the accomplishment of a specific goal. Further, a particular motor skill can be accomplished through a variety of different movements. The movements executed to run on an indoor running track, on a sandy beach, or on an incline are different, yet each contributes to the skill of running.

Ability is another term frequently used incorrectly to refer to motor skills. Abilities are stable and enduring traits that are genetically inherited. Abilities can be thought of as the building blocks of motor skills, because they underlie the execution of movements and play a significant role in determining a person's capacity to learn and perform motor skills. Examples of motor abilities are reaction time, hand-eye coordination, and speed of limb movement. (It should be noted that, as with the term *response*, the term *ability* also reflects specific theoretical assumptions, leading some contemporary theorists to disregard its use altogether.) We will consider the topic of abilities in more detail in Chapter 8.

response: A term used synonymously with motor skill, especially by those favoring a cognitive perspective of motor behavior.

action: A term used synonymously with motor skill.

movement: A change in the position of limbs or body segments; the behavioral components used to assemble motor skills.

ability: A genetically endowed trait underlying the performance of motor skills.

THE STUDY OF MOTOR SKILLS

The study of how motor skills are controlled, as well as what methods are the most effective when instructing them, is grounded in the way we conceptualize motor skills and in the kinds of questions we ask. In the following section, we examine the three components of motor skills studied by movement scientists.

The Three Components of Motor Skills

What are the components influencing the performance of motor skills? What can be observed and studied? Newell (1986) has offered an influential analysis of these questions. In his analysis, he suggests that three components of motor skills influence their performance, and that all three must be taken into account for the fullest understanding of motor skills. These components include the person performing the skill, the task that is performed, and the environment in which the skill is performed (see Figure 2.2). In the simplest terms, the conceptualization of motor skills must take into account the who, what, and where of skills. Although motor skills are a composite of all three components, each component addresses unique features of skill performance, and each therefore lends itself to the study of a unique set of questions.

The Person

The attributes of individual persons play a significant role in shaping the performance of motor skills. Each person brings a unique composition of innate abilities, physical characteristics, psychological traits, previous skill-learning experiences, age, and motivation to the performance of motor skills. Such personal features can interact in different ways with how individuals experience different practice arrangements, different types of instruction and feedback, and other training arrangements. By studying such individual and training differences, movement scientists can gain information concerning the properties of skills and of the processes responsible for their learning.

The Task

The nature of the task is the second component shaping the performance of motor skills. Motor skill tasks vary widely in their goals and in the movement demands placed upon performers. Some tasks must be performed under a variety of conditions, such as driving in traffic, whereas others are performed consistently from one performance context to the next, such as shooting basketball free throws. Tasks also vary relative to the perceptual demands they place upon individuals. Many motor

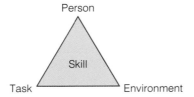

FIGURE **2.2** The Study of Motor Skills Encompasses Three Components Influencing Performance

skills have high perceptual demands. Baseball players must accurately determine the speed and path of a pitched ball when batting, and hockey goalies quickly discern the movement patterns of an opposing team rushing the net, for example. Other tasks require the manipulation of implements for successful performance. Bowling, hammering nails, and using a prosthesis all require coordinating bodily movements within constraints imposed by external objects. The rules of sports skills may also constrain a person's movements and influence the quality of task performance.

The Environment

The third component influencing skill performance is the environment in which a person executes the skill. Where will a motor task be performed? What is the environmental context of performance?

Skills may be performed within environments that are predictable or unpredictable, similar or dissimilar to practice conditions, recreational or competitive. Skills may also be performed alone or in the presence of others, who can include other performers as well as spectators. Physical conditions of the performance context may also influence performance characteristics. Lighting conditions, temperature, wind, and gravity can substantially alter the performance of many skills.

Ultimately, the fullest understanding of motor skills derives from an appreciation of the interaction of all three components contributing to their performance.

CHARACTERISTICS OF MOTOR SKILLS

Having defined motor skills, we next inquire into the characteristics common to motor skills. What features do all motor skills share in common? This is far from a question for mere speculation. In approaching the scientific study of motor skills, our assumptions, theories, and findings must remain embedded within the shared framework of such characteristics. Indeed, any theory or research finding must ultimately be tested by its ability to adequately address, and shed light upon, such shared characteristics. In identifying the characteristics common to all motor skills, Sheridan (1984) has proposed that any

---

BOX **2.3**   **Can You Identify the Components of Motor Skills That Influence Performance?**

The performance of any motor skill is influenced by three distinct skill components. The environment in which a skill is performed can both facilitate and limit performance possibilities. Likewise, the nature of the task, including equipment and rules, can assist as well as limit performance. Finally, qualities inherent in the person performing the skill, such as previous experience, physical fitness, and motivation, play a significant role in skill performance. For the following activities, can you think of something about each of these three components that would act to constrain or limit

performance, as well as something that would facilitate the quality of performance?

- Riding a bicycle
- Catching a Frisbee
- Walking on crutches
- Serving a volleyball
- Standing from a chair
- Driving a car

List one factor that might limit, as well as one that might enhance, performance of each skill for the skill components of environment, task, and person.

adequate theory of motor skills must address at least four essential characteristics common to all motor skills. These include motor equivalence, motor variability, motor consistency, and motor modifiability.

Motor Equivalence

Humans are highly flexible in the ways they can move to meet environmental demands (Lashley, 1930; Flash and Hogan, 1985). Flexibility of action is achieved by recruiting different muscles and joints to achieve the same skill goal (by organizing different movements to accomplish the same skill goals). For example, you can catch a ball with either your dominant or nondominant hand, turn on a light switch using your elbow when your hands are filled with packages (you can even use your nose), or sign your name holding a pen between your teeth while writing on a piece of paper. These are examples of skilled action accomplished with effectors we would not normally use to complete a given motor skill, but which nonetheless can often be done with great effectiveness even when we may never have attempted the action in exactly the same way before. This capacity to accomplish the same environmental skill goal in many

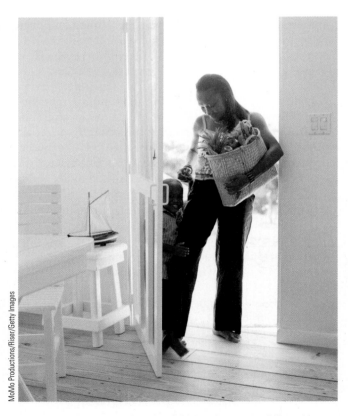

MoMo Productions/Riser/Getty Images

Humans are capable of accomplishing the same skill goal in many different ways, a capacity known as motor equivalence.

motor equivalence:
The capacity to produce many different movement patterns to accomplish the same action goal.

different, and often quite varied, ways is referred to as **motor equivalence,** and denotes the many equivalent ways we can move and still accomplish the same action goal. Although we typically accomplish such equivalent movements with considerable ease, the explanation of how we do so remains a complex and debated question among motor behavior theorists (Kelso et al., 1998).

Motor Variability

The uniqueness of human action—the fact that no two skills are ever accomplished in exactly the same way—is a second characteristic of human motor skills. Even when we watch a highly skilled performer completing successive repetitions of the same stereotypical skill—such as a tennis player hitting balls projected by a ball machine—the repeated actions are never completed in exactly the same way. Slight variations are evident, for example, in how the body is positioned prior to contacting the ball, in the kinematic patterns of limb movements during skill execution, and in the kinetic forces generated to accomplish the skill. More striking yet, the same neural pathways are never used successively in completing the same skill, nor are the same motor units recruited and patterned the same way to control muscular forces. Even when movement skills may appear nearly identical to an observer, at the neurological level they are markedly different, with movements organized and assembled through vastly different architectures of neural routes, synaptic impulses, and collectives of muscle fibers (see Chapter 3). This suggests that the movement patterns underlying motor skills are not rigidly constructed, but that new solutions to movement problems must be found each and every time a skill is

BOX **2.4**   **In How Many Different Ways Can the Goal of a Skill Be Accomplished?**

An old saying goes that "All roads lead to Rome." But can many movements lead to the same skill goal? Motor equivalence refers to the capacity of humans to recruit different effectors, and to organize movements in different ways, in order to accomplish the same movement goal. Most skill goals can be accomplished in an almost infinite variety of ways. In a first-round play-off game concluding the 2007 football season, the Green Bay Packers quickly gave up two touchdowns to the Seattle Seahawks and appeared on the verge of being eliminated from further competition. After rallying back, though, the Packers were down by only 4 points. Then Brett Favre, the Packer quarterback, drove his team to within 20 yards of a go-ahead score. But after three failed plays, and with a fourth down and still 20 yards to go to the end zone, the Packers' chances looked bleak. As the ball was snapped, the Packers' play-off hopes rode on a single play. Favre went back

to pass but was instantly surrounded by charging Seahawk defenders who chased him out of his protective pocket. Scrambling to avoid being tackled, Favre stumbled and was falling toward the turf. As he fell forward, he managed to twist his body a full 180 degrees so that his back was toward the ground and his body fully stretched out. A few inches before hitting the turf, Favre flipped the football across his body with a backhanded toss into the end zone, where a waiting receiver, Greg Jennings, caught it for a game-winning touchdown.

How many times do you suppose that Favre had practiced throwing the football in that particular way previously? The fact that he had almost certainly never done so, yet could organize his motor system to accomplish a well-learned skill in an entirely new and different way, a phenomenon called *motor equivalence*, is one of the most amazing movement characteristics that humans possess.

motor variability: No two movement patterns, even of the same skill, are ever produced in exactly the same way.

performed, even if that skill has been performed in more or less the same way thousands of times previously. This phenomenon is called **motor variability**, and is one of the most challenging problems in the study of motor skills.

Motor Consistency

Even though all motor skills are unique, as we have just seen, still we learn to move in skillful ways. That is, even though we never produce a skill in exactly the same way twice, in those skills for which we practice and become good, we are highly consistent from one time to the next in achieving the same outcome. A highly skilled baseball pitcher never uses the same neural pathways in throwing a fastball (even after throwing perhaps hundreds of thousands of fastballs), yet his fastball is consistent in striking out batters. This ability to accomplish the same movement goal, which is improved through experience and practice, is termed **motor consistency**. How we learn to produce such skilled actions, given the variability of each movement, is a problem motor learning specialists must answer if their theories of motor control and learning are to have the greatest explanatory power (see discussion of the skill acquisition problem in the following section of the chapter).

motor consistency: The capacity to achieve the goals of motor skills consistently; the capacity of the human motor system to learn.

Motor Modifiability

The final characteristic for which any theory of motor skills must account is that of a skilled performer's ability to modify an action once its execution has begun. Observing any athletic performance involving the need for athletes to quickly react to rapidly changing game situations will provide many examples of this characteristic. Examples could include, for instance, a baseball player who begins to swing at a pitched ball but then quickly lets up, stopping his swing when it becomes obvious the ball is not in the strike zone, or a basketball player starting to take a shot and then quickly changing her actions to pass the ball to a teammate when a defender covers her too closely. The ability to change an action quickly once it has begun is termed **motor modifiability**. Again, as with the other characteristics listed here, it is easily accomplished—often seemingly effortlessly—but a complex phenomenon when we begin to attempt a scientific explanation of it.

motor modifiability: The capacity to alter a movement pattern to achieve a new action goal.

In summary, the characteristics listed above and common to all motor skills present challenging problems in the study of motor skills, even when in practice their solution may seem achieved with considerable ease. This leads us to a consideration of the problems confronting us in the study of motor skills.

FOUR PROBLEMS IN THE STUDY OF MOTOR SKILLS

In the study of motor skills, four problems occupy a central place (Rosenbaum, 2010). None of the characteristics among motor skills presented above, for instance, can be adequately addressed without some explanation concerning these four persistent problems. Indeed, the major theories that guide research concerning motor behavior are largely attempts to provide satisfactory answers to these central questions. The fact that there are different theories is testimony to the complexity of these problems, and to the ongoing lack of a consensus in how they should be answered. These four persistent problems include (1) the degrees of freedom problem, (2) the perceptual-motor integration problem, the (3) serial-order (timing) problem, and (4) the skill acquisition problem.

The Degrees of Freedom Problem

One of the greatest challenges facing movement scientists concerns answering the question of how various **units of action** (e.g., joints, muscles, motor units, cells) are organized and controlled in order to accomplish skill goals. Specifically, how does a person, in response to his or her environment, coordinate and control a complex system of bony segments, linked by joints and layers of musculature, that is capable of moving in a variety of different ways. Recall that in the performance of any motor skill, there are many ways the motor system might be organized in order to produce movements capable of achieving skillful goals (i.e., motor equivalence). Only one of many alternative means of achieving a desired outcome must be selected, however. The question is: How is this accomplished?

The term **degrees of freedom** is used to describe the number of different ways in which any given unit of control is capable of being organized. Stated more precisely, it is the number of dimensions in which a system can independently vary. The term *independent* is critical to our understanding here. Simply, it means that regardless of the value one thing takes on (e.g., muscle A contracts a certain amount), another thing within the same system is still free to take on any of the values of which it is capable (e.g., muscle B is free to contract to any value, or to not contract at all—it is not limited by the value to which muscle A has contracted).

We can consider the degrees of freedom available to an individual as all of the possible choices for organizing desired motor skills. We can further specify these available degrees of freedom at various levels of analysis. If what we control during movement are the joints, then to move the arm, for example, would require seven degrees of freedom. Three degrees of freedom are available at the shoulder (it can move up and down, side to side, and rotate), two at the elbow (it can flex and extend and it can rotate), and two at the wrist joint (it can move from side to side and it can flex and extend). If we go a step further and consider muscles as the unit that is controlling movement, the number of degrees of freedom rises dramatically. In order to move the same arm successfully, we must now regulate a minimum of 26 degrees of freedom: 10 muscles at the shoulder joint, 10 more at the elbow joint, and 6 controlling the different movements of the wrist joint. If this analysis of an arm movement is extended to the unit of action of motor units, the estimated number for the degrees of freedom available rises exponentially—into the thousands (see Box 2.5). The greater the number of degrees of freedom that must be controlled, it should be pointed out, the greater the complexity of the problem that must be solved by the motor system.

Over half a century ago, the Russian physiologist A. N. Bernstein recognized that human coordination emerges from the accumulated involvement of many redundant degrees of freedom that underlie multijoint movements. The many different ways in which movements might be organized in order

unit of action: A specified component of movement that can be used repeatedly in various actions, producing essentially the same results.

degrees of freedom: The number of dimensions in which a system can independently vary.

to accomplish skill goals is made possible by a large surplus of degrees of freedom available. How one pattern of organizing these redundant degrees of freedom is selected rather than another has come to be referred to as the **degrees of freedom problem**. In initially formulating this problem, Bernstein argued that the computational demands placed upon the central nervous system were too great for it to be considered the sole executor of movement control. The degrees of freedom problem first formulated by Bernstein remains at the core of today's contemporary theorizing concerning the control of human movement.

degrees of freedom problem: How the many degrees of freedom available in the human motor system are controlled to produce a particular movement.

The Perceptual-Motor Integration Problem

Skills do not occur in a perceptual vacuum. Perception is the process of acquiring, selecting, interpreting, and organizing sensory information. Skill movements are guided by sensory information arising from both the environment and performer's body. How perceptual information is coupled with bodily movement in order to achieve skillful actions is one aspect of the perceptual-motor integration problem. For example, in order to catch a tossed object, the

---

BOX 2.5 How Many Ways Can You Touch Your Nose?

The large redundancy of degrees of freedom available in the human motor system makes possible tremendous flexibility in people's movement capabilities, but also presents a challenging problem to movement scientists attempting to understand the control of movement. This problem can be illustrated with a simple exercise (Rosenbaum, 1991). To perform this exercise, touch the tip of your index finger to the tip of your nose (go ahead and complete this).

No doubt, you performed this exercise with little effort, but consider the computational demands it placed upon your central nervous system. If we consider just the arm as our basic unit of analysis, and the unit of action as the joints involved in moving the arm, then there are seven degrees of freedom that must be controlled in touching your nose. That is, the shoulder is free to assume values in each of three dimensions (horizontal, vertical, and twisting), the elbow in two dimensions (it can bend and twist), and the wrist also in two dimensions (up and down and side to side). Consider, though, that each way a particular joint might vary can be coupled with every way both of the other joints

might vary, so that in reality there are 12 distinct movement combinations made possible by the degrees of freedom in the arm (i.e., the number of degrees of freedom for each joint multiplied through, or $3 \times 2 \times 2$). If we extend our analysis to the level of muscles, however, the challenge will appear to become somewhat greater. Now there are 26 degrees of freedom in the arm (10 muscles control shoulder movements, 10 for the elbow, and 6 for the wrist). Calculating the number of different muscle activation patterns possible, there are 600 different contraction/no contraction combinations among the 26 individual muscles ($10 \times 10 \times 6$). That is, there are 600 basic coordination patterns available to select from in touching your nose.

One final level of analysis must still be considered. Remember that the nervous system controls both joints and muscles indirectly; direct control is of motor units. If we take a conservative estimate and assign a value of 100 motor units to each muscle (there would be more in our example), then the 26 muscles controlling the arm represent 2,600 degrees of freedom at the motor unit level of analysis. Again, because motor units are also trajectory of the object must be determined and related to the current position of the hand that will be used to catch it. The position of the fingers, as well as the "firmness" with which the catching limb is maintained, must also be adjusted depending upon the perceived size, shape, and velocity of the tossed object. Moreover, these adjustments must be initiated prior to contact with the tossed object. Thus, the relevant aspects of a person's environment must be perceived and effectively coupled with movements of the catching limb and hand to successfully accomplish the goal of intercepting and grasping the tossed object. A persistent problem in the study of motor skills is to understand how the highly coordinated movements of limbs and bodily segments are effectively coupled with sensory information to produce the exquisitely executed skills of which humans are capable. This is referred to as the **perceptual-motor integration problem.**

Although perception guides movement, movement also influences perception. One obvious reason for this is that movement transports sensory receptors to new locations, thus benefiting perception. Turning your head supplies additional visual information concerning the environment, thus enriching and

perceptual-motor integration problem: The intellectual problems arising when attempting to explain how perception is coupled with human movement to produce motor skills.

free to take on any individual value in relation to any other motor unit (each can be "on" or "off" according to the all-or-none law), there are within the movement system of the arm *600 million* possible combinations available when recruiting motor units to touch your nose (1,000 × 1,000 × 600). How you

selected a particular combination from the many possibilities available is still debated by movement scientists, though fortunately it will not prevent you from scratching your nose should you have an itch. A summary of our calculations is shown in the accompanying table.

	Units of Action		
	Joints	Muscles	Motor Units
Shoulder	3	10	1,000
Elbow	2	10	1,000
Wrist	2	6	600
Degrees of freedom in three-joint system	7	26	2,600
Total number of possible combinations of degrees of freedom within three-joint system	12	600	600,000,000

benefiting perception. Walking to a new location allows you to see and hear more of what is present in the environment. Exploring objects with your hands allows you to better perceive their shapes and surface textures.

Movement affects perception in even more subtle ways, however. There is growing evidence that perception is altered by the movements that humans are capable of producing (Proctor and Dutta, 1995; Vickers, 2007). When people view a cluttered environment through which they must navigate, for instance, they are most likely to perceive those environmental features that afford the greatest opportunity for passage given their movement capabilities (such opportunities are called **affordances**). Individuals with poor or limited movement skills are most likely to perceive features within the environment that provide for the greatest ease of passage, whereas those with a greater repertoire of movement skills are the most likely to perceive features indicating a more difficult but shorter path across the cluttered space, for example. In other words, a person's movement capabilities play a role in what he or she perceives in the environment, supposedly providing the perceptual cues that will be of the greatest benefit.

affordances: The properties of an object or of the environment that offer opportunities for action.

Although perception and movement are intricately linked and mutually dependent upon one another, there is considerable debate concerning how they are linked. Some theorists posit that higher-order cognitive representations of skills mediate between perception and movement, viewing perception as "information" used to plan and carry out movements. Other theorists emphasize a direct link between perception and action, seeing little need for additional mediation (Gibson, 1966, 1979). Regardless of which theoretical perspective is assumed, however, the coupling between perception and movement remains one of the most challenging problems facing motor skill theorists and researchers.

The Serial-Order (Timing) Problem

Whenever skills require the sequencing of discrete movement elements, some means of organizing their execution is required (Proctor and Dutta, 1995). A dancer rhythmically linking dozens of individual movements into delicate routines of choreographed precision and grace, a typist whose fingers appear to fly from letter to letter on a keyboard without error, the competitive swimmer perfectly coordinating patterns of arm circles and leg kicks while racing through the water—all illustrate the human capacity for stitching individual threads of movement into the many patterns representing the fabric of motor skills.

serial-order problem: The problems arising in attempting to provide an adequate explanation for how the order and timing of movement elements forming motor skills are organized and controlled.

We need not look only to expertly performed skill examples such as those of the dancer, typist, or swimmer to observe the intricate timing involved in most motor skills, however. Daily activities such as walking, speech, and dressing are also comprised of the linkage of many precisely timed and ordered submovements. The **serial-order problem** consists in how the ordering and timing of the various subelements that comprise motor skills are controlled. One possible explanation is that skills rely on some sort of stimulus–response mechanism so that sensory feedback from one response acts to initiate the following response in a sequence. This notion is referred to as *linear chaining*. A major weakness in the linear chain notion, however, is that no single motor element acts to elicit the same response in every skill situation, but may indeed be followed by many different responses depending upon the particular situation. This weakness, first pointed out many years ago by Lashley (1951), has led to the search for alternative explanations for how motor acts are timed. Two major alternatives have been advanced, with both a hierarchical model based upon cognitive control and a constraints-led model based upon the interaction of the actor and environment proposed. Although theoretically different, both models have provided revealing insights and continue to advance our understanding of how the timing and sequencing components of human motor skills are controlled.

The Skill Acquisition Problem

In presenting the characteristics common to all motor skills, we have stated a seeming contradiction; that is, skills exhibit motor variability—even when performed in highly stereotypical fashion, they are never organized in exactly the same way twice. On the other hand, skills exhibit motor consistency. Through repeated experiences, people become more capable of meeting the goals of a skill—they become more skilled. How does such learning take place given the variability inherent in skilled behaviors? This question represents the **skill acquisition problem**.

skill acquisition problem: An intellectual or research problem arising in attempting to explain how motor skills are learned.

To the movement practitioner, this is probably the most critical problem in the study of motor skills. Certainly, an adequate understanding of how motor skills are acquired is critical to the design of effective practice experiences. To the movement scientist also, though, the question of how motor skills are acquired presents many research and theoretical challenges. The general problem of skill acquisition is really expressed as a series of subproblems. Among the most intriguing and widely researched are the following:

1. What are the underlying processes responsible for skill learning?
2. How are skills represented in the nervous system? Or are they?
3. Are some skills innate, or are all skills acquired through experience or practice?
4. Do people pass through identifiable stages when learning skills? If so, are they the same for everyone?
5. As motor skills are acquired, what changes occur within individuals?
6. What is the optimal way to schedule practice experiences?
7. What kind of instructions prove of the greatest benefit to learners? Of what information are learners in the most need?
8. Is there an upper limit to how proficient an individual can become in a given skill?
9. Why do individuals differ in their capacity for learning different skills?
10. How does the learning of one skill influence the learning of other skills?

Answers to these questions, as well as the broader question concerning the primary mechanisms responsible for skill acquisition generally, remain among the most challenging to movement scientists.

THE CLASSIFICATION OF MOTOR SKILLS

As is clear from our discussion in this chapter, motor skills represent a diverse collection of movement behaviors. Motor skills include activities as different as knitting and Olympic weight lifting, downhill skiing and brushing your teeth, or fly-fishing and ballet. Such striking differences among the behaviors defined as motor skills can easily lead to confusion, especially when we wish to communicate about important similarities or differences among motor skills. What is needed is a method of classifying motor skills based upon a limited number of relevant features that can provide for meaningful grouping as well as effective communication. In the study of motor skills, two methods of classification, one-dimensional and two-dimensional systems, are widely used.

One-Dimensional Classification Systems

In a one-dimensional classification system, the phenomena of interest are classified on a continuum between two polar opposites. For example, temperature can be classified on a continuum running between the polar opposites of hot and cold, mood between polar opposites of sad and happy, or political identity between polar opposites of liberal and conservative. When applying a one-dimensional system to the classification of motor skills, three dimensions of performance or of the performance context are identified. These include (1) the stability of the environment in which a skill is performed, (2) the temporal features of the skill relative to its beginning and ending, and (3) the precision of movement required in accomplishing the skill. All motor skills can be classified along each of these three dimensions.

The Classification of Motor Skills Based upon the Stability of the Environment

One system for classifying motor skills is based upon the stability of the environment in which they are performed. Here, environment refers to the context in which a person performs, as well as any object or objects upon which the person acts. Motor skills are classified as either closed or open, depending upon the predictability of the environment.

If the environment in which a person performs remains relatively constant from one time the skill is performed until the next, we classify the skill as a closed motor skill. Typing, for example, is a closed skill. The placement of the letters on a keyboard does not change from one keyboard to the next. Closed skills have the important feature that the environment or object acted upon waits, in effect, to be acted upon by the performer. You decide when to start typing, as well as when to stop and then start again. For this reason, closed motor skills are sometimes referred to as self-paced motor skills. Examples of closed skills include target shooting, writing, using a knife and fork, shooting basketball free throws, pitching horseshoes, and painting a wall.

As opposed to closed skills, an open motor skill is performed in a changing, unstable, and unpredictable environment. A person does not know from one attempt of a skill until the next how an object or the performance context may change and require modifications to the way in which the skill must be performed. Although free-throw shooting is a closed motor skill in the sport of basketball, dribbling down court during a basketball game is an open skill. In this case, the basketball player must react to movements of opposing players,

closed motor skill: A skill in which action occurs in a stable and predictable environment.

self-paced motor skill: A commonly used term denoting a closed motor skill.

open motor skill: A skill for which the object acted upon or the context in which action occurs varies from one performance to the next.

as well as those of teammates, all the while responding to constantly changing game situations. Proper skill execution, or even whether a skill should or should not be executed, cannot be accurately predicted and planned for in advance. For this reason, open motor skills are also referred to as reactive motor skills. Examples of open motor skills include open-field running in football, driving in traffic, chasing a dog, downhill snow skiing, dodging water balloons, and surf boarding.

How would you classify bowling? Is it a closed or an open motor skill? If you consider only the first ball in each frame, it is certainly closed because everything about the environment remains constant from one attempt to the next. But what about the second ball of each frame? For two kinds of bowlers, nothing changes: an expert bowler rolling a 300 game, and a beginner bowling all gutter balls. For both types of bowlers every attempt presents the same situation—all 10 pins are standing. For most bowlers, however, the second ball of each frame will present a somewhat different situation than the initial ball. Some of the pins will have been knocked down, although not the same ones each time. Sometimes nine pins will remain standing, and other times only a single pin; sometimes pins will remain standing on the right, sometimes on the left; and sometimes on both sides of the lane—a dreaded split! In each case, something has changed about the environment. How, then, should we classify the second ball in a frame?

Although some features of the environment in our example of second balls within frames of bowling may change, it should be clear that many more remain predictable. The ball is still the same. The lane on which the ball is rolled does

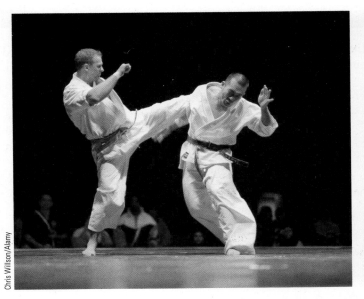
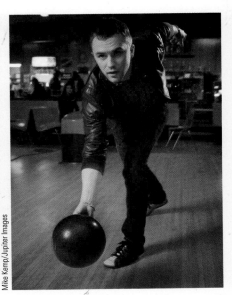

Chris Willson/Alamy

Mike Kemp/Jupiter Images

In open motor skills performers must react to unpredictable and changing conditions (left), while closed motor skills are performed within stable and predictable environments (right).

not change. And even though the exact arrangement of pins may vary, they do not do so in a way that drastically alters the movement pattern required to successfully bowl the ball and knock down each changing pin arrangement. More importantly, regardless of the number of pins standing, the skill is still self-paced—the performer can act when ready. So we can say that even a split presents a relatively closed environment where most features remain the same as for other balls thrown in the game. Thus, considering skills on a continuum ranging between closed and open environmental features, the second ball of a bowling frame remains closer to the closed end of the continuum than to the open end. Regardless of the particular arrangement of pins in the environment, bowling, in general, is considered a closed motor skill.

The closed–open classification system has been popular in instructional skill settings. An important reason is that it is relatively easy to classify skills in this fashion, and skills in each category follow common principles of instruction that teachers and therapists can readily apply. The closed–open distinction is also common in motor skills research, because findings relative to each category easily translate into real-world applications (see Figure 2.3).

The Classification of Motor Skills Based upon Temporal Predictability

A second way of classifying motor skills in a one-dimensional system is on the basis of the predictability of their beginning and ending points. Based upon these temporal features, motor skills are classified as being discrete, continuous, or serial.

Some skills, like hitting a baseball, have specific beginning and ending points. A batter must begin swinging as the ball approaches home plate, and once the swing is completed, all relevant action is over. Skills of this type, which have clearly identifiable beginning and ending points, are classified as **discrete motor skills.**

discrete motor skill:
A motor skill in which the beginning and ending points are clearly defined.

Unlike batting in baseball, not all discrete motor skills have both a forced beginning and ending point. Some, like hitting a golf ball rather than a baseball,

Closed Skills ←		→ Open Skills
Predictable performance context	Semi-predictable performance context	Unpredictable performance context
Basketball free throw	High jump	Mountain biking
Typing	Chopping wood	Wrestling
Springboard diving	Driving on a quiet road	Driving on a busy road
Painting a wall	Passing a basketball to a teammate in a game	Defending a goal in ice hockey

FIGURE **2.3** Classification of Skills as Closed or Open

Source: Created by author.

have arbitrary beginning points—the performer can wait until ready to hit the ball. The ending point to hitting a golf ball, however, is still forced by the completion of the swing and striking of the ball (this is, of course, the distinction between open and closed skills). Discrete skills are also typically completed quickly, usually lasting from a fraction of a second to no more than a few seconds.

A discrete skill is one that exhibits well-defined beginning and ending points, and is typically executed in a relatively brief period of time. We can add that the beginning point is not always temporally predictable, though the timing of the action is often rigidly fixed and highly predictable. Examples of discrete motor skills include serving a tennis ball, throwing darts, standing from a sitting position, ringing a doorbell, jumping over a fence, and flipping a coin.

continuous motor skill:
A motor skill in which the beginning and ending of action is arbitrary.

A **continuous motor skill** is one in which both the beginning and ending are arbitrary and unpredictable. Continuous skills are often (though not always) repetitive and rhythmic in nature—like walking and swimming, for example. A different but important class of continuous skills includes tracking skills, such as steering an automobile or keeping a stylus in contact with the target on a rotary pursuit task, which require the performer to continuously monitor the external environment and correct actions in an ongoing fashion. The point in either case is that the temporal dimensions of the tasks involved (beginning and, especially, ending points) are arbitrary and cannot be determined prior to the completion of an action. The individual decides when to end a continuous skill, and frequently when it will begin, also. Examples of continuous skills include riding a bicycle, running, tracking a moving target on a computer screen using a joystick, stirring hot coffee with a spoon, and flying a kite.

An interesting problem confronts us when deciding upon classifying motor skills on the basis of temporal considerations. Consider the skill of typing, for example. It is clear when watching a beginning typist that the actions involved are discrete in nature. That is, the beginning typist deliberately strikes a single key at a time—"C" for example—stops to search for the next key and then produces another discrete action—striking "A" in this example—then pausing to search again before striking another key—"T" to complete the example "CAT"—and so on and on. When those learning to type, it is clear that their actions represent a series of discrete acts. What about the same skill with an advanced typist? The expert's fingers seem to race effortlessly over the keyboard without pause. It is tempting to say the expert typist is performing a continuous skill. The problem is that a skill cannot be classified as two different types of skill, in this case both discrete and continuous, depending on a performer's skill level. (Remember that it is the skill itself, not the performer's skill level, that is classified in one-dimensional systems).

serial motor skill:
A motor skill composed of a series of discrete skills such that the integration of each discrete component into a continuous movement pattern is crucial to performance success.

The solution is a special classification for skills such as typing. Skills that require a series or sequence of discrete elements, like typing, are classified as **serial motor skills.** Serial skills are discrete skills that are linked together (often through a stimulus-response connection) and performed in a sequenced action, often so rapidly that they mimic a continuous skill. Examples of serial skills include hammering a nail, shifting gears in an automobile, a dance routine, playing the piano, brushing your teeth, and dribbling a basketball. It should be noted that some serial skills involve a simple repetitive or even rhythmic sequencing of the same action, such as dribbling a basketball or hammering a nail. Other serial skills involve the sequencing of different discrete skill elements in an exact order, such as typing or shifting gears in an automobile.

Although discrete skills have clearly predictable ending points, and the completion of continuous skills is arbitrary, the temporal predictability of a serial skill's ending point may be either predictable or arbitrary. For serial skills consisting of a series of different subskills, such as shifting gears in an automobile, the completion of the skill is highly predictable, whereas for highly repetitive actions like dribbling a basketball the performer decides upon the ending point (see Figure 2.4).

The Classification of Motor Skills Based upon Movement Precision

A third one-dimensional system for classifying motor skills is based on the precision of the movements required for completing the skill. (In defining this dimension, some writers prefer to focus upon the size of the primary musculature required in performing skills.) Within this one-dimensional system, motor skills are classified as being either fine or gross.

fine motor skill: A motor skill in which the precision of movement is the primary requisite for performance success.

Skills such as threading a needle that place primary emphasis on the precision of movement, rather than upon muscular effort, are labeled **fine motor skills**. Fine motor skills are typically accomplished by recruiting small muscle groups such as those of the fingers, hands, and forearms; may place a high premium on hand-eye coordination; and require little muscular force or energy to successfully accomplish. Examples of fine motor skills include handwriting, sewing, using chopsticks, buttoning a shirt, repairing watches, using precision tools, and operating a rotary-pursuit apparatus in a motor learning laboratory. In all of these cases, it is the precision of the movement itself, and not how forcefully it is done, that results in successful performance of the skill.

gross motor skill: A motor skill in which the contributions of muscular force are the primary requisite for performance success.

Gross motor skills are those that require the use of relatively large musculature in producing an action. Fundamental motor skills such as walking, running, leaping, jumping, throwing, balancing, and climbing are gross motor skills. Gross motor skills typically involve many muscle groups and, frequently, movement of the entire body. Although many sports skills classified as gross motor skills may require exquisite coordination to accomplish,

Discrete Skills	Serial Skills	Continuous Skills
Tennis serve	Triple jump	Water skiing
Flipping a coin	Paddleboarding	Flying a kite
Catching a ball	Shifting car gears	Brushing your teeth
Throwing a dart	Playing the drums	Rowing a canoe

FIGURE **2.4** Classification of Skills as Discrete, Serial, or Continuous

Source: Created by author.

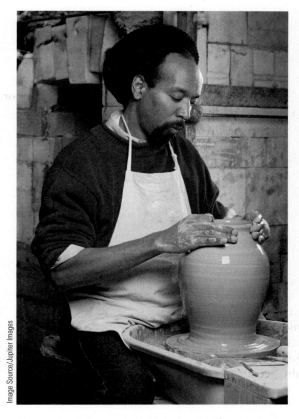

Image Source/Jupiter Images

Fine motor skills require a high degree of movement precision, and typically require the manual manipulation of objects and good hand-eye coordination.

the contributions of muscular force outweigh demands on movement precision in accomplishing the action. Examples of gross motor skills include standing from a chair, catching a football, doing somersaults, performing a *tour en l'air* in a ballet program, blocking in volleyball, and climbing a ladder.

Fine and gross skills form a continuum marked by the gradual shift of importance placed on either movement precision or force production in accomplishing the goals of a skill (see Figure 2.5).

Gentile's Two-Dimensional Taxonomy for Classifying Motor Skills

When making decisions about appropriate skill activities, motor skill instructors must frequently take into account the performance demands placed upon individuals. Although one-dimensional classification systems effectively discriminate among different classes of motor skills based on several important task considerations, they are less effective in delineating among skills based upon performance demands. What is often required is a system for grouping motor skills into categories based upon similar performance characteristics (recall here the analogous situation with the two definitions of motor skill

Fine Skills ◀———————————————————————▶ Gross Skills		
Knitting	Steering a car	Pole vaulting
Buttoning a shirt	Taping an athlete's ankle	Changing a tire
Drawing	Putting in golf	Weight lifting
Repairing a watch	Shooting pool	Playing tug-o-war

FIGURE **2.5** Classification of Skills as Fine or Gross

Source: Created by author.

discussed at the beginning of this chapter, with the classic definition assuming a task perspective and Guthrie's definition taking a performance perspective in defining motor skills).

In response to this need, Gentile (1972, 2000) broadened the categorization of motor skills into a two-dimensional system comprising a taxonomy having 16 skill categories (a taxonomy is simply a classification of things into groups having similar features). Gentile's original purpose in creating her taxonomy was to provide a tool for physical therapists to more effectively evaluate the motor skill proficiencies of their patients and to determine appropriate treatment protocols. Although Gentile's taxonomy was originally designed for use in physical and occupational therapy, its use has broadened to encompass instructional design considerations in many movement-related fields and today is used in sports, physical education, performing arts, and industrial settings. The taxonomy underpins evaluation and instructional decisions across a wide spectrum of applications and provides an important tool for movement practitioners in all fields involving the acquisition and performance of motor skills.

Gentile's taxonomy starts by classifying all skills on the basis of two dimensions influencing performance. These include the demands placed upon individuals by the environment as well as those requirements imposed by the task itself.

BOX 2.6   Can You Classify Skills According to the One-Dimensional Classification System?

The one-dimensional classification system for motor skills is widely used among professionals in many movement-related fields and provides a common vocabulary for communicating about motor skills. To test your ability to use this classification system, see whether you can classify the following skills into each of the three one-dimensional systems presented in this text. For each skill, decide whether it is a (1) open or closed skill; (2) discrete, serial, or continuous skill; and (3) fine or gross skill.

- Assembling a puzzle
- Playing billiards
- Chopping wood
- Dribbling a yo-yo up and down
- Playing a video game
- Playing the banjo
- Punting a football
- Texting
- Sport-wall climbing
- Walking on crutches

Environmental Demands

The first dimension in Gentile's taxonomy considers the demands placed upon individuals by the environment in which a skill is performed, and is labeled Environmental Demands in the taxonomy (see Table 2.2). Two characteristics of the environment are considered in the taxonomy. Gentile referred to these as regulatory conditions and intertrial variability.

Regulatory conditions refer to those features of the environment that are relevant to how a skill must be performed. Regulatory conditions specify and constrain the actions a person must execute. Features of the performance environment including spatial dimensions, obstacles and the arrangement of objects within the performance space, the nature of the supporting surface on which a skill is performed, wind and lighting conditions, and the presence of other people are examples. An important distinction in Gentile's taxonomy is whether regulatory conditions are stationary or in motion. As this description indicates, stationary regulatory conditions are stable and do not demonstrate relevant change within the environmental context. The initiation and timing of action is, given stationary regulatory conditions, under the control of the performer. In-motion regulatory conditions, also as the term implies, refer to those conditions in which relevant features of the environment change or are in motion during the performance of a skill, imposing how the initiation and timing of action must be controlled. The distinction between stationary and in-motion regulatory conditions in Gentile's taxonomy is, in this case, the same as the one-dimensional system distinction between closed and open skills. Gentile's taxonomy extends the distinction between closed and open skills further, however, by considering also the notion of intertrial variability.

A second feature of environmental context demands classified by Gentile is whether regulatory conditions remain the same or change from one performance attempt to the next, referred to as intertrial variability. Although many skills performed in stationary regulatory conditions show few if any environmental changes from one attempt to another (e.g., a basketball free throw), others are marked by both environmental stability and trial-to-trial environmental change (e.g., billiards). Likewise, in-motion regulatory conditions can also exhibit intertrial variability (e.g., driving on a busy street), probably the most typical situation, or little or no variability (e.g., stepping on to a moving escalator). In Gentile's taxonomy, intertrial variability is classified as being either absent or present.

Action Requirements

The second dimension classified by Gentile's taxonomy pertains to the actions required in performing a skill. Specifically, Gentile classified two aspects of a performer's bodily actions. These include what she termed *body transport* and *object manipulation* (see Table 2.2).

Body transport refers to whether a person must change location when performing a skill. Playing soccer and snow skiing both demand changes in a performer's spatial location. Some skills may involve bodily transport as the primary goal of performance (e.g., a 100-yard dash), whereas for others the requirement to change location imposes additional demands on other

---

regulatory conditions: Features of the performance environment that determine how a skill must be performed in order to be successful.

performance goals (e.g., moving to avoid a defender before taking a shot in basketball). Other skills require no change in location in order to accomplish the skill successfully (e.g., performing a sit-up, driving a golf ball).

In addition to considerations of body transport, a second essential feature of action requirements is whether the manipulation of an object, or of other individuals, is required when performing a skill. Many motor skills require the performer to manipulate objects (e.g., swing a golf club, throw a ball) or other people (e.g., wrestling, square dancing) when performing the skill. Although such manipulations are frequently accomplished using the hands, other body segments may also be involved (e.g., kicking a soccer ball, blocking in football). As with intertrial variability, object manipulation is classified as being either absent or present.

Gentile's 16 Skill Categories

To classify skills within Gentile's taxonomy, the four environmental demand conditions (stationary and in-motion regulatory conditions, the absence or presence of intertrial variability) are crossed with the four possible action requirements (body stability or transport, the absence or presence of object manipulation) to yield 16 skill categories. Table 2.2 illustrates the taxonomy along with examples of two skills in each of the 16 categories.

Each of the 16 categories into which skills can be classified imposes a different set of demands on performers. Gentile specified that as the number and complexity of environmental and task demands to which a performer must attend and control increases, the difficulty of task performance also increases (Gentile, 2000). In the taxonomy, environmental demands increase with movement down the categorical columns, whereas action requirements increase with movement from left to right across the categorical rows. Skills in the upper left-hand category represent the simplest and least difficult skills to perform, whereas those skills in the bottom right-hand category are the most complex and demanding. For ease of reference, categories are labeled by number from 1 to 4 down columns, and by letter from A to D across rows, with an increase in either direction indicating greater skill complexity. As skills move diagonally across the columns from left to right, and down the rows from top to bottom, performance demands increase, with skills in category 1A being the simplest, and those in category 4D the most complex.

Application of Gentile's Taxonomy

Because the categorical classification of skills in Gentile's taxonomy progressively increases in task difficulty with movement across columns and down rows, the taxonomy can be used to assess and compare different skills, or variations of the same skill, in regard to demands placed upon performers. This makes possible two important applications of the taxonomy. First, as Gentile originally intended when developing the taxonomy, it can be used to evaluate an individual's level of movement proficiency. As a diagnostic tool in physical therapy settings, the taxonomy provides an effective method for gauging a patient's movement capabilities and limitations (Huxham, Goldie, and Patla, 2001). For example, a therapist could evaluate a patient recovering from hip

TABLE **2.2**
Gentile's Taxonomy

			Action Requirements			
			Body Stability		Body Transport	
			No Objection Manipulation	Object Manipulation	No Objection Manipulation	Object Manipulation
Environmental Demands	Stationary Regulatory Conditions	No Intertrial Variability	**1A** Standing on a flat surface with arms held out to your sides Doing sit-ups on a flat surface	**1B** Playing the piano Practicing basketball free throws	**1C** Walking up a flight of stairs Practicing the same balance bar routine	**1D** Using crutches to walk down an empty hallway Throwing a javelin
		Intertrial Variability	**2A** Practicing the movements of various golf swings without using a golf club Using sign language	**2B** Cutting vegetables with a knife on a cutting board Polishing silverware	**2C** Competing in the high jump Carrying a plate of food from your kitchen to the dining room	**2D** Raking leaves in a yard Participating in a sack race
	In-Motion Regulatory Conditions	No Intertrial Variability	**3A** Standing on a moving escalator Timing your swing at baseballs pitched by a machine without using a bat	**3B** Standing on a moving escalator while drinking a cup of coffee Doing tricks with a yo-yo	**3C** Walking on a moving escalator Practicing a dance routine that must be timed with a partner with whom you have no contact	**3D** A game of bowling (first ball in each frame) Dribbling a soccer ball with no defenders
		Intertrial Variability	**4A** Standing in a moving bus Riding a horse on a country lane	**4B** Balancing a spinning basketball on the tips of your fingers Catching balls pitched to home plate	**4C** Playfully chasing a pet dog Swimming in a moving river	**4D** A game of bowling (all balls including spares) Surfing

replacement surgery by first assessing the patient's ability to stand on a flat surface and maintain balance while extending his or her arms in various directions (category 1A in the taxonomy). If the patient demonstrated sufficient confidence and capability performing these actions, the same activity could be tested with the patient holding and moving a beanbag from hand to hand (category 1B). Progressively, the patient could be asked to walk a short distance with hands free (category 1C), and then while carrying a beanbag in both hands (category 1D). If the patient were able to perform all of these actions successfully, the therapist could then repeat the same sequence but vary the intertrial regulatory conditions by having the patient attempt each skill progression on a flat unencumbered surface, a carpeted surface, and a flat surface where movement around a chair or other obstacle was required (progression in this sequence would be from 2A to 2D). By gradually varying task demands, the therapist can accurately evaluate a patient's level of movement proficiency, prescribe appropriate training activities for the patient's current level of movement capabilities, and meaningfully measure progress over the course of treatment.

In the example just cited, an important feature of the evaluation sequence can be observed. That is, beyond simply evaluating an individual's current movement capabilities, the taxonomy effectively charts a progression of increasingly challenging activities. This leads to a second major use of the taxonomy, which is the identification of systematically more demanding skill variations. In our example, if the patient was capable of standing on a flat surface while manipulating beanbags but was not able to maintain stability when attempting to walk, the taxonomy could be used by the therapist to effectively plan a progressive sequence of treatment activities. Because the patient starts at category 1B in the taxonomy, the most immediate goal of treatment would be to emphasize walking on a flat surface while remaining unencumbered by any demands for manipulating objects (category 1C). Progressively, as the patient could successfully meet the challenges of each new category, the therapist would devise activities representing the next category in order to continually, in gradual steps, increase the patient's movement capabilities.

The use of Gentile's taxonomy to plan meaningful instructional progressions in a variety of skills and performance settings has provided an effective

---

BOX **2.7**   **Using Gentile's Taxonomy**

Gentile's taxonomy provides an effective guide for systematically identifying meaningful skill progressions. Can you identify meaningful steps when teaching someone a new skill using the taxonomy? Try developing a description of progressive activities a person might practice to acquire one of the following skills. Begin with category 1A and describe practice activities for each category to 16D.

- Returning a serve in tennis
- Skiing a downhill slalom course
- Regaining the capability to ride a bicycle after spinal surgery
- Dribbling a soccer ball against defenders
- Learning a ballroom dance routine

tool for movement practitioners when planning instructional activities. When used in physical education settings, the taxonomy provides a coherent framework for curricular development (Adams, 1999). The teacher instructing a unit of softball, for example, may observe that a particular class of students is having difficulty learning to bat when thrown pitched balls. In this case, the instructor may decide students are not ready for the demands imposed by live pitches (i.e., both regulatory and intertrial variability) and could reduce these challenges to manageable levels by stabilizing environmental conditions. To do this, the teacher could have students learn correct movement patterns by hitting the softball from a batting tee set at an appropriate midbody level while maintaining both feet in place (category 1B). Progressions could then be planned to practice hitting movements without a bat but by moving the front foot toward the tee and "stepping into the pitch" (category 1C); by adding the bat and hitting the ball while stepping forward (category 1D); and then by repeating the same activities while varying the height of the tee on which the ball is placed (categories 2A to 2D). Once skill proficiency in these categories was attained, the progressions would be repeated with a pitcher throwing the same type of pitch on each trial (categories 3A to 3D) and finally with the pitcher throwing a variety of different pitches (categories 4A to 4D). The systematic and incremental increase in task demands made possible by using Gentile's taxonomy provides the instructor with a useful tool for meaningfully planning an effective series of progressively challenging, yet manageable, steps in meeting skill goals. It can also be noted that instructors may decide to begin progressions within any category of the taxonomy, depending upon an evaluation of student capabilities and readiness (progressions need not always begin with category 1A), and also that some categorical steps may be omitted depending on learner needs and progress.

SUMMARY

Skills of many and varied types make up a majority of the activities comprising daily life. Depending upon the requisite capabilities most critical in accomplishing their goals, skills are classified into cognitive, perceptual, and motor domains.

Motor skills, as a separate domain of skill, are defined in two ways:

- The classic definition of motor skills assumes a task perspective and defines motor skills as voluntary, goal-directed, learned behaviors accomplished primarily through contributions of the muscular-skeletal system.
- Guthrie's definition of motor skills assumes a performance perspective and defines motor skills as maximizing goal attainment while minimizing energy expenditures and movement time.

The study of motor skills comprises three components influencing performance, each of which plays a role in both facilitating and limiting performance capabilities:

- Environment
- Task
- Person

Four aspects of skilled behavior characterize all motor skills:

- Motor equivalence
- Motor variability
- Motor consistency
- Motor modifiability

Among the most persistent problems facing motor skill researchers, four in particular underscore differences in theoretical perspectives and are the most challenging to researchers:

- The degrees of freedom problem
- The perceptual-motor integration problem
- The serial-order problem
- The skill acquisition problem

Two systems for classifying motor skills are used today:

- One-dimensional classification systems assume a task perspective and classify skills along a continuum. One-dimensional systems have been developed based upon the stability environmental features (closed vs. open), temporal predictability (discrete, serial, and continuous), and movement precision (fine vs. gross).
- Gentile's two-dimensional system classifies skills into 16 categories representing combinations of environmental demands and action requirements. The taxonomy is particularly useful for purposes of evaluating movement capabilities and planning instruction progressions when teaching motor skills.

LEARNING EXERCISES

1. Observe a venue where people are performing various motor skills (it could be a sporting event, a work situation, a clinical setting, or even some public display where people are involved in different movement activities). Observe and describe the situation and the kinds of movement activities taking place. Look for examples of each of the seven one-dimensional categories of skill and specifically describe one example of each of these seven categories.

2. Keep a log of your movement activities for one day, recording specific examples of each of the four skill characteristics identified by Sheridan (you will obviously not record every motor skill you perform).

From your log, provide several examples of each of the four skill characteristics. Does any one type of skill characteristic appear to be more prevalent than others? What insights about your daily motor skill activities did you gain from your observations?

3. Select an example of a complex motor skill with which you are well acquainted (sports or recreational skill, occupational skill, daily life skill, etc.). For this skill, design an instructional progression based upon Gentile's taxonomy that could be used to instruct someone who was unpracticed or incapacitated relative to the skill; begin your progression at the simplest performance level and advance

to a stage in which the skill can be well performed. Describe the person (adult, child, specific remedial requirements, etc.) for whom you are designing the instructional progression, and identify specific practice conditions at each stage of your progression (identify the category number of Gentile's taxonomy for each of these progressive stages).

4. An acquaintance comments to you, "Motor skills are much simpler and less demanding than intellectual skills." How would you respond to this statement? Prepare a reply effectively refuting this position.

FOR FURTHER STUDY

HOW MUCH DO YOU KNOW?

For each of the following, select the letter that best answers the question.

1. Motor skills are comprised of elements from
   a. the motor domain of skill only.
   b. both the perceptual and motor domains of skill.
   c. all three domains of skill.
   d. all three domains of skill equally.
2. According to Guthrie's definition, motor skills result in all but which one of the following?
   a. They maximize certainty of goal-attainment.
   b. They minimize cognitive effort.
   c. They minimize energy expenditure.
   d. They minimize movement time.
3. The capacity to achieve the same skill goal using different movements is termed
   a. motor consistency.
   b. motor equivalence.
   c. motor variability.
   d. motor modifiability.
4. What term is used to describe the behavioral characteristics of a person's limbs, head, and other bodily segments?
   a. Abilities
   b. Actions
   c. Movements
   d. Responses
5. Which of the following categories of motor skills is based upon classification according to the predictability of the beginning and ending of action?
   a. Discrete skills
   b. Closed skills
   c. Self-paced skills
   d. Open skills

6. For the skill of driving an automobile on a busy city street during rush hour, the regulatory conditions would most likely be which of the following?
   a. Stable with no intertrial variability
   b. Stable with intertrial variability
   c. In motion with no intertrial variability
   d. In motion with intertrial variability

Answer the following with the word or words that best complete each sentence.

7. Deciding on which play to run in a football game is an example of the _____ domain of skill.
8. The capacity to change a movement once an action has begun is termed _____.
9. Individual genetic traits that underlie motor skills are called _____.
10. The number of ways in which a unit of movement analysis may independently vary is termed _____.
11. If a motor skill were classified based upon the stability of the performance environment, then roller-skating in a crowded skating rink would be classified as a(n) _____ skill.
12. Walking up a flight of familiar stairs daily carrying an armful of schoolbooks would be classified in which category of Gentile's taxonomy?

Answers are provided at the end of this review section.

STUDY QUESTIONS

1. Explain why motor skills are always composed of elements of each of the three different skill domains but are nevertheless classified into the motor domain of skills.
2. How are motor skills defined? What two definitions comprise the standard definitions? How do these definitions differ?
3. What is meant by degrees of freedom? Why is the redundancy in degrees of freedom in the human motor system a tremendous advantage to people? Given this advantage, why is there a degrees of freedom problem?
4. Define and provide examples for each of the four characteristics of motor skills.
5. Discuss ways in which attributes of the environment, task, and person each contribute to the performance of a motor skill. For each of these three components, list several examples of factors that may enhance, as well as factors that may limit, skill performance.
6. What three criteria are used in classifying motor skills into one-dimensional systems of classification? Define each of the seven broad categories into which motor skills can be classified, providing an example for each.
7. How does Gentile's taxonomy differ from one-dimensional classification systems? Why did Gentile develop her system for classifying motor skills and how can it be used for purposes of skill evaluation and the design of instructional progressions?

ADDITIONAL READING

Adams, DL. (1999). "Develop better motor skill progressions with Gentile's Taxonomy of Tasks." *Journal of Physical Education, Recreation, and Dance, 70*(8), 35–38.

Clark, JE (2005). From the beginning: "A developmental perspective on movement and mobility." *Quest, 57,* 37–45.

Gentile, AM. (2000). "Skill acquisition: Action, movement, and neuromotor process." In J Carr and R Shepherd (eds.), *Movement Science: Foundations for Physical Therapy and Rehabilitation* (pp. 111–188). Gaitherburg, MD: Aspen Publications.

Oglesby, CA (1968). "Movement and culture." In HM Smith, *Introduction to human movement,* pp. 37–48. Reading, MA: Addison-Wesley.

Rosenbaum, DA, Carlson, RA, and Gilmore, RO. (2001). "Acquisition of intellectual and perceptual-motor skills." *Annual Review of Psychology, 2001,* 453–470.

Sheridan, MR. (1984). "Planning and controlling simple movement." In MM Smyth and AL Wing (eds.), *The Psychology of Movement* (pp. 47–82). London: Academic Press.

Wulf, G, and Shea, C. (2002). "Principles derived from the study of simple skills do not generalize to complex skills." *Psychonomic Bulletin & Review, 9,* 185–211.

REFERENCES

Adams, DL. (1999). "Develop better motor skill progressions with Gentile's taxonomy of tasks." *Journal of Physical Education, Recreation and Dance, 70*(8), 35–38.

Adams, JA. (1987). "Historical review and appraisal of research on the learning, retention, and transfer of human motor skills." *Psychological Bulletin, 101*(1), 41–74.

Allman, JM. (1999). *Evolving brains.* New York: Freeman Publishers.

Anderson, JR. (1982). "Acquisition of cognitive skill." *Psychological Review, 89,* 369–406.

Billard, A. (2001). "Learning motor skills by imitation: A biologically inspired robotic model." *Cybernetics and Systems: An International Journal, 32,* 155–193.

Crammond, DJ. (1997). "Motor imagery: Never in your wildest dreams." *Trends in Neuroscience, 20,* 54–57.

Fiez, JA. (1996). "Cerebellar contributions to cognition." *Neuron, 16,* 13–15.

Fitts, PM, and Posner, MI. (1967). *Human performance*. Belmont, CA: Brooks/Cole.

Flash, T, and Hogan, KN. (1985). "The coordination of arm movements: An experimental confirmed mathematical model." *Journal of Neuroscience, 5*, 1688–1703.

Gardner, H. (1983). *Frames of mind—The theory of multiple intelligences*. New York: Basic Books.

Gentile, AM. (1972). "A working model of skill acquisition with application to teaching." *Quest, 17*, 3–23.

Gentile, AM. (2000). "Skill acquisition: Action, movement, and the neuromotor processes." In JH Carr and RB Shepherd (eds.), *Movement science: Foundations for physical therapy in rehabilitation*, 2nd ed. (pp. 111–188). Rockville, MD: Aspen Press.

Gibson, JJ. (1966). *The senses considered as perceptual systems*. Boston: Houghton Mifflin.

Gibson, JJ. (1979). *The Ecological approach to visual perception*. Boston: Houghton Mifflin.

Guthrie, ER. (1952). *The psychology of learning*. New York: Harper & Row.

Haywood, KM, and Getchell, N. (2004). *Life span motor development*, 4th ed. Champaign, IL: Human Kinetics.

Heathcote, A, Brown, S, and Mewhort, DJK. (2000). "The power law repealed: The case for an exponential law of practice." *Psychonomic Bulletin Review, 7*, 185–207.

Huxham, FE, Goldie, PA, and Patla, AE. (2001). "Theoretical considerations in balance assessment." *Australian Journal of Physiotherapy, 47*, 89–100.

Jeannerod, M. (1994). "The representing brain: Neural correlates of motor intention and imagery." *Brain Behavior and Science, 17*, 187–245.

Kelso, AS, Fuchs, A, Lancaster, R, Holroyd, T, Cheyne, D, and Weinberg, H. (1998). "Dynamical cortical activity in the human brain reveals motor equivalence." *Nature, 392*, 814–818.

Kramer, AF, Strayer, DL, and Buckley, J. (1990). "Development and transfer of automatic processes." *Journal of Experimental Psychology: Human Perception and Performance, 16*, 505–522.

Lashley, KS. (1930). "Basic neural mechanisms in behavior." *Psychological Review, 37*, 1–24.

Lashley, KS. (1951). "The problem of serial order in behavior." In LA Jeffress (ed.), Cerebral mechanisms in behavior: The Hixon symposium (pp. 112–136). New York: Wiley.

Neves, DM, and Anderson, JR. (1981). "Knowledge compilation: Mechanisms for the automatization of cognitive skills." In JR Anderson (ed.), *Cognitive Skills and Their Acquisition* (pp. 57–84). Hillsdale, NJ: Lawrence Erlbaum.

Newell, KM. (1986). "Constraints on the development of coordination." In MG Wade and HTA Whiting (eds.), *Motor development in children: Aspects of Coordination and Control* (pp. 341–360). Boston: Martinus Nijhoff.

Proctor, RW, and Dutta, A. (1995). *Skill acquisition and human performance*. Thousand Oaks, CA: Sage Publications.

Rosenbaum, DA, Carlson, RA, and Gilmore, RO. (2001). "Acquisition of intellectual and perceptual-motor skills." *Annual Review of Psychology, 2001*, 453–470.

Rosenbaum, DA. (2010). *Human motor control, 2nd Ed*. San Diego: Academic Press.

Schmidt, RA, and Bjork, RA. (1992). "New conceptualizations of practice: Common principles in three paradigms suggest new concepts of training." *Psychological Science, 3*, 207–214.

Sheridan, MR. (1984). Planning and controlling simple movements. In MM Smyth and AL Wing (eds.), *The psychology of movement* (pp. 47–82). London: Academic Press.

Singley, K, and Anderson, JR. (1989). *The transfer of cognitive skill*. Cambridge, MA: Harvard University Press.

Smyth, MM, and Haggard, P. (1999). "Movement and action: Introduction to the special topic." *British Journal of Psychology, 90*(12), 243–246.

Vickers, JN. (2007). Perception, Cognition, and Decision Training: The Quiet Eye in Action. Champaign, IL: Human Kinetics.

Answers to How Much Do You Know questions: (1) C, (2) B, (3) B, (4) C, (5) A, (6) D, (7) cognitive, (8) motor modifiability, (9) abilities, (10) degrees of freedom, (11) open, (12) 1D.

CHAPTER 3

The Neurological Bases of Human Movement

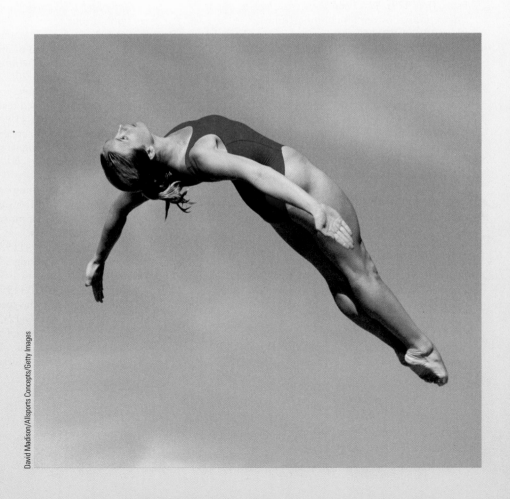

David Madison/Allsports Concepts/Getty Images

To move things is all mankind can do, and for such the sole executant is muscle, whether in whispering a syllable or in felling a forest.
Sir Charles Sherrington (1857–1952)

KEY QUESTIONS

- How are motor control and learning determined at the cellular level?
- What structures contribute to perception, and how does perception contribute to the learning and control of motor skills?
- What is kinesthesis?
- What two visual systems control movements and how do they differ?
- What are the major structures of the brain contributing to motor learning and control?
- How does the central nervous system coordinate movements?
- How are muscular contractions organized and controlled by the central nervous system?

CHAPTER OVERVIEW

If you wanted to tune up an automobile so that it ran more smoothly and efficiently, you would need to understand how the engine and other component parts of a car worked. You would not attempt to tune the engine, or be successful at it, if you did not know what the distributor was for or where the battery cables connected or what the alternator does. If the car you wanted to make run better was a race car, you would need even greater knowledge about the principles of how cars run. Whether your goal was to repair a broken car, tune up a family car so it would run efficiently on a daily basis, or build a race car capable of winning the Daytona 500, you would first need to have a good grasp of the workings of the engine and other important components of automobiles. You could not expect to effectively reach your goals apart from having first acquired knowledge critical to your understanding of what makes automobiles run in the first place.

The same principle applies to diagnosing and teaching motor skills. Without a basic understanding of the body's engine for movement, the design and instruction of motor skills is compromised. It is essential that in order to be most effective, motor skill practitioners must possess a basic understanding of the mechanisms controlling the skills they diagnose and instruct.

For something as important as people's movement capabilities, our understanding of how movement is controlled remains a patchwork of fact and conjecture, with some things well understood while others remain debated. To the casual observer, human movement may seem straightforward, and given the seeming ease with which many everyday movement skills are accomplished, even simplistic. We command our muscles to contract, they do, and we move. What could be more simple?

Of course, it is not simple. Human movements are far from simple acts, even those that have been repeated many thousands of times and easily performed with little or no thought. Movement involves the entire human organism, from structures deep within the brain, to various receptors monitoring and sensing our physical surroundings, to muscles that can in one instance tenderly wipe a tear from a child's eye, yet in another fell a tree with the mighty swing of an axe. The interplay of millions of nerve cells extending throughout the body, coordinating vast amounts of information that would overwhelm the most powerful of modern computers, harmoniously combine to accomplish the thousands of motor skills humans perform daily.

The control of this sophisticated orchestration of the body's muscular apparatus is the topic of this chapter. Although the control of human movement is the result of contributions from many systems and bodily components acting in concert, it will simplify our discussion significantly to focus on three distinct contributions to skilled movement: perception, functions of the human brain, and command of the muscular system. We will begin, however, by first considering the communication network of nerves that makes cooperation among these three areas possible.

THE COMMUNICATION OF INFORMATION: THE CELLULAR BASES FOR MOTOR LEARNING AND CONTROL

At the most fundamental level, the study of motor behavior is the study of connections. That is, the various systems of the body—perceptual, nervous, motor, muscular, and so on—must all communicate with one another. This communication is made possible through a vast and sophisticated system of nerve cells. These nerve cells, forming the human nervous system, are initially classified within two main divisions: the central and peripheral nervous systems. The **central nervous system** (CNS) includes all nerve cells within the brain and spine, whereas all other nerve cells make up the **peripheral nervous system** (PNS). Cells originating in the PNS communicate their information to the CNS, whereas those originating in the CNS carry their signals away from the CNS (though many may both originate and terminate entirely within the CNS).

Those nerve cells that form the communication network of the nervous system are called **neurons,** of which about 200 billion comprise the nervous system of the average person (with about an equal number comprising both the brain and the remainder of the nervous system). Neurons are responsible for sending and receiving information.

central nervous system: All of the nerve cells within or originating within the brain or spine.

peripheral nervous system: All of the nerve cells originating or contained entirely outside of the the central nervous system.

neuron: The basic cell for communication within the central nervous system.

cell body (soma): The metabolic center of a neuron containing the nucleus and other organelles.

dendrites: Branching fibers extending from the cell body of neurons that receive signals from other neurons.

axon: A long fiber extending from the cell body of a neuron ending in presynaptic terminals that send signals to other neurons.

glia: Supportive cells of the central nervous system.

As with all cells, neurons contain a **cell body** (or soma) containing the cell nucleus and other organelles that produce energy and direct the cell's activities. Branching from the cell's body are numerous tentacles called **dendrites** (a Greek word for "tree"), which receive messages directed toward the cell. Extending from the cell's body is an elongated, tubular shaped fiber called an **axon**, which carries messages away from the neuron and, through perhaps thousands of terminal branches, to the dendrites of other neurons. Axons are encased within a myelin sheath, a fatty covering important for both the conductivity and insulation of the neural messages traveling their length. The entire cell is encased within a thin, permeable membrane. The basic parts of the neuron are illustrated in Figure 3.1.

Besides neurons, the nervous system contains another essential cellular building block called the neuroglia, or simply **glia**. Glial cells support the activity of neurons, and there are many more glia than neurons (by about 10 to 1). Until recently, relatively little attention was paid to glia because it was believed that they played a scant role in the activities of the CNS apart from acting to insulate neuronal cells. Glial cells literally do provide the "glue" that holds the nervous system together, but neuroscientists are beginning to discover that they also fulfill other significant roles such as strengthening synaptic transmission, guiding neuronal development, and repairing damaged neurons. It is the neurons, however, that are the principle players in the control of movement.

The Neuron

Of the billions of neurons in the CNS, no two are exactly alike. They vary in size, shape, and functional capacity. Luckily, however, though they differ, all neurons can be classified into one of three basic types depending on their function. The functional classes of neurons found in the nervous

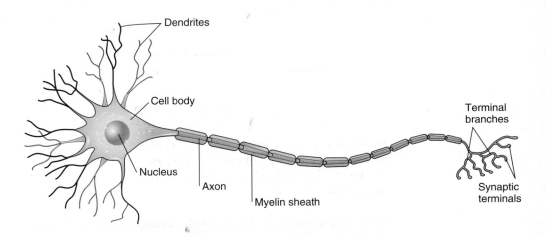

FIGURE **3.1** A Typical Neuron

Source: Adapted from Solomon/Berg/Martin, *Biology,* 8/e, p. 847.

system are sensory neurons, motor neurons, and interneurons (see Kandel et al., 2000).

Sensory Neurons

sensory neuron: One of three major types of neurons, they convey information about the environment from sensory receptors to the CNS.

afferent pathway: The path of a neural signal traveling toward the CNS (also referred to as the *ascending pathway*).

Sensory neurons convey information from both the environment and body toward the spine and brain. Communication toward the brain is said to follow an ascending or **afferent pathway,** and for this reason sensory neurons are also called *afferent neurons*. A sensory neuron is shaped somewhat differently than are motor neurons and interneurons. Projecting from the cell body, instead of dendrites, is a fiber called an *afferent fiber* that is typically located outside of the spinal cord and is attached, at its terminal ending, to a sensory receptor, often at some distance from the cell body. Sensory receptors generate messages in response to certain types of stimuli. We have sensory receptors for vision, touch, hearing, smell, heat, cold, pressure, pain, and the detection of changes in motion. Once a signal from the afferent fiber reaches the cell body of the sensory neuron, it is further conveyed over the cell's axon into the spine, where it may either continue toward the brain, or else connect to motor neurons in the spine or brain stem to form reflex arcs. Reflexes allow for quicker responses to certain kinds of stimuli than if signals from sensory receptors traveled all the way to the brain and a decision to act had to be made. It is in the higher centers of the brain that meaning is attached to afferent messages, however, and the perception and interpretation of sensations gained from experience allow for the control of more complex movements, and certainly all actions that can be classified as skills.

Motor Neurons

motor neuron: One of three major types of neurons; they form synapses with muscle cells conveying information from the CNS and converting it into movement.

efferent pathway: The path of a neural signal traveling away from the CNS (also referred to as the descending pathway).

Motor neurons send messages from the CNS to the effectors (muscles or glands) that they innervate, conveying the commands that the effectors are to carry out. Communication from the CNS to muscles is said to follow a descending or **efferent pathway.** The primary function of a motor neuron is to control muscle contraction. The motor neuron responsible for the contraction of skeletal muscle is called the *alpha motor neuron* (and is also frequently referred to as a *motoneuron*). Motor neurons do not generate the commands that they communicate to muscles; these commands are initially received from sensory neurons, interneurons, or brain structures, including especially the cerebral cortex. Motor neurons gather information from many places within the CNS and route it effectively to the muscles required to carry out movement skills. The orchestration of many motor neurons working harmoniously together can result in movement over a broad range of complexity, from the simplest to the most complex of movement skills.

Interneurons

interneuron: One of three major types of neurons; they connect and convey signals between sensory and motor neurons.

Embedded deep within the spinal cord and other brain structures and contained entirely within the CNS, **interneurons** comprise the large majority of neurons in the CNS. Interneurons play two primary roles. First, as their name suggests, interneurons link motor neurons, sensory neurons, and higher brain centers. Far from making simple connections, however, interneurons integrate the informational exchange between brain centers and sensory and motor neurons, making possible the tremendous amount of information and the degree of complexity that can be communicated within the CNS. The greater the number of interneurons interposed between afferent messages and efferent responses, the greater the complexity of the resulting movements that are possible. Second, the interconnections between interneurons themselves are believed to be responsible for the abstract features of the nervous system we call *mind*, such as thoughts, emotions, memory, creativity, intellect, and motivation (Sherwood, 2006). These activities, all of which play central roles in human movement, are still the least understood aspects of the nervous system, however.

The Neural Impulse and Synaptic Transmission

The primary function of a neuron is to transmit a signal, called the neural impulse, to another neuron. Any of the 200 or so billion neurons can communicate with any other neuron through the vast web of linkages among neurons (see Box 3.1). No neuron is more than two or three degrees of separation from any other neuron (Restak, 2001). With each act you perform, millions of connections are formed, and with each repetition of the act, those connections are strengthened. So each time you type a letter or hit a golf ball, you are literally rewiring your central nervous system and advancing your learning of the skill performed.

As complex as human movement can be, the messages between neurons are always simple "on" and "off" signals, much like flipping a light switch on or off. The complexity of human movement is not made possible because of the complexity of the signals between neurons, but by the complexity of many millions of on and off connections creating ever-changing patterns of chemically produced electrical flashes speeding across the neural landscape.

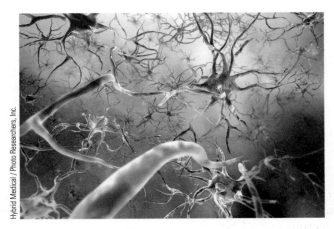

Hybrid Medical / Photo Researchers, Inc.

The human brain is composed of approximately 100 billion neurons, each capable of connecting directly with hundreds to thousands of other neurons.

polarization: A change in the membrane potential of a cell increasing its negativity and making it less excitable and less likely to generate an action potential.

depolarization: A change in the membrane potential of a cell, reducing its negativity and making it more excitable and likely to generate an action potential.

excitation: The depolarization of a cell, increasing the likelihood that an action potential will be propagated.

action potential: A temporary electrical signal that propagates along the axon of a neuron and at the presynaptic terminal triggers the release of a neurotransmitter to target neurons.

synapse: The site of communication between two neurons consisting of a presynaptic terminal, postsynaptic cell, and synaptic cleft.

The on or off connection between two neurons is determined by the distribution of ions (i.e., charged particles) inside and outside of the neuronal cells. Located on either side of a cell's membrane are charged ions of sodium (Na+), potassium (K+), and chloride (Cl−). When the ions on both sides of the cell membrane result in a more or less equal charge, the neuron is said to be in a resting state, or state of **polarization**. This is the "off" position; transmission of a signal between neurons will not occur. However, if more negatively charged ions become concentrated on the inside of the cell, while more positively charged ions cluster on the outside of the cell, an imbalance of electrical charges results. This condition results in an electrical tension across the cell membrane. If the tension becomes great enough, positive ions will cross the membrane wall and rush inside the cell, a condition referred to as a state of **depolarization** or **excitation**. The positive ions entering the cell will then be quickly pumped out of the cell by a mechanism known as a *sodium pump*, so that a resting potential of more or less equally charged ions is once again established on either side of the cell walls. The process of depolarization will continue long enough, however, to transmit a charge, called an **action potential**, down the entire length of the axon and toward other neurons to which it may connect.

The Synapse

At the end of the axon, the action potential reaches a seeming impasse in its travels called a **synapse**—the juncture between neurons (the neuron in which the action potential is initially conveyed is called *the presynaptic neuron*, while the neuron on the other side of the synaptic cleft with the potential of receiving its signal is called the *postsynaptic neuron*). Two neurons never touch; although very small (on the order of only 100 to 200 angstroms) (Kluka, 1999), there is always a space, called the *synaptic cleft*, between neurons. Movement across this gap, called *synaptic transmission*, must be accomplished if messages are to be propagated among neurons.

When the action potential reaches the end of a presynaptic neuron's axon, called the *synaptic knob*, its transmission across the synaptic cleft can be

---

BOX 3.1   **The Number of Synapses in the Brain Exceeds the Total Number of Atoms in the Known Universe**

Neurons are responsible for the communication of information within the central nervous system. In the brain alone, 100 billion neurons, along with their supporting glia, communicate information involved in the planning and execution of movements. The neuroscientist Richard Restak (2001) has pointed out that to connect this vast array of neurons requires at least a million billion synaptic connections. If you could count one of these synapses every second, it would take 32 million years to count them all. If you calculate the number of different connections possible given this number of synapses, the number is even more astonishing: 10 followed by a million zeros. To put that number in perspective, "Consider," says Restak, "that the number of particles in the known universe comes to only 10 followed by 79 zeros. Finally, consider that the glia, which exceed the number of neurons by at least a power of ten, are also believed to be capable of communication. If this is true, then the number of possible brain states exceeds even our most extravagant projections."

neurotransmitter:
A chemical substance
that is released from one
neuron and binds with
receptors in another
neuron to either convey
or inhibit transmission of
a signal.

facilitated, blocked, or changed. Within the synaptic knob are vesicles (tiny fluid filled sacs) that are capable of releasing chemicals known as **neurotransmitters** as a result of the action potential's arrival. These neurotransmitters influence the transmission of the neural impulse, increasing or decreasing the likelihood of depolarization across the synaptic gap (see Figure 3.2). When properly stimulated, neurotransmitters facilitate transmission of the presynaptic neuron's signal across the synaptic gap to the receiving dendrites of a postsynaptic neuron, stimulating depolarization within that neuron and, as this chain of events is repeated, encompassing more neurons to assemble a final command structure capable of activating complex arrangements of muscular activity.

acetylcholine: A
neurotransmitter released
by motor neurons.

A number of different neurotransmitters have been identified. The most common, relative to the command of muscular activities, is **acetylcholine** (abbreviated as ACh). ACh is the primary neurotransmitter working on skeletal muscle. When released into receptors of skeletal muscle, it stimulates contraction. Other important neurotransmitters involved in muscular activity include nonepinephrine, epinephrine (also called adrenalin), dopamine, serotonin, glutimate, and GABA (gamma-aminobutyric acid).

Research into the roles of the various neurotransmitters holds considerable promise for uncovering the causes of, and developing treatments for, many motor-related problems and diseases. As an example, a primary cause of

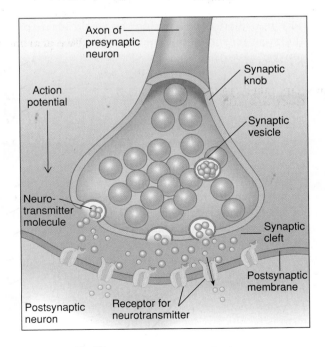

FIGURE **3.2** Synaptic Transmission

Source: Adapted from Solomon/Berg/Martin, *Biology*, 8/e, p. 858.

Parkinson's disease, a progressive inability to coordinate bodily movements, has been identified as the destruction of dopamine secreting neurons in one region of the brain. Treatment of this disease using the drug L-Dopa, an amino acid precursor of dopamine that can help to facilitate effective synaptic transmissions in affected brain areas, has provided an effective method of slowing the progression of this disease in many cases (Keltner, 1996; Stelmach and Phillips, 1991). Research is also beginning to uncover significant benefits from the effects of regular physical activity on the regulation and maintenance of neurotransmitter functioning, and this appears especially true as people age (Meeusen, 2006; Piacentini et al., 2004).

PERCEPTION

perception: The process by which sensations arising from within or outside of the body are brought to conscious awareness.

Everything that we experience, from a subtle breeze brushing across the cheek, to the total exhaustion of body and limbs after the physical exertions of an athletic contest or strenuous bout of exercise, depends on perception. **Perception** is the process by which humans interpret, give meaning to, and orient themselves to the world. The environment in which we live and move is constantly bombarding us with sensations about conditions both within and outside of our bodies. Perception involves making sense of this vast and constantly changing array of sensory information. In the control of human action, the transformation of sensations into meaningful perceptual information primarily involves two perceptual systems. The somatosensory system provides information concerning the world inside of our body, whereas the visual system tells us about the outside world in which our body is located and moves.

Somatosensory Perception and Kinesthesis

proprioceptors: Sensory receptors located in the body that supply information about forces within muscles, joint and limb position, movement, and general body orientation.

kinesthetic system: The system composed of muscle spindles, Golgi tendon organs, joint receptors, and the vestibular apparatus, which together provide the sense of kinesthesis.

kinesthesis: Sense of position and movement of the body and limbs and of external forces acting on the body.

The somatosensory system is comprised of receptors located in muscles, tendons, joints, the vestibular apparatus, and the skin. Those receptors located in or near layers of the skin are called cutaneous receptors, while those found in muscles, tendons, joints, and the inner ear are called **proprioceptors**. Cutaneous receptors and proprioceptors are a class of receptors known as mechanoreceptors, which is a type of receptor specialized to detect forms of mechanical energy in the environment (i.e., changes in pressure, position, and acceleration). Four proprioceptors—muscle spindles, Golgi tendon organs, joint receptors, and the vestibular apparatus—in addition to being classified as part of the somatosensory system, also form the **kinesthetic system**. The kinesthetic system makes possible the perception of body and limb positions and movements, as well as the general orientation of the body in space, a collective sense known as **kinesthesis**.

The kinesthetic sense is frequently referred to as *muscle memory*, though this term is technically incorrect (muscles do not remember). The proprioceptors constantly send information to the brain concerning the body's position and movements. Every body part that contains a muscle, joint, or both, is constantly sending moment-to-moment information to the brain about its state. Close your eyes and you can still tell where your arms are located. This is because of your kinesthetic sense. Additionally, kinesthesis conveys a global sense of the body's position in space and its overall movement (primarily due to activities of the vestibular apparatuses, as we will see shortly). Our general sense of our body's configuration and movement, as well as specific awareness of the position and movement of individual limbs, is a function of kinesthesis.

The kinesthetic sense provides the information that athletes rely on in order to accomplish their highly skilled performances or that we all rely on to perform the perhaps more ordinary, yet still highly skilled, activities of daily life such as standing, walking, getting dressed, eating, climbing stairs, and driving automobiles. The ability to perform daily activities is, of course, different in extent, though not kind, from the ability to perform highly complex athletic skills. There does appear to be considerable variation in kinesthetic sensitivity among people. Almost everyone possesses sufficient kinesthetic sensitivities to perform needed daily activities, and probably a significant number of complex activities at a high skill level. But kinesthetic sensitivity is specific to the performance of motor skills, and not everyone will possess the degree of kinesthesis required to excel at every activity or to become an Olympic champion. The kinesthetic sense is also age dependent (Colavita, 2006). Evidence suggests that a person's maximum kinesthetic sensitivity peaks at about the age of 12, remaining fairly stable until the mid to late 20s, at which time very slight decrements in overall kinesthetic sensitivity begin to appear. By their 40s, most people involved in motor skills requiring the precise execution of movements, such as golfers, professional dancers, and recreational skiers, will have noticed some differences in their skill levels. In normal aging, however, the gradual decline in

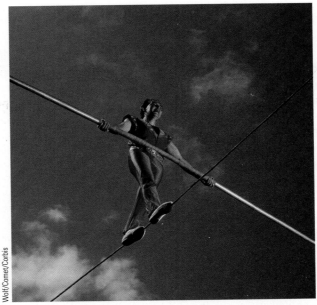

Acute awareness of body position and movement is made possible by the kinesthetic system.

Wolf/Comet/Corbis

kinesthesis poses no real problem with the performance of daily skills into the eighties or nineties for most people, and there is mounting evidence that even these declines can be greatly reduced through the maintenance of an active lifestyle.

The kinesthetic sense that sustains our most basic daily acts, as well as making possible the most complex and exquisite expressions of skilled human movement, arise from the sensory information supplied by the four proprioceptors. We turn next to a consideration of each of these.

Muscle Spindles

muscle spindle:
A proprioceptor found in all skeletal muscles that supplies information concerning stretch and changes in the length of muscle.

Muscle spindles tell us about the state of contraction of a muscle. They provide moment-to-moment information concerning the length of muscles and the rate of change (i.e., velocity) in their length as they contract and relax (Burke, 1985; Leonard, 1997). They are sensitive to the state of muscular contraction and provide information across the entire spectrum of contraction from "fully relaxed" to "maximally contracted."

Muscle spindles are located within all skeletal muscles. As receptors, they are unique in that they are composed of both a cellular structure (the receptor site) and muscle fibers. Skeletal muscles are composed of two types of fibers—the "ordinary" **extrafusal fibers** that provide the contractile forces necessary for moving joints, and **intrafusal fibers** that make up the muscle spindles. It is the extrafusal fiber that we normally think about when we consider muscles, the fibers that make up the bulk, or "meat," of a muscle. Intrafusal fibers, on the other hand, are relatively tiny and make up a small proportion of a muscle; they have few contractile elements and do not contribute to the overall contractile forces produced by skeletal muscles. Their function is to act as transducers of information about the stretch and rate of change within the muscle's extrafusal fibers.

extrafusal muscle fiber:
Skeletal muscle attached to bones and capable of generating significant contractile forces; responsible for purposeful movements and under voluntary control.

intrafusal muscle fiber:
Muscle fiber making up part of the muscle spindle, the deformation of which initiates afferent signal stimulation.

Muscle spindles monitor the contraction of muscles through a simple mechanical mechanism. The intrafusal fibers of the muscle spindles are attached to extrafusal fibers, so that when those fibers are stretched or contracted, they in turn stretch or contract the intrafusal fibers attached to them,

---

BOX **3.2**   **The Role of Kinesthesis**

For the skills listed below, think about the specific contributions of kinesthetic awareness that are most important in performing the skill. Are there specific limb positions that must be maintained or monitored? How precisely must various limb movements be executed? Must the timing between or among the movement of limbs be coordinated? Must the body's stability be maintained during the execution of the skill, or must the skill be executed while moving? What sources of information must

be monitored moment to moment while performing the particular skill?

- Bowling
- Bicycling
- Climbing a ladder
- Twirling a hula hoop
- Walking through your house at night in the dark
- Participating in your favorite recreational activity or sport

which in turn activates the muscle spindle receptor. Imagine a small elastic ball to which rubber bands are attached on either side. Now imagine that those rubber bands are attached, on either side of the ball, to a single muscle, and that they have just the right amount of tension to keep the ball a certain shape. What will happen if the muscle is stretched? The rubber bands will pull in opposite directions, stretching the elastic ball held between them. When the muscle goes back to its original state, the rubber bands also return to their normal tension, and the ball in the center to its normal shape. If the muscle contracts, however, the rubber bands become relaxed, and the elastic ball, which was being held in its normal shape by the rubber bands, also relaxes and becomes deformed. Muscle spindles work in the same way. The receptor site in the center is stretched and deformed as the intrafusal fibers connecting it to extrafusal fibers stretch and contract depending on the state of contraction of the muscle. Specialized afferent neurons originating in the receptor site of muscle spindles constantly convey information to the brain concerning the tension and rate of change of contraction within the extrafusal muscle fibers. Depending on the size and sensitivity of a muscle, hundreds or even thousands of muscle spindles may monitor its contractile state. Assembled together, this information gives a clear picture of the overall forces acting within a muscle at any specific time.

gamma motor neuron:
A motor neuron that innervates the fibers of a muscle spindle.

Extrafusal muscle fibers are innervated by the alpha motor neuron system discussed earlier in this chapter. The intrafusal fibers of muscle spindles are also innervated by motor neurons, in this case a specialized type called **gamma motor neurons** (γ-motor neurons). The fact that both extrafusal and intrafusal fibers can be innervated at the same time, a condition called *coactivation*, allows for the fine-tuning of how tension is maintained between the two fiber types. This has a number of advantages, including increasing the sensitivity and rate of response of the muscle spindles concerning muscular contractions.

The sensory information supplied by the activity of muscle spindles underlies three primary functions of these important receptors. First, as we have seen, muscle spindles send their signals about the tension and movement of skeletal muscles to the brain, thus supplying an important source of kinesthetic information. An individual's sense of limb position and movement is highly dependent upon afferent signals from muscle spindles. Most of the daily activities that we take for granted would not be possible if it were not for the activity of muscle spindles and the critical information they supply about the ever-changing state of our body's muscular system.

A second important function of muscle spindles is to initiate the stretch reflex. Whenever a whole muscle is passively and quickly stretched, neural impulses from muscle spindle afferents synapse in the spinal column with the alpha motor neurons that innervate the extrafusal fibers of the same muscle, resulting in contraction of the muscle. The classic example of a stretch reflex is observed in the knee-jerk reflex. This reflex is normally tested as part of a routine assessment of nervous system function. A normal knee jerk is an indication that a number of neural and muscular components—muscle spindle, afferent input, motor neurons, efferent output, and muscles themselves—are functioning normally (Sherwood, 2006).

Although the stretch reflex plays an important protective role in correcting quick and unanticipated lengthening of skeletal muscles, it also has a subtler role in responding to gravitational forces that constantly act to undermine the maintenance of upright body position. The constant initiation of very slight stretch reflex corrections to body position, as the muscles of the legs, back, abdomen, and neck in particular are acted upon by gravitational forces, goes largely unnoticed but is essential to the maintenance of an upright body position and stability.

The third major function of muscle spindles is to allow for adjustments in muscle responses to external loads and perturbations. This is made possible because of the coactivation capacity of the alpha and gamma motor neuron systems. Under normal activity, coactivation results in a coordinated firing pattern that allows a muscle to maintain its sensitivity to stretch and relaxation over its entire range of movement, a process entirely under the control of spinal reflexes. Higher centers in the brain, however, can "set" the level of spinal reflex coactivation to best meet the desired goals of voluntary movements (i.e., of motor skills). That is, the gamma motor system can be programmed to maintain a predetermined stretch of a muscle's intrafusal fibers (called *gamma bias*), which causes the afferent signals from muscle spindles to synapse in the spine with alpha motor neurons to the muscle's extrafusal fibers in order to maintain a "pre-set" tension in the muscle. This process is termed the *gamma loop*. In this fashion, a steady tension in a muscle can be maintained through constant, quick, and automatic reflexive corrections. Such reflexive corrections allow individuals to maintain a predetermined joint angle when external loads are constantly changing and causing perturbations to a limb. Maintaining a steady hold on an armful of library books as a friend piles additional books on top of those you are already holding; keeping a glass of milk to your lips as you drink and the weight of the glass constantly becomes lighter; safely cradling a wriggling child in your arms; or maintaining your position on the line of scrimmage as a charging lineman attempts to drive you back are all possible because of the gamma loop activity of muscle spindles.

Golgi Tendon Organs

Golgi tendon organ:
Mechanoreceptor located in the muscle-tendon junction of all skeletal muscles providing information about tension.

The **Golgi tendon organ** (typically abbreviated GTO), like the muscle spindle, is a mechanoreceptor contributing to the kinesthetic sense. The GTO monitors the tension on tendons caused by muscular contraction. Unlike muscle spindles in the muscle itself, GTOs are located in the tendons that attach muscle to bone. They provide information about the state of tension that a contracting muscle is putting on the tendon. Although it might seem that the contraction of a muscle would pull on the muscle's tendons and that muscle spindles would, therefore, be good indicators of the tension placed on tendons, in fact most of the force (the tension) of a muscle's contraction stretch is absorbed by the muscle itself rather than by the tendons attaching muscle to bone. A number of factors influence the tension developed in a muscle during contraction beside its length, such as the rate of motor unit recruitment, making it essential that some mechanism for monitoring the actual tension developed in muscles and pulling on tendons be available. GTOs provide this mechanism.

GTOs are cells consisting of a single axon of relatively large size sending its signals into the spine and ascending toward the brain. A number of afferent fiber endings containing receptors connect to the GTO axon. Each of these endings is entwined within bundles of connective tissue fibers that make up the tendon. When the extrafusal fibers of the muscle contract, they pull on the tendon, tightening these connective tissue bundles and causing the GTO afferents to fire, with the frequency of firing directly proportional to the degree of tension developed in the muscle.

clasp-knife reflex:
A protective reflex initiated by Golgi tendon organs, resulting in the relaxation of a muscle stretched beyond a familiar load.

Golgi tendon organs have a protective function. If an unusually heavy load on a tendon is detected, a protective reflex called the **clasp-knife reflex** is triggered. In a clasp-knife reflex, the contracting muscle suddenly and completely relaxes. The clasp-knife reflex may be seen, for example, in the initial phases of strength training. A person beginning a new weight lifting program who attempts to force just one last repetition with a heavy weight may suddenly experience a collapse of the involved muscles. This is because GTOs, having detected an unusually heavy load on the tendons of the muscles being exercised, initiates a clasp-knife reflex to protect the exercising muscle and its tendons.

An important point in the example of the person starting a weight training program, is that the detected load triggering the clasp-knife reflex does not have to be particularly heavy or dangerous, it just has to be unfamiliar. Over time, with repetition after repetition of training, GTOs adapt to the imposition of greater loads; we might even say that they "learn" from experience that they can safely tolerate increasing amounts of tension on the involved tendons before triggering a protective clasp-knife reflex. One goal of exercise training in particular is to get the GTOs to accept higher and higher loadings without collapsing exercising muscles.

Another issue involving the GTOs has to do with the forces on tendons that result from extreme joint angles. When the joints of a limb approach maximal extension, the tendons are pulled and stretched. If, additionally, the muscle to which the tendon is attached is contracted, increased tension is placed upon the tendon, a situation seen in a number of sports that require a broad range of motion on limbs. Sports like golf, tennis, and bowling, for example, require considerable backswing or follow-through, or both, when executing skills. Beginners in these activities are typically observed to truncate the extent of these motions, such as the golfer who takes a short backswing with his club when driving the ball, or the tennis player who executes "choppy" shots with her racquet when returning serves. As practice continues, GTOs adapt to increasing loads in these activities, and a greater range of motion when executing backswings and follow-throughs is possible. GTOs play an important role in gaining skill proficiency in a number of sports and other activities.

Joint Receptors

joint receptor:
Mechanoreceptors located in the capsules of all synovial joints and which provide information on joint angle.

A third type of mechanoreceptor is the **joint receptor**. Joint receptors are located in the joint capsules and ligaments of all synovial joints in the skeletal system. Several types of joint receptors have been identified, but all send their sensory endings into either the ligaments or tissue around joints and include a single axon conveying information from these endings to the CNS. The exact function and role of joint receptors in kinesthesis remains somewhat debated. At one time, they were believed to provide the primary source of information concerning joint angle and movement, but that function is now attributed to the coordinated input of muscle spindles and GTOs. Certainly joint receptors play some role in the monitoring of the angle of joints, and probably of static joint angles in particular, though they fire their afferent signals too slowly to be the main source for information concerning dynamic joint movements.

It has been observed that joint receptors increase their signaling activity dramatically as joints are placed in extreme angles and when they are rotated, though they remain fairly quiet in mid-range and lesser angles. Based upon this observation, it is now suggested that joint receptors may play an important role in assessing distressful and potentially injurious movement of joints. This conclusion must be somewhat tempered, because joint receptors do not form spinal synapses with alpha motor neurons in initiating protective reflexive responses. The fact that afferent signals from joint receptors do ascend to the brain and are consciously mediated, however, may mean that they nevertheless perform a protective role, but one under conscious control. Probably the best that can be stated authoritatively at present is that joint receptors are involved in monitoring the angle of joints, and in this regard contribute to kinesthetic awareness. More research is needed before a fuller explication of the function and role of joint receptors is available.

The continuing debate concerning the exact function of joint receptors has led to divergent opinions regarding the outcomes and treatment options for individuals undergoing joint replacements. When a joint is removed and replaced with an artificial one, all or most of the joint receptors are also removed. Theoretically, at least, this would suggest that individuals having undergone these procedures would demonstrate less sensitivity to both the position of a replaced joint and to pain or stress associated with acute rotations or displacement of the joint. Although this issue is far from settled, current research does not support this assumption, leaving the exact function of joint receptors unclear. Perhaps the best conclusion at present is that because all three mechanoreceptors discussed so far appear to work in concert, muscle spindles and GTOs are capable of taking on some of the functions of joint receptors if they are damaged or removed.

Vestibular Apparatus

When you think of the ears, you probably think about hearing. The mechanism of the ear is unique in that it is both a proprioceptor and an exteroceptor. **Exteroception** is the awareness of the environment outside of one's body, and hearing, along with vision, is an important source of information about our external environment necessary for movement control. But the ear also serves as a proprioceptor. In this case, a mechanoreceptor called the *vestibular apparatus* is located within the inner ear.

Muscle spindles, GTOs, and joint receptors, as we have just seen, provide specific information about the body's system of muscles and joints. They do not, however, provide a global sense of the body's movement or of its changing position in space. These functions are fulfilled by the vestibular apparatus.

exteroception:
Perception of information in the environment external to the body.

Although the outer and middle ear contain auditory structures concerned with hearing, the inner ear contains a complex grouping of interconnected canals and sacs devoted to providing proprioceptive information. These structures include two saclike chambers called the *saccule* and *utricle*, and three semicircular canals. Collectively, these structures are called the **vestibular apparatus** (see Figure 3.3).

The saccule and utricle are both fluid-filled chambers that contain tiny hair-like nerve endings on their inner surfaces. These tiny endings are covered with a membrane enclosing a gelatinous fluid. Within this gelatinous fluid and lying among the thicket of bristle-like nerve endings are small calcium carbonate ear stones called *othliths*. When the head moves, the hairs bend within their fluid-filled membrane covering in a direction directly opposite to the head's movement. The othliths, however, being influenced by the pull of gravity, do not move with the hairs but rather literally bump into the hairs and press against them. In turn, the hairs initiate afferent signals indicating both the direction and intensity of the head's movement. Because the thicket of hairs is compacted to a greater degree in the horizontal plane in the utricle and in the vertical plane in the saccule, combined information from both structures provides a complete picture of the head's position with respect to three-dimensional space (i.e., with respect to gravity). The primary information supplied by the saccule and utricle is the position of the head with respect to gravity. Because other proprioceptors supply information about limb and joint movements and position, the addition of sensory input from the vestibular system, along with these other sources of information, is combined within the CNS to supply an

vestibular apparatus: Region of the inner ear that provides sense of equilibrium and controls head movements, as well as coordinates head and eye movements; it consists of the utricle, saccule, and semicircular canals.

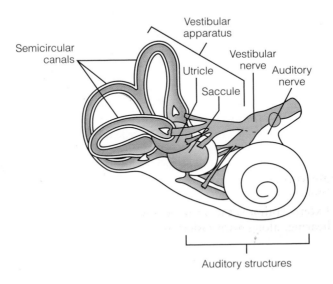

FIGURE **3.3** The Vestibular Apparatus

Source: Adapted from McLester/Pierre, *Applied Biomechanics: Concepts and Connections*, p. 50.

integrated, global awareness of the entire body's position relative to the gravity (i.e., relative to the earth).

Although the saccule and utricle signal information about the head's position, the semicircular canals are specialized to monitor the head's movements, particularly angular movement and acceleration and deceleration of the head (remember that the rest of the body moves along with the head). Each ear contains three semicircular canals arranged three-dimensionally in planes that lie at right angles to one another (which are also the three planes of body movement—i.e., sagittal, transverse, and horizontal). Like the saccule and utricle, the semicircular canals enclose a gelatinous fluid that washes against the inner surface of the canals from which nerve endings protrude. As a person's head moves, the fluid within the canals presses against the nerve endings that, in turn, initiate signals to the CNS. Again, the greatest pressure within the three canals will occur in a direction directly opposite to the direction of movement. Taken together, the semicircular canals supply information about movement in any direction, as well as about acceleration and deceleration of movement. It must be noted, however, that these structures supply information only about changes in the direction of movement, or in acceleration. This is because only such changes in body movement result in the shifting waves of fluid within the canals that stimulate nerve endings to signal movement. Once a steady state of movement is obtained, the fluid within the semicircular canals ceases to wash over the inner canal surface and, so, depolarization and signaling by the nerve endings ceases. That is why you are aware of accelerating during takeoff in a jet plane, but have no sense of moving when traveling at a steady 500 mph in route to your destination.

Taken together, the structures of the vestibular apparatus supply information essential to maintaining one's sense of balance (indeed, a loss of balance is an initial sign of damage to the inner ear). They supply kinesthetic information concerning the head's position with respect to gravity, as well as changes in angular movement or in acceleration or deceleration. For reasons that are not well understood, some people are especially sensitive to particular motions that activate the vestibular system and that cause feelings of dizziness and nausea, a condition we know as *motion sickness* (see Box 3.3).

There is one other important role that the vestibular system plays, and that is in its contributions to the guidance of visual activities. Whenever a person is tracking an object moving across his or her field of vision, or when the person is moving while attempting to maintain visual fixation on a stationary object, a problem arises in that the head and eyes must move in opposite directions. Because the eyes must fixate temporarily on an object to identify it, the eyes move in a series of quick, small, alternating movements and fixations known as *nystagmus*. As the head moves, the eyes remain a step behind. What is needed is some sort of compensatory mechanism to coordinate the activities of the eyes and the head. The vestibular system supplies just such a mechanism. As the head moves, vestibular inputs synapse in the brain with neural pathways commanding effectors controlling the ocular muscles to initiate a reflex called the **vestibulo-ocular reflex (VOR)** (Nakamagoe, Iwamoto, and Yoshida, 2000). The VOR coordinates the timing between the eyes and head so that the center

vestibulo-ocular reflex: A reflex initiated by the vestibular system in which head and eye movements cooperate in compensatory actions designed to maintain visual focus on moving targets.

of the eyes' focus remains on the object of interest. The control of eye movement occurs much more quickly than would be possible if conscious control were relied upon. In fact, for most visual tasks involving the tracking or identification of moving objects, or of objects when one's own body is moving—or a combination of both—conscious control is too slow to allow for effective visual activity.

A similar relationship among the eyes, head, and hands also appears to exist (Schmidt and Lee, 2005). Electromyographic studies have shown that the onset of eye and head movements occurs almost instantaneously with movements involving the arm and hand, such as when reaching for or grasping objects. The suggestion, though unconfirmed as yet, is that the vestibular system may well play a role in many more bodily activities than was once believed.

cutaneous receptors: Receptors located in the dermis and epidermis throughout the body and specialized to monitor one of several types of sensory stimulation, including pressure, heat, cold, pain, and chemical stimuli.

Cutaneous Receptors

A number of different receptors, collectively called **cutaneous receptors**, are grouped just under the skin in a layer called the *epidermis*, or in deeper layers of the skin called the *dermis*. Cutaneous receptors provide information

---

BOX 3.3   When Movement Makes You Sick

Motion sickness is a common condition experienced by many people in response to certain movements, though it can occur while remaining perfectly still also. Usually, the condition is experienced when riding in an automobile (*car sickness*) or airplane (*air sickness*), on a boat (*sea sickness*) or train (*train sickness*), or even while flying in the space shuttle (*space sickness*). Whatever the initiating situation and by whatever name it is called, motion sickness is typically accompanied by feelings of dizziness, fatigue, queasiness in one's stomach, sweatiness, and, as the condition worsens, full-blown nausea.

Age and sex appear to play a significant role in susceptibility to motion sickness. Infants under 2 years of age rarely experience motion sickness, whereas children between 2 and 12 years of age are especially susceptible. By their 20s, about one-third of the population continue to periodically experience the condition, with the number dropping to about 10 to 15 percent of those in their 30s. The percentage continues to decrease, until by age 50 motion sickness is rare among people, Apparently because of female-specific hormones, women have greater susceptibility to motion sickness at all ages.

For such a common condition, the causes of motion sickness remain a mystery. What brings on the condition, however, is well understood. Motion sickness results from the discontinuity of two difference sources of perceptual information. Specifically, motion sickness occurs when the vestibular and visual systems report a confused mix of information to the brain. Think, for example, of someone sitting in the cabin of a boat reading a book. The windows are closed and all that the person can see when looking up from reading is the interior of the cabin. Now think of the signals being sent to the person's brain by vestibular and visual receptors. The vestibular system is sensitive to movement with respect to gravity, and so faithfully monitors the up and down rocking of the boat on the sea. The visual system, however, not only fails to detect motion but reports that the person is sitting motionless in the cabin. Because the inside of the cabin is moving up and down in perfect sync with the person, it visually appears as though the boat is not moving at all. There is a conflict in the perceptual information the person's brain is receiving, with one source reporting movement, and the other no movement. Although its underlying causes may remain a mystery, it is this conflicting perceptual information that initiates motion sickness.

about stimulation of the skin and deeper tissue and structures within the body. The various types of cutaneous receptors supply different information, including information concerning pressure (touch), heat, cold, pain, and chemical stimuli.

Although cutaneous receptors certainly play an important role in keeping individuals apprised of the external environment, their role in kinesthesis appears limited at best. Probably those receptors that provide information on pressure, and to some extent those signaling pain, contribute to the functions of motor control and learning. Pressure-sensitive receptors are concentrated in especially high numbers in areas where fine motor control is essential, such as the fingertips, palms of the hands, and lips and tongue (remember that speech is a motor activity). (To test your understanding of the proprioceptors supporting kinesthesis, see Box 3.4.)

Visual Perception

Although the somatosensory system supplies information about the internal world of the body, the visual system supplies information about the external world outside of the body. The eyes, the lone source of visual information, are roughly spherically shaped receptive organs set in deeply cupped cavities in the skull called *orbits*. Each eye rotates within these protective cavities under the control of tiny muscles, called *orbital muscles*, capable of orienting its gaze across a broad visual field.

rods: Visual receptors specialized for detecting movement and subserving ambient vision.

cones: Visual receptors specialized for discerning detail and color in objects and subserving focal vision.

fovea: Central area of the retina comprised entirely of cones and responsible for both focal and color vision.

The eyes convert the physical energy of light waves (called *electromagnetic radiation*) entering them into electrochemical impulses that are then transmitted by sensory neurons to the brain. As light enters the opening of the eye, it passes through a series of structures (cornea, iris, pupil, and lens) focusing its waves and directing them through a clear gel-like supportive filling (the vitreous humor) toward the receptor-rich areas covering the rear half of the eye's inner wall. This area is called the *retina* and contains the photoreceptors receiving the focused light waves. Two types of photoreceptors, called rods and cones, convert light energy into neural impulses. A central area of the retina, called the fovea, is made up entirely of cones, whereas the more peripheral retinal area outside of the fovea is comprised of all of the eye's rods and only a few cones. The axonal projections from the receptors in these two areas of the retina follow

BOX 3.4   The Sources of Kinesthesis

The performance of motor skills requires a constant supply of information concerning the position and movement of various limbs and body parts, as well as of internal and external forces acting on the performer's body, which together comprise the person's awareness of his or her body that is called *kinesthesis*. Without the kinesthetic sense, movement skills would be impossible.

In the following example, think of specific information supplied by each of the four proprioceptors (muscle spindles, Golgi tendon organs, joint receptors, and the vestibular apparatuses) that make performing the skill possible: keeping an egg balanced in a spoon, with the spoon's handle clutched between your teeth, while racing in a straight line on a grassy park surface, at a family picnic.

distinct pathways in ascending to the brain where, after crossing, they converge in the brain's occipital lobes (Palmer, 1999). From these two-dimensional retinal images, the brain constructs three-dimensional perceptions of the world.

The photoreceptors of the eye, the rods and cones, are specialized to project distinctively different types of sensory information to the brain. The more numerous rods, of which there are about 100 million in each eye, or more than 30 times the number of cones, are, as already mentioned, abundant in the periphery of the retina outside of the fovea. Cones, with their smaller number, are compacted in the fovea, although a relatively small number are also found in the periphery.

Rods and cones have distinctive visual properties. Rods provide vision only in shades of gray, whereas cones provide color vision. Rods have a high sensitivity to light, needing relatively little to be stimulated sufficiently to propagate sensory signals. Rods therefore provide good vision in low light and are the source of good night vision, but they lack acuity (the ability to discern between two nearby points; sharpness of vision). Cones require high illumination for effective sensory input but are capable of high degrees of acuity. Cones provide sharp vision with high resolution and fine detail. Though cones provide better information concerning details in the visual field than do rods, rods provide greater discernment concerning movement within the environment of the visual field.

Two Visual Systems

Recalling that the fovea, which is made up exclusively of cones, and the retinal periphery with its abundance of rods follow two distinct ascending pathways to the brain's visual centers, it should not come as too great a surprise that humans have two distinct visual systems. These are the **focal visual system** and the **ambient visual system.** Because only the focal visual system is consciously perceived, most people are not aware of the activities of the ambient system (and, indeed, are often surprised to learn that they have two separate visual systems constantly guiding their behaviors and actions).

Neural tracts from the fovea supply focal vision. Because the fovea is limited to sensory information supplied by cones, focal vision provides detailed information for object identification and bathes the world in a rich pallet of colors. It is degraded in low illumination, though, and limited to objects in the center of vision. Focal vision is under conscious control; it provides the only visual information of which we are aware.

In contrast to the tracts for focal vision, neural pathways coming from the retina's periphery are composed almost entirely of rods. These pathways stimulate the ambient visual system, and its abilities reflect the properties of rods. Ambient vision provides information about the location of objects in the visual field, especially in the periphery, but little detail concerning those objects. Though poor at identifying details, ambient vision is an excellent source of information concerning movement within the visual field, even under conditions of low illumination. Ambient vision is not under conscious control, and its sensory input serves automatic and nonconscious responses. Whereas focal vision is primarily concerned with object identification, with answering questions about "what" something is, the properties of ambient vision provide for

focal visual system:
Conscious visual system specialized for object identification.

ambient visual system:
Nonconscious visual system specialized for movement control.

its primary purposes in movement control, with answering the question about "where" something is, whether the "where" in question is of an object in space or of the individual's body moving through space. A comparison of the ambient and focal systems is seen in Table 3.1.

The Ambient System and Movement Control

The idea that two separate visual systems underlie behavior could lead to the misguided conclusion that information from each is separately processed and independently used. In fact, the two systems work in tandem, each providing essential aspects of a single unified perception of visual reality. Although we may focus conscious attention on specific features of the environment supplied by focal vision, we do so against the backdrop of information from ambient vision locating those features in relation to our body and its movement within the environment.

The American psychologist J. J. Gibson (1904–1979) was the first to point out that patterns inherent in the visual field could influence perception directly. The way in which information from the ambient system is used to interpret location and movement within our visual environment is related to the way in which light waves entering the eye strike and sweep across the retina. Light waves enter the eye from different angles, with those coming from objects in the center of the eye's focus entering in a straight line and those from the periphery entering at angles. The further off center an object is in our visual field, the greater the angle with which light waves from it enter the eye. In a similar way, as objects move closer or further away from us, the light waves from their edges, crossing through the eye's lens, form an angle that expands on the retina as the object moves closer and contracts when it moves away. As objects move in our field of vision or as we move, changing our relationship to the visual images entering our eyes, the light waves focused on the back of the eye dance across retinal receptors in a complex calculus of shifting patterns of angles and spaces. Even though these patterns are extremely complex and may change rapidly, they nevertheless adhere to the mathematical regularities

TABLE **3.1**

Comparison of Focal and Ambient Visual Systems

Focal Vision	Ambient Vision
Color vision	Vision in shades of gray
High visual acuity	Low visual acuity
Central visual focus	Peripheral vision
Needs good illumination (Day vision)	Good in low illumination (Night vision)
Conscious awareness	Nonconscious perception
Moderate discernment of movement limited by conscious awareness	High movement discernment under quick and automatic control

of lines and angles (though far beyond what most of us learned in beginning trigonometry). In ways not fully understood, the brain is able to compute and interpret these shifting patterns of light waves flowing over the retinal surfaces of the eyes. This source of sensory information concerning the location and movement of objects in the visual field is called **optic flow** and is critical for many aspects of motor control (Vaina, Beardsley, and Rushton, 2004). Hence, the optic flow of visual images joins the detailed images arising from focal vision, resulting in a unified perception of what an object is, how it is moving, and where it is located in relation to the perceiver.

As a source for guiding movement behaviors, focal vision, for all of its obvious advantages, also has the disadvantages of being attention demanding (it is under conscious mediation) as well as being limited by the types of

optic flow: The patterning of light rays moving across the retina that supplies information concerning the speed and direction of the movement of objects in the environment.

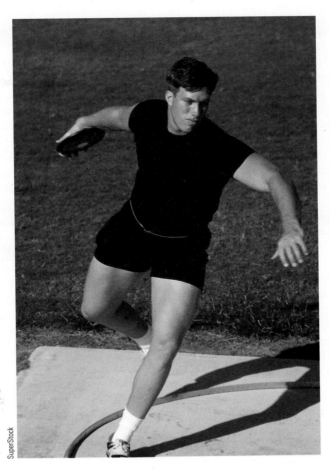

Though not under conscious control, the ambient visual system supplies an important source of information helping people maintain bodily balance and stability by initiating postural corrections to changes in body position.

information available from cones as its exclusive receptive source. Ambient vision, with its rich array of optic flow information, is quickly and automatically processed through nonconscious channels, thus allowing decision making to be focused on other aspects of movement control.

Sensory input from the ambient system plays a critical role in providing the motor framework upon which specific skills can then be constructed. That framework includes a rich source of information concerning how a person's body is located and moving relative to the environment (from slight, almost imperceptible perturbation while standing, to dynamic changes in body orientation during gymnastics or dance routines), to how one's limbs are positioned and moving relative to the body (see Box 3.5). A listing of some of the functions subserved by the ambient visual system include the following: postural stability and balance, maintenance of stability and balance during locomotion, guidance of limb movements during reaching and grasping, guidance of limb motions when propelling (i.e., throwing) objects, orienting the body in space, and assessing the velocity and direction of moving objects in the environment or of one's own body in relation to the environment.

The role played by ambient vision during activities from walking, to reaching for a glass of water, to hitting baseballs is critical. Because of the essential part it plays in the awareness of body position and movement, ambient vision underlies the expression *visual proprioception*, often used to denote vision's contributions to bodily orientation and movement control.

The Perception of Affordances (Perceiving Opportunities for Action)

In discussing the properties of vision in the preceding section, we alluded to the concept of optic flow as a direct source of movement information supplied through perceptual mechanisms. The idea that perception can directly supply movement-related information is part of a larger psychological approach called **ecological psychology**, developed in the 1960s and '70s by Gibson. Ecological psychologists focus attention on perceptual processes. In particular, they study the ways in which perceptual sources provide direct information about opportunities for action without the necessity of cognitive intervention. According to this view, perception is much more than a shadow

ecological psychology: A branch of psychology emphasizing the role of the environment in human behavior, especially the interface between perception and action.

BOX **3.5**   The Illusion of Movement

Everyone has had the compelling feeling of moving when, in reality, remaining stationary. This happens, for instance, when, seated on a stationary train, you observe a train on the next track start to pull away from the station, or when you are stalled in heavy traffic and a large truck observed out your side window begins to creep forward. The problem in cases like these arises because your entire peripheral visual field is moving, which your ambient system interprets as being stationary, because no other visual cues are present. Your brain then interprets this to mean that it is you who must be moving. Even though your focal vision signals that the view in front of you is stationary, this information is overridden by your nonconscious ambient system. This phenomenon is referred to as the *illusion of bodily self-motion*, and demonstrates the powerful influence that the ambient visual system has on movement control.

of the sensory world, which must be illuminated by cognitive representations such as memory to give it meaning. Rather, perception directly conveys information about movement possibilities to the central nervous system. This information about the opportunities for action within the perceived field is called an **affordance**.

affordance: The properties of an object or of the environment that offer opportunities for action.

Affordances refer to both the actual and the perceived qualities of things, primarily those qualities of objects or environments that determine how they can be used and what actions they allow us to perform. A chair affords support of the body and therefore affords the action of sitting. A chair could also, though, afford standing on to reach a book on the top shelf of a tall bookcase. The seat of the chair might also afford a convenient surface on which to place an armful of books for which you cannot find storage space in the bookcase. A ball affords throwing. Some balls afford both throwing and bouncing. A stick might afford hitting a ball if it is solid enough, or tying a string to for fishing, or poking into a hornets' nest to see whether the nest is active. A grassy field affords sitting on, running on, and an area suitable for flying a kite. Water affords swimming, wading, or diving into, depending upon its extent and depth (see if you can identify affordances in Box 3.6).

An important principle of ecological psychology is that in examples like those above, perception and action are linked. We do not perceive a chair and then decide that it affords sitting; the action of sitting is implicit in the perception of the chair. For ecological psychologists, perception and action are coupled (recall the problem of perceptual-action coupling discussed in Chapter 2). Indeed, according to this view, we see the world in terms of our action possibilities (see Figure 3.4). An implication of this is that we see the world differently depending upon our movement capabilities (our potential for action). Although a healthy teenager may perceive a long flight of stairs as providing easy access to the top floor of a building, an individual with arthritic knees may see steps as preventing access. In this view, an important goal of athletic training, for instance, is to enhance the athlete's movement capabilities so that he or she views the perceptual landscape of the sport in a new way, a way providing more opportunities for taking advantage of affordances. The athlete is said to become "attuned" to opportunities for action, as his or her perception of available affordances becomes greater (a concept we will take up in more detail in Chapter 7).

BOX **3.6** Identifying Affordances

How many affordances can you think of for the following objects or environments?

- Brick
- Empty plastic bottle
- Snow-covered hill
- Tennis racquet

- 10 feet of 6-inch elastic band
- Wheelchair
- 20-lb barbells
- Apple
- Sandy beach
- Beach ball

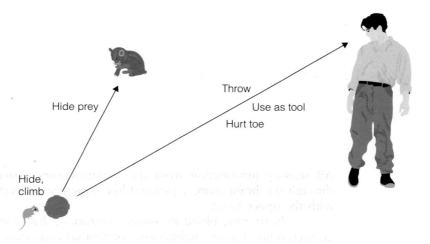

Hide prey

Throw
Use as tool
Hurt toe

Hide,
climb

FIGURE **3.4** Affordances Tell About Opportunities for Action

Source: © Fraunhofer Institute for Intelligent Analysis and Information Systems IAIS.

THE BRAIN

brain: The organ that mediates all mental functions and all behaviors.

The human **brain,** weighing no more than about three pounds yet comprised of more than 100 billion neurons making possible trillions of neural connections, integrates sensory input from the somatosensory and visual systems with processes in the brain controlling the actions of the muscular system. Given the complexity of the human brain, any complete appraisal of its role in motor control would require many volumes (but for good introductions, see Aamodt and Wang, 2008; Berthoz, 2000; Latash, 1998; and Leonard, 1997). In this chapter, we will be able to sketch only the major structures and functions of the brain as they relate to the control and learning of movement. (We should always keep in mind, though, that the entire brain, including those components we are more likely to typically associate with cognitive functions, is involved in the learning and control of movement.) Some foundational grounding concerning the brain's structure and most basic functions in motor control and learning is necessary in order to fully grasp the mechanisms and complexities involved in the development and acquisition of motor skills.

The various structures and regions of the brain can be grouped according to anatomical, functional, or developmental distinctions, depending on purpose. For our purposes, we will first identify the gross external regions of the brain, those you could see if you were to hold a brain in your hand and look at it. We will then identify and locate major structures and parts of the brain involved in the control of voluntary movement (this will actually take us through most of the brain's major structures). We will also follow a conventional "bottom up" arrangement in our consideration of brain regions.

Figure 3.5 shows two representations of the human brain. Figure 3.5a on page 94 presents the external features of the brain. It identifies the major structures and cortical lobes mapping out the terrain of the brain's surface features, naming the regions that help us navigate our way around the brain. Figure 3.5b shows the location within the brain of those major structures and components related to motor control, which we will examine in greater detail (see Restak, 1984, for an approachable and authoritative overview of the structures of the human brain). Referring to these figures as we proceed will help orient you to the relative locations of the structures we will be learning about. We will begin our tour of the brain on the ground floor, with the brain stem.

The Brain Stem

brain stem: Part of the brain just above the spinal column housing the medulla, pons, and reticular formation.

medulla: Part of the brain stem responsible for regulation of respiration, blood pressure, and heart rate.

pons: Portion of brain stem responsible for integrating sensory signals and routing them forward to higher brain centers.

All sensory information from the somatosensory system enters the brain through the **brain stem**, a pedestal-like structure connecting the spinal cord with the upper brain. The brain stem controls essential autonomic functions such as heart rate, blood pressure, respiration, digestion, sweating, glandular secretions, and the maintenance of arousal and attention levels. These are all functions vital to life and are controlled through nonconscious processes in the brain stem. The brain stem includes the medulla, pons, and reticular formation.

The **medulla**, which sits just on top of the spinal column, is primarily responsible for regulating respiration, blood pressure, and heart rate. Just above the medulla is the **pons**. The pons is an important structure for integrating signals from the lower body, such as those from muscles and joints. In fact, *pons* means "bridge," and the pons is indeed the bridge where sensory information from the body "crosses over" on its way to higher brain centers. Sensory information from the left side of the body crosses here to connect with centers in the right half of the brain, whereas information from the body's right side crosses to continue on to the left half of the brain. In a similar fashion, the pons reverses these steps for descending signals, with motor commands from the left hemisphere of the brain being routed to the right side of the body, and vice versa. The pons also receives afferent signals from the vestibular apparatus, where they synapse with motor neurons to initiate reflexive controls concerned with head and eye movements (the VOR discussed earlier is one example).

BOX **3.7**   **The 10 Percent Myth**

Among the most widely entrenched popular beliefs about the brain is that people use only 10 percent of their brains. This idea continues to be promoted by popular books and self-improvement programs promising to unlock the 90 percent of the brain's untapped potential.

As seductive as the idea that the brain harbors a vast reserve of untapped potential waiting to be tapped may be, it is unfounded. Scientific evidence, especially brain imaging research, has shown that there is no part of the brain that is inactive. In fact,

almost every part of the brain is involved in normal daily activities. There are no unused parts in our brain.

The 10 percent myth probably stems from a misinterpretation of the writings of William James, a founder of American psychology, who mused at the turn of the twentieth century that people used only a small portion of their intellectual potential. In a reference to this in the 1936 best-selling book *How to Win Friends and Influence People* by Dale Carnegie, James's observation was turned into the 10 percent figure and became part of modern lore.

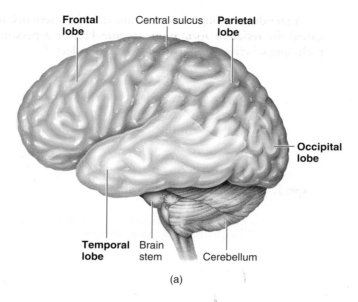

(a)

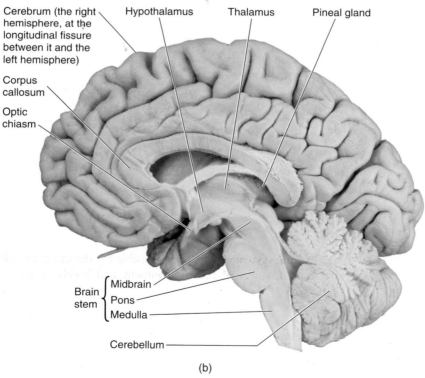

(b)

FIGURE **3.5** The Human Brain

Source: From Sherwood, *Human Physiology*, 7/e, p. 146.

reticular formation:
Area of the brain stem that acts to filter out irrelevant sensory input from further processing activities.

Extending throughout the brain stem is a network of interwoven neurons called the **reticular formation,** responsible for a person's degree of alertness, including whether the person is awake or asleep. You are reading this page now because your reticular formation is sufficiently activated to keep you awake and, hopefully, sufficiently alert. When you are asleep, the reticular formation is at rest, maintaining only minimal physiological activities such as respiration. When an alarm clock sounds, though, an excitation wave of action potentials spreads quickly upward to the conscious cortical areas of the brain waking you up, then initiating signals to the motor system so that you can spring out of bed alert and ready for the challenges of a school day. All of this happens quickly because the organization of cells in the reticular formation is designed to spread rapidly to the whole brain. The interneurons comprising the reticular formation are short and therefore fan out rapidly over a wide area of the brain, making possible the swift changes in levels of alertness we have all experienced. Activity of the reticular formation also goes in two directions. Not only does it send its signals into higher regions of the brain, but once there they stimulate descending waves of excitation to the muscles controlling action. The reticular formation is the general alertness center for both brain and body.

Remembering that all proprioceptive sensations enter the brain through the brain stem, another task of this portal to the upper brain is to decide which of the many signals coming from the body are important and should be passed along for conscious processing, and to which no further attention need be paid. Approximately 99 percent of ascending sensory signals are filtered out by the reticular formation, with only those that are important to ongoing activities projected into higher regions of the brain. Without this moment-to-moment filtering system, conscious attention would easily become overwhelmed and an individual's ability to make decisions and to control actions compromised. Indeed, the cacophony of disparate sensory signals flowing into conscious resources, if all sensory input entering the brain stem were allowed to continue its journey to higher conscious brain centers, would make any decision-making—or meaningful awareness—impossible. How the reticular formation identifies what is important and what can be ignored remains one of the unsolved mysteries of the brain (though certainly the direction of conscious and nonconscious attentional resources are involved).

reticular activating system: A grouping of cells within the reticular formation responsible for general alertness and arousal levels.

A grouping of cells within the reticular formation, called the **reticular activating system** (RAS), is responsible for directing an individual's attention to specific features of the environment and bodily states. The RAS regulates neural activity throughout the central nervous system. It does this by releasing chemicals called *neuromodulators*. These neuromodulators alter the release of neurotransmitters, or the response to neurotransmitters, in a wide region of the brain and spinal cord, thereby blocking the communication of some information while facilitating the communication of other information. These activities of the RAS have the effect of focusing attention, either more broadly or more narrowly, on sources of environmental and bodily information. The RAS plays the primary role in how, and to what extent, we direct conscious attention, and on our general level of arousal. It allows individuals to muster their cognitive and physical resources and direct them toward specific needs at any one point in time.

It is the RAS that controls the level of arousal, and attentional focus, of athletes and artistic performers as well as all of those who must perform motor skills at high levels of expertise. This system, in fact, plays a significant role in the performance of sports skills, or any motor skill where arousal levels may be influenced by performance conditions. As an individual's level of arousal increases, the RAS responds by progressively filtering out incoming sensory information from being transmitted further. In filtering out incoming stimuli from somatosensory sources, the RAS prioritizes information judicially to be either excluded or conveyed upward to higher brain regions. It first blocks further transfer of sensory information irrelevant to skills being performed. This is a good thing because it allows higher brain regions involved with the direct processing of information to be dedicated more exclusively to pertinent sensory input and to direct increased attention to important features of the environment. As arousal levels continue to increase, additional sensory input is blocked and eliminated from further processing. There reaches a point, however, at which only relevant sensory input remains. What happens if arousal levels continue to increase after this point is reached? In this case, only relevant information important in continued processing activities remains to be excluded. Continued increases in one's level of arousal begin eliminating necessary sources of sensory information, which in turn begins to degrade performance levels. This description of the RAS's function is called the **inverted-U theory**, because it assumes arousal improves performance to a point (the top of the "U" when shown as inverted, after which continued arousal levels progressively hinder performance. An important function of the RAS is to maintain optimal levels of arousal in order to maximize skilled performance. The nature of the skill performed is also important in this perspective. Some skills, especially fine motor skills requiring a high degree of movement precision involving the hands or digits, require low arousal levels that allow significant flows of information from the hands and digits to be transmitted unimpeded to the brain. Other skills, usually gross skills in which the production of force is more critical than movement precision, benefit from higher levels of arousal, arguably because such high levels eliminate the need for overprocessing of sensory input from smaller muscles.

The RAS, as the gate either blocking the passage of sensory information or allowing it entrance to higher brain centers, works in two ways. On the one hand, it is responsible for establishing a person's general level of alertness and attention. But individuals also have the ability to mediate the activity of the RAS through both physical and cognitive means. Taking a relaxing bath, listening to calming music, recalling a pleasant experience can all shift RAS activity toward lower levels of arousal, just as worrying about an upcoming exam or harboring a grudge can increase RAS activity and arousal level. The use of psychological techniques for the enhancement of athletic performance in recent years is in reality a method of manipulating RAS activity in order to optimize attentional focus and associated arousal levels controlled by the RAS. An instructor counseling a student learning golf to breath deeply and mentally rehearse putting before she attempts it in practice, or a football coach urging a player to imagine the intensity and physical power he will exert to make a

inverted-U theory:
A psychological theory that increases in the state of a person's arousal are beneficial to performance up until a point when they then begin to detract from performance.

perfect block, are both attempting to take advantages of the workings of the reticular activating system (see Box 3.8).

The Cerebellum

cerebellum: One of the major parts of the brain involved in motor control; involved in motor coordination, muscle tone, balance, and the learning of motor skills.

Next in ascending order from the brain stem is the **cerebellum**. Together, the brain stem and cerebellum are sometimes called the *hindbrain*. The cerebellum consists of two wrinkled-appearing hemispheres at the back of the brain just below the large cerebral hemispheres and behind the pons. Although it makes up only about 10 percent of the brain, the cerebellum contains over half of all the brain's neurons, a devotion of resources indicative of its essential functions. The cerebellum can be considered a sort of traffic control officer at a busy intersection, in this case a neural intersection between higher command centers and lower control functions. Much of the neural traffic directed from other parts of the brain to the effectors and muscles controlling movement passes through the cerebellum. The role of the cerebellum is to make sure that neural messages are routed correctly and to reroute any that are misdirected. Far from being a passive observer of this passing neural traffic, however, the cerebellum serves an important role in the planning and evaluation of motor activities.

BOX 3.8   Mighty Casey's Reticular Activating System

Perhaps the most famous sports poem ever written, "Casey at the Bat," was penned in 1888 by Ernest Lawrence Thayer. The poem tells of a championship game between the Mudville Nine and an unnamed opponent. In the final inning of the game, the Mudville team is on the brink of defeat with two men out. Their only chance is if somehow Casey, Mighty Casey, can get to bat. But the odds of that are long because Flynn and Blake both come up first, and "the former is a pudd'n," and the "latter a flake." But to everyone's astonishment, both players safely reach base. "Then from the gladdened multitude went up a joyous yell—It rumbled in the mountaintops, it rattled in the dell." Mighty Casey was advancing to bat.

As he advanced to home plate, Casey smiled, he doffed his hat to his cheering fans, he strolled with ease and unconcern in his manner. At bat, Casey watched the first pitch go by. "Strike one." Casey smiled. "That ain't my style," he called to the crowd. Casey calmly ignored the second pitch altogether. He waved off the booing of the crowd as the umpire called, "Strike two." Casey was confident in his talent, expressing no worry or concern. Only now was he ready to save the game.

We pick up the poem with Casey at bat, two strikes, at last ready for the next pitch.

The sneer is gone from Casey's lips, his teeth are clenched in hate,
He pounds with cruel vengeance his bat upon the plate;
And now the pitcher holds the ball, and now he lets it go,
And now the air is shattered by the force of Casey's blow.

Oh, somewhere in this favored land the sun is shining bright,
The band is playing somewhere, and somewhere hearts are light;
And somewhere men are laughing, and somewhere children shout,
But there is no joy in Mudville—Mighty Casey has struck out.

What is your opinion of how Casey's attitude and behavior influenced the activity of his reticular activating system? Were his actions appropriate from what you know about how this system influences skilled performance? How might the activities of Casey's reticular formation explain the outcome of his performance? What might he have done differently?

In regard to this last point, the cerebellum acts as a comparator between outgoing signals from the brain and incoming signals from sensory receptors, evaluating the effectiveness with which higher brain center commands are being carried out by the muscular system. When outgoing and incoming signals are in discord, the cerebellum initiates corrections as needed. The coordination and timing of movements, as well as the ongoing correction of movement errors, are essential tasks of the cerebellum. From seemingly ordinary activities such as regulating muscular activities involved with maintaining upright posture, to the synchronization of limbs during highly complex athletic skills, the cerebellum plays a key role in coordinating, evaluating, and correcting action. When you reach for a bottle of cold water after an exhausting workout, coordinating your hand and arm movements to lift the bottle smoothly to exactly, but lightly, reach your lips is a result of the cerebellum's activities. The cerebellum, in a phrase, is responsible for the smooth coordination of muscular activities, from the simplest to the most complex skills. As one neuroscientist has well put it, "A ballet dance represents perfect cerebral functioning in which thousands of muscles are controlled with exquisite precision" (Restak, 1979, p. 144).

Coordinated, highly skilled movements would be impossible without the activities of the cerebellum. Indeed, damage to the cerebellum can result in a number of movement disorders. These include the conditions of hypotonia (a reduced resistance to passive displacement of the limbs), taxia (lack of coordination or impaired ability to execute voluntary movements), and tremor (oscillation of the limbs which may occur during movement activities) (Rose and Christina, 2006). An inability to consciously identify and correct movement errors can also result from disease or damage to the cerebellum (Leonard, 1997).

Although the cerebellum has always been recognized for its major role in coordinating motor activities, recent research has begun to reveal additional functions performed by the cerebellum. Because of its role in evaluating ongoing movement errors, the cerebellum has recently received considerable attention concerning its contributions to learning. There now appears to be strong evidence of an important role it plays in the learning of motor skills (Thach, 1998). Analogous to its role within the motor system, the cerebellum has also been shown to play a role in coordinating the timing of cognitive functions as well, directing one's cognitive attention as situational requirements make necessary (Ratey, 2002).

The Cerebrum

cerebrum: Composed of two large hemispheres comprising the majority of the brain, it functions as the center for learning, emotional control, memory, and voluntary movement.

Sitting on top of the brain stem is the cerebrum. The cerebrum makes up the majority of the brain—about 80 percent by weight—and is devoted to the two large hemispheres that are the most obvious visual feature of the brain and gives it the shape that most people think about when envisioning the brain (see Figure 3.5a). These two structures, divided almost evenly longitudinally into right and left cerebral hemispheres, are connected by a thick band of neurons (about 300 million of them) forming a communication bridge between the

corpus callosum: The
thick band of neurons
connecting the two
cerebral hemispheres
and acting as a
communications bridge
between them.

hemispheres called the **corpus callosum** (Figure 3.5b). When viewed from the outside, only the two large hemispheres are seen. Below this cortex, however, in the central regions of the brain, are a number of structures having importance to movement control and learning. We will present these structures in the order they ascend from the brain stem, which can be followed by referring to Figure 3.5b.

Hippocampus

hippocampus: Part
of the limbic system
especially responsible for
the formation of long-
term memories.

The **hippocampus**, a horseshoe-shaped structure, is vital to the storage of short-term memories as well as to the consolidation of memories into permanent stores. It is believed that the hippocampus retains new memories temporarily until they can be transferred to other cortical sites associated with long-term memory. Damage to the hippocampus is manifested by extreme forgetfulness. The hippocampus therefore plays a critical role in the learning of motor skills.

Hypothalamus and Thalamus

diencephalon: The
part of the cerebrum
containing the
hypothalamus and
thalamus.

hypothalamus: The
brain structure just below
the thalamus that is
responsible for regulating
body temperature and
energy use.

thalamus: Brain
structure just above the
hypothalamus responsible
for relaying sensory
inputs to sensory areas of
the cerebral cortex.

Two structures in the cerebrum's interior, the hypothalamus and thalamus, make up an area called the **diencephalon**. The **hypothalamus** controls body temperature as well as energy use and efficiency by regulating the use of carbohydrates and fats. It also plays a role in emotional and behavioral patterns. The **thalamus**, just above the hypothalamus, integrates incoming sensory information from all parts of the body. It cooperates with the reticular formation as part of the reticular activating system already mentioned. All sensory information from the body passes through the thalamus on its way to sensory receiving areas in the cortex, and it plays an important role in routing these sensory signals to the correct higher processing areas. The thalamus is also involved in reinforcing correct voluntary motor behaviors (in communication with the cerebellum).

Basal Ganglia

basal ganglia: A group
of four brain structures
lying within the central
region of the brain that
help regulate motor
activity.

The **basal ganglia**, the final structure of the inner cerebrum we will discuss, is made up of a collection of cells connected to sensory and motor areas of the cerebral cortex. The basal ganglia play an important role in the planning and execution of motor skills. They regulate background muscle tone in preparation for movement activities. When you write, for example, the basal ganglia prepare for hand movements by tensing the muscles of the upper arm in order to stabilize your hand (Shea, Shebilske, and Worchel, 1993). In similar fashion, shifts in one's center of gravity are also initiated by the basal ganglia in preparation for the execution of movements. These preparatory actions occur either just prior to, or simultaneously with, the onset of planned movement acts (and are accomplished nonconsciously). The basal ganglia are also involved in controlling *motor set*, the preparation of the motor system to control actions in specific ways as circumstances change and dictate, such as the setting of a specific level of gamma bias for the gamma loop, as we have previously observed. As should be obvious, the basal ganglia have a critical role in planning and preparing the motor system for movement.

The basal ganglia, together with the cerebellum, play a major role in coordinating all voluntary movements. Motor commands from the motor cortex, where movements are initially planned, are passed through both the cerebellum and the basal ganglia on their way to affected muscles. As we have already seen, the cerebellum monitors sensory input from the muscles to detect compliance with these outgoing commands, initiating corrective actions when the outgoing and incoming information is in conflict. The basal ganglia perform the same function, comparing the sensory responses of movements with the commands originally sent and initiating moment-to-moment corrections as needed. The difference between the functions of the cerebellum and basal ganglia is in the nature of the corrective actions that they control. The cerebellum initiates excitatory commands to muscles, exciting greater muscular activity, whereas the basal ganglia initiate inhibitory commands, reducing or inhibiting muscular activity. We might think of these two structures as "on" and "off" values, increasing or reducing the amount of muscular activity as required. The basal ganglia specifically signal the motor cortex to inhibit muscular commands when ascending sensory signals indicate a need for the motor cortex to reduce or correct its descending muscular commands. Signals from the basal ganglia to the motor cortex are routed through the thalamus, where they can be combined with information from the cerebellum and integrated into appropriate bundles of information for the cortex (remember that to get to the cortex, signals must go through the thalamus). Figure 3.6 illustrates combined activities of the basal ganglia and cerebellum in the control of voluntary movement skills (with the " − " sign representing inhibitory activities, and the " + " excitatory activities of the muscular system).

Because of its importance in movement preparation and planning, disease or damage to the basal ganglia has profound effects on an individual's ability to control bodily movements. The most widely known of the diseases of the basal ganglia include Parkinson's and Huntington's diseases, which

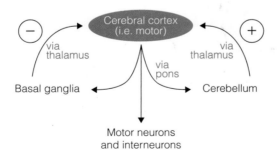

FIGURE **3.6** Balancing between Inhibitory Signals from Basal Ganglia and Excitatory Signals from the Cerebellum to Achieve Muscular Coordination

Source: Adapted from **www.wustl.edu/course/cerebell.html**.

both begin with manifestations of muscle rigidity and resting tremor, and progressively result in an almost total inability to control body movements. A number of new treatments aimed at the basal ganglia are currently being studied for their possible benefits in slowing or halting the effects of these diseases.

The Limbic System

limbic system:
Composed of a number of structures deep within the cerebrum, this system plays a critical role in motivation, emotions, value judgments, and the control of movements.

Within the cerebrum the hippocampus, hypothalamus, thalamus, and basal ganglia (along with a number of other structures including the amygdale and pituitary) form the **limbic system.** The limbic system functions on a nonconscious level and operates by influencing the endocrine system and autonomic nervous system. It is associated with motivational levels and the desire to act.

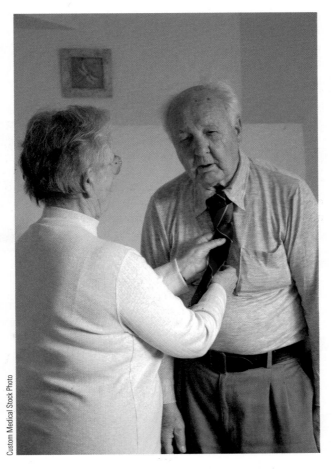

Custom Medical Stock Photo

Disease or damage to the basal ganglia, critical in the planning and execution of movement, results in the severe loss of coordination, such as observed in Parkinson's and Huntington's patients.

It interacts with higher cortical structures, therefore, in the initiation of movement skills, with the desire to act generated within the limbic system transformed into a specific action plan within the prefrontal cortex. The limbic system is also the seat of emotional life. A wide range of emotions are regulated by the release of excitatory and inhibitory neurotransmitters. Feelings of pleasure, for example, are highly linked to the regulation of serotonin and dopamine. The release of these neurotransmitters, and associated feelings of pleasure, during the performance of physical skills may play an important role in the limbic system's motivational directives, reinforcing the desire to engage in the skilled behaviors eliciting pleasurable responses.

The limbic system also plays an essential role in the formation of new memories, perhaps the most critical aspect in the learning of motor skills (and the subject of Chapter 6). One of the roles of the limbic system in the formation of memories appears to be prioritizing relative to some measure of salience and relevance for an individual. That is, the limbic system plays a role in determining how an individual acts on information within memory when it again appears. The limbic system is involved in reinforcing some behaviors—but not others—giving it an important role in the processes of learning.

The Cerebral Cortex

Each hemisphere of the cerebrum is composed of a thin outer layer of gray matter consisting predominantly of compacted neuronal cell bodies and their dendrites. Below the gray matter is the white matter, made up of tracts of myelinated axon fibers from the cells of the gray matter (it is white because of the lipid composition of the myelin). The gray matter might be viewed as the "computers" of the CNS, and the white matter as the "wires" connecting them to one another (Sherwood, 2006).

cerebral cortex: Outer layer of the cerebrum composed of gray matter, and the major site of higher brain functions such as abstraction, reasoning, decision making, and voluntary motor control.

The layers of outer gray matter of the cerebral hemispheres are called the cerebral cortex. The cerebral cortex represents the highest center of brain activity, where the processes of abstract reasoning, memory storage, and decision making occur (though we will see in Chapter 4 on theory that a fundamental debate exists about this interpretation). Each half of the cerebral cortex is divided into four functionally different areas, as shown in Figure 3.5a. These areas are called *lobes*, and include the frontal, occipital, parietal, and temporal lobes. The occipital lobes, located at the back of the head, are specialized for initial processing of visual input. The temporal lobes, located on each side of the head, receive and organize initial auditory sensations. The parietal lobes, on the top and toward the rear half of the hemispheres, primarily receive and process sensory information. The frontal lobes, located on the top and toward the front half of the hemispheres, are devoted to abstract reasoning, language, and voluntary motor activity. We will look more closely at the functions of receiving sensory input and organizing motor responses involving the parietal and frontal lobes.

somatosensory cortex: Band of neurons on cerebral cortex where sensory information is organized and brought to perception.

Transversing the front portion of the parietal lobes of both hemispheric cortices is a band of neurons forming the **somatosensory cortex** (Figure 3.7). This is where sensory input from proprioceptors ultimately projects and is brought to perception. When you become aware of sensory information from your body, it is because signals from the affected body regions have reached the somatosensory cortex.

Just how various bodily sensations are organized on the somatosensory cortex remained a mystery for some time, however. In the 1950s, neuroscientists were able to unravel this mystery (see Kandel, 2006, for the interesting story of how this mystery was solved). The entire surface of the body, as well as many deeper tissues and structures involved in the kinesthetic sense, is represented on the somatosensory cortex in the form of a point-for-point neural map. Every part of the body has a specific location where its sensory information is received and brought to perception. The location of various body parts and regions on the somatosensory cortex is illustrated in Figure 3.7. As can be seen in the figure, parts of the body are represented on the somatosensory cortex configured in more or less the same way as the human body. What was most remarkable, though, is that the width of the neural band (i.e., its size) devoted to bodily areas is proportional to the relative sensitivity of the body part or area rather than to the body part's actual size. The largest areas on the somatosensory cortex represent parts of the body that have the greatest sensitivity. That is, significantly more neural resources are devoted to areas of the body for which keen sensory information is critical (hands, fingers, lips, tongue, feet, genitalia) than to those for which sensitivity is not as critical as is gross awareness (back, thighs, shoulders, trunk, etc.). These size differences closely mirror the requirements of fine and gross motor skills. The hands, which are often used for fine skills, as an example, require the input of precise amounts of sensory information, whereas the legs may play the most essential role in gross skills such as running and lifting, but do not require the same degree of sensory precision in order to accomplish these tasks.

In fact, all types of sensory information (visual, auditory, information from joints and muscles, etc.) are represented topographically in the brain, though in different regions of the cerebral cortex. These sensory maps are easiest to understand, however, by representing the sense of touch in the somatosensory cortex. The relative size differences in the sensitivity to touch of each area of the body as represented on the somatosensory cortex can be illustrated by a **homunculus** (meaning "little man"). The homunculus, which appears as a dramatic distortion of the body form, nevertheless visually highlights the brain's view of the human body and its allocation of its neural resources (Figure 3.7).

The knowledge that body regions are faithfully represented in the brain at specific locations, and that they differ in sensitivity, has been useful in the identification and treatment of neurological disorders. By testing for bodily sensitivity (even in simple ways such as using a pin to test for pain or a feather to discern relative sensitivity of various parts of the body), specialists can accurately identify regions of the brain responsible for any sensitivity deficits and that may signal the need for further testing.

Just as the somatosensory cortex is organized to receive and prioritize incoming sensory signals, the **motor cortex** is topographically arranged to prioritize motor command resources. The motor cortex is a band of neurons at the rear of the frontal lobe and lying just in front of the somatosensory cortex (see Figure 3.7). It organizes and initiates the signals responsible for controlling

homunculus: A bodily representation indicating size of body regions as proportional to area devoted to them by either the somatosensory cortex or motor cortex.

motor cortex: Area of the cerebral cortex where afferent signals directly controlling each of the body's skeletal muscles originate.

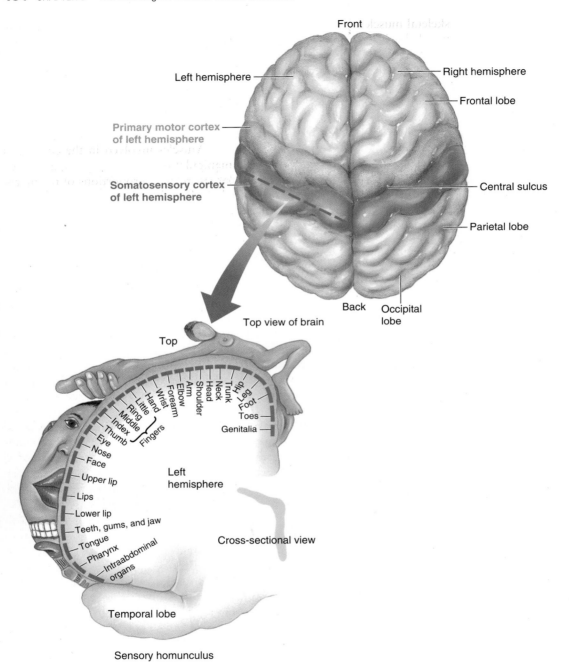

Front

Left hemisphere

Right hemisphere

Frontal lobe

Primary motor cortex
of left hemisphere

Somatosensory cortex
of left hemisphere

Central sulcus

Parietal lobe

Back   Occipital
        lobe

Top view of brain

Top

Hip
Leg
Foot
Toes
Trunk
Neck
Head
Shoulder
Arm
Elbow
Forearm
Wrist
Hand
Little
Ring
Middle
Index
Thumb
Fingers

Genitalia

Eye
Nose
Face
Upper lip
Lips
Lower lip
Teeth, gums, and jaw
Tongue
Pharynx
Intraabdominal
organs

Left
hemisphere

Cross-sectional view

Temporal lobe

Sensory homunculus

FIGURE **3.7** Allocation of Cortical Resources (the "Little Man in the Brain")

Source: From Sherwood, *Human Physiology*, 7/e, p. 148.

skeletal muscles. Neuronal tracts originating in the motor cortex directly trigger skeletal muscle contractions (though going through the basal ganglia and cerebellum first). In similar fashion to the somatosensory cortex, bands of neurons along the motor cortex are responsible for activating specific muscles. That is, each muscle in the body is represented by a specific location on the motor cortex. Also analogous to the somatosensory cortex, the motor cortex is topographically arranged according to the cortical sensitivity required for each body region. Those muscles requiring the greatest control precision are represented by the largest areas on the motor cortex. Muscles involved in the control of speech (lips, tongue, pharynx), object manipulation (hands, fingers), and body stability (ankles, feet, toes) receive the largest relative proportions of the motor cortex's neural space. Comparatively, relatively little space on the motor cortex is devoted to the trunk, arms, and lower extremities, which therefore are not as capable of precise movements. Like the somatosensory cortex, the relative area devoted to each muscle by the motor cortex can be represented by a motor homunculus (which appears almost identical to its twin sensory homunculus).

The organization of the somatosensory and motor cortex maps—the sensory and motor homunculi—is the same for everyone. This general pattern is governed by genetic and developmental processes, and cannot be greatly altered. Indeed, until fairly recently it was believed that these cortical maps were fixed and immutable. An important clue to the processes underlying learning occurred, however, with the discovery that this cortical architecture is influenced by habitual motor behaviors. In a classic study first demonstrating this, monkeys were trained to use their middle fingers to make complex rotary movements of a disk in order to receive a food reward. After several months, the area of the cortex devoted to each monkey's middle fingers had expanded—the area of the cortex used in the skill grew as learning occurred (Kandel, 2006)! In another widely reported study, this one using human subjects, modern neural-mapping techniques revealed the left hand of right-handed string musicians, the hand used to manipulate the strings, was represented by larger areas on the somatosensory and motor cortices than the right hand. Other studies have shown that learning of visual discrimination skills also leads to changes in brain anatomy and improved perceptual skills. The learning of new motor skills appears to result in at least some reprioritization of neural space along the sensory and motor cortices. There would appear to be a sort of "use-dependent competition" (Sherwood, 2006) for space on these two cortices, with more frequently used areas expanding their influence and stealing underused space from their less active neighbors.

Even though signals from the motor cortex directly activate the descending pathways stimulating muscular contractions, it is not the only brain region involved in commanding voluntary movements. Two regions of the cerebral cortex, the supplemental motor cortex and the premotor cortex, are especially involved with decision-making activities and coordinate their functions closely with the motor cortex. The supplemental motor cortex lies on the medial (inner) surface of each of the frontal hemispheres just in front of the motor cortex, and appears especially involved in preparing the motor system for action. The premotor cortex, located on the lateral surface of each hemisphere in front of the motor cortex, plays an important role in the temporal organization of movements. Although each of these individual regions of the motor control system has its specialized functions, it can be difficult to separate their activities from each other. All three motor areas of the cerebral cortex (the motor cortex, supplemental motor cortex, and premotor cortex) are intricately involved in the planning and execution of motor skills. These processes are called motor programming, and the resulting plan of action a motor program (as previously stated, theoretical debate remains concerning this, which we will take up in Chapter 4). The decision making involved in producing skilled motor activities relies highly on memory, and it should be noted that the frontal lobe of the cerebral cortex is also the seat of learning and memory.

The various brain components discussed here, along with their contributions to motor control and learning, are summarized in Table 3.2.

Where Does Learning Occur in the Brain?

Having completed our tour of the human brain, one final question remains regarding its role in motor control and learning: Exactly where in the brain does learning take place? That is, how do the neural mechanisms of the brain that are responsible for the control of movement change in ways that improve the effectiveness and quality of those movement activities, especially for activities that are deliberately practiced?

Answers to these questions are the focus of much contemporary work being carried out in diverse fields of scientific inquiry. To begin to glean those answers, we must return to where we began—with the individual nerve cell. Whatever answers are finally arrived at, it is clear to scientists by now that the answers must be grounded in the activity of neurons. That is, motor learning and control ultimately have a cellular basis (Kendal, 2006; Sousa, 2001; Sylwester, 1995).

To better appreciate this, we can start with the observation that both functional and physical changes occur in neurons during the course of learning. There is a change in the synaptic strength of neurons, in fact. More amazingly, the actual numbers of synapses in neural circuits change as the neurons underlying practiced skills grow. As individuals learn new motor skills, the neurons participating in the neural networks for those skills may more than double the number of connections they make with other neurons. Sensory neurons grow new terminal endings to their axons, and motor neurons branch out with more dendritic endings to receive the greater number of messages conveyed. The result, even for simple skills, can easily be millions of new neural routes for organizing messages between sensory and motor neurons. As we have seen, this neural growth can result in the expansion of areas of the brain to accommodate greater processing efficiency. The metabolic mechanisms involved in the cell's interior nucleus for producing neurotransmitters may also change, as does the cell's control of ion concentrations facilitating or inhibiting action potentials.

When added together, these microscopic changes to individual cells continually reorganize and restructure the brain. Depending on one's theoretical perspective, the brain gains new resources for the storage and processing of

TABLE **3.2**

Structures and Motor-Related Functions of Major Components of the Brain's Motor System

Brain Component	Major Functions
Medulla	• Regulates respiration, blood pressure, heart rate
Pons	• Routes ascending signals to upper brain components ("cross-over" relay station)
Reticular formation	• Prioritizes incoming sensory signals and eliminates irrelevant information from further processing activities • Controls alertness and arousal levels
Cerebellum	• Coordinates and plans voluntary muscular skills • Maintains balance • Monitors feedback from ongoing movements and initiates corrective actions • Maintains muscle tone • Helps with synchronization of limb movements
Hippocampus	• Retains working memory of ongoing movements • Plays essential role in consolidation of long-term memories
Hypothalamus	• Controls body temperature • Regulates energy use • Links brain and endocrine systems • Helps regulate emotions and behavioral patterns
Thalamus	• Relays all sensory inputs to somatosensory cortex • Reinforces voluntary motor behaviors initiated by higher brain centers
Basal ganglia	• Plays role in the planning and execution of motor skills • Is involved in preparing and stabilizing body for movement • Works in concert with cerebellum to coordinate voluntary movements • Coordinates slow, sustained movement
Somatosensory cortex	• Sensory perception • Routes sensory information to motor centers of cortex • Prioritizes sensory sensitivity of bodily regions
Motor cortex	• Directly controls skeletal muscle contractions • Prepares and executes the "motor program" • Prioritizes complexity of motor control available to the bodily regions
Supplemental cortex	• Is intricately involved in planning and control of all voluntary movements
Premotor cortex	• Plans and controls all voluntary movements • Especially is involved in temporal organization of limb and body movements

information, adaptation, and self-organization. This neuronal organization, which includes multiple centers and levels of the brain, is eventually expressed in movement. As changes to cells continually rework neural networks and pathways, these expressions of movement become more effective in accomplishing desired actions, the outward manifestation of learning having first occurred within the recesses of the brain's hidden interior. Learning, even of the most complex skill involving movement of the entire body, starts with the tiny neuron.

NEURAL CONTROL OF THE MUSCULAR SYSTEM

Humans have approximately 600 muscles, including cardiac muscle, smooth muscles lining blood vessels and the intestinal tract, and skeletal muscles. Although cardiac and smooth muscle actions are controlled almost entirely automatically, skeletal muscles (of which the average person has 326 by most accounts) control all voluntary actions and, therefore, underlie the performance of movement skills.

The Motor Unit

alpha motor neuron: A motor neuron that innervates skeletal muscle (also called a *motoneuron*).

motor unit: An alpha motor neuron and all of the muscle fibers that it innervates.

Every muscle fiber in every muscle is controlled by a motor neuron. Neurons that innervate skeletal muscles are called **alpha motor neurons** (α-motor neurons). Because the axonal endings of these nerves branch, one alpha motor neuron can innervate many individual muscle fibers. A single alpha motor neuron and all of the muscle fibers that it innervates are called a **motor unit.** As with all communication between neurons, the alpha motor neuron conveys its messages to muscle fibers across a synaptic gap called the *neuromuscular junction*; this occurs at a location on the muscle's fiber called a *motor end plate*. As we have already seen, acetylcholine is the neurotransmitter responsible for conveying an action potential across this neuromuscular junction from the neuron to the skeletal muscle fibers. A typical motor unit is illustrated in Figure 3.8.

motor unit pool: All of the motor units controlling a specific muscle.

Every muscle in the body is controlled by a number of motor units, with the exact number varying depending on the size and functional requirements of the particular muscle. All of the motor units controlling a specific muscle are referred to as a **motor unit pool.** The number of motor units within a muscle's motor unit pool is a function of both the need for movement precision and the generation of force typical of the muscle's actions (Leonard, 1997). For movements of the eye, which must be precise and finely tuned, extraocular muscles have a nerve-to-muscle fiber ratio of between 1:10 and 1:50. That is, a single alpha motor neuron controls only a relatively small number of muscle fibers, somewhere between 10 and 50, making fine gradations of movement possible and contributing to precise and finely controlled eye movements. Muscles controlling the digits of the hand are in the 1:100 to 1:200 range. The nerve-to-fiber ratio for the large muscles of the leg (e.g., *rectus femoris, vastus lateralis*) varies from approximately 1:200 to 1:2,000. That is, a single alpha motor neuron can innervate as many as 2,000 muscle fibers within an individual leg muscle, contributing to the demands for muscular power needed in activities such as running, lifting, and jumping. Altogether, the average person has around half

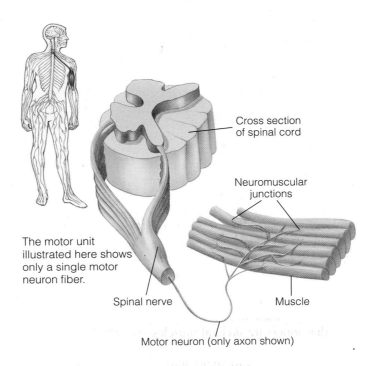

Cross section
of spinal cord

Neuromuscular
junctions

The motor unit
illustrated here shows
only a single motor
neuron fiber.

Spinal nerve

Muscle

Motor neuron (only axon shown)

FIGURE **3.8** The Motor Unit

Source: Adapted from Solomon/Berg/Martin, *Biology*, 8/e, p. 840.

a million individual skeletal muscle fibers that must each be controlled effectively to meet the goals of the many and diverse skills performed each day.

Regardless of the exact number of muscle fibers innervated by the arrival of an action potential from an alpha motor neuron, all movements require muscular contraction. Indeed, the only influence that an alpha motor neuron has on the muscle fibers of its associated motor unit is to cause them to contract maximally (called a twitch) for a brief instant (about 1/10th of a second). When an alpha motor neuron's signal is sufficient, all of the fibers in the motor unit contract (twitch) maximally; if the signal is insufficient to cross the synaptic cleft from the neuron to the muscle fiber at the neuromuscular junction, none of the fibers in the motor unit will be activated. This is known as the all-or-none law; that is, all of the muscle fibers in a motor unit contract maximally, or none contract at all.

Different skilled movements, however, require different amounts of contractile force. If all of the muscle fibers in a muscle contract maximally when an alpha motor neuron delivers a sufficient action potential, how are gradations in force production controlled? The answer to this question is both simple and elegant. The motor system specifies exact force requirements in two different ways. The first is through a process known as *motor unit recruitment*, and refers to the specification of the number and type of motor units innervated.

all-or-none law: Law stating that all of the muscle fibers of a motor unit will contract maximally when the motor neuron propagates sufficient stimulation, or none of the muscle fibers will contract in the absence of a sufficient action potential.

rate modulation: The frequency with which action potentials are propagated between a motor unit and its associated muscle fibers, affecting force produced by the muscle fibers.

size principle: Mechanism for motor unit recruitment where motor units with smallest axons are recruited first and those with largest axons recruited last; the order is reversed in deactivation.

slow-twitch muscle fiber: Muscle fibers that produce low contractile forces and that are relatively slow in responding, but capable of maintaining sustained work loads.

fast-twitch muscle fiber: Muscle fibers capable of producing quick, high contractile force responses.

The second mechanism is called **rate modulation** (or rate coding), and refers to the process of varying the rate or frequency at which each active motor unit generates action potentials.

Motor Unit Recruitment

Motor units are not activated randomly. They are activated and deactivated in a predictable sequence or order described by the **size principle** (Gardiner, 2001). Most simply stated, the size principle states that the alpha motor neurons with the smallest diameter axons will typically have the lowest threshold for synaptic activation and will therefore be recruited first within a given motor unit pool. As more force is required for an action, sequentially larger and larger motor neurons will be recruited until at the highest activation levels the alpha motor neurons with the largest diameter axons will be recruited. The order of deactivation is just the opposite. As activation levels decrease, the largest motor neurons are deactivated first and the smallest deactivated last.

This sequence of contraction activations is significant because although all motor units function similarly, they have different contractile and metabolic characteristics. Some motor units are more suited for aerobic metabolism, whereas others are more appropriate for anaerobic activity. Two distinctive muscle fiber types can be classified based upon their contractile and metabolic characteristics (Reggiani and Bortolotto, 2006). These are generally termed **slow-twitch** and **fast-twitch muscle fibers**, or more specifically referred to as *type I* and *type II muscle fibers*, respectively. Fast-twitch or Type II fibers are further subdivided into two distinct types identified as *type IIa* and *type IIb*. Type I fibers possess a high aerobic metabolic capacity. Type IIa fibers have a well-developed capacity for both aerobic and anaerobic metabolism, whereas type IIb fibers possess the greatest anaerobic capacity. The characteristics of these fiber types are presented in Table 3.3.

As can be seen in Table 3.3, slow-twitch muscle fibers (type I) are specialized for prolonged, low-to-moderate intensity activity, whereas fast-twitch muscle fibers are advantageous for high force production, short-duration, high-intensity activity. Within the fast-twitch fibers, type IIb can typically

TABLE **3.3**
Comparison of Muscle Fiber Types

Fiber Characteristic	Type I (slow twitch)	Type IIa (fast twitch)	Type IIb (fast twitch)
Force Production	Low	Intermediate	High
Contraction Speed	Slow	Fast	Fast
Fatigue Resistance	High	Moderate	Low
Endurance Capacity	High	Moderate	Low

produce higher levels of contractile force than the type IIa fibers, although for significantly shorter time durations. In recent years, further subdivisions of these muscle fiber types have been postulated (see Hoffman, 2002), but we will not consider them here because they do not alter the basic premises of the size principle of motor unit recruitment, and their separate classification is still open to debate. The average person possesses roughly an equal number of both slow-twitch and fast-twitch muscle fibers (i.e., 50% of each type) distributed proportionally across all the muscles of the body, although individual differences are evident, with some people having a greater bodily percentage of one or the other type (Gardiner, 2001). A person's percentage of each fiber type is genetically determined and can play a significant role in determining the motor skills for which a person has the greatest potential (see Box 3.9).

Returning to our consideration of motor unit recruitment, the importance of muscle fiber type is evident when it is observed that fiber type is highly associated with the size of motor neurons. Generally, those motor neurons with the smallest axons are connected to slow-twitch (type I) muscle fibers; as axonal size becomes larger, the proportion of motor units comprised of type IIa fast-twitch fibers increases, and finally those motor neurons with the largest axons innervate motor units comprised almost entirely of type IIb fast-twitch fibers. The ordering of the most appropriate muscle fibers for a specific movement, whether task requirements are for low-energy demanding but prolonged activity, or short-duration but high-energy activity, becomes greatly simplified. The size principle provides a simple mechanistic solution to the problem of recruitment order. At low levels of activation within a motor unit pool, slow-twitch type I fibers are initially innervated; but as the level of activation increases over the entire collection of motor units within a muscle, fast-twitch fibers are progressively recruited in an orderly gradient of fiber type. This arrangement greatly simplifies the command structures needed within the CNS to exactly control levels of muscular contraction required for specific movement demands. Moreover, the size principle also confers a "computational benefit" (Rosenbaum, 1991). Because hundreds or even thousands of motor units may be recruited in the activation of a muscle group, the recruitment order of these motor units can become very large (larger, it can be mathematically demonstrated, than the number of neurons in the brain's motor system). A sequential recruitment order based on size greatly simplifies and reduces the computational demands

---

BOX **3.9**   **Muscle Type and Athletic Performance**

Muscle fiber type is one factor that influences the sports and motor skills for which people possess a natural tendency to excel. Although most people have a body percentage of approximately 50 percent for both fast- and slow-twitch fibers, studies have revealed that Olympic athletes are strongly disposed to possessing an overabundance of the fiber type matching the characteristics of their particular competitive skill. For example, Olympic sprinters have been shown to possess at least 80 percent fast-twitch fibers, whereas Olympic marathoners possess 80 percent or greater slow-twitch fibers.

on the CNS, providing one solution to the degrees of freedom problem discussed in Chapter 2.

Rate Modulation

A second method of controlling muscle force is rate modulation. Muscular force depends not only on the number and type of motor units recruited, but also on the rate at which they discharge their action potentials (Shea, Shebilske, and Worchel, 1993). Generally, large increases in muscular force are generated by recruiting more motor units, whereas varying the rate at which muscle fibers are contracted is the preferred mechanism of providing for smaller increases in force.

The force produced within a muscle increases as the discharge rate of action potentials at the neuromuscular junction increases. As previously stated, the activation of a muscle fiber results in a twitch, a contraction of the fiber for a brief time, as the term implies. How long the twitch lasts depends on the type of fiber and the load imposed upon it. If a muscle fiber is innervated again before the previous twitch is completed, it twitches once more. The strength of contraction is a function of how far a twitch response has proceeded by the time a second signal arrives. The effect of the second contraction is added to that of the first, producing greater tension in the fiber than a single twitch, a phenomenon called **temporal summation**. With additional signals, the strength of the contraction increases even further. If several twitches are summed in this fashion, the muscle fiber reaches a point of producing a maximal contraction, a condition called **tetany**, upon the summation of several twitches. Temporal summation is possible because the duration of an action potential (1 to 2 msec) is much shorter than the duration of a typical muscle twitch (about 100 msec). The modulation of motor unit activation rates, along with the recruitment of motor units based on specific fiber and size characteristics, makes possible the gradation of muscular forces necessary for the many movement skills in which humans engage.

temporal summation: The summation of several postsynaptic action potentials on the contraction of an extrafusal muscle fiber because of the rapid successive firing of a single presynaptic alpha motor neuron.

tetany: The maximal contractile force that can be produced by a muscle and that results from rapid frequency of stimulation from presynaptic motor neurons.

SUMMARY

- The neurological bases for human movement include contributions of an extensive system of sensory receptors; processes within the brain, including the motor control system; and a vast network of nerve cells connecting the many aspects of the central nervous system with the muscular system.
  - The control and learning of motor skills depends, fundamentally, on the communication of information at the cellular level.
  - Neurons convey information to and from the central nervous system.
  - Communication between neurons occurs through the process of synaptic transmission.
- Perception of the body's movements, location, and muscular states (i.e., kinesthesis) is supplied by the somatosensory system.

- Muscles spindles, Golgi tendon organs, and joint receptors monitor body movement, joint angles, and contractile forces within muscles.
- The vestibular apparatus monitors general body position, orientation with respect to gravity, and changes in movement.
- The visual system supplies perception of the environment external to the body. Humans have two separate visual systems, the focal and ambient visual systems.
- Relative to motor control and learning, the human brain is responsible for detecting and interpreting sensory information, planning appropriate movements, executing movement commands, correcting movement errors, and learning movement skills.
  - The brain stem regulates vital functions including respiration, blood pressure, and heart rate; controls general alertness; and routes sensory signals from the body to appropriate higher levels of processing.
  - The cerebellum contains feedback loops responsible for coordinating and correcting movement skills and plays a critical role in maintaining muscular tone.
  - Structures in the midbrain relay sensory information from higher brain centers to appropriate effectors, coordinate slow movements, and are involved in the consolidation of memories for movement skills.
  - The cerebral cortex is concerned with sensory perception, decision making, organizing motor commands, and the memory of motor skills.
- The brain's control of muscles is conveyed through motor units.
  - The precise control of muscular activity is accomplished through the recruitment order and rate modulation of motor units.

LEARNING EXERCISES

1. For this exercise, select a moderately complex motor skill that involves whole body movement (i.e., sports, recreational, or everyday skill). Analyze the perpetual needs involved in the skill and then prepare a written report detailing the specific contributions of each of the following proprioceptors to the performance of the skill: muscle spindles, Golgi tendon organs, joint receptors, vestibular apparatus, and cutaneous receptors.

2. For this exercise, you are to observe an athlete, dancer, or performance artist (e.g., acrobat, circus performer, rodeo performer, etc.) performing for approximately 15 minutes under conditions in which you are able to closely monitor the person's actions and record notes (television is acceptable if these conditions can be met). The skill observed should be fairly complex and involve at least some sustained activity. Based upon your observations and analysis, your task is to prepare a written report comparing the contributions of the focal and ambient visual systems to the performance of the skill you observed. Your report should include a description of the activity you observed (including a description of the performer, location, and date of the observation), your method of collecting data (what you watched for and how you took notes), and the comparative analysis

of the two visual systems. Complete your report with a comparative analysis of the importance and role of both visual systems in performing the skill you observed.

3. In completing this exercise, you will interview an individual having a neurological deficit limiting their movement capabilities. This could include individuals who have sustained a traumatic brain injury, suffer from some form of tremors, or who have Parkinson's or Huntington's disease. During your interview, inquire about the limitations in movement control that the person experiences (you might also observe these, at least in part, during your interview). Describe these as part of your written report for this exercise. After the

interview, analyze, based upon your study of this chapter, the brain areas (or major structures) responsible for the movement limitations you reported for the subject that you interviewed. Complete your written report with your analysis.

4. Think of a situation in which you sometimes become anxious, worried, or overly excited and do not perform well (you may describe either a motor or a cognitive skill). Describe how you feel in this situation and how it affects your performance. Describe the role that your reticular activating system most likely plays in this situation, how it influences your performance, and what you might do to better moderate the activity of your RAS and perform better in the future.

FOR FURTHER STUDY

HOW MUCH DO YOU KNOW?

For each of the following, select the letter that best answers the question.

1. Sensory neurons send their signals to the CNS over _____ pathways.
   a. efferent
   b. ascending
   c. sensory
   d. descending
2. The clasp-knife reflex is initiated by which sensory receptor?
   a. Muscle spindle
   b. Joint receptor
   c. Golgi tendon organ
   d. Vestibular apparatus
3. The utricle and saccule are components of which sensory receptor?
   a. Muscle spindle
   b. Joint receptor
   c. Golgi tendon organ
   d. Vestibular apparatus
4. Which of the following brain structures has as one of its primary functions the maintenance of alertness?
   a. Thalamus
   b. Cerebellum

   c. Reticular formation
   d. Hippocampus
5. In which lobe of the brain is the motor cortex located?
   a. Frontal
   b. Temporal
   c. Occipital
   d. Parietal
6. When a motor unit discharges, all of its associated muscle fibers contract maximally, a condition specified by the
   a. summation of forces principle.
   b. rate modulation principle.
   c. law of fiber size recruitment.
   d. all-or-none law.

Answer the following with the word or words which best complete each sentence.

7. The cell structure that receives synaptic transmissions from other cells is the _____.
8. The visual receptors responsible for color vision are _____.

9. A(n) _____ is the property of a thing or of the environment which provides a person with an opportunity for action.
10. Two brain structures that work closely together in coordinating voluntary movements, one exciting muscular contractions and the other inhibiting contractions, are the _____.
11. Where are impulses from sensory receptors brought to perception?
12. The highest contraction speed and greatest force production occur in which type of muscle fiber?

Answers are provided at the end of this review section.

STUDY QUESTIONS

1. Why is the study of the neurological bases of motor control important for those involved in instructing motor skills?
2. What is the function of neurons and what are their components? What are the three primary types of neurons?
3. Describe the processes involved in synaptic transmission.
4. What is somatosensory perception? What is the primary function of each of the four somatosensory receptors (i.e., muscle spindles, Golgi tendon organ, joint receptors, and vestibular apparatus)?
5. How does the gamma loop explain the maintenance of standing posture?
6. What is kinesthesis and why is it essential to the performance of motor skills?
7. Explain the structural and functional differences between focal vision and ambient vision.
8. How does ambient vision play an essential role in movement control and balance?
9. What are affordances and how do they expand the concept of perception?
10. What is the reticular activating system and how does it influence the performance of motor skills?
11. What are the functions of the hippocampus, hypothalamus, and thalamus?
12. How do the cerebellum and the basal ganglia cooperate in promoting the smooth, coordinated movements required in performing most motor skills?
13. What are the main functions of the brain associated with the cerebral cortex?
14. How do the sensory and motor homunculi explain differences in the sensitivity and movement precision found in different parts of the body?
15. Where does the planning of motor skills occur in the brain?
16. What are the different types of skeletal muscle fibers found in the human body, and how do they differ in their functional characteristics?
17. Describe the motor unit and the All-or-None Law.
18. How do motor unit recruitment order and rate modulation contribute to the effective performance of motor skills?

ADDITIONAL READING

Aamodt, S, and Wang, S. (2008). *Welcome to your brain: Why you lose your keys but never forget how to drive and other puzzles of everyday life.* London: Bloomsbury Publishers.

Hubel, DH. (1995). *Eye, brain, and vision* (Scientific American library No. 22). New York: W. H. Freeman.

Klawans, HL. (1996). *Why Michael couldn't hit: And other tales of the neurology of sports.* New York: W. H. Freeman.

Kluka, DA, and Knudson, D. (1997). "The impact of vision training on sports performance." *Journal of Health, Physical Education, Recreation and Dance*, 68(4), 17–24.

Laskowski, ER, Newcomer-Aney, K, and Smith, J. (1997). "Refining rehabilitation with proprioception training: Expediting return to play." *The Physician and Sportsmedicine*, 25(10), 89–102.

Meeusen, R. (2006). "Physical activity and neurotransmitter release." In EO Acevedo and E Panteleimon (eds.), *Psychobiology of physical activity*. Champaign, IL: Human Kinetics.

Park, S, and Toole, T (1999). Functional roles of the proprioceptive system in the control of goal-directed movement. Perceptual and Motor Skills, 88(2), 631-47.

Ratey, JJ. (2002). *A user's guide to the brain: Perception, attention, and the four theaters of the brain.* New York: Vintage Books.

Thach, WT. (1998). "A role for the cerebellum in learning movement coordination." *Neurobiology of learning and memory*, 70, 177–188.

REFERENCES

Aamodt, S, and Wang, S. (2008). *Welcome to your brain: Why you lose your keys but never forget how to drive and other puzzles of everyday life.* London: Bloomsbury Publishers.

Berthoz, A. (trans. by G. Weiss) (2000). *The brain's sense of movement.* Cambridge, MA: Harvard University Press.

Burke, D. (1985). "Muscle spindle function during movement." In EV Evarts, SP Wise, and D Bousfield (eds.), *The motor system in neurobiology* (pp. 168–172). Amsterdam: Elsevier.

Colavita, FB. (2006). *Sensation, perception, and the aging process.* Chantilly, VA: The Teaching Company.

Gardiner, PF. (2001). *Neuromuscular aspects of physical activity.* Champaign, IL: Human Kinetics.

Hoffman, J. (2002). *Physiological aspects of sport training and performance.* Champaign, IL: Human Kinetics.

Kandel, ER. (2006). *In search of memory: The emergence of a new science of mind.* New York: W. W. Norton & Company.

Keltner, NL. (1996). "The basal ganglia and movement disorders." *Perspectives in Psychiatric Care*, 32, 30–32.

Kluka, DA. (1999). *Motor behavior: From learning to performance.* Belmont, CA: Wadsworth.

Latash, ML. (1998). *Neurophysiological basis of movement.* Champaign, IL: Human Kinetics.

Leonard, CT. (1997). *The neuroscience of human movement.* St. Louis, MO: Mosby-Year Book.

Meeusen, R. (2006). "Physical activity and neurotransmitter release." In Acevedo, EO, and E Panteleimon (eds.), *Psychobiology of physical activity*, Champaign, IL: Human Kinetics.

Nakamagoe, K, Iwamoto, Y, and Yoshida, K. (2000). "Evidence for brain stem structures participating in oculomotor integration." *Science, 288*, 857.

Palmer, SE. (1999). *Vision science: Photons to phenomenology.* Boston: MIT Press.

Piacentini, MF, Meeusen, R, Buyse, L, De Schutter, G, and De Meirier, K. (2004). "Hormonal responses during prolonged exercise are influenced by a selective DA/NA reuptake inhibitor." *British Journal of Medicine*, 38, 129–133.

Ratey, JJ. (2002). *A user's guide to the brain: Perception, attention, and the four theaters of the brain.* New York: Vintage Books.

Reggiani, C, and Bortolotto, S. (2006). "Cellular and molecular basis of heterogeneity to contractile performance of human muscle." In K Davids, S Bennett, and K Newell (eds.), *Movement system variability*, Champaign, IL: Human Kinetics.

Restak, RM. (1979). *The brain: The last frontier.* New York: Warner Books.

Restak, RM. (1984). *The brain.* New York: Bantam Books.

Restak, RM. (2001). *Mozart's brain and the fighter pilot: Unleashing your brain's potential.* New York: Random House.

Rosenbaum, DA. (1991). *Human motor control.* San Diego, CA: Academic Press.

Schmidt, RA, and Lee, TD. (2005). *Motor control and learning: A behavioral emphasis*, 4th ed.. Champaign, IL: Human Kinetics.

Shea, CH, Shebilske, WL, and Worchel, S. (1993). *Motor learning and control*. Englewood Cliffs, NJ: Prentice-Hall.

Sherwood, L. (2006). *Human physiology: From cells to systems*, 6th ed. Belmont, CA: Brooks/Cole.

Sousa, DA. (2001). *How the brain learns: A classroom teacher's guide*, 2nd ed. Thousand Oaks, CA: Corwin Press.

Stelmach, GE, and Phillips, JG. (1991). "Movement disorders—limb movement and the basal ganglia." *Physical Therapy*, 71, 60–67.

Sylwester, R. (1995). *A celebration of neurons: An educator's guide to the human brain*. Alexandria, VA: Association for Supervision and Curriculum Development.

Thach, WT. (1998). "A role for the cerebellum in learning movement coordination." *Neurobiology of Learning and Memory*, 70, 177–188.

Vaina, LM, Beardslay, SA, and Rushton, SK. (2004). *Optic flow and beyond*. Boston: Kluwer.

Answers to How Much Do You Know questions: (1) B, (2) C, (3) D, (4) C, (5) A, (6) D, (7) dendrite, (8) cone, (9) affordance, (10) cerebellum and basal ganglia, (11) somatosensory cortex, (12) Type IIb.

CHAPTER 4

Theoretical Perspectives

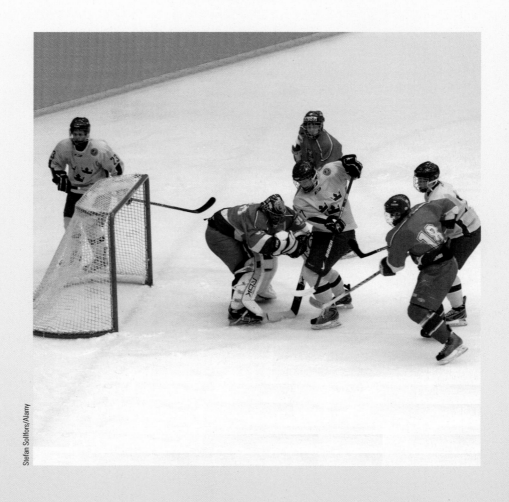

Stefan Sollfors/Alamy

If the facts don't fit the theory, change the facts.
Albert Einstein (1879–1955)

KEY QUESTIONS

- What is a scientific theory, and why are theories important in the study of motor skills?

- What two theoretical approaches underlie the contemporary study of motor skills?

- What are closed control approaches to theory building? What are the major theories comprising this approach in the study of motor skills?

- What are open control approaches to theory building? What are the major theories comprising this approach in the study of motor skills?

- What are the relative strengths and weaknesses of each of the major theories underlying the study of motor skills?

- How can differing theories be useful in explaining motor skill behavior, even when they are based on seemingly contradictory theoretical assumptions?

CHAPTER OVERVIEW

Most people have experienced the modern painting technique called *op art*. Comprised of dots, lines, and other shapes of various colors and sizes, these paintings appear a confused jumble of abstract images when initially viewed. Each individual painting element is clearly discernable, but how it relates to other elements of the painting remains unclear.

If you study such a painting long enough, however, focusing your vision in different ways, a single image eventually springs into focus. What at first seemed a collection of unrelated elements suddenly becomes a clear picture—a flower, a face, a flag, a map of the United States. It can then be seen that all of the individual elements are really part of a single image, but one had to assume the correct perspective, to look in just the right way, before this became obvious.

Theories are like ways of looking at op art. They can provide a perspective that brings a collection of individual facts into a single coherent framework. As in op art, a theory provides the perspective that connects individual elements into a unified picture. A theory, in the case of human movement, allows us to see how the many individual elements comprising motor skills are connected. It refocuses our intellectual perspective—rather than a crazy quilt patched together from many isolated facts, a single blended fabric of unified meanings is discernable. As you study the individual elements of motor skills, a solid grasp of theory will place them in a broader and more meaningful perspective.

———————

Human motor skills are amazingly complex. The body contains over 600 muscles and more than 200 bones, forming an intricate system of levers and pulleys capable of producing the extensive variety of movements underlying human motor skills. This mechanical arrangement of bone and muscle is further connected through the networking of a vast array of nerves, making possible the infinite patterning of actions seen in human movement.

Although the degrees of freedom available in the human motor system make possible the great flexibility inherent in motor skills, they also inform a significant intellectual problem for those attempting to understand the acquisition and control of such skills. How is this intricate system of interconnected bones, muscles, and nerves coordinated so that the movements underlying skilled actions are controlled? How can the contributions of millions of individual nerve and muscle cells be harnessed to act in unison toward the accomplishment of specific skills? How do humans adapt and learn to control their movements in new ways? To begin answering such questions, researchers embed their thinking within scientific theories capable of connecting the many facets concerning motor skills revealed through research. A theory provides perspective, allowing us to see how individual facts are connected to form a single, meaningful picture of human movement.

SCIENTIFIC THEORIES

theory: A coherent statement or set of statements relating a large number of observations into a logical and testable framework; a theory must be open to empirical verification and prediction of future observations within its conceptual area of phenomena.

A scientific **theory** is a statement or set of statements that relates observations about a specific phenomenon of interest in a coherent, logical, and testable way. A good theory does two things (see Hawking and Mlodinow, 2005). First, it accounts for a significantly large class of observations on the basis of only a few simple, though powerful, propositions. Second, it makes definite predictions about the results of future observations—it is testable.

For example, Einstein's theory of special relativity is based upon two simple propositions: that the speed of light is the same for any observer regardless of his or her relative speed, and that the laws of physics as described by Newton will always be the same for observers in the same inertial (i.e., non-accelerating) frame of reference. Given these two simple statements, Einstein's theory has successfully predicted the expansion and structure of the universe, the properties of subatomic particles, the principles of nuclear power, and provided the necessary guidelines for sending space vehicles to other planets in our solar system.

The results of over a century of scientific experimentation concerning motor skills have led scientists to develop theories designed to explain the many and often seemingly contradictory observations concerning how movements are acquired and controlled. Today, two major theoretical approaches dominate thinking and scientific inquiry (Summers, 2004). The oldest of these focuses upon the workings of the central nervous system and is what scientists refer to as a **closed control system.** Closed systems are those in which control is explained entirely by processes inherent within the control system itself and which are capable of meeting system goals in isolation from the surrounding environment. We will refer to this approach to the study of motor behavior as a cognitive-based perspective, for reasons we will see shortly.

closed control system:
A system in which the mechanisms of control are internal and closed to influences outside of the system itself.

The second approach taken in explaining human motor learning and control focuses not on the central nervous system, nor on any bodily system exclusively, but rather on the interaction of various bodily systems with the surrounding environment, taking environment in the broadest sense to include both its physical and cultural aspects. Such control systems are referred to as **open control systems,** because the system under consideration, in this case the human body and its various subsystems, interacts with—is open to—the surrounding environment. In this theoretical approach, the body and its various systems, including the central nervous system, hold no privileged position in controlling bodily actions, with the larger environment playing just as important of a role in the emergence of motor skills. We will refer to this approach, which is the more recent of the two, as the *dynamical systems perspective* (this choice of terminology will be explained later in the chapter).

open control system:
A system that interacts with the environment outside of itself and responds to external influences in its mechanisms of control.

BOX 4.1   **Is a Theory, "Just a Theory"?**

You often hear people say that something is "just a theory," by which they mean it is a supposition that might or might not be true (and, in fact, the implication is usually that it cannot be trusted and should not be considered true). In science, however, a theory is an explanation for which there is considerable support and which is therefore generally considered to be true.

In science, a sort of hierarchy of claims to validity exists (scientists never claim to have arrived at absolute truth). This hierarchy is expressed by the terms *hypothesis*, *theory*, and *law*. A closer look at each of these important terms follows.

Hypothesis

A hypothesis is an educated guess based upon previous observations. It usually describes how one thing is guessed to have an effect on another thing, which is then tested experimentally. A hypothesis can be proven false, but never proven to be true—it is accepted, however, until it may be disproved in future experiments.

Theory

A theory summarizes a significant group of hypotheses that have supported the same conclusions about something through repeated testing. One way to consider a theory is to define it as the acceptance of a large number of hypotheses. A theory is considered to be valid as long as there is no evidence to dispute it (this can be a point of major contention between scientists of competing views).

Law

A law generalizes a large body of scientific observations, usually of many experiments over a substantial period of time, that have tested something in a broad diversity of ways. At the time it is postulated, no exceptions have been found to the law. Scientific laws explain things rather than describing them as do theories. One way to distinguish a law from a theory is that if it answers the question of why something is as it is, then it is a law.

Can More Than One Theory Be Correct?

To the movement science student, it may seem that because the two dominant theoretical perspectives concerning motor control and learning differ so drastically, one being a closed system and the other an open system, one approach must be incorrect and, presumably, the other correct. Such an assumption would be unwarranted, though. Both cognitive-based and dynamical systems perspectives meet the criteria of being good scientific theories. That is, both explain in fairly parsimonious yet elegant terms a large and diverse set of observations concerning human movement. Both also have proved successful in predicting new observations, thereby expanding our understanding of the factors responsible for human movement control and learning.

How can we make sense of this seeming enigma? Remember that a theory explains a large and significant number of observations but that it does not explain all of them. Human movement is extremely complex, and fully explaining it is not only beyond our present state of knowledge, but probably our knowledge in the foreseeable future as well. This does not mean that we should give up in our quest to understand the workings of the motor system, however. The very fact that we have competing theories—that a new theory has evolved to challenge existing assumptions—is a strong sign that we are indeed advancing in our quest for knowledge and understanding. It is reasonable to assume that both theoretical perspectives offer much toward advancing our knowledge, though each in its own way. That is, each theory has both strengths and weaknesses, and together each might provide perspectives that neither can alone. Of even greater significance is the potential that taken together, each perspective might help point the way for future researchers to develop a more powerful and explanatory theory encompassing the insights of both present perspectives. Just what potential for a workable synthesis of the two theories there may be, however, for the present remains a contested area of debate. We should take assurance in the belief, though, that each perspective provides unique insights into human motor control, as well as specific guidelines for the effective instruction of motor skills (see Box 4.2).

BOX 4.2 It All Started with Descartes

The seventeenth-century French philosopher Rene Descartes (1596–1650) set the stage for how scientists conceive of human nature when he argued that the mind and body are two entirely different kinds of things, with the body being purely physical and the mind purely mental and nonphysical. Descartes further argued that the mind was superior and therefore controlled the body. His position, called dualism, has influenced how we think—both scientists and nonscientists alike—not just about human nature but also about human movement ever since. His ideas also raised a great scientific and philosophical debate that has continued to this day:

How can something nonphysical, mind, control something physical, body? The two theories presented in this chapter are really a continuation of this debate. Cognitive-based theories assume that mind (or cognitive processes, as we are more apt to conceive of mind today) controls bodily actions. Dynamical systems theory, on the other hand, is an attempt to put mind and body back together as really representing different aspects of a single reality—the individual human person. As we consider these two theories of motor control and learning, we are also taking part in one of the greatest scientific debates of the past three-and-a-half centuries.

COGNITIVE-BASED THEORIES

The oldest and probably most intuitive approach to understanding how movement skills are acquired and controlled is to consider them as products of mental activity, or in more psychological terms as products of cognitive processes. What kinds of cognitive processes underlie motor skills? Scientists working in fields as diverse as cognitive psychology, neural physiology, artificial intelligence, computer science, education, and kinesiology have been studying this question intensely for many years. Across these various disciplines, the term **motor program** has come to indicate the cognitive structures responsible for skilled movements.

motor program:
A procedural memory comprised of the rules commanding muscular activity for producing specific skills.

Central to the concept of the motor program is that because skills can be learned and retained, they must somehow be represented within memory. The motor program, most broadly viewed, (1) is a structure that is centrally located (i.e., in the central nervous system); (2) consists of a hierarchical arrangement of elements (i.e., the brain, and specifically higher centers in the brain such as those involving memory, commands lower levels of action, ultimately muscle); and (3) is sufficient to explain the learning and control of movement skills (i.e., it is a closed control system—no further explanation is needed). Given these assumptions, motor programs represent a top-down system of control. Higher elements in the control system (higher cortical areas of the brain) control lower elements (lower brain regions, brain stem, spinal cord, motor units, muscle). Think of the hierarchical arrangement of a factory. A boss decides what is to be made, how much, and on what schedule. The boss's orders are then issued to senior managers, who instruct lower-level managers, who then command the workers who actually implement the boss's original decisions. In analogous fashion, movement plans are drawn up within higher cortical centers of the brain, and motor programs prepared commanding descending levels of control, ultimately resulting in muscles, the "workers" in our analogy, carrying out the brain's commands.

The idea of a motor program, taking a good deal of license with the concept, is so immediately intuitive that it goes back at least 25 centuries, to the time of the ancient Greeks and the philosopher Plato. Plato believed that before a movement could be performed, a person first had to form an idea, a mental picture, of the movement. This idea could then be actualized in the real world. Plato went further, though, in his belief that there existed an ideal form for every skill—that is, a perfect image of every skill existing in an otherworldly and perfect realm of ideas. Humankind being imperfect, any person's mental picture of a movement skill was also imperfect, always only a shadowy likeness of the perfect or ideal skill. Plato believed that as a person practiced, though, his or her picture of the skill gradually came closer and closer to the ideal skill, although never fully reaching it.

Plato's notion of mental images controlling movement skills, a distant approximation of the idea of motor programs, was barely advanced over the centuries until the development of psychology in the latter third of the nineteenth century. Early leaders in the field of psychology, such as William James in America and Wilhelm Wundt in Germany, began theorizing about the kinds of cognitive structures responsible for human action (James, 1890, alluded to Plato as prompting his thinking in this regard). As the study of motor skills advanced during the early decades of psychology, the concept of the motor program became the primary theoretical framework against which research findings concerning practice and other instructional variables were ultimately explained. The actual term *motor program* was first used in the psychological literature in 1917 (Lashley).

The Information Processing Model

An important advancement in modern concepts of motor programs occurred in 1948, when Craik, an English psychologist, first proposed that the brain be considered as a type of computer in which information is received, processed, and an output generated (Craik, 1948). This idea soon led to the development of the **information processing model,** which since then has continued to influence all cognitive-based theories of motor control and learning. The information processing model provides a framework describing the various cognitive processes associated with the workings of motor programs. It describes three distinct stages of cognitive processes underlying the events responsible for the production of motor skills. These are the perceptual stage, the decision-making stage, and the programming stage (see Figure 4.1).

Perceptual Stage

In the first stage of the information processing model, called the **perceptual stage,** sensory information from the environment is received and processed. Higher brain centers are constantly bombarded with neural transmissions from thousands of sensory receptors located throughout the body, including visual, auditory, proprioceptive, and cutaneous receptors (see Chapter 3). Taken together, this combined sensory input forms a continuously shifting pattern of signals concerning events in both the external physical and internal bodily environments. So much sensory information is continuously transmitted to the brain about conditions within body and environment that humans lack sufficient processing capabilities to act on all of it. Thus the function of the perceptual stage is to select from among the many sources of informational input the most critical and important information and to bring this to the individual's awareness so that it can be acted upon.

information processing model: A model of cognitive processes occurring in the central nervous system underlying the production of motor skills; three stages are identified, including the perceptual, decision-making, and programming stages.

perceptual stage: The first stage of information processing in which sensory information is detected and identified.

BOX **4.3**   **Karl S. Lashley on the *Motor Program***

Karl S. Lashley (1890–1958), a researcher famous for first developing the idea that specific areas of the brain could be identified as centers for motor control (which he called *motor localization*), was also the first to significantly develop and coin the use of the term *motor program*. Writing in 1917, Lashley stated his belief in the existence of motor programs;

"I believe that there exist in the nervous organization, elaborate systems of interrelated neurons capable of imposing certain types of integration upon a large number of widely spaced effectors elements....These systems are in constant action. They form a sort of substratum upon which other activity is built."

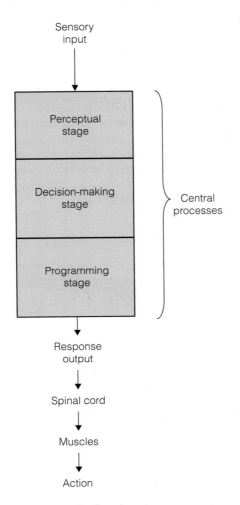

FIGURE **4.1** The Information Processing Model

Source: Created by author.

sensation: Sensory information that reaches the cortex and is capable of being perceived and acted upon.

perception: The process by which sensations arising from within or outside of the body are brought to conscious awareness.

In performing this function, two primary tasks comprise the perceptual stage. The first of these is called **sensation** and involves detecting and selecting for further processing relevant information from the environment. The second task is called **perception**, in which sensations are given meaning, a process involving comparison of sensations to information stored within memory (dynamical theorists, in contrast, view perception as a direct process not relying upon memory). For example, within this stage a person might assemble a series of changing visual features and colors forming the sensation of an object moving toward him or her. Combined with previous memories, these sensations form the perception of a baseball that will cross home plate at a specific location and a specific time. This perceptual information will then be transmitted to the next stage of information processing, where it will form the basis for deciding whether to take a ball or to swing away.

Decision-Making Stage

In the second or **decision-making stage** of information processing, the individual uses information transmitted from the perceptual stage to decide upon a course of action. In this stage, information from the perceptual stage is compared to past information (memory) to determine an appropriate action. Continuing with the example described in the perceptual stage, the individual batter must decide whether to swing at the approaching ball, and if so, when and how. Depending on the number of possible responses stored in memory relative to the characteristics of the approaching pitch, selecting the correct action may be easy or difficult (this difficulty, at least in terms of the time needed to select a correct response, can actually be quantified by a fundamental principle in movement science known as Hick's Law).

Programming Stage

The third stage of information processing involves preparing the appropriate motor program to carry out the action decided upon in the decision-making stage. It is in this **programming stage** that the motor program is prepared for issuance to lower levels to be carried out. Again continuing with our batting example, assuming that the decision has been made to hit away, the individual must prepare and execute the required action. At least five distinct processes can be identified in this programming stage. First, the appropriate motor program must be retrieved from memory. Second, changes in posture necessary before action is initiated must be made (e.g., commands to stabilize the shoulder joint and legs must be made in preparation for the dynamic movement patterns involved in swinging a bat). Third, the order and timing of muscular commands for the upcoming action (i.e., batting) must be prepared. Fourth, the various sensory systems must be oriented appropriately for the upcoming action (i.e., steadying one's visual focus appropriately for batting). Fifth, the action is initiated when appropriate. These processes are carried out in the programming stage and then conveyed to the appropriate effectors.

Closed-Loop Systems of Information Processing

Within the information processing model, two different methods of control have been identified. The original models of information processing borrowed from engineering concepts of servo-mechanisms. A *servo-mechanism* is a closed system in which an error detection device constantly monitors the system for discrepancies between desired and actual conditions and automatically makes adjustments to correct detected errors. A thermostat is an example of a simple servo-mechanism. When the thermostat controlling the heater in your home is set at 72 degrees, for example, it constantly monitors room temperature and makes adjustments by turning the heater on or off as needed to maintain the desired temperature.

In the case of a home heating system, the thermostat uses feedback concerning current room temperature, which is then compared to a desired temperature in order to detect any discrepancies and control the on/off output of the heating system so as to correct temperature errors. In a closed-loop

closed-loop control:
A system of control in which feedback is compared to a reference of correctness during the course of action and errors corrected when necessary.

system of control, feedback plays an essential role. In closed-loop control, corrections are made on the basis of feedback. Adams (1971), a leading proponent of closed-loop theories of motor control, defined a closed system as one having "feedback, error detection, and error correction as key elements." In such a system, he continued, there is "a reference that specifies the desired value for the system, and the output of the system is fed back and compared to the reference for error detection and, if necessary, corrected" (p. 116).

Closed-loop systems are believed to underlie the control of movements that are relatively slow and deliberate. Driving a car, threading a needle, running to catch a fly ball, maintaining one's balance while standing still, and tracking a moving target on a video screen are all examples of closed-loop control. In steering a car, for example, visual feedback concerning the direction in which the car is moving relative to road conditions ahead is transmitted to the brain. There it is interpreted in the perceptual stage of information processing and forwarded to the decision-making stage. If one's car is safely aligned with upcoming road conditions, no corrective actions are taken. If, however, the car's direction of travel is beginning to veer away from the course of the road ahead, a decision concerning movement adjustments is made and forwarded to the programming stage, where new commands are organized and transmitted to shoulder, arm, and wrist muscles to change the steering pattern and correct the car's direction of travel. Once the car is traveling safely down the road again, corrective signals to the musculature controlling steering cease, and the current direction of travel is maintained until a new error is detected, when the corrective process begins again.

Closed-loop control does not depend upon detailed movement instructions. Rather, a more general set of controlling guidelines, coupled with task-specific goals, initiate action, and feedback is then used to adjust muscular commands in compliance with task goals. Thus, closed-loop control is a hierarchical system with one important distinction. Although control centers responsible for initiating, monitoring, correcting, and commanding lower levels of the musculature entail central processes within the brain, information necessary to these central processes is derived through sensory feedback. Motor programs need not contain complete information necessary for movement production, but only that required to initiate action and guide its ongoing progress, for which the motor program is dependent upon external sources of information.

Advantages and Disadvantages of Closed-Loop Control

Closed-loop control has both advantages and disadvantages as a system for explaining motor control. Three specific advantages and two disadvantages are frequently cited in the literature (see, for example, Shea, Shebilske, and Worchel, 1993). The first advantage is that closed-loop control is especially appropriate when performing unpracticed skills. Learning new skills often proceeds on a trial-and-error basis, accompanied by many errors, so that continuous correction of ongoing movement is required. Second, closed-loop control has the obvious advantage of allowing movements to be corrected once they have begun, rather than having movement errors continue until action is completed (open-loop control systems, which we will next describe, are not capable of correction during movement execution). Third, closed-loop control, because of its constant error detection and correction processes, can result in precise and accurate movements. Motor skills such as threading a needle, cutting a diamond, or docking a space shuttle require the precision of movement made possible only by constant attendance to feedback and corrective processes.

There are also two major disadvantages to closed-loop control systems. First, they are attention demanding. Because of the requirement to monitor feedback and generate new movement commands in response, individuals must use much of their conscious and attentional resources in maintaining the quality of their movements. Because these resources are limited, they may therefore become unavailable for other important tasks, such as those required by athletes who must execute skills while also attending to the movements of their opponents and determining correct response strategies. Second, and the greatest disadvantage of closed-loop control, is the time required to prepare and execute successive corrections to an ongoing action. Most humans are incapable of generating corrective responses to perceived action errors in less than 200 ms, and the execution of complex corrective responses may take 400 to 500 ms. For dynamic or reactive skills that must be completed quickly (typically in half a second or less), there is simply too little time to allow for the preparation of corrective actions.

From our discussion here, it should appear clear that closed-loop control is a good candidate for the control of continuous and fine motor skills. Skills of a relatively long duration or that require high degrees of movement precision are well suited to closed-loop control processes. On the other hand, skills that are executed and completed relatively quickly, such as many discrete and ballistic skills, are poor candidates for a closed-loop system of control. This latter difficulty led to the conceptualization of open-loop theories of motor control.

Open-Loop Systems of Information Processing

open-loop control: A system of control in which movement commands are prestructured and executed without corrective intervention from feedback.

Theories of open-loop control represent the most faithful adherence to notions of the motor program and have, in one form or another, been advanced for many years. Their greatest development, though, began in the 1970s in response to perceived weaknesses of closed-loop control explanations. In an open-loop system of control, there is no mechanism for monitoring sensory feedback and correcting ongoing movements, as in a closed-loop system. Rather, perceptual sensing mechanisms detect information in the environment and act to determine whether a response is required. Assuming perceptual processes indicate the need for a response, an appropriate motor program is selected and executed. In an open-loop system, the motor program is held to contain all of the information needed for forming and executing an appropriate response without the further input of sensory feedback to initiate corrective commands. Commands initiated by the motor program are, presumably, sufficient to respond appropriately to the environment. Rather than using sensory information as feedback during the performance of a skill, open-loop systems use environmental information in order to prepare the motor system (i.e., the motor program) for action. Sensory information used in this fashion is called **feedforward**. In open-loop control systems, motor programs are viewed as being prestructured, their

feedforward: Sensory information related to the production of an action prior to the initiation of the action.

movement commands completely (or nearly completely) set prior to the initiation of movement.

Computer programs offer a good analogy of open-loop systems. Once a specific computer program is commanded to run by an appropriate mouse click, it will be retrieved and executed exactly as programmed without correction. Like computer programs, motor programs are believed to entail all of the commands necessary for completing the desired action.

Open-loop control appears to underlie many skills that individuals perform everyday. Skills that are performed quickly (with insufficient time available for attending to feedback) and automatically (with little or no conscious attention paid to them) are excellent candidates for open-loop control. Discrete skills executed quickly, usually in less than half a second, are believed controlled through open-loop processes. The key to understanding the control and performance of such skills is that their motor programs contain a complete set of instructions for their execution. If the environment in which a skill is performed is accurately perceived and an appropriate motor program is available within memory, then once that program is selected and executed, the resultant action should be effective in meeting environmental goals without the necessity of intervening corrective processes.

Advantages and Disadvantages of Open-Loop Control

As with closed-loop control systems, open-loop systems have both advantages and disadvantages. With open-loop systems, two major advantages and two major disadvantages are typically reported (e.g., Shea, Shebilske, and Worchel, 1993). The first advantage is probably obvious and readily apparent. Open-loop

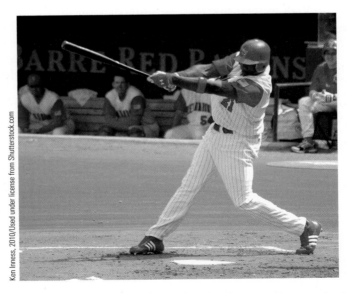

Ken Inness, 2010/Used under license from Shutterstock.com

According to information processing theories, open-loop mechanisms of control underline the execution of rapidly performed skills.

control is capable of producing quick movements because the commands for action are prestructured and, once initiated, carried out without the need for further major modification. Second, because movement commands are prestructured, attentional resources can be directed toward other tasks rather than being diverted to the conscious control of ongoing movement.

The disadvantages of open-loop control are also somewhat obvious. First, because open-loop control critically depends on the availability of an appropriate motor program, it is not effective for skills which are unpracticed or not well learned. The motor programs for such skills would be either insufficiently developed or absent altogether. It should be remembered that motor programs are a type of memory, and until such memories are sufficiently developed through repetition and practice, sufficient motor commands for effective skill production are unavailable. Second, because motor programs anticipate particular environmental conditions, open-loop control is not effective in changing environments.

From the foregoing discussion, we can conclude that discrete skills performed in closed environments are particularly good candidates for open-loop control, whereas continuous and open skills would not be well performed using this mode of control. A comparison of the advantages and disadvantages of closed-loop and open-loop control is shown in Table 4.1.

The Open-/Closed-Loop Control Continuum

By the mid-1970s, two major information processing theories of motor control and learning had gained wide acceptance and dominated the theoretical landscape of movement science. These were a closed-loop theory proposed by Jack Adams at the University of Illinois, and an open-loop theory proposed by Richard Schmidt at the University of Southern California. A major difference in these two theories was the role accorded sensory feedback in the production of motor skills. Adams' closed-loop theory provided a central role for feedback, whereas in Schmidt's theory feedback had little role in the completion of an action once initiated (though feedback played an important role in learning).

TABLE **4.1**

Comparison of the Strengths and Weaknesses of Closed-Loop and Open-Loop Control Mechanisms

Closed-Loop Control	Open-Loop Control
Advantages 1. Good for unpracticed skills 2. Ongoing corrections during performance possible 3. Allows for a high degree of movement precision	*Advantages* 1. Good for reactive, quickly executed skills 2. Not attention demanding
Disadvantages 1. Attention demanding 2. Requires greater planning and execution time	*Disadvantages* 1. Not effective for unpracticed skills 2. Not effective in unpredictable, changing environments

Throughout the 1970s, researchers debated the merits of both approaches. Those favoring closed-loop models tended to conduct research investigations utilizing relative slow, self-paced skills such as tracking tasks to demonstrate the explanatory efficacy of closed-loop models. Supporters of open-loop systems, on the other hand, typically designed their investigations around rapid, discrete tasks, which generally favored open-loop explanations of control. By the 1980s, most researchers had come to view both approaches as having merit, but differing on the relative contributions which feedback made to each mode of control. This led to the conclusion that open- and closed-loop control systems could be viewed as forming a continuum based upon the utilization of sensory feedback. These two types of control can be viewed as describing different ways in which the central and peripheral nervous systems initiate and control actions, with the nature of the task determining which mode of control has priority. Both control systems provide useful models for understanding the various processes responsible for the control and learning of motor skills. It can be presumed that based upon the nature of the task, the central nervous system selects the appropriate mode of control when commanding motor skills. An illustration of these two systems of control as related to the information processing model is presented in Figure 4.2.

An Example of the Open-/Closed-Loop Continuum—Fitts' Law

An example of the symbiotic cooperation between closed-loop and open-loop control processes is observed when considering how individuals balance between speed and accuracy when performing rapid tasks. In many motor skills, there is a trade-off between how quickly the skill can be performed on the one hand, or how accurately performed on the other. Pitching a fastball, a parry in fencing, and speed typing all require speed as well as accuracy to achieve successful performance, but if executed too rapidly, performance will suffer as the number of errors increases. In many skill performance situations an excessive emphasis on speed will result in an increased rate of error. The opposite is also true, with movement speed having to be reduced in order to increase accuracy. Thus for many skills, a **speed–accuracy trade-off** exists, where an optimal speed which minimizes errors must be determined in order to achieve performance success.

speed–accuracy trade-off: The observation that in the performance of many skills an increase in the speed with which the skill is performed is accompanied by a decrease in performance accuracy, and vice versa.

| BOX **4.4** | **Can You Classify Skills as Executed through Closed-Loop and Open-Loop Control?** |

For the skills listed below, decide whether closed-loop control, open-loop control, or a combination of both would be required for best meeting task goals (and if a combination, at what point a switch from one control method to the other occurs).

- Returning an opponent's tennis serve
- Typing a letter on a keyboard
- Braking to slow your car when approaching a stop sign

- Braking to avoid hitting a deer that suddenly runs in front of your car
- Brushing your teeth
- Catching a Frisbee
- Making a pool shot
- Striking a match
- Casting a fishing line
- Reaching for a cup of coffee

Open-loop control   **Closed-loop control**

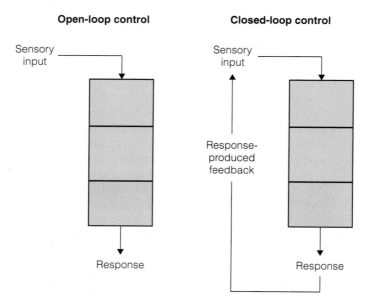

FIGURE **4.2** Open-Loop and Closed-Loop Systems of Control in the Information Processing Model

Source: Created by author.

Fitts' law: Law expressing the mathematical relationship between speed of movement and accuracy for discrete aiming tasks.

The trade-off between speed and accuracy is described by **Fitts' law**, one of the oldest and most important laws of motor control. Fitts' law (Fitts, 1954) quantifies the relationship between speed and spatial accuracy for rapid aiming tasks based upon distance moved and target size (see Box 4.5 for a description of Fitts' law). Although its original application was to continuous aiming tasks, the predictions of Fitts' law have been shown to hold for discrete as well as continuous skills, for individuals of all ages, for skills using different effectors (fingers, hands, arms, legs), and for skills performed underwater as well as on land. The conclusion that a speed–accuracy trade-off exists across a wide spectrum of skilled behaviors, individuals, and environmental contexts is well established and it forms one of the most important general laws of motor control.

For our current purposes, Fitts' law raises an interesting question concerning the roles of open-loop and closed-loop control in the production of rapid discrete tasks, and of the mechanisms underlying the achievement of both speed and accuracy in such tasks. Rapidly performed tasks would seem on first blush to require open-loop control processes, because the motor programs controlling rapidly performed skills can be preprogrammed and do not rely on the need for ongoing feedback. Open-loop processes do not explain, however, the accuracy that can be achieved in rapidly performed tasks, especially those requiring precise movement outcomes. How is a balance between speed and accuracy achieved in fast, discrete tasks?

Attempts to reconcile the implications of Fitts' law with the notions of open and closed-loop control mechanisms eventually led to the conclusion that both control systems play essential roles when both speed and accuracy are important in achieving task goals (an example of the role played by theory in resolving specific motor behavior questions). Working within a cognitive-based theoretical framework, it has been hypothesized that both open-loop and closed-loop control processes are related to the speed–accuracy trade-off. Three phases of control have been proposed. The first phase involves movement preparation. In this phase, an individual evaluates the environmental conditions present, determines that the appropriate action requires a rapid response, selects the appropriate motor program from memory, and programs the needed motor commands. The second phase, called the initial flight phase, is the first movement phase. In this phase, the preprogrammed motor program is initiated through open-loop control. The purpose of this phase is to move the requisite body part toward a target or final location quickly (i.e., a ballistic movement). The third phase, called the termination phase, occurs toward the end of the movement, comprising perhaps as little as five percent, in some cases, of the total distance moved. This phase is under closed-loop control. In this phase, the individual uses feedback (primarily visual) to assess the accuracy of the initial flight phase and makes any needed final corrections necessary for completing the task successfully.

BOX 4.5   Fitts' Law

The relationship between movement speed and outcome accuracy in rapid aiming tasks is described by Fitts' law. In a classic study in the motor control literature, Fitts (1954) had subjects perform a repetitive tapping task by moving a handheld stylus as rapidly as possible between two targets (shown in the accompanying figure). In the experiment, Fitts varied both the width of the targets (W) and the amplitude or distance between the targets (A). Subjects were scored by the number of correct taps (those within the target area) achieved in a prescribed time (usually 20 seconds).

Fitts observed, not surprisingly, that accuracy improved as either the amplitude (A) decreased, or the target width (W) increased. The opposite was also observed; accuracy decreased as amplitude increased, or target width decreased. Based upon these observations, Fitts derived an equation expressing the effects of target width and amplitude on movement accuracy. This equation

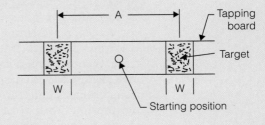

Fitts' Task.

has become known as Fitts' law, and is expressed mathematically as: $MT = a + b [\log_2 (2A/W)]$. In the equation, MT equals movement time, a and b are constants, and A and W are amplitude and target width as already specified. Stated simply, this equation specifies, with mathematical precision, that the average time it takes a person to tap between targets increases as the person must move further, hit a smaller target, or both.

As an example, consider a person ringing a doorbell. As the person approaches the door, he or she assesses the location and configuration of the doorbell relative to his or her body, assesses the accuracy needed for the task and which effectors should be used (i.e., single finger, joined fingers, palm of hand, etc.), readies for the action (i.e., stops at an appropriate distance from the door), and preprograms commands for the second phase of action. The second phase is an open-loop ballistic movement of the arm to get the hand (and finger) close to the doorbell. Finally, in the third phase, he or she shifts to closed-loop control, using feedback that has been monitored as well as ongoing visual feedback, to make final corrections to the spatial or temporal aspects of the moving limb (and finger) as needed to successfully contact and push the doorbell.

By combining both closed and open-loop control, the advantages of both control systems (including both speed and accuracy) can be applied to a wide variety of movement situations. We turn next to a further consideration of these two control mechanisms as viewed by the most prominent theory for each.

Adams' Closed-Loop Theory

The most completely developed closed-loop theory of information processing was proposed by Adams in 1971. Adams held that learning involved the forming and strengthening of neural traces in the brain's cortex. In his conception, a motor program consisting of two separate traces was responsible for the learning and control of all voluntary motor skills. The first of these traces was called the *memory trace*. The role of the memory trace, according to Adams' theory, is to select and initiate the desired action. Once initiated, the primary responsibility for the ongoing control of a movement is assigned to a second cortical trace called the *perceptual trace*. The perceptual trace evaluates the correctness of the action executed by the memory trace. It continually monitors and compares response-produced feedback from ongoing movement with a reference of correctness representing the feedback qualities expected in a correct response. If sensory feedback from the ongoing action does not match the perceptual trace, then new muscular commands are generated to bring sensory feedback into alignment with desired action goals. This process of detection and correction continues until the system is back in balance with its desired state (recall our previous analogy of a thermostat and heater).

In Adams' theory, the perceptual trace is not a single structure, but a complex series of traces produced over many practice experiences. As an individual practices a skill, sensory feedback is evaluated against expected consequences on every practice attempt. Over the course of practice, an individual learns which corrective actions (which perceptual traces) best maintain continuity between the actions initiated by the memory trace and the sensory feedback produced as a result. Eventually, the collective of individual traces becomes more aligned with desired outcomes, the individual performs more consistently, and learning can be said to have occurred.

The theoretical implications of Adams' closed-loop model supported several conclusions concerning the practice of skills, placing especially considerable emphases on the roles of practice repetitions and augmented feedback. Because the memory trace is specific to each skill (and to each way a skill might be executed), it follows that it is best developed through repetitive practice attempts performed as faithfully as possible relative to the target skill. Adams' theory lent considerable support to the **specificity of practice hypothesis**, the notion that skills should be practiced as exactly as possible to the way in which they are intended to be performed. Adams' theory also focused renewed attention on the instructional feedback learners received during practice, because in his theory such feedback played a significant role in guiding a learner's evaluation of outcome errors and therefore development of the perceptual trace.

specificity of practice hypothesis: The notion that the best learning experiences are those that most closely approximate the movement components and environmental conditions of the target skill and target context.

Problems of Novelty and Storage

Although Adams' theory provided an especially influential analysis of the role and uses of feedback in the execution of motor skills, it was not without criticism. In essence, these criticisms were not with the closed-loop assumptions posited by Adams, but with his assumptions about motor programs, which were never fully developed in his theory. Two specific problems, which came to be called the novelty problem and storage problem, came in for particular criticism by those involved in the study of motor skills.

The first of these problems, the **novelty problem**, concerns how a specific motor act is performed for the first time. Because the memory trace is a result of practice, how is an unpracticed skill performed for the first time? Technically, in Adams' theory the memory trace is nonexistent because it has not been developed through previous practice. Similarly, even when a skill is well learned, how could it be performed in a different manner? A second aspect of this problem is that Adams' theory holds that the perceptual trace is strengthened as a function of practice. If the conditions under which a skill is performed are novel, what mechanism is responsible for controlling action once initiated by the memory trace? Both the memory trace and perceptual trace in Adams' theory are specific to exact ways of executing motor skills.

novelty problem: A deficiency of simple motor program theory based on the notion that individuals should be unable to effectively produce unpracticed variations of learned movements because they have not developed specific motor programs for them.

Apart from scholarly criticism, the novelty problem is immediately recognizable in many everyday situations. Watching the athlete who has performed a well-practiced skill one way thousands or even hundreds of thousands of times then execute the same skill flawlessly under completely novel conditions during a sporting contest is an event recognizable to every sports fan. Likewise, after years of driving experience, people may unexpectedly experience new situations or road conditions they have never previously encountered, yet to which they are easily able to adapt their driving behaviors.

You will recall from Chapter 2 that one of the characteristics of motor skills that we said any adequate theory of motor control must be able to explain is the phenomenon of motor equivalence. That is, people are often able to accomplish motor skill goals effectively through unpracticed and completely novel movements when required to do so by changing environmental conditions. In this regard, Adams' theory proved inadequate because it holds that until a skill has been sufficiently practiced in the specific ways it is to be performed, neither the memory nor perceptual trace would have been sufficiently developed to allow for effective equivalent skilled performance.

storage problem: A deficiency of simple motor program theory based on the notion that a vast memory capacity would be needed to store all of the separate programs for controlling the nearly countless movement skills people are able to produce.

The second criticism of Adams' theory was coined the **storage problem**. If specific memory and perceptual traces were recorded for every way in which a particular skill had been practiced, as proposed by Adams, then a large repertoire of separate representations of movements would have to be stored in memory. Even slight differences in how a skill was practiced would require a separate and specific memory or motor program. It is difficult to explain how the vast number of individual memory structures needed, given the nearly countless skills and skill variations people are capable of performing, could be stored in the central nervous system. Certainly a much more parsimonious way of providing for the representation of motor skills within the central nervous system seemed demanded by these inadequacies in explaining storage mechanisms.

Schmidt's Schema Theory

In 1975, Richard Schmidt proposed a new theory of the motor program. Schmidt recognized that the deficiency with contemporary theories, such as that proposed by Adams, was the idea that a separate motor program was necessary for every variation of a particular skill, thus the problems of novelty and storage. Schmidt's solution to this problem was simple yet elegant. He proposed that every unique expression of a skill does not require a separate motor program, but that the motor program is more general in nature and adaptable to a wide variety of different ways in which a specific skill might be performed. Schmidt postulated that a motor program is generalized to represent an entire class of similar actions or skill variations and that this single motor program, which he termed a **generalized motor program** (abbreviated GMP), could be modified to yield various action outcomes (Schmidt, 1975, 1982).

The theory that Schmidt developed from these ideas is called **schema theory** (Schmidt, 1975, 2003). Schema theory provided a new and useful framework for studying motor skills. It ushered in several new lines of research that have significantly advanced our current understanding of how skills are learned and controlled. Although challenges have been made to the theory in the years since its introduction, and some continuing problems pointed out, today it remains the most influential and widely accepted theory of motor control and learning from a cognitive-based perspective (for an excellent collection of critiques of this theory, see Schmidt, 2003; Sherwood and Lee, 2003; and Newell, 2003).

Invariant Features of the GMP

Before proceeding further, attempt the writing exercise shown in Exercise 4.1.

generalized motor program (GMP): The concept of a motor program as proposed by schema theory; an abstract representation of rules generalized to control an entire class of actions.

schema theory: A theory of motor programs first proposed by Schmidt in 1975 that assumes that motor programs are made up of an abstract set of rules that can be generalized to control an entire class of actions.

EXERCISE 4.1　　　**A Writing Experiment**

At the top of the page of a blank piece of paper write the following phrase: "Learning about motor control is fun!" You should use your dominant hand and write just as you normally would.

Next, below this first line rewrite the same phrase—"Learning about motor control is fun!"—in the following additional ways.

1. Pressing down very hard
2. Pressing down very softly

3. Slowly, while maintaining legibility
4. Quickly, while maintaining legibility
5. With your nondominant hand
6. Holding the pen/pencil in your mouth
7. If you are inclined and adventurous, holding the pen or pencil between your toes

---

invariant features:
The components of a movement that remain the same, or constant, regardless of the timing, force, muscles used, or other features of a movement. Three invariant features are recognized in schema theory, including muscle sequencing, relative timing, and relative force.

In the writing exercise, regardless of how you wrote the phrase "Learning about motor control is fun," several underlying features of your writing remained constant. Those features that did not change from one writing method to another are called **invariant features**. To date, researchers have identified three sources of invariance in human motor skills. These are (1) the sequencing of actions or components, (2) relative timing, and (3) relative force.

In the writing exercise, for example, regardless of the way in which you wrote, you sequenced the components of the written phrase in the same order each time. That is, relative to the first word in the phrase, the letter "e" always followed the "L" and preceded the "a." And the word *about* always followed *Learning* and preceded the word *motor*. Any disruption of this particular order of letters and words would result in an error in writing. Not only do the letter and word components of the phrase occur in a specific order, but they are also related to one another in the timing and force features used to produce the various lines of the phrase. Whether you wrote the phrase slowly or quickly, pressed down hard or softly while writing, and regardless of which effector you used (hand, mouth, toes), the proportion of time you took to complete each letter remained constant (we say that the ratio of timing remains constant). The same is also true of the forces used to produce the various lines of the phrase. If EMG recordings were taken for the different muscles involved in writing the phrase, they would result in proportionally the same relationship of forces used to produce the written sentence whether you were writing softly or pressing down hard on the paper.

Invariant features as "rules" of the GMP   These three "rules" can be seen to apply to any given movement skill. In performing a volleyball spike in a game, for example, regardless of where the ball is set, the same sequence of actions is observed (i.e., the approach, the jump, the arm swing, hand contact, etc.) This sequencing rule does not change from one spike attempt to another (and this would be true whether the right or left hand were used to hit the ball). Relative timing features also remain constant and form a general timing rule of action. In essence, relative timing refers to the internal rhythm of a skill. The arm motion for a freestyle stroke in swimming, for example, can be broken down into five components. Of the total time needed to complete one cycle, let us say that 35 percent is accounted for by the entry, 13 percent by the catch, 8 percent by the mid-pull, 12 percent by the finish, and finally 32 percent by the recovery. Because relative timing is considered invariant, these percentages should remain the same regardless of whether an athlete is swimming slowly or quickly, even though the actual time involved would be different in each case.

Considerable research on the timing features of many motor skills has consistently demonstrated this to be the true (e.g., Shapiro et al., 1981). A similar internal relationship can also be seen with respect to force production. When the overall force used to execute a skill is changed, the actual force characteristics of each component (and each muscle used) also change proportionately. Thus, relative force is also an invariant feature of the GMP. These three rules—sequencing, relative timing, and relative force—are fixed (invariant) features of the GMP, which in turn are adaptable to variations in environmental conditions and goal requirements.

The implications of having to store only a single motor program for a particular skill rather than separate motor programs for every variation of how the skill might be performed are obvious. First, the problem of storage is neatly solved. Rather than a vast number of individual motor programs, only a single motor program is needed. The problem of novelty is also solved. Because one motor program is sufficient for execution of a skill in a wide variety of different ways, the GMP is readily adaptable to novel situations and changing environmental conditions, even when not having been previously practiced.

GMPs form rules for a "movement class." In Schmidt's theory, the problems of novelty and storage are solved because a single motor program contains a set of generalized rules for a wide variety of ways in which a particular skill might be performed. Schmidt termed all the different ways a skill might be performed while relying on the same rules of sequence, relative timing, and relative force, as a **movement class**. Throwing objects like softballs (or rocks or wadded-up paper balls) various distances, for example, can be considered as a movement class. This is because regardless of the distance one wants to throw (at least within a certain range), the rules governing the sequence of muscle activation, relative timing, and relative force remain constant. Regardless of the distance thrown, even to an unpracticed distance, the throwing action is still accomplished by the same rules and so can be effectively accomplished by the GMP. Throwing in this example entails a movement class.

Although there remains some debate about what constitutes a particular movement class, it is believed that movements having similar coordination patterns are controlled by the same motor program. Movement classes include basic skills such as running, grasping, throwing, catching, kicking, and jumping as well as specific learned skills such as the javelin throw, an overhead serve in volleyball, typing, a dance step, using a fork to eat, and brushing your teeth (see Box 4.6).

movement class:
All of the possible movements controlled by a single generalized motor program, typically sharing common coordination patterns.

BOX **4.6**   **Characteristics of a Movement Class**

Richard Schmidt, who developed schema theory for motor skills, has stated that a movement class is characterized by the following elements.

- Common sequencing among the elements of the action

- Common temporal, or rhythmical, organization (i.e., relative timing)
- Variable parameters, or surface features (e.g., speed) that people specify before each movement attempt, depending on goal requirements

Variant Features of the GMP

According to schema theory, rather than a specific motor program, an abstract representation of rules generalized across an entire movement class is stored in memory in the form of the GMP, as we have seen. But how can general rules guide movements? After all, you really do throw a ball a specific distance, and so the motor program must, at some level, specify the particular forces and timing of muscles necessary to throw at the specified distance. This brings us to the concept within schema theory of **variant features**, those features like environmental conditions, body and limb positions, and movement goals that change (or are potentially changeable) with every specific performance of a skill.

The features of a motor program that are flexible and define how to execute the program under differing variant feature conditions are termed **parameters**. Parameters are easily modified from one performance to another to produce variations of a motor response. This adaptability of parameters enables a center fielder, for example, to throw to third base from different areas of the field, as well as allowing an individual to walk up and down steps of varying heights. Three parameters are identified in schema theory; these are overall duration, overall force, and muscle selection (note that these correspond to the three rules of invariance).

The time taken to perform a well-learned skill, for example, can be increased or decreased as a unit according to changes in the overall duration parameter. Similarly, the overall force and amplitude (size of the movement) can be modified. Finally, as was demonstrated in our writing experiment (Exercise 4.1), the various effectors that can be used to perform the same movement (hand, foot, mouth in writing) can be modified (i.e., the specification of muscles and/or limbs to perform a movement is considered a parameter). The selection of the appropriate values for timing, force, or of the specific muscles used in a particular situation is referred to as *scaling* the generalized motor program.

Specifying Parameter Values—The Schema

According to the generalized motor program concept, an individual is able to perform a skill in a variety of different ways by assigning appropriate parameter values to the generalized motor program (scaling the GMP). But how does an individual know exactly what parametric values to assign? According to Schmidt's theory, the answer lies in the development of a **schema**.

A schema is a rule (or set of rules) that directs decision making when a learner is faced with a movement problem. Each movement attempt provides the learner with information about the movement that is translated into a relationship (i.e., invariant features) that will then be used to guide future attempts. The more performance attempts executed within a movement class, the more developed the rules or schema become.

Suppose that you go to the county fair and come across a ball toss game whose prize is a huge stuffed teddy bear. The object of the game is to toss a softball into a basket in such a way that it does not bounce out. Feeling confident, you purchase three chances. Having observed the attempts of some of the previous patrons, you decide that the best approach is to use an underhand toss. On your first toss, the ball ricochets off the bottom of the basket and bounces out.

variant feature: The aspects of a motor program that change from one performance attempt to another, including bodily states, environmental factors, and task goals.

parameters: Features of a skill that must be added to the invariant features of a generalized motor program to meet the specific demands of a situation. Parameters include overall duration, overall force, and muscle selection.

schema: A set of rules relating the various outcomes of an individual's actions (e.g., short distance of a throw) to the parameter values the individual chooses in order to produce those outcomes (e.g., small amount of force).

On your second attempt, you decide to lean over the barrier and adjust the toss, decreasing the height of the arc and aiming more toward the front of the basket. Again, the ball bounces out of the basket, but this time with less force. On your third attempt, you again lean over the barrier as far as possible and throw the same low-arcing toss, but this time with a little less force. Your parents/wife/husband/girlfriend/or boyfriend loves the stuffed teddy bear!

How was it that you corrected the motor program on each of the three attempts so that you could eventually accomplish the task goal and win the teddy bear? According to schema theory, on each attempt you subconsciously abstracted and evaluated four pieces of critical information. The first piece of information involves the initial conditions that were present at the start of the movement. This information includes limb and body position as well as environmental conditions when the movement was performed. Leaning over the barrier as far as possible is an example of an initial condition. The second piece of information involves the *response specifications*, or the parameters, used in the execution of the movement, such as the speed and force of your throw. Next, the sensory consequences of the movement consisting of sensory feedback are abstracted. Information regarding what the throw felt like, for example, would be assessed. Finally, the success of the response in relation to the original intended goal or outcome is obtained. This is known as the *response outcome*. In the example, the response outcome of each of the three attempts was different. In the first attempt, the ball ricocheted out of the basket, indicating that it had too great a force. In subsequent attempts, the magnitude of that force was gradually reduced, indicating that the movement produced was coming closer to the movement needed to achieve the goal.

These four sources of information are briefly stored in working memory following each attempt, allowing the learner to abstract the relationship

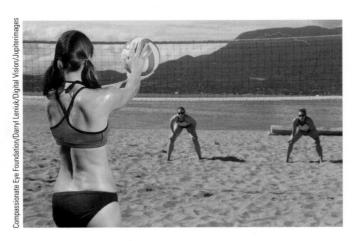

According to Schema Theory, motor programs are generalized so that a single program is capable of controlling an entire class of actions. This volleyball player can adjust the same motor program to serve the ball to various locations on her opponents' side of the net.

among them. What remains constant for each movement attempt, the invariant features, is preserved and stored in long-term memory in the form of a GMP, whereas what changes on every attempt (parameters) is discarded from memory and plays no further part in learning.

Schema Learning and the Variability of Learning Hypothesis

As we have just seen, four types of information contribute to the learning of schema, including initial conditions, response specifications, response outcome, and sensory consequences. From this information, the performer theoretically abstracts the relationships among them. This evaluation (which occurs subconsciously) forms the basis for the development of the GMP (Figure 4.3).

As the process of post-response evaluation occurs over the course of practice, the schema becomes more established and the individual can more accurately select the appropriate response specifications (parameter values) to accomplish a movement goal (i.e., learning occurs). Determining the most effective type of practice schedule is essential in almost all instructional situations, and the implications of schema theory have significantly altered our contemporary understanding concerning effective practice arrangements. Although a detailed discussion of this topic is left for later (especially Chapter 11), a brief introduction is appropriate here.

An important factor that has been shown to affect learning is the amount of variability in a practice sequence. In one sense, this is obvious. For many skills, variability is an inherent feature (open skills), such as fielding ground

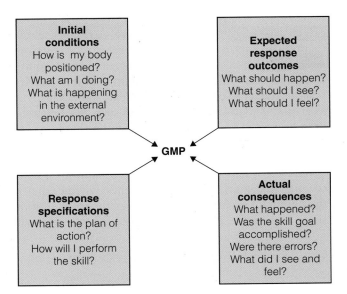

FIGURE **4.3** The Generalized Motor Program Is Abstracted from Four Sources of Information

Source: Created by author.

balls in baseball or steering a car down an unfamiliar road. An important part of learning such skills is acquiring the capacity to cope with novel situations; practicing under constant (unvarying) situations would typically not be appropriate, at least beyond an initial stage of learning. What about closed skills, though, where environmental conditions are always quite similar (e.g., archery, bowling, taping an athlete's ankle)? Here, because the skill to be learned is always performed the same way, it would seem that practice under conditions closely duplicating expected performance conditions would be the most beneficial. Yet the implications of schema theory are that, even for closed skills, varied practice should prove more effective. This is the case because, according to schema theory, the greater the variability in practice (the broader the range of parameters practiced), the more information available for abstracting relationships among the invariant features underlying a specific movement class of skill. Although we will leave the detailed discussion of these implications until Chapter 11, it can be stated that abundant research has confirmed this **variability of practice hypothesis** (Sherwood and Lee, 2003).

variability of practice hypothesis: The notion that the best learning experiences are those that vary the movement components and environmental conditions of the target skill and target context.

PRELUDE TO DYNAMICAL SYSTEMS THEORY— THE BERNSTEINIAN PERSPECTIVE

Cognitive-based theories, in one form or another, have dominated thinking about motor learning and control throughout most of the history of the scholarly study of motor skills, and they continue to exert a significant influence on such study and theorizing today. By the 1980s, however, an entirely new theoretical approach to the study of motor behavior began to offer new insights into our understanding of how motor skills are controlled and learned. Today such theoretical approaches, which we refer to collectively as **dynamical systems theory,** have gained wide acceptance as both a competing and in other ways complementary alternative to cognitive-based theories. The role of dynamical systems theory in contemporary research and scholarship is as influential today as is that of cognitive-based theories such as schema theory, and it is also beginning to exert a pronounced influence on the design of practice schedules and instructional methods (Davids, Button, and Bennett, 2008; McMorris, 2004; McMorris and Hale, 2006). Being relatively new, it remains to be seen whether dynamical systems approaches will remain an influential and balancing perspective to cognitive-based approaches; whether they might eventually become the dominant theoretical approach to the study of motor behavior; or whether some as yet undeveloped synthesis of the two approaches might arise.

dynamical systems theory: A theory of motor control and learning having as a major assumption that the human motor system interacts with the larger environment surrounding it and reacts to organize movement patterns establishing internal system stability.

The Genesis of Dynamical Systems Approaches to the Study of Motor Skills—The Insights of Bernstein

Dynamical systems theory arose because of a conceived weakness with cognitive-based theories that had troubled a number of movement scientists over the years. This weakness was seen as the perceived inability of the central nervous system, particularly the cortical areas of the brain, to control movement in isolation from other significant control agents. Remember that cognitive-based theories are closed and top-down theories, meaning that the brain, in this case, commands all lower regions of action production without the need for outside help. As computationally powerful as the brain is, to many scientists this seemed too great a task to assign to the brain alone. Critics often referred to this as the **problem of the homunculus,** or, in less technical terms, as the problem of the "little man in the brain." In this analogy, a little man residing in the brain plays the part of a movement musician who takes in information, decides upon a course of action, prepares a musical score of muscle activations, plays the score on the motor cortex (conceived of as a piano in the analogy), which then produces the desired tones (muscular contractions) and melody (action). In the analogy, the little man is in charge of the entire process involved in selecting and playing the correct musical score (like the conductor directing all the members of an orchestra). In the view of many movement scientists, this was too great a task to ask of the little man; in fact, in the view of many, there was no little man.

> **problem of the homunculus:** A criticism of cognitive-based theories that the brain alone is incapable of controlling all aspects of an action.

The first movement scientist to offer a convincing alternative to the problem of the little man in the brain was a Russian physiologist named Nicolai Bernstein (1896–1966). Bernstein, who can be considered the progenitor of modern dynamical systems approaches to the study of motor control and learning, devoted his life's work to unraveling the mysteries surrounding the complexity of human movement. He was the first to identify the problems with cognitive-based approaches that are the impetus for dynamical systems theory (for an overview of Bernstein and his work, see Gurfinkel and Cordo, 1998).

For Bernstein, two major problems inherent in a strictly cognitive understanding of motor control were evident. First, he recognized that the control of movement could not be reduced simply to a central mechanism of control responsible for commanding all muscle actions directly, but must take into account other forces acting on the moving body such as inertia, reactive forces, and gravitational and centripetal forces. Because the human body is subject to the laws of physics, just as is any moving physical object, outside forces acting on it will influence resultant bodily movements in addition to, and independent of, internal muscular forces. This obvious fact, Bernstein saw, only added to the almost limitless different combinations of forces that could act on limbs and body in producing actions to achieve desired movement goals. This highlighted a second problem with purely cognitive theories. How could the large number of ways in which various bodily and environmental variables interact, Bernstein asked, be organized meaningfully to produce coordinated action? These two problems, first recognized by Bernstein and, following his terminology, called the *context-conditioned variability problem* and the *degrees of freedom problem,* are of primary concern in all dynamical systems theory approaches.

The Context-Conditioned Variability Problem

If a central control mechanism, such as a motor program, is responsible for producing desired movement outcomes, then any specific outcome will be dependent upon a set of specific commands found within the control mechanism (i.e., the motor program). However, what if the context in which the movement is produced changes? In this case, will producing the same muscular commands result in the same outcome? Bernstein (1967) observed that the relationship between muscular forces used to generate a movement and the movement outcome is a variable one, and that this variability is context conditioned.

Suppose, for example, that you wish to lower your arm against a resistance (see Figure 4.4). To accomplish this action requires the contraction of the latissimus dorsi muscle; in fact, for any but the least resistance it is the prime mover used in completing this action. Now suppose, however, that resistance against the arm is removed. Does the same contraction of the latissimus dorsi muscle result in the same movement outcome? In this case, the latissimus dorsi muscle is not involved in the movement at all. An eccentric contraction of the deltoid muscle is necessary instead to accomplish the same movement outcome. So, although the same kinematic features are evident in both cases, and the movement goal remains the same, the muscles required to produce the desired outcome change because of the differing context in which the two movements are

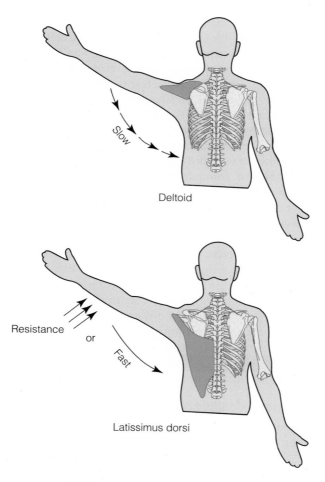

FIGURE **4.4** One Example of Context-conditioned Variability

performed—in this case because of either the presence or absence of resistive forces acting upon the limb in question. A motor program that controlled muscles independently would be insensitive to contextual variation (and this would be especially true for quick, dynamic actions where there would be insufficient time for sensory feedback to mediate centrally controlled commands). Bernstein identified a number of examples of context-conditioned variability of various types for which he argued that the motor program concept was insufficient as an explanation (see Turvey, Fitch, and Tuller, 1982, for a good discussion of various types of context-conditioned variability).

The Degrees of Freedom Problem

degrees of freedom:
The number of dimensions in which a system can independently vary.

In Chapter 2, we presented the degrees of freedom problem (see pp. 47–48). Bernstein was the first to formulate this problem. Recall that **degrees of freedom are defined as the number of ways in which a system can independently vary.** That is, how many different values can the components of a system assume without violating any geometric or physical laws? As we saw in Chapter 2, when the degrees of freedom available for any movement are specified from the macro to micro level of analysis, the available patterns of joint, muscular, and cellular combinations become exponentially large. At the cellular level, considering the motor unit as the basic unit of motor control, the redundancy of possible patterns of motor unit recruitment for complex skills can easily reach into many millions. For Bernstein, the many redundant degrees of freedom available for accomplishing skilled actions presented a problem of sufficient complexity to negate any exclusive role for cortical structures such as motor programs (see Box 4.7). If central control processes were incapable of organizing and commanding such a vast array of possible neural patterns, how did people effectively harness and control the many degrees of freedom accessible to them? The obvious solution, Bernstein reasoned, was that somehow humans must reduce the degrees of freedom needing control when performing complex skills. But how was this accomplished? Bernstein's solution was to focus, at least in part, on the spinal contributions to action. In this regard, perhaps his most enduring contribution to our understanding of motor control and learning is his concept of the **synergy.**

synergy: A grouping of joints, muscles, and cells that temporarily cooperate in acting together as a single collective action unit; can be assembled and unassembled as the need arises; also called a *coordinative structure.*

BOX **4.7**   The Centipede's Dilemma

Bernstein's ideas concerning how the large number of degrees of freedom available for controlling movements can be problematic if reduced to some cortical control mechanism (i.e., "little man in the brain") is well illustrated in an old children's rhyme about a centipede and a frog. Notice in the rhyme that the centipede is unable to control the complex coordination required of her walking patterns when she must think about them (i.e., rely upon cognitive processes alone).

The centipede was happy quite
Until a frog in fun
Said, "Pray which leg goes after which?"
And worked her mind to such a pitch,
She lay distracted in the ditch
Considering how to run.

Synergies

Before describing the mechanism of the synergy, it will be helpful to first consider an example. Imagine a person learning a golf swing (a good description of this is offered by Button, 2007). Producing an effective golf swing requires simultaneously coordinating actions of the arms, trunk, and legs, involving well over a hundred muscles that must be effectively controlled. When initially learning a golf swing, learners are unable to coordinate the large number of degrees of freedom this places at their disposal. Instead, they will typically adopt a strategy of locking their wrists and elbows and simply swinging their arms downward in a stick-like fashion as they rotate at the hips, all the while also keeping their knees locked and their lower body rigid. In this fashion, only rotation at the hips and shoulders must be controlled, dramatically reducing the number of joints and muscles (i.e., the number of degrees of freedom) that must be controlled in the swinging action. Of course, this inevitably results in a golf swing that is rigid, jerky, and inefficient. Nevertheless, in the early stages of practicing a new skill, and especially a complex one, learners are simply not able, cognitively, to simultaneously control all of the joints and muscles necessary to produce efficient actions, and so must limit in some way the number of elements they must control. Bernstein referred to this initial strategy of limiting the movements of some joints when learning a new skill as **freezing the degrees of freedom.**

freezing the degrees of freedom: Limiting the movement of limbs and joints.

Over time, as a consequence of practice, learners begin to relax some muscles and allow some joints to move more freely. As seen in our golfing example, they allow flexion and extension of the right elbow, as well as hyperextension of the wrists effectively timed to accelerate the club more powerfully into the ball. The knees also become free to rotate, allowing for more effective timing of trunk rotation and adding both greater velocity and precision to the trajectory of the club head's arc before striking the ball.

This example of learning a golf swing illustrates two important premises of dynamical systems theory, which may, at first, seem contradictory. First, learning a skill is characterized by a gradual increase in the use of available degrees of freedom. Second, because of the gradual increase in available degrees of freedom, learning must also be accompanied by the ability to increasingly control more degrees of freedom. This second point may seem obvious, but it begs the question of how individuals come to control greater numbers of degrees of freedom as a product of learning. Bernstein's insight was to see that the degrees of freedom available for a skill could be increased as a function of learning, whereas the number of those degrees of freedom that must be controlled was at the same time reduced. Or, simply stated, as people learn and acquire new skills, they have more degrees of freedom available to them but fewer that they must directly control. But how did Bernstein arrive at this seeming contradiction?

To return to our golfing example once more, the golfer must produce precisely timed and executed bodily movements in order to translate his or her movements to the club head and strike the ball with effective precision and force. To hit the ball effectively, different movement patterns are required on each swing. Also, each person is unique with respect to body build, strength, flexibility, and physical conditioning, which also interact with the most appropriate movement pattern for different swings. A wide array of environmental conditions interacts with each golf swing. Learning involves more than being able to adapt to these changing conditions. It also involves learning how to take advantage of, or as dynamical theorists put it, "exploit," changing environmental conditions. By freeing joint movements ("unfreezing" muscles) and releasing more degrees of freedom, the golfer has more movement choices available to him or her to meet changing environmental conditions. Freeing joint movements increases the range of motion available for generating angular rotation of the club head and, therefore, greater distances the ball can be hit.

So, learning involves increasing the degrees of freedom available for coordinating bodily movements, thereby increasing the possible movement patterns available to exploit changing environmental conditions. But if more degrees of freedom become available through learning, meaning that more units of action (joints, muscles, motor units) must be simultaneously controlled, how does the learner learn to control this ever-increasing number of movement options available to him or her, given the limitations of cognitive capabilities? Bernstein's answer was that one of the most important products of learning is a clustering of degrees of freedom into cooperating collectives called *synergies* (also referred to as *coordinative structures*) that can be controlled as single units of action rather than each degree of freedom operating independently. (We will see later in this chapter that this idea anticipated one of the most important concepts in modern dynamical systems theory, known as *self-organization*.)

According to Bernstein, over the course of practice task-specific groupings of joints, muscles, and motor units become operative that effectively reduce the number of degrees of freedom that need to be controlled. That is, movement elements that are specific to a given task become linked as temporary collectives for purposes of task execution. These elements are constrained to act as a single unit during the execution of the task, thereby greatly reducing the number of separate action units that must be controlled. Saltzman and Munhall (1992) have defined synergies as "temporary and flexible assembled functional organizations that are defined over a group of muscles and joints and that convert those components into task-specific coherent multiple-degrees-of-freedom ensembles" (p. 50). Rather than many separate elements, each controlled individually, only a single unit needs to be under cortical control (this aspect of synergies anticipated another central idea of dynamical systems theory called *emergence*).

Further, synergies are capable of being assembled and unassembled as needed. Their collective action only operates when needed in the execution of a specific task (such assemblies are referred to as *soft assemblies*). Presumably, in Bernstein's (1984) thinking, these linkages take place in the spinal column among the myriad patterns possible in synaptic connections.

Many questions about the exact nature of synergies, however, still remain and are debated among modern dynamical systems theorists, and their exact configuration is still somewhat of a mystery (Latash, 2008). Nevertheless, Bernstein's identification of context-conditioned variability problems inherent in cognitive-based theories about motor skills, his analysis of the degrees of

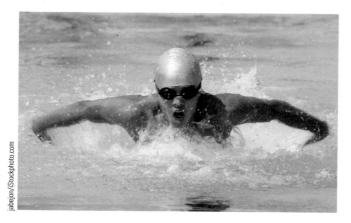

The development of synergies offers one solution to the degrees of freedom problem, helping to explain how individuals can control the actions of many limbs and joints simultaneously.

freedom problem and identification of synergistic structures, and his description of learning processes are important, and even foundational, contributions to modern dynamical systems theory concerning motor control and learning.

MODERN DYNAMICAL SYSTEMS THEORY

Because of political tensions between the former Soviet Union and Western countries during the period we now call the Cold War, Bernstein's seminal work on motor behavior and synergies was not translated from the Russian for almost three decades after its original publication (cf. Bernstein, 1967). At about the same time as his work was coming to the attention of movement scientists in the West, however, a larger scientific revolution was fortuitously underway. This was a revolution across physical, social, and biological sciences in the way dynamical systems are scientifically studied. In the vocabulary of science, a system refers to any collection of interacting parts functioning as a whole, such as the motor system comprised of bones, muscles, and nerve cells; the solar system comprised of the planets; or collectives of people forming communities (Meadows, 2008). Dynamical systems are systems in motion, or systems that change over time. Neither a rock nor an airplane is a dynamical system, but the geological evolution of rocks and the flight of airplanes are dynamical. The many ways in which humans can harness various movements in order to produce diverse patterns of skill are also dynamical.

Science, from its beginnings, has studied systems displaying regular (that is, predictable) dynamics. A key to all of these systems is that changes occur in a linear fashion. Linear systems allow scientists to make certain mathematical assumptions, such as that 1 + 1 always equals 2, 1 + 2 always equals 3, 1 + 3 always equals 4, and so forth. That is, the mathematics of linear systems is also linear. This means that such systems are highly predictable—in fact, if you know

system: A collection of interacting parts that functions as a single entity.

dynamical system: Any system that is in motion or exhibits change over time.

the correct mathematics and have sufficient information, you can always predict exactly what a system will do under any given circumstances.

A major challenge for scientists is that many systems do not act linearly. In fact, many systems are notoriously nonlinear in their behavior. They change in abrupt and unpredictable ways. They may act in a linear, predictable way up to some point but then abruptly change—they act nonlinearly. Water, for example, remains in the same state as temperature varies over many degrees, but at 32° F it abruptly and nonlinearly changes to ice. Although the change from one state to another is predictable in the case of water to ice, shifts from one condition or state to another for most complex systems are highly unpredictable. Many systems, in fact, seem to behave chaotically.

Dynamical Systems and Complexity

Dynamical systems that act in nonlinear ways share an important characteristic: They are complex. In this case, complex does not mean complicated or difficult, though complex systems may certainly be that. Rather, **complexity** refers to systems that are comprised of diverse constituent parts that are connected, interdependent, and capable of adapting (Miller and Page, 2007; Mitchell, 2009). In order to be considered complex, a system must exhibit all four of these qualities:

- Diversity (comprised of many elements differing in kind)
- Connection (form a linked network)
- Interdependence (a change in one element affects all other elements)
- Adaptation (capable of change, i.e., of learning)

Examples of complex systems include areas as diverse as weather and climate, economics, biological systems, chemical reactions, bird migration patterns, population growth, highway traffic flow, social fads, and baseball records. Human movement skills also possess the qualities of complexity (Mayer-Kress, Liu, and Newell, 2006). Movement skills are the result of many diverse elements (muscles, neurons, bone, motor units, enzymes, etc.) connected and regulated through neural, chemical, and physical processes and capable of adaptation (i.e., of learning).

Systems that exhibit complexity, such as human movement, produce bottom-up, emergent phenomena. This is expressed by two essential and cooperating features of dynamical systems theory—emergence and self-organization. **Emergence** entails the creation of something new that transcends the parts from which it is produced. Wetness, for instance, is an emergent property of water. Water is made up of individual molecules of hydrogen and oxygen, neither of which possesses the quality of wetness. When combined to form water, however, a new quality, wetness, which is not inherent in individual hydrogen and oxygen molecules, emerges—it is something new that could not have been predicted from its parts. Consciousness, as another example, is an emergent property. Consciousness does not reside, even in the smallest part, within individual neurons. When millions of neurons are organized together in the human brain, however, consciousness, in some way wonderfully mysterious but as yet far from understood, emerges. How such a new phenomenon as consciousness

complexity:
A characteristic of systems that are comprised of diverse elements that are connected and interdependent, and capable of adaptation.

emergence: The spontaneous creation of a new state or pattern resulting from the self-organization of the elements of a complex system.

arises can never be explained from studying individual neurons. This is because consciousness is simply not a component of neurons—it is the product of a neuronal collective, something that results from the interaction of neurons, but not from the neurons themselves! Therefore, an important aspect of emergence is that the macro (the whole, e.g., consciousness) differs from the micro (the parts, e.g., neurons). Something new is created, and the whole is greater than the sum of its parts.

An important aspect of emergence is that it is part of an adaptive process. Emergence is the spontaneous creation of order and functionality from disorder. Emergence results from diverse system components seeking order and stability. This brings us to the concept of **self-organization.** Remember that in closed systems top-down control is established. The boss commands the workers in a factory. The orchestra conductor directs the individual musicians. A motor program commands lower levels of muscular activity. In open systems, however—and complex systems are by definition open—control is from the bottom up. Many diverse connected components organize together to form a new whole. There is no overall command structure—no boss, no orchestra leader, no motor program—in fact, no predetermined plan for overall control at all. The individual components of a system each adapt to changing circumstances in their own unique ways, contributing to the emergence of new structures and patterns. In a sense, it is the individual parts that command the final whole. The collective dynamical systems result of the contributions of the various parts to the whole, of the micro to the macro, is termed *self-organization* (see Box 4.8).

self-organization: The tendency for elements within a complex system to synergistically adapt so that new states or patterns emerge.

A New Paradigm for the Study of Motor Skills

In dynamical systems theory, a motor skill is viewed as an emergent property of diverse systems exhibiting complexity. Recall that Bernstein's work, coming to the attention of Western researchers just as dynamical systems theory was becoming established within scientific communities, postulated that movement coordination exhibited the essential features of complex systems (Bernstein, 1967). Bernstein, breaking with cognitive theorists, saw human movements as emerging from the interaction of many systems and subsystems, including both biological and environmental systems, which were both connected, interdependent, and adapting. He further focused attention, through the ideas of context-conditioned variability, on the ways in which changes in environmental and physical properties could accumulate within biokinematic chains, resulting in very different patterns of action—that is, movement manifests emergence. Finally, Bernstein's conception of synergies matched perfectly to dynamical systems concepts of self-organization—that is, that systems spontaneously organize into cooperating collectives. What Bernstein's ideas and observations lacked, however, was a larger theoretical context within which they could be explained and from which new ideas could be developed and tested. Dynamical systems theory provided just such a framework.

Today, the ideas of dynamical systems theory are applied by movement scientists working across a broad range of subdisciplinary areas. Although different names may be given to the theories employed across various subdisciplinary communities (i.e., nonlinear dynamics, action theory, dynamical theory, movement dynamics, constraints-led approach, etc.), they all share common assumptions that we shall mean to imply by the more generic (and widely understood) term *dynamical systems theory*. A psychological approach to the study of perception that was first advanced by Gibson in the 1960s (1966, 1979), called *ecological psychology*, has played such an integral role in addressing issues concerning perception within dynamical systems approaches that it is also probably acceptable to consider it as part of dynamical systems theory approaches to the study of motor skills (we addressed this perspective when discussing perception in Chapter 3 and will have more to say about it in Chapter 6 when discussing the concept of memory for affordances).

BOX **4.8**   The Complexity of Fireflies and Movement Systems

For over 300 years, travelers to Southeast Asia returned home with stories about vast congregations of fireflies stretching for many miles along riverbanks blinking on and off in perfect unison against night skies (Strogatz, 2000). For many years, these stories were considered only fanciful flights of imagination, or as exaggerations at best. But in the early years of the last century, scientists begin to study and measure these flashing displays of millions of fireflies moving together along riverbeds, blanketing them in perfectly synchronous displays of light and darkness. They were at a loss to explain this strange phenomenon, however. How could millions of individual fireflies orchestrate their brilliant light display so perfectly over such vast distances?

For many decades, scientists could come up with no answer to how the fireflies choreographed their rhythmic nighttime displays. The problem, which only became clear in hindsight, was that everyone assumed that the fireflies must represent a closed system and that the mechanism underlying their synchronous behavior had to be some higher-order factor controlling each individual firefly—perhaps some atmospheric condition, or lead firefly signaling all the others, or even some property inherent in the human visual system that interacted with the light from this particular type of firefly to create the illusion of flashing.

All of these theories proved inadequate for one reason or another, however. Then, in the 1960s, some scientists begin looking more closely at the contributions of individual fireflies to the behavior of the collective. What they discovered was one of the first demonstrations of how complex systems work. When fireflies were separated from one another, their flashes were chaotic and nonrhythmic. It was only when they were brought back together in a large enough collective that their synchronous displays began to return, among small groups at first, but which then spread until all of the individual fireflies had joined into a common illumination chorus. There was no higher-order mechanism contolling the behavior of individual fireflies. Rather, something inherent in each firefly combined with all the others in the firefly community to form a new collective behavior—the mechanism of control went from the bottom up. What scientists were seeing were the processes of self-organization and emergence. The colony of fireflies, numbering in the millions, self-organized their individual behaviors into a new, emergent pattern for the whole colony.

Today we understand that the same kind of synchronous patterning is found in all living systems—flocks of birds, schools of fish, cities of people, colonies of neurons in the human brain, and structures of coordination among diverse colonies within the human movement system. It is in these final colonies, those found in human brains and muscular systems, that the greatest degree of self-organized emergence is to be found, and they are of a magnitude of complexity many times greater than the flashing illuminations of fireflies along distant riverbanks.

Regardless of the specific theoretical model one applies, all dynamical systems theories assume basic, common premises. Three in particular are critical to the study of motor behavior. The first of these is that systems are always constrained to act within certain boundaries. The second, as we have mentioned, is that new patterns emerge from the interaction of systems in a manner referred to as *self-organization*. Thirdly, the new patterns that emerge are organized around preferred behaviors or patterns that are called *attractors*. Taken together, the application of these three premises to the study of movement coordination has revealed many new insights into how motor skills are controlled and acquired. We will look more closely at each of these themes and consider how they help explain the characteristics of motor behavior.

The Emergence of Motor Skills—A Dynamical Systems Analysis

Any analysis of human movement from a dynamical systems perspective includes, among other aspects, consideration of three premises about the control and learning of all motor skills:

- Various constraints impose boundaries on movement possibilities.
- Diverse movement system components self-organize into emergent patterns.
- Self-organization directs emergence toward preferred, attractor states.

We will turn our attention to a discussion of each of these premises.

Movement Constraints

Although dynamical systems are characterized by change, they are also limited by the amount of change that is possible. Water, as we have seen for example, is limited to temperatures between 32° F and 212° F. Below 32° F it turns to ice; above 212° F it becomes steam. Water is therefore constrained, or bounded, by temperature: It cannot go below or above a certain temperature and remain water. In dynamical systems terminology, temperature is a **constraint** for water. Constraints establish the limits or boundaries of the states that a system can assume. All of the states that a system is free to assume within the boundaries of its constraints (i.e., all of the values that it can assume) are called its **state space**. The state space for water includes all of the temperatures between 32° F and 212° F.

Human movement, as a dynamical system of many bodily and environmental subsystems interacting, is limited by both biological and environmental constraints. Clark (1995) has observed that constraints are the boundaries limiting the movement capabilities of individuals. Newell (1986) has identified three categories of constraints; these are constraints imposed by the organism (i.e., the person), the environment, and the task itself. All three can also act together to impose new forms of constraint.

Organismic constraints Organismic constraints refer to characteristics of the individual, including both structural and functional characteristics. These include not only physical characteristics such as height, weight, and body type, but also behavioral characteristics, including cognitive, motivational,

---

constraint: Boundaries that limit the possible values or patterns that a system can assume that are imposed by the organism, physical environment, and task itself.

state space: All of the possible patterns or states that a system is capable of assuming.

organismic constraint: Characteristics of an individual that act as constraints on movement, including structural characteristics such as height, weight, and body shape, as well as functional characteristics such as intelligence, motivation, and psychological states.

emotional, and other psychological attributes of the individual. Factors such as physical condition and existing skill level are included in this category.

The effects of organismic constraints on motor skills are usually obvious, as are the strategies for developing resources to deal with such constraints more effectively. Structural constraints such as poor flexibility, for example, would limit an individual's range of motion and ability to take advantage of (to "exploit") physical forces in many movement skills such as gymnastics or reaching for objects on the floor. So engaging in stretching exercises to increase range of motion would allow an individual to increase the state space available for movement production. Likewise, organismic constraints may set boundaries curtailing movement possibilities. A 150-pound college freshman probably will be unable to generate the force required of an offensive lineman to successfully overcome the physical constraints imposed by a 300-pound defensive lineman. Generally, efforts to take advantage of organismic constraints—to increase the state space in which the individual is able to functionally perform—are gained through making changes in physical conditioning and/or knowledge and motivation directed at performance. These are, of course, typical categories addressed in skills practice.

Environmental constraints   Environmental constraints arise in both the physical and the sociocultural environments of individuals. The most obvious environmental constraints are physical in nature. These would include gravity (perhaps the most influential environmental constraint upon moving individuals), ambient light, temperature, features of the terrain, and the movement medium (i.e., air, water, etc.). Other environmental constraints are social in nature, although these act more subtly than do physical constraints (Clark, 1995). Sociocultural factors such as family support networks, peer groups, and social expectations and values also shape behavior. Reed (1993) has referred to these sociocultural constraints as *promoted actions,* that is as actions which a culture promotes and values.

Physical forces in the environment place considerable constraints upon motor performance. When throwing a javelin, wind condition is an important consideration because of the aerodynamics of the javelin, and failure to take wind velocity and direction into consideration as constraints on performance will have negative consequences (Coker, 2009). As mentioned above, gravity acts as a particularly critical constraint on movement in all tasks. Consider, for example, a skier skiing down a steep mountain slope. The visual flow of information presented by the surface moguls (i.e., bumps in the snow pack) ahead of the skier can be used to regulate muscular tension across the hip, knee, and ankle joints. Larger mounds of snow will require the skier to bend more at the hips and knees in order to cushion the impact on the joints caused by reactive forces as he or she passes over the moguls (Araujo et al., 2004). Walking and running patterns, as another example, are significantly influenced by surface features. Walking on a flat hard surface requires a different coordination pattern than when walking on sand or snow or up an incline. Additionally, social constraints such as family support and social approval may facilitate or hinder performance through the marshaling of motivational and instructional resources.

environmental constraint: Features of the physical environment such as gravity, temperature, and light that act to constrain movement patterns; also includes social features such as cultural norms that constrain movement behavior.

task constraint:
Constraints on human movement imposed by the task performed, including task goals, equipment used, and mandated rules and procedures.

Task constraints   Task constraints, the third category of constraints Newell (1986) identified, are specific to the task itself. Newell identified three types of task constraints, including (1) the goal of the task; (2) rules governing performance when imposed (e.g., game rules and boundary markings in a sporting contest), as well as instructional aids when provided (e.g., augmented feedback and visual demonstrations); and (3) the implements, tools, or equipment used in performing the task.

In response to organismic and environmental constraints, the task itself imposes the final shape of the coordination patterns that will prove most effective. The goal of the task when driving a golf ball, for example, will force the golfer to adopt a long swing of the club because the laws of physics dictate this as the most effective method of hitting the ball down the fairway. The rules of an activity also impose constraints on movement patterns. In tennis, the rules of the game force a player to search for opportunities to hit the ball past an opponent, for instance. The constraints imposed by the use of implements or equipment also significantly alter the effectiveness of movement patterns. Changing the weight of a hammer will affect the amount of muscular force needed when driving nails. Effective gait patterns will change depending on whether an individual is walking on a treadmill or a Stairmaster, or using crutches. The size and weight of sporting equipment relative to body size also often places considerable constraints on movement, as can most readily be seen in children using equipment designed for adults.

The combined effects of constraints   Each category of constraints and each individual constraint within those categories imposes its particular boundaries upon movement options. Taken together, the combined effects of all constraints acting upon the moving person are synergistic. Although environmental constraints may support a broad range of movement possibilities when performing a specific skill, for example, a particular individual may

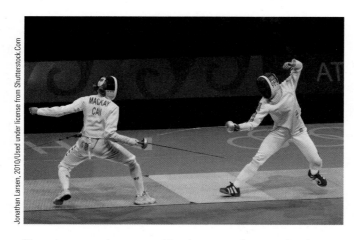

Jonathan Larsen, 2010/Used under license from Shutterstock.Com

The rules governing competition in sports, the use of various types of sporting equipment, and an athlete's physical characteristics all combine to constrain movement into particular patterns influencing skill level.

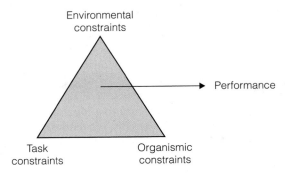

FIGURE **4.5** The Triangular Effect of Constraints on Learning

Source: Adapted from Newell, KM. (1986). "Constraints on the development of coordination." In Wade, MG, and Whiting, HTA (editors), *Motor development in children: Aspects of coordination and control.* Dordrecht, Germany: Martinus Nighoff, 341–360.

lack the physical capacity (organismic capabilities) to take full advantage of the entire range of available environmental options. In this case, it is where environmental and organismic constraints overlap that available movement options are to be found. Even in considering only two types of constraints, it becomes clear that interaction among constraints functions to narrow movement options (state space) dramatically. As illustrated in Figure 4.5, skilled movement arises as an outcome of the interactions of organismic, environmental, and task constraints.

Awareness of the three ways in which movement is constrained and of the interactions among the task, person, and environment is also critical to effective practice and learning (to test your knowledge, see Box 4.9). Newell (1986) claimed that there is a triangular effect on learning from the interaction of all three constraints and that the design of effective practice requires consideration of this combined influence. In terms of dynamical systems theory, the management of constraints in practice designs is an attempt to impose the most beneficial state space in which the most effective movement patterns can emerge. How those patterns emerge leads us to the next major theme of nonlinear dynamics, the self-organizing of systems.

BOX **4.9**   **Identifying Movement Constraints**

Classify each of the following as being either an organismic, environmental, or task constraint.

- Being poorly motivated
- A prosthetic limb
- Body weight for a pole vault
- The height and size of opening of a basketball basket
- The height and width of individual steps in a flight of stairs

- A regulation bat for a 9-year-old Little League player
- The firmness of a snow pack when skiing
- Looking into the sun when attempting to catch a football
- Genetically determined ratio of fast- and slow-twitch muscle composition
- The skill level of one's partner in a dance routine
- An older sibling who excelled at a particular sport

Self-Organization

The concept of self-organization is one of the most intriguing to come out of dynamical systems theory and one of the most important and far-reaching concepts in modern science. As previously defined, self-organization refers to a process whereby the organization of a system spontaneously increases and becomes more stable because of inherent properties within the system itself. Self-organization is the counter-intuitive idea that something left to itself tends to become more organized. Normally, we tend to think that things left to themselves become more disorganized, that they decay or run down, but nature is filled with examples of self-organizing systems. The synchronized flashing of fireflies on a summer's eve, the coordinated movements of flocks of birds and schools of fish, the spontaneous formation of crystals, the homeostatic self-maintaining nature of cells, and the formation of galaxies all exhibit the properties of self-organization. Indeed, examples of self-organization are found in all of the sciences, and have in recent years become central to the description of biological sciences, including human movement studies (Erdi, 2007; Holland, 1998).

As we saw earlier, an important feature of self-organizing systems is that they are adaptive; they change and evolve within themselves in response to their environments. Self-organizing systems, regardless of the type of system involved, exhibit two major characteristics, namely openness and self-reference. Openness means that the system is open to its environment, that it actively seeks information from its environment and makes that information widely available to all parts of the system. Self-reference refers to deterministic principles inherent within the system itself that guide the organization of the system (within bodily systems these self-referencing principles are believed to be genetically established). When information is received by the system concerning changes in the external environment, the system always adapts in a way that remains consistent with its own inherent guiding principles.

Systems manifesting the properties of self-organization are in constant contact with their surrounding environment. When conditions in that environment threaten the stability of the system, it reconfigures its component parts into new organizational patterns capable of functionally adapting to the changing external conditions. Though such reorganization is in response to the environmental surround, it is not controlled by it but rather restructures around internally self-regulating processes. From this self-organizing process, a new organizational pattern spontaneously emerges. These emergent properties, resulting from reorganizing processes, tend toward maintaining the stability or coherence of the system.

In the dynamical systems perspective of motor control, the coordination of movement is viewed as an emergent property. External constraints (organismic, environmental, and task-specific) interact with the muscular-skeletal system which in turn organizes itself into appropriate patterns of coordination among its component parts in order to most effectively meet movement goals within the limits of its state space, available degrees of freedom, and inherent guiding principles. Over time, the movement system is capable of reorganizing itself even further into collectives of synergies that are increasingly capable of effectively adapting to external demands constraining the system. Further, the guiding principles directing these processes of self-organization are attracted to (i.e., directed toward) patterns maximizing the stability and movement effectiveness of the system. We will next turn to a consideration of these optimal coordination states known as *attractor states*.

Attractors and Phase Shifts

Systems self-organize into new patterns in response to changes outside of the system that threaten its stability. Any change in a system's environment that causes disequilibrium in the system is called a *perturbance*. The spatial-temporal patterns of gait involved in walking on a flat surface are perturbed, for instance, when the grade on which a person is walking changes from a flat surface to an incline. When this happens, the system of muscular actions controlling the person's gait pattern becomes unstable and no longer efficient in meeting the task goal of continuing to move the body forward. In response to this perturbance, the muscular-skeletal system self-organizes into a new spatial-temporal pattern of muscular activity to reestablish the stability of the system and adapt to the new environmental constraints imposed upon it by the increased incline. The emergence of a new pattern of walking occurring spontaneously in response to such perturbations is called a **phase shift** (a phase is a specific pattern of organization within a system, and a phase shift is a spontaneous transition from one phase to another). Sudden phase shifts (often referred to colloquially as *tipping points*) are seen throughout nature—in the sudden breakup of a smooth flowing stream into a rushing turbulence of whorls and eddies, a single plume of smoke rising smoothly from a chimney until it reaches a certain velocity and then instantly splintering into a thousand wildly swirling puffs, and a kernel of corn popping.

The question arises, When a phase shift occurs, what does the system shift toward? What makes one new phase more likely to occur than others? What are the self-organizing principles that guide the shift? The key to answering these questions is that systems prefer states of stability. When one phase becomes unstable because of external perturbations in system constraints, the system self-organizes into a new phase that is stable in meeting the new conditions imposed upon it. These preferred states or patterns of stability are known as attractors, or attractor states. An **attractor** is an organizational arrangement that keeps a system's component parts working in harmony to fulfill the system's mission. A system may have a number of attractors, each one being more effective than the others under given environmental conditions. Relative to human movement systems, attractors are states of spatial-temporal muscular organization that are able to maintain stable movement patterns with the greatest efficiency in specific situations (Huys, Daffertshofer, and Beek, 2004; Wallace, 1996).

An experiment demonstrating attractor states and phase shifts   One of the first experiments to demonstrate the role of attractors and phase shifts in the coordination of human movement was reported by Kelso and Schoner in 1988. In their experiment, Kelso and Schoner had subjects place their hands on a tabletop, as shown in Figure 4.6a. They were then instructed to move the index finger

---

phase shift: In a dynamical system, the spontaneous transition from one organizational pattern to another as a result of self-organization.

attractor: A preferred pattern of stability toward which a system tends.

of each hand in a synchronous fashion to either the right or left in keeping with the beat of a metronome, as shown in Figure 4.6b. Although it might at first appear that both fingers were doing the same thing at the same time, they were actually doing opposite things. The muscles controlling the fingers were operating simultaneously, but in opposite ways relative to the midline of the body. When the right finger was abducted, the left finger was adducted, and vice versa. This is termed an antiphase pattern because the two fingers are actually out of phase with one another doing opposite things. As subjects performed these timed finger movements, the speed of the metronome was gradually increased. When a critical speed of the metronome was reached, an abrupt change occurred in the subjects' finger movements. They spontaneously shifted from the antiphase pattern to a new pattern in which the fingers kept time to the metronome in opposite directions, as illustrated in Figure 4.6c. That is, in the new pattern, known as an in-phase pattern, both fingers abducted or adducted at the same time.

In the Kelso and Schoner experiment, two attractors were observed, one that organized finger movements in an antiphase manner and the other that organized them in an in-phase manner. At the lower speeds of the metronome's beat, both attractors provided the system with sufficient stability that either could be freely chosen. As the speed of the metronome increased, however, a critical point was reached in which the antiphase pattern could no longer be maintained, in this

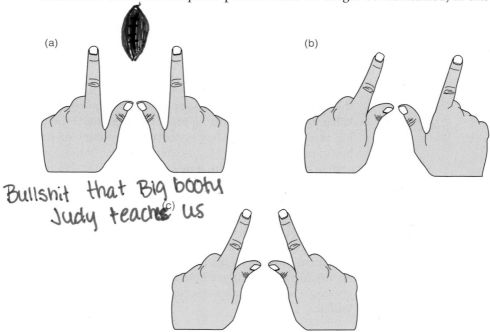

FIGURE **4.6** Kelso and Schoner Experiment

Source: Adapted from Coker, C., *Motor Learning & Control*, 2e, pg. 170–172. © 2009 Holcomb Hathaway Publishers.

case because the speed of the metronome caused the system to become unstable. In response to this perturbation, the system reorganized and made a phase shift into the optimally effective in-phase pattern that could best maintain the system's integrity. Although such phase shifts are spontaneous rather than gradual, we should point out that there is a transitional period in which the old pattern becomes less and less effective, until the new pattern finally emerges. In the Kelso and Schoner experiment, the researchers observed that as the speed of the metronome increased, there was a point at which subjects maintained the antiphase pattern even though it was becoming more and more difficult for them to do so. It was only when a critical speed was finally reached, however, that the new and more effective in-phase pattern spontaneously emerged.

The strength of attractor states—shallow and deep basins   The fact that subjects in Kelso and Schoner's study could maintain movement around a relatively ineffective attractor until finally forced by a sufficient perturbance to shift into a new phase has significant implications for understanding the development of motor skills. We have previously stated that a number of attractors likely operate on a system relative to specific task goals and that individuals are sometimes drawn to viable but relatively inefficient attractors. That is, individuals can choose among many movement patterns that may accomplish a task, but some will be more effective than others. Said another way, individuals can override a system's inherent tendency to self-organize around optimal attractor states for several reasons, including the person's stage of learning, or lack thereof, and the extent to which constraints act to perturb the system into a phase shift.

In regard to the role of learning in the organization of system behaviors around various attractor states, Ennis (1992) has suggested that attractors act much like basins (see Figure 4.7). The patterns toward which a system tends as it is drawn toward a specific attractor are said to collect as water collects in a basin, with the depth of the basin a function of the strength of the attractor in

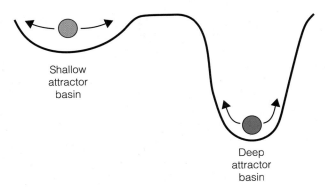

FIGURE **4.7** **Shallow and Deep Attractor Basins**

Source: Adapted from Ennis, C. (1992). "Reconceptualizing learning as a dynamical system." *Journal of Curriculum and Supervision, 7*(2), 173–183.

maintaining the system's stability. In place of water, however, attractor basins collect patterns of behavior used in controlling a system. Some basins are shallow and therefore relatively weak in maintaining system stability, and easily susceptible to change. Other basins are deep, being characteristic of stable systems and difficult to change. Small perturbations do not dislodge such systems from their region of state space, and once perturbed they quickly return to their original state. Relative to human movement, the depth of a basin, a preferred state of muscular-skeletal organization, is, broadly speaking, a function of genetics and, perhaps most importantly, learning. Some basins are genetically determined and very deep. For example, given the perturbance of an external force dynamically stretching particular muscles, the system will always self-organize into a new pattern we know as the *stretch reflex*. Well-learned skill patterns may not be quite as deep as such genetically determined reflexes, but they are still deep, functionally strong, and difficult to overcome. The motor system is strongly drawn to such deep basin attractors. Other basins, characteristic of movement patterns that are not well learned, will be relatively shallow, easily disturbed, and unstable in their application. Individuals will have difficulty maintaining these movement patterns when even small changes in any of the system constraints perturb the organizational waters of the basin.

The state space for a particular motor skill, all of the ways in which movement might be organized to accomplish the goals of the skill, is really made up of a diverse and intertwined collection of many attractors. Some attractors will form deep basins, whereas others will be shallow in comparison. In the early stages of learning a skill, most, if not all, of the attractors available for controlling action will be represented by shallow basins. These attractors will be relatively unstable in maintaining their associated behavioral patterns and easily disturbed by even a slight perturbation in the environment. Small changes in environmental conditions, including cognitive uncertainty and shifting emotional and motivational states, will disrupt the controlling attractor, causing frequent phase shifts to other attractor states as individuals search for more effective movement patterns. As individuals continue to learn, however, well-learned behaviors will pool into deeper and deeper basins. These new deeper basin attractors will exert a stronger draw on muscular organizational patterns, and be more stable and resistant to external perturbations. Movement behaviors will become more consistent and stable, and phase shifts to other attractors will emerge only when sufficient environmental changes occur to warrant new movement patterns.

Learning from a Dynamical Systems Perspective

The process of learning from the perspective of dynamical systems theory involves structuring the learning environment in ways designed to (1) promote the learners' exploration of the state space, and (2) develop deep basins of attraction which can be exploited under various environmental conditions in order to optimize stable and effective movement patterns. Learning is seen as a balancing of exploration and exploitation of the performance landscape. Although this strategy shares many similar instructional implications with schema theory, such as an emphasis on the variability of practice, it also entails distinct differences such as placing a greater emphasis on providing learners with opportunities for the self-discovery of movement options. In chapters dealing with various practice and instructional designs, we will be examining these similarities and differences in greater detail. Both theoretical approaches provide useful conceptualizations about how learning occurs, with each, in its own way, adding to our understanding of how best to approach the teaching and learning of motor skills.

SUMMARY

- Scientific theories explain a broad range of diverse facts and observations by a few encompassing principles, and they allow for the prediction and testing of future observations.
- Two major theoretical approaches dominate motor learning and control scholarship today. The oldest of these approaches are cognitive-based theories, whereas more recent challenges have come from dynamical systems theory.
- Cognitive-based theories are closed system theories in which the central nervous system is held to be responsible for all elements of motor control, with the primary agent of control being a motor program. The dominant expression of cognitive-based theories are information processing models.
  - Information processing models assume either closed-loop or open-loop control mechanisms. The most successful information processing models have been
    - Adams' closed-loop theory
    - Schmidt's schema theory (open-loop)
- Dynamical systems theories are a response to criticisms of cognitive-based theories. Bernstein first identified the degrees of freedom problem with cognitive-based theories and proposed the concept of the synergy as one solution.
- Modern dynamical systems approaches are open system theories assuming interaction among subsystems. Movement scientists applying dynamical systems theories view movement coordination and skilled performance as arising from the synergistic interaction of complex systems. Movement systems are
  - Diverse
  - Connected
  - Interdependent
  - Adapting
- Motor skills, from a dynamical systems perspective, result from emergence, from the cooperating organization of system elements guided by the activities of
  - Movement constraints
  - Self-organization
  - Attractors
- Learning, from a dynamical systems perspective, results from a balancing of exploration and exploitation of the movement environment.

LEARNING EXERCISES

1. Select an open motor skill for which you are both skilled and knowledgeable, and design a set of instructional guidelines based upon principles derived from schema theory for teaching the skill to a beginner.

2. Identify a situation in which you can observe two people performing the same skill at a noticeably different level of expertise, with one person being relatively unskilled and the other person at least fairly well skilled (examples can be found in school and recreational settings, clinics, and training programs for various skills). Observe both individuals for at least 20 minutes each and record your observations of constraints influencing their activities. Record examples of organismic, environmental, and task constraints for each person, indicating how each either limits or facilitates performance. Prepare a table comparing the various constraints you observed between the two individuals. Discuss the results of your observations with reference to how they help explain each person's skill level.

3. For this exercise, you will prepare to take one side in debating the following question: Which offers the better explanation of human movement skills: schema theory or dynamical systems theory? This exercise may be part of a class activity suggested by your instructor, or you might offer it as a suggestion for the class. You may also structure the debate between yourself and another opponent, or for two teams of two or three individuals each. The following debate format is suggested: 5-minute opening arguments (both debaters or team), 5 minutes for rebuttal to opposing arguments (both sides), 5 to 15 minutes for questions from the audience (for either or both sides as directed), 2 minutes for closing statement (both sides). If desired, a vote of the audience can be taken to declare a winning side.

FOR FURTHER STUDY

HOW MUCH DO YOU KNOW?

For each of the following, select the letter that best answers the question.

1. Theories of motor control and learning that assume that processes entirely within the central nervous system are capable of explaining movement phenomena without consideration of factors external to the CNS are termed
   a. closed control systems.
   b. open control systems.
   c. complex systems.
   d. dynamical systems.

2. In order to be truly scientific, a good theory must explain a wide variety of observations through relatively few simple principles, and it must also
   a. be reducible to mathematical formulas.
   b. be incapable of being refuted by future observations.
   c. be supported by a majority of scientists in the area.
   d. make predictions about future observations that can be tested.

3. One advantage of open-loop control mechanisms is that they are good for
   a. relatively slow, precise tasks.
   b. unpracticed tasks.
   c. reactive tasks that must be performed quickly.
   d. tasks that must be performed in unpredictable environments.

4. Which of the following is *not* an invariant feature of generalized motor programs?
   a. Relative timing
   b. Parameter selection

     c. Sequencing

     d. Relative force

5. All but which of the following are characteristic of complex systems?

     a. Connectedness

     b. Adaptability

     c. Diversity

     d. Linearity

6. A sudden spontaneous change from one fixed pattern or state to a new pattern or state within a dynamical system is called a

     a. manifold conversion.

     b. phase shift.

     c. nonlinear conversion.

     d. state-space transition.

Answer the following with the word or words that best complete each sentence.

7. In the information processing model, the stage in which information from the environment is initially received is called the _____ stage.

8. Schema theory offered solutions to two problems with previous motor programming theories, which were the problems of _____ and _____.

9. The implications of schema theory support the _____ of practice hypothesis.

10. First identified by Bernstein, groupings of muscles that can be temporarily constrained to act as a single action unit are called _____.

11. A physical characteristic of an individual, such as flexibility or upper-body strength, which acts to limit the person's action possibilities is called a(n) _____.

12. The quality of complex systems to self-organize to produce new patterns or states not inherent within the system's constituent parts is termed _____.

Answers are provided at the end of this review section.

STUDY QUESTIONS

1. What are scientific theories, and why is their use critical in the study of motor skills? What are the two major divisions among the types of scientific theories?

2. What are the three stages in the information processing model? What processes occur in each of the stages?

3. What are the advantages and disadvantages of both closed-loop and open-loop control processes of information processing?

4. Define Fitts' law and explain how both movement speed and accuracy can be maximized through a blending of both open-loop and closed-loop control processes.

5. Discuss Adams' closed-loop theory of motor control and learning, defining both the memory trace and the perceptual trace, and the theory's implications for instruction and learning.

6. Discuss Schmidt's schema theory. Explain the concept of the generalized motor program, and identify invariant and variant features of the GMP.

7. Delineate the implications of schema theory for instruction and learning, explaining how it supports the variability of practice hypothesis.

8. What kinds of phenomena are studied using dynamical systems theories? Why is human movement considered a dynamical system?

9. What criticisms of cognitive-based theories of human movement and action have led some scientists to adopt dynamical systems approaches as an alternative to the study of motor skills? What are the basic theoretical assumptions of these scientists concerning the nature of human movement skills?

10. What does it mean to say that motor skills are "emergent properties?"

11. How might the insights from both cognitive-based and dynamical systems theories be combined in order to better understand human movement?

ADDITIONAL READING

Clark, JE. (1995). "On becoming skillful: Patterns and constraints." *Research Quarterly for Exercise and Sport*, 66(3), 173–183.

Johnson, S. (2001). *Emergence: The connected lives of ants, brains, cities, and software.* New York: Scribner.

Schmidt, RA. (1982). "More on motor programs." In JAS Kelso (ed.), *Human Motor Behavior: An Introduction* (pp. 189–218). Hillsdale, NJ: Lawrence Erlbaum Associates.

Schmidt, RA. (2003). "Motor schema theory after 27 years: Reflections and implications for a new theory." *Research Quarterly for Exercise and Sport*, 74, 366–375.

Stelmach, GE. (1982). "Information-processing framework for understanding human motor behavior." In Kelso, JAS, *Human motor behavior:*

An introduction (pp. 63–92). Hillsdale, NJ: Lawrence Erlbaum.

Summers, J. (2004). "A historical perspective on skill acquisition." In M Williams and N Hodges (eds.), *Skill acquisition in sport: Research, theory, and practice* (pp. 1–26). London: Routledge.

Turvey, MT, Fitch, KL, and Tuller, B. (1982). "The Bernstein perspective: I. The problems of degrees of freedom and context-conditioned variability." In JAS Kelso (ed.), *Human motor behavior: An introduction* (pp. 239–252). Hillsdale, NJ: Lawrence Erlbaum.

Wallace, SA. (1996). "Dynamic pattern perspective of rhythmic movements: An introduction." In HN Zelaznik (ed.), *Advances in motor learning and control* (pp. 155–194). Champaign, IL: Human Kinetics.

REFERENCES

Adams, JA. (1971). "A closed-loop theory of motor learning." *Journal of Motor Behavior*, 3, 111–150.

Araujo, D, Davids, K, Bennett, SJ, Button, C, and Chapman, G. (2004). "Emergence of sport skills under constraints." In AM Williams and NJ Hodges (eds.), *Skill acquisition in sport: Research, theory and practice* (pp. 409–433). New York: Routledge.

Bernstein, NA. (1967). *The co-ordination and regulation of movement.* London: Pergamon Press.

Bernstein, NA. (1984). "Some emergent problems of the regulation of motor acts." In HTA Whiting (ed.), *Human motor actions: Bernstein reassessed* (pp. 343–371). Amsterdam: North-Holland.

Button, C. (2007). "Enhancing skill acquisition in golf—Some key principles." (http://www.coachesinfo.com/article/?id=55).

Clark, JE. (1995). "On becoming skillful: Patterns and constraints." *Research Quarterly for Exercise and Sport*, 66(3), 173–183.

Coker, CA (2009). *Motor learning and control for practitioners*, 2nd edition. Scottsdale. AZ: Holcomb Hathaway.

Craik, KJW. (1948). "The theory of the human operator in control systems: II. Man as an element in the control system." *British Journal of Psychology*, 38, 142–148.

Davids, K, Button, C, and Bennett, S. (2008). *Dynamics of skill acquisition: A constraints-led approach.* Champaign, IL: Human Kinetics.

Ennis, C. (1992). "Reconceptualizing learning as a dynamical system." *Journal of Curriculum and Supervision*, 7(2), 173–183.

Erdi, P. (2007). *Complexity explained.* New York: Springer.

Fitts, PM. (1954). "The information capacity of the human motor system in controlling the amplitude of movement." *Journal of Experimental Psychology*, 47, 381–391.

Gibson, JJ. (1966). *The senses considered as perceptual systems.* Boston: Houghton Mifflin.

Gibson, JJ. (1979). *The ecological approach to visual perception.* Hillsdale, NJ: Lawrence Erlbaum.

Gurfinkel, VS, and Cordo, PJ. (1998). "The scientific legacy of Nikolai Bernstein." In ML Latash (ed.), *Progress in motor control, vol 1: Bernstein's traditions in movement studies.* (pp. 1–20). Champaign, IL: Human Kinetics.

Hawking, S, and Mlodinow, L. (2005). *A briefer history of time.* New York: Random House.

Holland, JH. (1998). *Emergence: From chaos to order.* Reading, MA: Addison-Wesley.

Huys, R, Daffertshofer, A, and Beek, PJ. (2004). "The evolution of coordination during skill acquisition: The dynamical systems approach." In AM Williams and NJ Hodges (eds.), *Skill acquisition in sport: Research, theory and practice* (pp. 351–373). New York: Routledge.

James, W. (1890). *Principles of psychology.* New York: Holt.

Kelso, JAS, and Schoner, G. (1988). "Self-organization of coordinative movement patterns." *Human Movement Science, 7,* 27–46.

Lashley, KS. (1917). "The accuracy of movement in the absence of excitation from the moving organ." *The American Journal of Physiology, 43,* 169–194.

Latash, ML. (2008). *Synergy.* New York: Oxford University Press.

McMorris, T. (2004). *Acquisition and performance of sports skills.* West Sussex, UK: John Wiley and Sons.

McMorris, T, and Hale, T. (2006). *Coaching science: Theory into practice.* West Sussex, UK: John Wiley and Sons.

Meadows, D. (2008). *Thinking in systems: A primer.* White River, VT: Chelsea Green.

Miller, JH, and Page, SE. (2007). *Complex adaptive systems: An introductory computational model of social life.* Princeton, NJ: Princeton University Press.

Mitchell, M. (2009). *Complexity: A guided tour.* New York: Oxford University Press.

Newell, KM. (1986). "Constraints on the development of coordination." In MG Wade and HTA Whiting (eds.), *Motor development in children: Aspects of coordination and control* (pp. 341–360). Dordrecht, Germany: Martinus Nighoff.

Newell, KM. (2003). "Schema theory (1975): Retrospectives and prospectives." *Research Quarterly for Exercise and Sport, 74,* 383–388.

Saltzman, EL, and Munhall, KG. (1992). "Skill acquisition and development: The role of state-, parameter-, and graph-dynamics." *Journal of Motor Behavior, 24,* 49–57.

Schmidt, RA. (1975). "A schema theory of discrete motor learning skill learning." *Psychological Review, 82,* 225–260.

Schmidt, RA. (2003). "Motor schema theory after 27 years: Reflections and implications for a new theory." *Research Quarterly for Exercise and Sport, 74,* 366–375.

Schmidt, RA, and Lee, TD. (2005). *Motor control and learning: A behavioral emphasis.* Champaign, IL: Human Kinetics.

Shapiro, DC, Zernicke, RE, Gregor, RJ, and Diestel, JD (1981). "Evidence for generalized motor programs using gait pattern analysis." *Journal of Motor Behavior, 13,* 33–47.

Shea, CH, Shebilske, WL, and Worchel, S. (1993). *Motor learning and control.* Englewood Cliffs, NJ: Prentice Hall.

Sherwood, DE, and Lee, TD. (2003). "Schema theory: Critical review and implications for the role of cognition in a new theory of motor learning." *Research Quarterly for Exercise and Sport, 74,* 376–382.

Strogatz, S. (2000). *Sync: The emerging science of spontaneous order.* New York: Hyperion.

Summers, J. (2004). "A historical perspective on skill acquisition." In M Williams and N Hodges (eds.), *Skill acquisition in sport: Research, theory, and practice* (pp. 1–26). London: Routledge.

Turvey, MT, Fitch, KL, and Tuller, B. (1982). "The Bernstein perspective: I. The problems of degrees of freedom and context-conditioned variability." In JAS Kelso (ed.), *Human motor behavior: An introduction* (pp. 239–252). Hillsdale, NJ: Lawrence Erlbaum.

Wallace, SA. (1996). "Dynamic pattern perspective of rhythmic movements: An introduction." In HN Zelaznik (ed.), *Advances in motor learning and control* (pp. 155–194). Champaign, IL: Human Kinetics.

Answers to How Much Do You Know questions: (1) A, (2) D, (3) C, (4) B, (5) D, (6) B, (7) perceptual, (8) storage and novelty, (9) variability, (10) synergies, (11) organismic constraint, (12) emergence.

CHAPTER 5

The Learning of Motor Skills

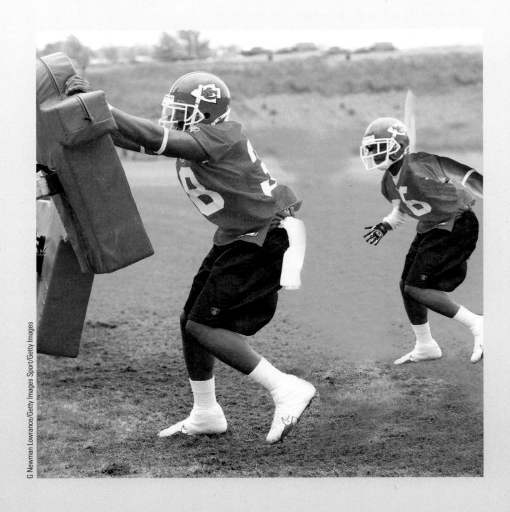

G Newman Lowrance/Getty Images Sport/Getty Images

"Learning is not attained by chance, it must be sought for with ardor and attended to with diligence."
Abigail Adams, 1780

KEY QUESTIONS

- How is learning defined?

- How do performance and learning differ?

- How is learning measured? Are all improvements in performance indications of learning?

- What is the law of practice?

- Is there an upper limit to how much a person can learn?

- Is it necessary to continue practicing a skill once a desired level of performance is achieved?

- When does learning one skill benefit the learning of a second skill?

CHAPTER OVERVIEW

If you were planning a trip by car to a new city you had never visited before, perhaps one in another state, what would be the first thing that you would do? More than likely, you would look at a map. You would want to get a general idea of where the city was located. Where is it in relation to other cities that you know, and have perhaps visited? How far, and in what direction, is it from where you presently live?

Because you are driving, you would also want to identify the major routes you could take in your travels, and determine which would be the best ones to follow. You probably know from experience that starting on a trip without a clear plan for getting to where you want to go, is not a good idea. Without knowing the major routes leading to your destination, you are likely to get lost along the way. Without knowing the major highways to take, all roads are as likely to look inviting, and it becomes easy to take incorrect turns and follow roads that lead in the wrong direction from the intended city. You may even eventually become so disoriented and lost, that you give up on your travels altogether.

Starting on the journey toward understanding what constitutes the most effective methods for learning motor skills is a lot like starting on a journey to a new city. Just as you would not consult a city street map to determine the best way of reaching the city, so we cannot accurately comprehend the specific methods for best learning motor skills without first understanding the major principles, laws, and assumptions that underlie such learning. As a road map shows the best way of reaching a new city, fundamental principles in the domain of motor learning reveal the most effective methods for attaining new movement skills. In this chapter, we will examine fundamental principles and laws that guide decisions about practice. Just as first consulting a road map prevents you from getting lost when traveling to a new city, understanding the fundamentals of learning can prevent you from drawing false conclusions about how to best help people learn motor skills. In this chapter, we explore those essential fundamentals.

Motor skills, as we saw in Chapter 2, entail an extensive variety of human behaviors. Activities as diverse as walking across a street to driving on a busy highway, typing a letter to playing a musical instrument, or performing a triple axial in ice skating to crashing through the line in football are all examples of motor skills. Although such diverse activities may appear on their surface to have little in common, a central feature of all of them is that each is acquired through learning. Recall again from Chapter 2 that an essential component of the definition of skills is that they are learned behaviors. All skills, from the simplest to the most complex, are learned through either practice or experience.

Even though motor skills encompass a broad diversity of behaviors, extensive research spanning more than a century has revealed common principles underlying their learning (Anderson, 1981; Lane, 1987; Lee and Swinnen, 1993; Proctor and Dutta, 1995; Rosenbaum, Carlson, and Gilmore, 2001). So normative are the patterns of skill acquisition, in fact, that highly predictive principles and laws have been identified to describe the processes underlying skill learning. The same fundamental principles of learning apply to a child learning to take his or her first steps, a dancer learning a new ballet routine, a track and field athlete learning to put the shot, and a stroke patient relearning to grasp objects.

The ability to learn a wide variety of new motor skills throughout life is one of the most essential capacities possessed by humans. Understanding how people learn motor skills, and how they can learn them most effectively, is a particularly critical and useful area of human knowledge. In this chapter, we will look at the ways in which movement scientists study skill learning, as well as the fundamental principles of motor learning that derive from such study.

DEFINING LEARNING

Any attempt to define learning must begin with the important distinction between performance and learning. Far from simply being a definitional consideration, this distinction is critical. As we will see in this chapter and in others to follow, a failure to appreciate the distinction between performance and learning can lead to many false conclusions concerning instructional and practice methods, the assessment of learning, or even whether learning has occurred at all. Such conclusions can, and frequently do, lead directly to less than optimal learning outcomes.

Performance

performance: Qualitative or quantitative assessment of what can be observed during the execution of a skill.

Simply stated, **performance** is observable behavior. If you see someone bicycle across campus, serve a tennis ball, or swim laps in a pool, you are observing their performance of these skills. Performance refers to the execution of a skill at a specific time and in a specific location or situation. In speaking of performance, we may refer to a single execution of a skill ("She drove the ball 200 yards down the fairway."), to a single manifestation of skills within a specific context ("He was really on his game and played well today."), or even to the evaluation of an extended series of performance observations ("The Bobcats played poorly this season.") Additionally, performance may be measured and specified quantitatively (a 200-yard drive), or referred to in a more evaluative qualitative fashion (the Bobcats had a poor season). In each case, however, the evaluation of performance is based upon observations of skill level at specific places and times.

Learning, on the other hand, cannot be observed directly but must be *inferred* from the characteristics of a person's performance. What we observe is always performance—never learning.

Learning

learning: A relatively stable change in performance resulting from practice or experience.

Learning, the process by which people acquire a new capacity to perform a skill, is inferred from performance observations. We infer that learning has occurred (or has not) based upon observations of performance. We should not be surprised, for example, to hear that someone had "learned" to play tennis if we observed him or her unable to hit the ball during an initial practice season, and then returned some months later to see the same person placing ball after ball precisely in an opponent's court. Clearly, he or she has acquired a new capacity to perform tennis skills that indicates that learning must have taken place. We would further expect that if we inquired about the person's activities during the intervening months, we would be told about many hours of practice devoted to improving tennis skills. We would be surprised, and probably more than a bit skeptical, to be told that no practice had occurred between the first and second time we observed the person playing tennis. We know from experience that improvements of such magnitude cannot occur without practice.

Finally, if asked whether we thought that the tennis player would perform more like the first or second time we observed him or her play if we returned tomorrow, we would obviously respond by saying more like the second time—skills are not just lost overnight. In fact, we would expect that if we returned in several months, or even after several years, our tennis player would never completely revert to his or her original inability to hit the ball, even if some skill level was lost due to nonpractice. More than likely, we would assume that further practice would continue and lead to even better performances of tennis skills in the future.

In our example, we inferred that the tennis player had demonstrated his or her learning of tennis skills in three ways: (1) The player's performance improved over time, (2) the improvement resulted from practice, and (3) the player's improved skill level was stable and, to some degree at least, permanent. If we forge these common-sense observations of learning into a definition, we can then define learning as a change in the capacity to perform a skill that is inferred from a relatively permanent improvement in performance as a result of practice or experience. It should be carefully noted in our example that learning is not (and never is) observed directly, but rather is inferred from performance observations. We infer that learning has occurred when the following three conditions are observed, which comprise the definition of learning:

1. Learning is a change in performance or the capacity to perform.
2. Learning results from practice or experience.
3. Learning is relatively stable or permanent.

The Learning–Performance Distinction

Considerable misunderstanding concerning the degree of learning attained during practice results from failing to fully appreciate the distinctions between learning and performance. At the root of this misunderstanding is the assumption that performance is an accurate reflection of learning, a mirror in which is displayed the true image of learning. The problem with this assumption is that what we see when observing performance is not always an accurate reflection of learning. Indeed, the mirror of performance from which we are prone to draw such conclusions frequently reflects a distorted image of learning, just as mirrors found in carnival fun houses distort one's true body image.

The major problem with assuming that performance is an accurate reflection of learning is that such thinking leads to the further assumption that learning is best facilitated when it is accompanied by good performance. The better the performance, the better the learning. It follows from this that enhancing performance within practice should be a major goal of the motor skills practitioner. Similarly, practice resulting in performance that is less than that of which a learner is capable is assumed to also be less effective in promoting optimal learning. But although it is true that performance often does mirror learning accurately, it is just as true that it can, and frequently does, mask the true quality and extent of learning. The effective practitioner must therefore understand when performance is, and when it is not, a reliable guide for assessing learning.

The problem in relying too exclusively on performance observations when assessing learning is that performance is a *temporary* expression of a learner's ability to execute a skill. As such, it is a reflection both of the person's learned capacity to perform the skill *and* of the presence of temporary features inherent within the practice or performance context. These temporary factors are called *performance variables*, and include instructional, environmental, and learner characteristics.

Instructional characteristics include such factors as type of practice schedule, the order in which various skills are sequenced, the relative intensity or restfulness of practice, the use of simplification techniques such as part practice,

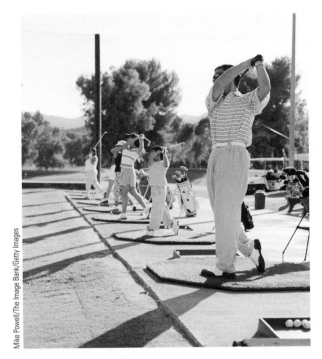

Mike Powell/The Image Bank/Getty Images

An individual's performance during practice may not always be a good indicator of how effectively he or she is learning.

type of instructions provided to learners, and the amount and type of feedback given to learners. Environmental characteristics include the physical characteristics of the practice setting as well as any equipment that is used in executing skills. Learner characteristics include such factors as anxiety, fatigue, motivation, physical condition, the use of stimulants or drugs, and whether practicing alone or in the presence of others.

Each of the factors just listed, as well as many not listed, can have pronounced effects on practice performance. Some factors may help learners perform well during practice, but such performance enhancement is not permanent and quickly dissipates once practice is over. Some factors, on the other hand, may depress a learner's capacity to perform during practice, but once the temporarily imposed practice conditions are removed, the learner may be able to demonstrate an improved capacity to perform (i.e., can demonstrate having learned to perform better than he or she was capable of performing during practice). The effective motor skills instructor must understand this **learning–performance distinction**, and be able to discriminate between temporary effects on performance and more permanent influences on learning. We will especially consider the influence of a number of such performance variables in Chapters 11 and 12. Basic distinctions between performance and learning are summarized in Table 5.1.

learning–performance distinction: Refers to the well-established finding that performance measures during acquisition may mask the true degree of learning that has occurred.

TABLE **5.1**
Differences between Performance and Learning

Performance	Learning
• Observable behavior—What we can see	• Inferred from performance—cannot be observed directly
• May represent only temporary changes in behavior	• Relatively permanent changes in behavior
• Influenced by performance variables	• Not influenced by performance variables

ASSESSING LEARNING—MEASURING ART

Learning, as we have seen, cannot be directly observed but must be inferred from performance observations. But as we have also seen, the presence of different performance variables may obscure the true quality of learning occurring during practice. How do researchers study the effects of various performance artifacts and disentangle their differing effects on performance and learning? How can they tell the degree to which learning has actually occurred?

There are three methods for determining from observations of performance if, and the degree to which, learning has occurred. These three methods are (1) measurements of acquisition, (2) retention tests, and (3) transfer tests. All three methods require repeated observations of performance. It is typical in motor learning research to use all three methods in combination because each provides different but equally important information on the extent and nature of learning. For simplicity, we can refer to these three types of measurement as **ART measures** (i.e., short for acquisition, retention, and transfer measurements).

ART measures:
An acronym for the acquisition, retention, and transfer measurements used in assessing learning in an experiment.

acquisition: Those practice experiences of a skill designed to influence the learning of the skill.

Acquisition

Acquisition refers to the direct measurement of performance experiences. In a laboratory experiment, for example, a series of practice trials may be observed and the results for each trial measured and recorded. These measurements represent any changes in performance observed over the course of practice, which could entail a single laboratory session of a specified number of trials or a significantly longer period of time encompassing many practice sessions. In a sense, acquisition measures are analogous to practice periods, because they are designed as the method for "acquiring" (i.e., learning) a skill. Acquisition trials include all of the practice attempts designed specifically for purposes of skill learning. Acquisition measurements are direct, faithful recordings of observed performance. A series of acquisition measures may be graphed to illustrate changes in performance over the course of practice and is referred to as a *performance curve* (about which we will have more to say later in this chapter).

The important point to recognize about acquisition measurements is that they are measurements of performance rather than of learning. Although not direct measurements of learning, acquisition measurements do, however, illustrate important features of learning such as the effect of various performance variables on skill attainment.

Retention

retention test: A measurement of performance conducted subsequent to acquisition trials and after sufficient time has elapsed to allow any effects of performance variables to dissipate.

retention: The persistence of improvement in the performance of a skill over a period of no practice; it is interpreted as a measure of learning.

performance variable: A variable influencing performance measures during acquisition, but which has little or no influence on learning.

retention interval: The time elapsed between the completion of acquisition trials and a retention test in a learning experiment.

Retention tests refer to performance measurements conducted subsequent to acquisition trials or observations. They provide sufficient time for any effects of performance variables acting during acquisition to dissipate. Remembering that one of the three key elements in the definition of learning is that it is a relatively permanent improvement in performance, then performance that has been *retained* over a period of nonpractice can be said to have been learned. **Retention** refers to the persistence of original learning over a period of no practice.

During acquisition, a number of variables may influence performance. Although it is tempting to assume that the only (or at least primary) variable influencing performance during acquisition is learning, this is not always the case, as we have previously stated. Many **performance variables,** such as instructional methods, the practice environment, and subject motivation can influence performance. Performance variables may influence performance both positively and negatively, but their effects are temporary. Such temporary effects mask the real effects of learning. To measure retention, these temporary effects of performance variables during acquisition must be allowed to dissipate. After some period of time, called a **retention interval** (which experimentally could vary between as little as 10 minutes to as long as several days, weeks, or even months), a new performance measurement is taken of a small slice of performance capability (e.g., either a single or relatively small number of trials). This method allows for only the relatively permanent changes in performance that result from practice to influence performance measurements (as long as a limited number of trials are measured before performance variables can again "build up" to influence performance). In this way, presumably only the permanent influences affecting performance are retained and measured, and these then allow for the inference that learning has occurred. For this reason, retention is typically considered a more accurate measure of learning than are acquisition measures.

Transfer Tests

transfer test: A type of retention test in which the object is to measure the amount of learning that can be transferred to a similar but different skill, or to the original skill in a new context.

The third method for measuring learning is the **transfer test.** Simply stated, a transfer test measures how effectively a person can transfer the learning of a skill from one condition to another. Does learning to shoot a basketball from a set position directly in front of the basket transfer to an ability to make angled corner shots of an equal distance? Does learning to dribble around cones placed on a basketball floor transfer to effectively dribbling against live opponents? In both examples, transfer is a measure of the strength of learning in terms of how adaptable the learning is to novel, nonpracticed conditions. Such conditions can represent performance of the skill in a new way (side corner shots rather than those made directly in front of the basket), or performance of the skill in the manner practiced but within a new context (against live opponents rather than statically placed cones). In either case, the ability to adapt the practiced skill to performance in a novel way is a measure of the strength of learning. Unlike retention tests that measure learning in terms of improvement of a skill as practiced, transfer tests measure learning effects in terms of the adaptability, or generalizability, of learning, which in many circumstances is an essential goal of learning. If performance in the new situation is "high," then transfer is considered to have taken place and therefore learning to have occurred "robustly" in the original practice situation. At this point, however, we will merely mention transfer tests and their place in assessing learning; later in this chapter we will discuss the concept of transfer more thoroughly.

Taken Together, "ART" Measurements "Paint" a Complete Picture of Learning

Each of the ART measures contributes something unique to our understanding of the learning process. Acquisition measurements allow us to determine the "shape" and "rate" of learning; that is, we can investigate factors that influence performance and, presumably, the rate of learning. Retention tests tell us about learning independently of temporary performance variables; they help us identify whether learning is occurring even when comparatively poor performance would seem to indicate otherwise. Retention tests also tell us about the permanence of practice effects. Transfer tests allow us to measure the influence of practice on the strength of learning such that it can be readily transferred to other settings and conditions.

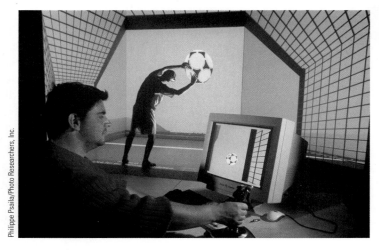

Philippe Psaila/Photo Researchers, Inc.

In order to accurately assess the effects of different variables on learning, researchers typically perform acquisition, retention, and transfer tests.

ASSESSING LEARNING—A "CLASSIC" MOTOR LEARNING EXPERIMENT

In order to understand the influence of various practice conditions on learning, researchers are interested in how various experimental manipulations affect the acquisition, retention, and transfer of motor skills. It is therefore typical for researchers to test all three ART measurements in their experimental investigations. To see how these three types of measurements are used in motor learning research, we will describe an important study in the history of motor learning. Two researchers, John Shea and Robyn Morgan, conducted the study in 1979, and their findings subsequently influenced the way motor skills are taught in many different settings.

The question that interested Shea and Morgan concerned the effects of two different methods of scheduling practice. Traditionally, and certainly at the time Shea and Morgan reported their research findings, instructors in various motor learning settings believed that **blocked practice** scheduling was the best way to teach (and to learn) motor skills. For example, if three different skills were scheduled for instruction during a practice session, then it was believed that they should be blocked into three *independently presented units* for instruction. All of the first skill would be practiced and completed before moving on to the second skill, which would then be completely practiced before moving on to the third skill. In this fashion, each skill was practiced in a block for the total number of trials instructed before instruction and practice were provided for the next skill. This is a traditional method of teaching motor skills that is still widely used today (although in too many instances, it is not the *best* method).

Shea and Morgan questioned this traditional approach. They hypothesized that, compared to a blocked presentation of skills, a random ordering of skill presentation might be more effective for learning. In a **random practice** schedule of three different skills, for example, all three skills are mixed and randomly presented in the practice order, such that the learner does not know from one practice trial to the next which skill is to be performed. (Shea and Morgan had theoretical reasons for believing that random practice might be beneficial; they did not decide to compare these two instructional methods on a whim.)

To test their idea, Shea and Morgan developed a laboratory task in which the research subjects sat in front of a small table-like device with six upright barriers (three on each side) that could be knocked down with a blow from the subject's hand (see Figure 5.1). Three colored lights were attached to the front of the device. As a subject sat in front of the device, one of the three lights would be lit. Depending on the color of the light, the subject was to knock down three of the barriers in a prescribed order as quickly as possible—each color light indicating a different order, or pattern, for knocking down the barriers. Shea and Morgan split their subjects into two groups—a "blocked" practice group and a "random" practice group. Each group was presented exactly the same number of practice trials—54 in all—but in a different order. The blocked group practiced one pattern for 18 trials before moving on to practice the second pattern, again for 18 trials, and then finally the last pattern for

blocked practice:
A practice schedule in which the same skill is rehearsed in repetitive fashion.

random practice:
A practice schedule in which different skills are rehearsed in an unpredictable trial-to-trial order.

18 trials. The random group also practiced 18 trials of each pattern, but in a random order. Subjects in the random group did not know from one trial to the next which color light would be lit and therefore which pattern they were expected to duplicate in knocking down the barriers.

To compare the acquisition scores of the blocked and random practice groups, the researchers averaged scores into six blocks of 6 trials each. The less time subjects needed to complete a block, the better their performance. The results of the acquisition performance are presented in Figure 5.2. Viewing the figure, we can observe that the two practice schedules resulted in markedly different acquisition patterns. The blocked group improved quickly compared to the random group, and in fact performed better on all blocks of trials. The random group appeared to acquire performance capabilities at a much slower rate initially and never to attain the same performance level as did subjects in the blocked group (although they did get closer in the final trials).

Based only upon observations of performance during acquisition, we could easily conclude from these experimental results that blocked practice is superior to random practice for learning (because of the mistaken assumption that methods promoting the best practice performance must be the best for learning, as has been previously stated). But remember that performance is influenced by various performance variables that may mask the true nature of learning. In this case, the effects of scheduling (i.e., blocked and random) may have acted as performance variables influencing performance and learning in different ways. To investigate this possibility, a retention test was required.

To conduct their retention test, Shea and Morgan had subjects rest for 10 minutes before performing a final block of retention trials. This period

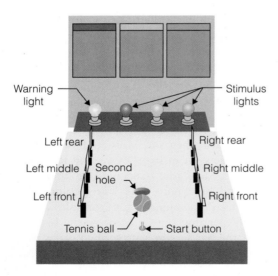

FIGURE **5.1** Apparatus Used in Shea and Morgan Experiment

Source: Adapted from Shea, JB and Kohl, RM. (1991). "Composition of practice: Influence on the retention of motor skills." *Research Quarterly for Exercise and Sport, 62,* 187–195.

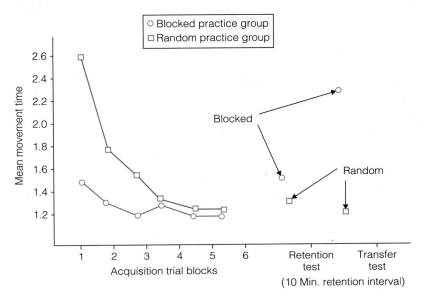

FIGURE **5.2** **Results of Shea and Morgan Experiment**

Source: Adapted from Shea, JB and Kohl, RM. (1991). "Composition of practice: Influence on the retention of motor skills." *Research Quarterly for Exercise and Sport, 62,* 187–195.

of nonpractice, the retention interval, allowed for any temporary acquisition effects on performance to dissipate so that the measurement of performance after the rest period was most likely to capture a true measure of learning uncontaminated by other performance factors, in this case those attributed to scheduling effects. In this experiment, for instance, one important performance variable associated with the two practice schedules was believed to be short-term memory. Subjects in the blocked practice group were advantaged by the relatively reduced demands placed upon memory compared to those subjects in the random practice group. Blocked subjects simply had less of a demand placed upon their memories, which may have facilitated their better acquisition performance. In contrast, the greater demand placed on the memories of the random practice subjects, although hindering their performance, may have actually led to superior learning. This was one of the possibilities that Shea and Morgan conducted their experiment to investigate. A retention interval of 10 minutes was used because this period is sufficient to allow short-term memory effects to dissipate. (In many cases, researchers will employ not only a relatively short retention interval of 10 or 15 minutes, but will also conduct a second retention test after a longer interval of anywhere from a day to several months in order to examine both immediate and long-term influences on learning. In fact, Shea and Morgan also included a second retention test after a 10-day retention interval. Because the results of this second retention test supported the findings of the more immediate 10-minute test, however, we will exclude it for the sake of simplifying our discussion.)

After the retention interval, half of the subjects from each practice group performed a final block of practice trials (we will see why Shea and Morgan used only half of the subjects from each group shortly). Subjects from the blocked practice group performed all six trials of the same pattern, with one-third of the subjects presented the red-ordered pattern, one-third the blue pattern, and one-third the green pattern. The subjects in the random practice group were presented two trials of each of the three patterns, though the order of presentation was mixed among the subjects.

Again viewing Figure 5.2, we see that the random practice group performed better on the retention test than did the blocked practice group. That is, even though the subjects in the random group failed to perform at the same level as subjects in the blocked group during acquisition, they retained a greater capacity to perform once the acquisition phase ended and the influence of performance-only factors were allowed to dissipate. Remember that an essential part of the definition of learning is that it is a permanent change in performance, or in the capacity to perform. In this case, the inclusion of a retention test revealed something unobserved when looking at performance during acquisition alone, which was that random practice led to better retention outcomes than did blocked practice.

To further investigate the comparative effects of blocked and random practice, Shea and Morgan included a transfer test. Remember that transfer tests may be conducted in different ways. One type of transfer test is to have subjects perform the same skill, but under new conditions. Another type of transfer test involves performing a variation of the originally practiced skill. In either case, the goal is to assess the strength of learning by assessing the effectiveness of the original acquisition conditions in transferring either to new performance conditions or new variations of the skill. Often the type of transfer test is made based upon ecological considerations. That is, skills are often practiced in conditions differing from those in which they will ultimately be performed. An important aspect in assessing the strength of learning is to determine how effective acquisition conditions prove in promoting the adaptability of performance in these intended new conditions (we will discuss specific factors influencing transfer later in this chapter).

In Shea and Morgan's experiment, they assumed a rather broad and general transfer paradigm. Remember that the dominant practice schedule design at the time Shea and Morgan conducted their study (and perhaps even still) was blocked practice. Shea and Morgan realized, however, that even when skills were practiced under blocked conditions, they were not always intended to be performed in a prescribed order. Practicing three different tennis strokes in blocked fashion, for example, is not really ecologically valid, because the intention of practice is to learn to perform any of the three skills quickly and effectively as game conditions dictate. Other skills are practiced with the intention that they will always be performed in a single and predictable way, such as shooting a free throw in basketball or performing a forward somersault in a gymnastics floor routine. How does the intention of practice relate to the strength of learning for both blocked and random practice, then?

Given that the random practice group showed better retention performance than the blocked practice group, can the effectiveness of random practice be generalized to skills regardless of the intended performance conditions, or should skills be practiced using either a random or blocked practice depending on how they will ultimately be performed? To help answer these questions, Shea and Morgan used a transfer test in which subjects from the blocked practice group were transferred to a randomly presented block of six trials as a transfer test, whereas subjects from the random practice group were presented with a block of six trials of the same pattern as their transfer test (with an equal number of each of the three patterns distributed among them). The remaining half of the subjects in both the blocked and random practice groups, those not receiving the retention test, were then transferred to a transfer test of the opposite condition from that under which they had practiced. In this fashion, the strength of learning under both blocked and random acquisition conditions could be assessed for differing conditions of transfer.

Results of the transfer test revealed a marked difference in performance between the two groups (see Figure 5.2). When the random practice group was transferred to a blocked performance condition, they demonstrated a pronounced ability to perform, and in fact were able to perform at a better level than they had under either acquisition or retention conditions. The blocked practice group, however, proved particularly ineffective at performing under the random conditions. Indeed, their performance in the random transfer conditions was worse than their initial block of acquisition trials.

Given the results of their experiment, Shea and Morgan concluded that even though skill performance was better under a blocked practice schedule than under a random practice schedule, retention and transfer were better for those practicing under a random schedule of skill order. Based upon these results, Shea and Morgan concluded that random practice results in better learning than does blocked practice, at least for conditions similar to those of their experiment. This was also one of the first experiments in motor learning (there have been many more since) to clearly demonstrate the learning–performance distinction.

Although our discussion here is limited to illustrating the use of ART measurements in the assessment of learning, it should also be pointed out that Shea and Morgan's study has had profound ramifications on our understanding of practice effects in motor skill learning. Researchers are still investigating the extent of the benefits of random practice that Shea and Morgan were the first to report. There is still some question, for instance, concerning why random practice is so beneficial, as well as questions concerning what type of skills benefit most from random practice scheduling. Nevertheless, random practice effects are widely accepted—and used—today, and it was through the assiduous application of acquisition measurements, retention tests, and transfer tests that their benefits were first identified. This study also cogently demonstrated the distinction between performance and learning, especially highlighting how observations of performance only (i.e., what we see) can be misleading indicators of the amount of actual learning taking place.

THE SHAPE OF LEARNING—PERFORMANCE CURVES

When discussing acquisition measurements, we alluded to the fact that the plotting of individual performance observations could yield graphic representations called performance curves. Although performance curves may be influenced by performance variables distorting their accuracy as valid depictions of learning (such as we saw in the Shea and Morgan experiment), they nevertheless are particularly useful in determining several important aspects of learning. Performance curves tell us a great deal about the specific pattern (the "shape") and the rate of learning during acquisition, for example. (Performance curves are so useful in this regard that they are frequently, if inappropriately, referred to as "learning curves").

performance curve:
A two-dimensional graph of the changes in performance measures over time as a result of practice.

The **performance curve** is a line graph made up of a series of performance observations. Typically, a performance measurement (some measure of accuracy or speed) is plotted against a sequence of trials (or blocks of trials). The units of the performance are represented on the ordinate (i.e., vertical or Y-axis) of the graph, and the trials on the abscissa (i.e., horizontal or X-axis). Once these data are plotted, a "line of best fit" can be drawn through the individual data points to represent the general pattern or shape of performance (there are also mathematical methods for doing this). The resulting performance curve is a general representation of changes in performance over practice trials. From this general curve, the rate and nature of learning can be assessed.

As an example, consider a person performing a tracking task on a rotary pursuit device (see Figure 5.3). This laboratory device consists of an illuminated target that rotates at a prescribed speed forming a circle pattern (square and triangle patterns are also possible). The research subject holds a light sensitive wand in his or her hand and attempts to track (follow) the target by keeping the point of the wand over the illuminated target. Accuracy in this task is measured by "time on target," or the time a subject can maintain the wand over the target for a prescribed period. Assuming a simple experiment where a subject attempts 15 trials at 30 seconds each, we could plot the resulting acquisition measurements as shown in Figure 5.3. Notice that from the individual trial scores, a smoothly curved line of best fit is drawn. This curved line represents the general shape or trend of the individual measurements plotted, as well as all other acquisition measurements that could have been made during the acquisition period. That is, it graphically illustrates the general course of performance over time during the acquisition phase of learning.

Observing Figure 5.3, we can see two features of the performance curve from which we might reasonably infer that learning has occurred. First, the general direction of the graph is upward, which in this case indicates an improvement in performance over the acquisition trials. From these improved performance observations, we can infer that learning has occurred. Remember, though, that the presence of any number of performance variables may be clouding the true degree of learning, which could be either greater or less than indicated by the performance curve alone.

The second apparent feature observed is that the performance trials become more consistent over time. In the early trials, there is a relatively large difference between trials, whereas in the latter trials the differences become

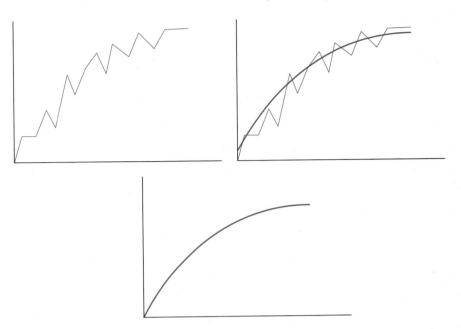

FIGURE **5.3** Acquisition on a Rotary Pursuit Task

Source: Created by author

linear performance curve: A performance curve in which equal amounts of time or number of trials during practice correspond to equal increases in performance measures.

negatively accelerating performance curve: A performance curve exhibiting diminished improvements in performance measures as a function of time or trials of practice.

positively accelerating performance curve: A performance curve exhibiting increasing improvements in performance measures as a function of time or trials of practice.

smaller—performance becomes more consistent. Both improved performance scores and greater consistency of scores indicate that learning has occurred. The curve, however, is called a "performance" rather than a "learning" curve because its shape is still subject to influences of performance variables unrepresentative of learning. (It should be noted, though, that the more trials, or longer the acquisition period, the more stable performance appears to become over time, and the more accurately the performance curve can be considered representative of learning.)

Types of Performance Curves

In assessing learning through performance curves, researchers have identified four general patterns among the types of performance curves possible. These four types of performance curves are shown in Figure 5.4 and are labeled linear, negatively accelerating, positively accelerating, and S-shaped or Ogive (Adams, 1977; Rudisill and Jackson, 1992).

The first of the general performance curve shapes, the **linear performance curve**, suggests that learning occurs proportionally over time. That is, equal amounts of practice yield equal results in skill improvement regardless of the point during acquisition in which it occurs. A **negatively accelerating performance curve** illustrates learning occurring more rapidly early in acquisition and then slowing as practice continues. In contrast, a **positively accelerating performance curve** illustrates greater improvement in performance later, rather than early, in

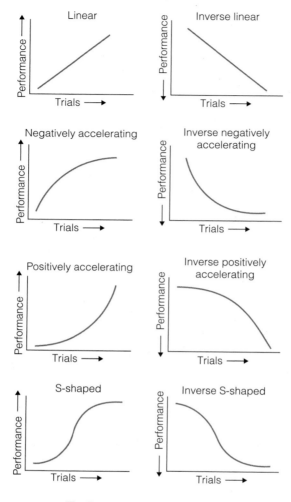

FIGURE **5.4** Performance Curves

Source: Created by author

S-shaped performance curve: A performance curve exhibiting relatively slow rates of improvement both early and late during acquisition, but accelerated rates of learning during the middle phase of acquisition.

acquisition. Finally, an **S-shaped performance curve** (also called an *Ogive* curve) demonstrates learning occurring slowly both early and later during acquisition but accelerating during the middle phase of practice. It should be noted that Figure 5.4 represents performance curves where learning is indicated by increasing performance scores. If learning were indicated by a decreasing performance measure, such as many skills in which reduced time indicates improved performance, the performance curves would be labeled "inverse," and reversed 180 degrees from their positive orientation (as seen in Figure 5.4.). You can test your understanding of performance curves by completing the exercise in Box 5.1.

Is There a "Normal" Performance Curve?

Of the four general types of performance curves, the most commonly observed is the negatively accelerating curve. That is, when acquiring motor skills, most individuals experience their greatest rate of improvement early in learning, whereas once the skill has been learned to some moderate level of performance, further improvements become increasing diminished and difficult. When initial performance requires the learning of particularly difficult—and perhaps novel—movement patterns, or the acquisition of complex cognitive skills before efficient practice of motor elements can be performed, a positively accelerating or S-shaped performance curve is more likely to result. In this case, the learner experiences difficulty in acquiring prerequisite skills necessary to successfully practice desired motor skills, so that initial performance is hindered until these requisite skills are sufficiently gained. After acquiring the requisite skills or knowledge, however, the continued learning of the motor skill will resemble the typical negatively accelerating pattern. In many cases, the demands inherent during early practice experiences may actual lead to beneficial learning outcomes, even when initial performance measures may be depressed. (If initial measures of depressed performance persist, however, it may be an indication that the level of practice is too challenging to be effective in promoting learning.)

In most situations, however, and certainly when performance is measured over extended periods of time, the negatively accelerating performance curve is considered the "typical" or "normal" curve relating performance to practice (Lane, 1987). Curves do deviate from this common shape, but usually as the result of one or more well-understood task characteristics or practice conditions. The negatively accelerating shape is sufficiently regular to form a baseline, or target curve, for learning, with major deviations often representing undetected aspects of the practice or training program.

Performance Curves May Represent Only Initial Phases of Learning

It is important to make one final observation about performance curves. Performance curves are representations of learning patterns only during early and intermediate phases of learning. At some point after an intermediate stage of learning

---

BOX 5.1   **Can You Identify the Performance Curve**

Decide which type of performance curve (linear, negatively accelerating, positively accelerating, or S-shaped) would most likely result in each of the following examples of skill learning. Also consider whether the curves would be regularly or inversely oriented.

- A teenager learning to drive a car with a stick shift on city streets
- A post-surgery knee-replacement patient relearning to walk in a clinical setting

- Learning bowling for the first time
- Learning to type (with performance measured by the number of words per minute correctly typed)
- A worker on an egg-packing line learning to sort various grades and sizes of eggs into correct cartons as quickly as possible
- An experienced dancer learning a new routine
- Learning to pole vault for the first time
- Learning tennis Wii for a novice gamer

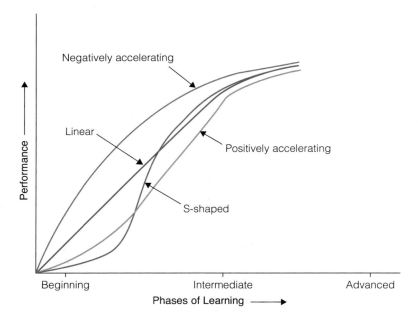

Performance

Negatively accelerating

Linear

Positively accelerating

S-shaped

Beginning   Intermediate   Advanced

Phases of Learning ⟶

FIGURE **5.5** Merging of Performance Curves

Source: Created by author

has been achieved, all four curves merge into a negatively accelerating pattern (see Figure 5.5). If this were not the case, then two of the curved patterns—linear and positively accelerating—would continue unabated in performance gains (and presumably learning gains as well), becoming exponentially larger as practice continued. Obviously, this cannot happen. Three of the performance curve types (linear, positively accelerating, and S-shaped) are considered representative of learning patterns observed only in beginning to intermediate phases of skill acquisition, which might range from a few trials to many months of practice, depending on a number of factors including skill complexity and quality of practice. (In Chapter 7, we will label this intermediate phase of learning more technically as the *associate stage* of learning.) The negatively accelerating performance curve, whether it is observed in these initial phases of learning or not, eventually becomes the pattern of acquisition in all learning situations. It is, in fact, so predictive that its pattern can be stated as being lawfully predictive, an important feature of learning to which we will next turn.

WHAT PERFORMANCE CURVES REVEAL ABOUT THE NATURE OF LEARNING

No doubt when learning many new motor skills, you have experienced rapid improvements in performance during the initial periods of practice, but as practice continued the rate at which you improved slowed down; you did not notice such large changes in performance as before, and the time between periods of noticeable change began to take longer and longer. This is, of course, the exact experience predicted by the negatively accelerating performance curve that captures the normal or typical pattern of learning most new skills. Regardless how small or large the actual improvement in performance, this pattern of change in the rate of learning is observed across virtually all motor skills (if not always in the initial stages of learning, eventually as learning progresses).

The Law of Practice

The regularity of the pattern for the rate of improvement during practice has long been recognized. Its first scientific recognition came in 1926, when an industrial psychologist named George Snoddy was attempting to determine differences in the time that it took workers to learn a number of different occupational skills (Snoddy, 1926). Industrial psychology was a new field at that time and no one had yet thought about investigating how the rates of learning might change for different kinds of physical work skills, though there was considerable interest in differences in training time that it took employees to acquire proficiency in occupationally related manual skills. After collecting large amounts of data from employees learning several different types of manufacturing and assembly skills, Snoddy noticed that even though the time to learn these different skills might greatly vary, there was nevertheless a consistency in the pattern of how the rates of learning changed as a result of experience. As a result of these observations, Snoddy formulated a mathematical expression of these consistent rate changes that became known as the **law of practice**.

law of practice: Improvement in performance continues as long as practice continues, but the rate at which it occurs gradually and predictably diminishes over time or number of practice trials; it can be expressed mathematically as a power function.

The law of practice is one of the most ubiquitous and highly reliable laws in learning theory. According to it, changes in performance during early practice are relatively large. As practice continues, however, the amount of improvement (its rate) becomes progressively smaller in comparison to previous rates of improvement (recall here that the negatively accelerating performance curve represents the normal shape of learning). This change in the rate of improvement over practice is so regular and predictable that it can be mathematically expressed. The formula for the law of practice is a type of mathematical expression called a *logarithmic power function*, meaning that performance continues to improve toward an upper limit, but at a progressively diminishing and predictable rate. This lawful pattern of change shows regularity for virtually all motor skills (although, of course, the exact rate will change depending on the skill, context, and learner).

The Monotonic Benefits Assumption

monotonic benefits assumption: The notion that learning occurs at the same rate as long as practice continues, though its manifestation in performance decreases at a predictable rate.

A significant conclusion of the law of practice is that as long as practice continues, learning never really stops. This conclusion is known as the **monotonic benefits assumption**. In the 1950s, a classic experiment was reported by another industrial psychologist, William Crossman, who tested predictions of the power law by examining the rates of improvement in a simple motor skill as a function of the number of years of practice. To test the monotonic benefits assumption that learning rates continued to improve as long as practice continued—though the rate of improvement might abate considerably over time—Crossman (1959) obtained the pay records of women employed in Cuban cigar-making companies for periods of time ranging up to 40 years. Because the women were paid daily based on the number of cigars they produced, these payment records were also accurate day-by-day indicators of the rate of improvement in the skill of cigar making. The skill itself was rather simple and could be done quickly. More importantly, in terms of the research question, if learning did continue to occur, as predicted by the law of practice, then it might reasonably be observed in this skill because neither physiological changes (muscular strength, reaction time, etc.), nor motivational changes (motivation could be considered constant because pay was based on the number of cigars made) would unduly affect performance levels.

Crossman's data included literally tens of millions of practice trials (production of one cigar) over many years of practice (study involving such vast amounts of data only became possible in the late 1950s because computers became available). After compiling the results of all of this data, Crossman observed that improvement in cigar-making performance did indeed follow the mathematical predictions of the law of practice, with almost all of the improvement occurring during the first two years of a worker's experience. However, even after as many as 40 years on the job, workers continued to show improvement, even though the rate of improvement was smaller and smaller with each passing year.

The Asymptotic Nature of Learning

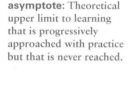

asymptote: Theoretical upper limit to learning that is progressively approached with practice but that is never reached.

Crossman's work was the first scientific demonstration (there have been many others since) that there exists some upper limit to learning that is approached, but never reached, as long as practice continues. Though this upper limit is never reached, it can be mathematically calculated by observing the rate of improvement over a sufficient amount of practice, and is called an **asymptote**

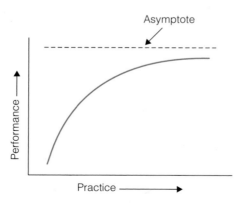

FIGURE **5.6** The Rate of Learning Changes as a Function of Approaching an Asymptote

Source: Created by author

(see Figure 5.6). An asymptote is an upper limit to performance that is considered the "best possible level of performance" (Lane, 1987, p. 21). As long as an individual continues to practice a skill, learning will also continue getting ever closer to this upper limit (asymptote), though never completely reaching it (see Box 5.2 for an interesting illustration of this principle).

"Wait a minute," you may be saying to yourself, "isn't it obvious that at some point people obtain a skill level above which further improvements no longer take place, or even a time when aging results in diminished levels of skill performance?" Of course, you would be correct in these observations. But remember from our earlier discussion that learning is a change in the "underlying capacity to perform a skill," and not in the actual level of performance that is observed. That is, the underlying control factors that improve with practice (motor programs, synergies, self-organizing adaptive networks, etc.) and that determine learning, continue to improve as long as practice continues, even when other factors may limit or even impede the actual performance level of the skill.

A number of factors influence performance, even when the underlying capacity to perform (i.e., learning) is otherwise not impacted. Psychological factors, for one case, have been known for some time to act as upper barriers to performance (see Box 5.3). Physiological limitations exert an even more powerful influence on performance limits. Although there is no "forced" upper limit on how much a competitive weight lifter can press overhead, for example, it is unlikely that his (or her) performance will improve beyond a certain point. Although there is no logical reason why a competitive weight lifter might not press 1,000 pounds overhead, the physiological limitations imposed by human biomechanical and muscular structures make such an outcome unlikely. More realistically, the athlete recognizes some upper limit

---

BOX 5.2   Asymptotes and Zeno's Paradox of the Arrow

The asymptotic nature of learning as expressed by the law of practice states that as long as practice continues, learning continues, though improvement becomes incrementally smaller and smaller over time as learning approaches, but never completely reaches, an upper limit. This idea was illustrated in an interesting way by the ancient Greek philosopher Zeno in his paradox of the arrow, which provides a good analogy when thinking about the law of practice.

Imagine, said Zeno, that Homer shoots an arrow at Aristotle. Although this may seem threatening, Aristotle need not really worry because, Zeno argued, the arrow can never actually hit Aristotle. This is because once Homer lets the arrow fly,

before it can reach Aristotle it must first cover half the distance between Homer and Aristotle; therefore, Aristotle is at that point in time safe. Aristotle continues to remain safe, though, because before the arrow can travel the remaining distance, it must travel half of that distance as well (or one-quarter of the original distance). Before it travels the remaining one-quarter distance, it must travel half of that (or one-eighth the original distance). In fact, the arrow must always travel half of the remaining distance between its present location and Aristotle before it can hit him. Because this means that some distance between the arrow and Aristotle will always remain, even though it gets progressively smaller and smaller, the arrow can never hit Aristotle.

to which he or she might reasonably aspire, and then performance, over time, reflects those limits.

Perhaps the most extreme forms of physiological limitations are imposed, of course, through maturational processes. Decreased levels of strength, endurance, and reaction time that inevitably accompany aging all have an effect on performance. Diminished levels of performance imposed by physiological limitations, however, do not mean that learning is not still occurring with practice. This is especially obvious when we note continued improvements in skill level, often well into senior years, for activities in which physiological variables are less limiting. Olympic gold medal winners in sailing and pistol shooting, for example, have been seen well into their 50s and 60s (see Box 5.4). Because learning these skills is not unduly limited by physiological factors like strength and speed, and because learning continues to improve over the course of practice, these older athletes may actually have an advantage over their younger peers because of the many years of additional practice they have accrued (meaning they have more closely approached the asymptotic limit of their potential).

Beyond psychological and physiological limitations, motivational factors may also limit, and in some cases even cause detriments to, continued improvements in performance. Individuals may simply lose interest in a sport or other motor activity after a period of time, which may range from minutes in laboratory settings to years in occupational and sport settings. Other life activities may also become more important and avert a person's attention and effort from continued practice of a particular motor skill. Because motivation plays such an essential role in skilled performance, any decline in it will almost certainly be attended by diminished levels of performance. Finally, in the absence of continued practice, memories underlying skill production may fade (though the actual memory does not fade, only the capacity to retrieve it; see Chapter 6).

Structural factors of a task (e.g., you can only score 100 points in the task, you cannot perform in a time less than 0 seconds) may also limit performance and act as an upper limit beyond which performance is impossible. But the

BOX 5.3 Psychological Limits and the Four-Minute Mile

Performance is limited by many factors, including physiological, anatomical, developmental, cultural, and training factors. Psychological factors can also play a major role in limiting performance. In fact, psychological factors can create a performance ceiling every bit as difficult to overcome as do physiological and mechanical factors. For example, it was at one time believed that humans could never run a mile in under four minutes, and that such a performance was simply beyond the physiological capacity of humans. Then in 1954, English miler and medical student Roger Bannister ran the mile in under four minutes. Within weeks of Bannister's world record, several other runners had broken the "impossible" four-minute barrier. Today's track athletes have even forgotten that the four-minute barrier ever existed, but at one time it acted as powerfully as any concrete physical barrier in preventing performance beyond a certain point.

point remains, as cogently demonstrated by observations of learning across a wide range of motor skills, that as long as practice continues, the underlying control factors (memorial, synergistic, adapting properties within systems, etc.) responsible for learning will continue to develop, even if other factors limit one's actual performance capabilities. The practical implication of the law of practice is that all motor skill learning has some upper limit (individually as well as generalized for groups) that will be approached though never exceeded, and exhibits smaller and smaller incremental increases over time, as long as practice continues. An old adage in skill learning is that "Practice makes perfect," but it would be more correct to say that "Practice never makes perfect." That is, as long as practice continues, learning still occurs, though a person's asymptotic potential is never fully realized.

BOX 5.4   Learning and Aging

Research on the brain is continuing to support the predictions of the law of practice that the learning of motor skills can continue well into middle and even advanced years. The list below identifies a number of athletes who have continued to compete at high levels (either professionally or in the Olympic Games) into their middle years and beyond. Even if some physical capabilities they possessed in younger years might have abated, the additional years of practice these athletes acquired may well have provided them an edge in learning over younger opponents.

Athlete	Sport	Age in Last Year of Competition	Last Year of Competition
Buddy Helms	Auto racing	87	2003
Satchel Page	Baseball	59	1966
Robert Jaworski	Basketball (men's)	52	1998
Nancy Lieberman	Basketball (women's)	50	2008
George Foreman	Boxing	50	2000
Hiroshi Hoketsu	Olympic equestrian events	61	2008
Tom Morris	Golf	74	1895
Gordie Howe	Ice hockey	52	1980
Jeff Hartwig	Olympic pole vault	41	2008
Fred Davis	Snookers	78	1992
Martina Navratilova	Tennis	49	2006
Carle Pace	Olympic track (distance events)	90	2008
Karch Kiraly	Olympic volleyball	46	2008

OVERLEARNING

overlearning: The concept that practice of a newly acquired skill beyond the point of mastery benefits long-term retention of the skill.

In the previous section, we mentioned that the capacity to perform a learned skill may decrease over the course of time if the skill is not adequately practiced. Everyone is familiar with this phenomenon. Although we may remember how to perform some skills even over long periods of nonpractice (like never forgetting how to ride a bicycle), other skills may readily be lost, or at least our ability to perform them severely diminished, if they are not practiced with some degree of regularity. That is, we forget. Forgetting does not mean that our underlying capacity for performance is lost, but that we are unable to retrieve and utilize that capacity (for reasons we will discuss in the next chapter).

There is a long history of research devoted to discovering methods by which levels of learning, once attained, can be maintained or at least optimized (Driskell, Willis, and Copper, 1992). Primary among these methods is the use of overlearning schedules. **Overlearning** refers to the continued practice of a skill beyond the point at which some desired level of mastery is reached. The goal of overlearning is not to increase the learner's level of performance, but to make the original level of performance more resistant to forgetting. Overlearning is employed to help maintain a desired level of skill performance over periods, sometimes prolonged, of little or even no actual performance of the skill.

mastery level:
A predetermined performance level established as the goal of practice.

Most skills are practiced with the intent of achieving a specific performance criterion as a level of mastery. A basketball instructor may have students practice free throws until they can make 15 out of 25 baskets, a physical therapist may have a client practice standing from a chair until the task can be accomplished unaided, or a flight instructor may require pilots to complete 10 perfect landings in a flight simulator before they are allowed to attempt the real thing. Notice that the **mastery level** does not need to be 100 percent; basketball students in our example did not have to make all 25 free-throw attempts. Though 100 percent mastery may be a target of practice in some situations, in most situations a more arbitrary mastery level is the goal of practice.

original learning: The amount of practice required to attain a specified level of mastery.

Overlearning is defined as the amount of practice (number of trials or amount of time) devoted to the continuation of practice once a desired mastery level has been achieved. The amount of practice required to attain such mastery is called **original learning**. Overlearning, which may occur immediately after original learning or incrementally over some relatively short period of time, is then specified as a percentage of the original learning. That is, 50 percent overlearning means that half again as many practice trials (or as much time) as taken to achieve original learning is devoted to overlearning practice beyond the mastery level.

How much overlearning is required to maximize retention of learned skills? Though this is an important question, it has received relatively little research attention. In a review of the literature on overlearning, Driskell, Willis, and Copper (1992), in the most comprehensive review to date, found only 15 studies on overlearning reported between 1929 and 1982. Their review did, however, lead to the conclusion that overlearning schedules

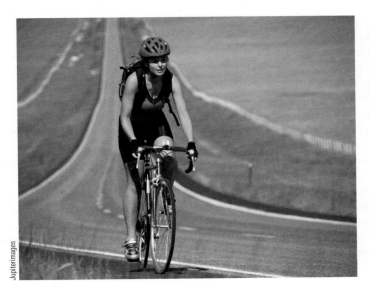

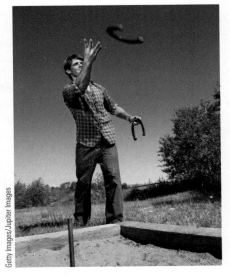

People maintain their performance levels of continuous skills for significantly longer periods of nonpractice than they do for discrete skills.

ranging from 50 to 200 percent were effective in promoting higher levels of retention (insufficient research with overlearning beyond 200% exists to draw any valid conclusions). The lower percentage of overlearning was reported for motor skills that are continuous and relatively simple, whereas the higher percentage was found for discrete, complex skills. As a general guideline, motor skills that are simple or continuous in nature, or a combination of both, appear to require about half as much additional practice as that originally engaged in, whereas complex or discrete skills, or those which are a combination of both, require double the original practice to maintain a high degree of retention over periods of little or no performance (see Box 5.5). Regardless of the type of skill, the advantages of overlearning in maintaining levels of original learning are believed to be due to the effects that such additional practice has on memory consolidation. Additional practice promotes the deeper encoding of a skill in memory, making it in turn more resistant to forgetting (Schendel and Hagman, 1982).

BOX **5.5**   **Applying the Principles of Overlearning**

The legendary football coach Bear Bryant, whose University of Alabama teams won six national championships and whose players were known for their levels of skill attainment, was once asked what he did to get his players so highly skilled. "It's easy," Coach Bryant reportedly replied, "We just practice until every player gets it perfect. And then, how ever much practice it took us to get perfect, we do that again!"

automaticity: The capacity of individuals to access and operate on procedural memory without the need for conscious attentional resources when executing well-learned skills.

Perhaps the real advantage of overlearning, however, is not so much with its effect on increasing retention levels, but with its effect on the automaticity of performance. **Automaticity** is the capacity, developed within procedural memory structures, to respond quickly, adapt readily to changing situations, and perform skills with little or no conscious attention. Automaticity is the hallmark of skills that are well learned, such as many everyday skills like driving a car or brushing your teeth, or more specialized skills like playing a sport or a musical instrument. The amount of practice for a skill is directly related to the development of automaticity (Logan, 1985; Schmidt and Wrisberg, 2008). In fact, automaticity is believed fully developed only given large amounts of practice. Even if overlearning does not result in dramatic increases in the performance level for a given skill, it may still lead to the ability to perform the skill more automatically in a variety of different and changing situations and with the need for fewer conscious resources and less effort.

refresher practice: A form of overlearning in which continued practice of a skill is carried out beyond the attainment of the original performance goal in incrementally spaced practice intervals as a method of maintaining achieved performance levels.

On a final note before leaving our discussion of overlearning, it should be pointed out that an alternative form of overlearning is the technique called **refresher practice** (or sometimes *retention practice*). Although overlearning implies continued practice immediately or shortly after the attainment of original learning, refresher practice refers to overlearning practice that is spread out over incremental practice sessions. Airline pilots who have completed a course of training in emergency procedures, for example, may return every few months to their training facility for a day or two of refresher training on these procedures, because it is critical to maintain their original levels of training, and hopefully they have not had to practice these skills in actual performance situations. Athletic coaches intuitively apply refresher practice when they have their players practice important but seldom used skills or plays to help refresh the players' memories of how to perform. Whether supplemental practice is supplied through overlearning or refresher practice schedules, though, does not appear to be a particularly critical factor. The introduction of additional practice is far more important than the time at which it is provided in enhancing retention (Druckman and Bjork, 1991; Schendel and Hagman, 1982).

Considering the advantages overlearning may have in a given situation, there is, of course, one major disadvantage. Overlearning takes more time. In many situations, the time available for practice is limited. The advantages of overlearning practice must be weighed against that of devoting practice time to other skill-learning activities. Instructors must carefully analyze the need for instructing skills in ways that lead to automaticity and that are especially resistant to forgetting over time when deciding upon the most appropriate allocation of practice in any particular situation. Overlearning is especially critical for skills that will be practiced for a specific time period, and then not performed for some length of time, particularly if a skill must be performed at a high level of proficiency when called upon (Hagman and Rose, 1983). As with every practice variable, there is no single correct answer to how much practice should be provided in any specific situation. Each new practice situation requires a careful analysis of the goals of practice along with an application of principles based upon a solid understanding of the research literature and principles derived from it.

THE TRANSFER OF LEARNING

transfer: The influence of practicing one skill on the learning of another skill or of the same skill in a new context.

One of the oldest topics in skill learning is the study of the transfer of learning. **Transfer** refers to the influence of learning one skill on the performance of another skill. We first learn our numbers in elementary school, for example, because experts tell us that doing so will transfer later to doing problems in algebra or other higher mathematical problems. We frequently make predictions about how well someone might learn a new sport based upon how well they have learned another sport. Our assumption is that something about the learning of one skill will transfer to a new skill or at least influence how well we can learn the new skill (but see Chapter 8 concerning individual differences for a discussion about the validity of making such inferences).

The practice of any motor skill typically assumes some degree of transfer. Recall that one of the ways for assessing learning is through a transfer test, because transfer to other skills or contexts is often a primary goal of practice. Baseball players hit balls from a pitching machine because they believe doing so will help them to better hit live pitched balls. Therapy patients practice assisted walking exercise in a clinical environment because they expect such practice to help them better navigate about their homes. Pilots practice in simulators because experience tells them skills learned doing such practice will transfer to flying real airplanes.

target skill: The task a person wishes to be able to perform as a result of practice.

The kind of transfer that is of interest to a learner may be that from one skill to another or from one context to another. When we practice one skill believing it will influence a second, different skill, we are typically interested in the amount of transfer to the unpracticed target skill. By **target skill**, we mean to imply the real skill of interest during practice. Basketball players may practice a jumping drill during practice, for example. The intention of this drill is not to learn to jump, however, but to improve one's rebounding skill in a game. Rebounding is the target skill, the real skill of interest for which we assume jumping drills will transfer. We may also practice a skill with the intention that practicing it in one context will transfer to another context. In the above example of practicing walking in an unencumbered clinical setting, the real intent of practice is the **target context** of a patient's home with all of the carpets and furniture found there. In either case, though, we expect practice to have an influence (to transfer) to the target skill or target context of real interest.

target context: The environmental situation in which an individual wishes to perform a particular skill as a result of practice.

We may also be interested in how experience with one skill or context may transfer to a different skill or context. Do good swimmers make good springboard divers? Is someone who is good with power tools more likely than someone who is not to also be good with hand tools? Does watching a film about road safety make one a safer driver?

positive transfer: When learning one skill positively influences the learning of another skill or of the same skill in a new context.

When experience in one skill or in one context enhances the level of performance in another skill or context, transfer is said to be positive. **Positive transfer** means that some part of learning one skill, or of learning a skill in one context, has a beneficial effect on the performance of a different skill or of the same skill in a different context. The degree of influence could be strong or minimal, but as long as some improvement results in the new skill or context, transfer is referred to as being positive.

negative transfer:
When learning one skill negatively influences the learning of another skill or of the same skill in a new context.

Transfer of learning can also be negative. Though **negative transfer** is a somewhat rare phenomenon, it can and does occur. Perhaps the classic example of negative transfer is from tennis to badminton, or vice versa. Though the two skills seem similar and one might indeed expect positive transfer, the influence of learning one of these skills typically depresses learning of the other, at least initially. In badminton, the wrist must be snapped when hitting the birdie, whereas in tennis one must keep the wrist rigid throughout the racquet swing, including at contact with the ball. This difference can lead to initial confusion when performing one of the skills as new, because the strong influence of the wrist action in the other skill causes confusion and readily leads to performance errors in wrist control. Such a dampening effect of experience in one skill on the performance of another skill leads to negative transfer.

Of course, there may well be no influence between two skills of two different context conditions. Learning to play the violin would have no influence on

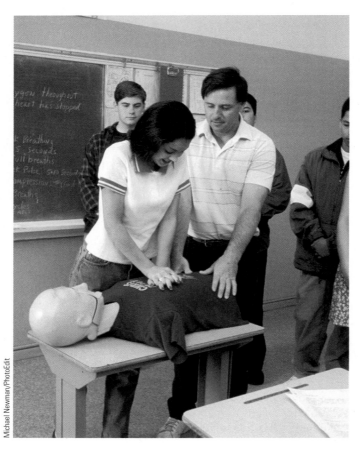

Michael Newman/PhotoEdit

Whenever practice conditions deviate in any way from the target conditions for learning, the amount of transfer between the practice and target environments is critical.

one's ability to hit a fastball or to drive a car. In such cases, transfer is considered nonexistent and is termed **zero transfer** (some authors prefer to term this as *neutral* transfer). The effects of experience in one skill or skill situation have no effect on another skill or on the skill in a different context.

Measuring Transfer

In measuring transfer, two paradigms are frequently employed. There are others, but we will limit our discussion here to the two most commonly used (see Ellis, 1965; and Haskell, 2001, for good reviews of different transfer designs). The first and most frequently employed of the two is known as a *proactive transfer design* (see Figure 5.7). In this design, two groups, an experimental and a control, are compared on the transfer criterion. The experimental group practices one skill or skill variation (Task A), and then a second skill or skill variation (Task B) is practiced. The control group practices only Task B. The only difference between the two groups is that the experimental group has first practiced Task A for some specified number of trials or period of time. The question of interest is whether practice of Task A will have an influence on the experimental group's performance when practicing Task B. The design is termed proactive because the potentially influencing task A comes before practicing the criterion task B (the prefix *pro* is from Greek meaning "before"). A second transfer design is called *retroactive* (the prefix *retro* means behind or after), because in this design the research question of interest is whether a skill A practiced after the criterion skill B will influence subsequent performance of task B (Figure 5.7).

It is typical to report the results of research using either the proactive or retroactive designs as the percentage of performance improvement in the criterion task B as a result of practicing the transfer task A. The formula for this score follows:

$$\text{Percentage of transfer} = [(E - C) / (E + C)] \times 100$$

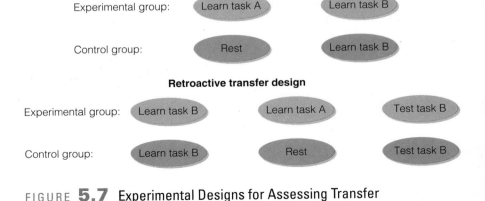

Proactive transfer design

Experimental group:	Learn task A	Learn task B
Control group:	Rest	Learn task B

Retroactive transfer design

Experimental group:	Learn task B	Learn task A	Test task B
Control group:	Learn task B	Rest	Test task B

FIGURE **5.7** Experimental Designs for Assessing Transfer

Source: Created by author

E is the mean average score on practice of task B for the experimental group, and C the mean average score for practice of task B for the control group.

As an example, consider the effects of first learning to track a triangle pattern on the rotary pursuit (we described this laboratory equipment earlier in this chapter) on performance in tracking a circle pattern on the same apparatus. In this case, we would employ a proactive transfer design, meaning that the experimental group would first practice a specified number of trials of the triangle pattern and then switch to some number of practice trials (typically the same number) with the circle pattern. Let us say that we carry out this experiment and find the average score on task B (the circle pattern) for the experimental group is 15 seconds for a series of 30-second trials. The control group also performs the same number of trials with the circle pattern and they average 10 seconds on their trials. Using the formula above, we would calculate that Percentage Transfer = $[(15 - 10)/(15 + 10)] \times 100 = 20\%$. This 20 percent figure represents the percentage of the difference between the experimental and control groups' performance scores on Task B. Percentage scores can only range between 100 percent for perfect positive transfer, and −100 percent for perfect negative transfer. A score of 0 represents neutral transfer. The greater the percentage score in either direction, the greater the transfer effects. In the case of our experiment, we would conclude that the learning of tracking triangle patterns in a rotary pursuit task transferred positively to learning to perform tracking of circle patterns, with 20 percent transfer representing a significant but probably rather minimal benefit (although this conclusion would depend greatly upon how much practice on the transfer task was required to gain benefits on the target task).

Theories Explaining Transfer Effects

Why does transfer occur (or fail to occur)? Two theories have been advanced: identical elements theory and transfer-appropriate processing theory.

Identical Elements Theory

identical elements theory: The theory that transfer is positively related to the number of elements that two skills share in common.

The first of the two dominant theories of transfer, **identical elements theory**, has a long history and much intuitive appeal. In fact, it was originally proposed by Thorndike and Woodworth in 1901. According to this perspective, transfer occurs to the degree that two skills share common elements. The greater the number of common elements, the stronger the transfer.

Although identical elements theory is intuitively appealing and certainly has merit as a theory, the problem has been that Thorndike and Woodworth never specified what might be included as common elements. Such a lack of definition has made the theory difficult to test and open to wide interpretation. A number of characteristics have been suggested over the years as common elements, including various motor traits, movement kinematics, perceptual demands, and general timing characteristics among others. Still, no consensus has emerged, and research has lead to disagreement concerning what might constitute relative elements. Although it remains logical to argue that transfer is facilitated by common elements shared by skills, our lack of understanding concerning which elements are relevant, and exactly how they might influence transfer, has made it difficult to apply this perspective in more than a general manner.

Transfer-Appropriate Processing Theory

A second theory of transfer called the **transfer-appropriate processing theory** (TAPS for short) was first put forward by Bransford et al. in 1979. This theory is somewhat analogous to identical elements theory but argues that instead of skill elements, what is important to transfer is the similarity of the cognitive processing elements between skills. Although movement patterns are viewed as irrelevant, cognitive demands such as problem-solving skills, speed of decision making, attentional focus, and the application of rules that are shared between skills determine the degree of transfer possible. The more the cognitive elements involved in two skills are similar, regardless of similarities among actual kinematic patterns, the greater will be the degree of transfer. In perhaps an oversimplification, we might say that identical elements theory suggests that two skills will transfer to the degree that they look alike, while transfer-appropriate processing theory suggests that two skills will transfer to the degree that individuals must engage in similar processing activities.

A Comparison of Theories of Transfer

As an illustration of the application of these two theories, let us consider an experiment conducted by Smeeton, Ward, and Williams (2004). These researchers were interested in the degree to which the recognition of patterns of play might transfer between sports skills. In many team sports, it is important to be able to recognize and quickly respond to changes in an opponent's team movement patterns. To test whether this capacity might transfer between sports, the researchers studied players from soccer, field hockey, and volleyball teams. Subjects included six players from each sport who were highly skilled (meaning that they had participated on high level national teams for five or more years) and six players from each sport who were recreational club players (all having played less than two years) and considered low skilled. All of the subjects had experience only in their sport, having never played or received instruction in either of the other sports.

After viewing a general introductory film on all three sports, each subject viewed 32 ten-second clips of actual game play in each sport. Half of the clips for each sport demonstrated a particular movement pattern of the players (focusing on one team side only). Each of these patterns was different. The other half of the clips showed playing conditions in which no movement patterns were evident. Once this original phase was completed, each subject was shown another 32 ten-second film clips of play in each sport. This time, however, one-half of the clips in each sport were new, while one-half had been included in the original group of clips shown. The task for subjects was to identify, as quickly as possible, when a film clip in the second group was the same as one they had viewed in the first group.

The results showed that both the skilled soccer players and field hockey players were highly successful in identifying team movement patterns in all

transfer-appropriate processing theory: The theory that transfer between skills is positively related to similarities in required mental operations shared by the skills.

three sports, while the skilled volleyball players, although as good as the soccer and field hockey players in identifying patterns in their own sport, were not able to transfer this capability to either soccer or field hockey. All of the unskilled players were unable to significantly transfer ability in their skill to either of the other two skills. The skilled soccer and field hockey players, showed significant transfer of pattern recognition skills from their respective sport to the other sports. Said another way, they were able to positively transfer pattern recognition skills among sports. Learning to recognize an opponent's team movements in their respective sport influenced their learning of pattern recognition in other sports. Skilled volleyball players and low-skilled players in all three sports were not significantly capable of transferring learning in one sport to other sports.

In this example, we can make a strong case for both the identical elements and transfer-appropriate processing theories. In both soccer and field hockey, the physical movements of players are varied yet similar, as are many offensive and defensive techniques that are shared by both sports. Theoretically, it could be argued that many of these physical movement patterns are shared by all three sports, and learning them in one of the sports would transfer to their recognition in the other two. Similarly, the patterns in all three sports also represent rules concerning strategy that are shared by all three (using some movement patterns for purposes of "faking," for example), and these cognitive elements might also be transferred.

It would appear that both theories might offer some explanation for the transfer effects observed in the Smeeton, Ward, and Williams study. After all, both movement and cognitive elements are present in all of the movements patterns studied. Perhaps the volleyball players, because their sport involves fewer players and movements confined to a more restricted playing area, do not benefit from as rich an array of different movement patterns as the soccer or field hockey players and, although excelling in their own sport, are not as able to transfer aspects of pattern recognition specific to volleyball to other sports.

The analysis of this study, as well as the ability to focus meaningfully on different specific elements that may be involved in transfer among the sports, suggests two things: First, both theories may be useful in explaining transfer, each capturing something of importance that the other lacks. In fact, it can be argued that transfer-appropriate processing theory is really an extension of identical elements theory that comes into play when similarity of skill components is minimal. Second, the study illustrates that even though the notion of something similar transferring between sports is an old one and has much internal logic, we simply do not understand what kind of elements may be the most crucial in transfer or how different elements may interact in the transfer of learning from one activity to another. In perhaps the most extensive review of transfer phenomena to date, Schmidt and Young (1987) concluded that we still do not know much about what factors account for transfer. Until more research is conducted aimed directly at exploring the elements most responsible for the transfer of motor skill learning, experience and intuition will remain important guides in assessing the exact causes for why one activity does or does not influence performance in a second activity. It is important to keep in mind, though, that we can assess the strength of that influence, even if we cannot fully explain it.

General Conclusions Concerning Transfer

In concluding our discussion of transfer, we might make two general observations: The first is that the actual amount of transfer observed between motor skills is really quite small. Schmidt and Young (1987) conclude that research does not support strong transfer effects except when two skills (or skill variations) are fairly similar. The term **near transfer** is often used to denote such transfer effects between similar skills. Although these terms are somewhat subjective, *far transfer* then refers to transfer effects between skills that are fairly dissimilar (i.e., do not share many common elements).

This leads to our second observation. The "nearer" two skills are in shared common elements, the greater will be the amount of transfer between the two. It is interesting, however, that although the literature typically shows some degree of transfer between two skills sharing common elements, with the degree of transfer becoming more pronounced as similarity between the skills increases, the results for near transfer remain somewhat ambivalent. Generally, similarity between skills facilitates transfer, at least to some degree. When two skills are similar in common elements, however, negative transfer is frequently observed between them at least initially (recall the example of badminton and tennis).

near transfer: Positive transfer between similar skills.

BOX 5.6   Transfer and "Wax On, Wax Off"

In the popular 1984 movie *The Karate Kid*, the character of Daniel LaRusso is a high school student being bullied by a group of his classmates belonging to a karate club, who threaten to use their skills against Daniel. In self-defense, Daniel seeks out the help of a neighborhood man who just happens to be a former karate champion. Mr. Kesuke agrees to help Daniel learn karate but tells the young man that he must follow his instructions explicitly and without question.

When Daniel arrives at Mr. Kesuke's home for his first lesson, he is surprised when Mr. Kesuke puts him to work washing and waxing his many antique cars. In a famous scene from the movie, Mr. Kesuke instructs Daniel on the correct method for waxing. Grasping a sponge in both hands, Daniel is to apply the wax making precise circular patterns with his sponges, first circling outward with the right hand, and then circling outward with the left

hand, all the while keeping the circling motions of both hands in rhythm by repeating the phrase "Wax on, wax off."

After several days of waxing on and waxing off, Daniel expresses his concern to Mr. Kesuke that he is not learning karate and wonders if Mr. Kesuke has just been deceiving him in order to get his cars polished. Daniel is in for a surprise, though, when he learns that he has completed his first lesson and has already acquired important new karate skills. As Mr. Kesuke demonstrates by throwing various karate punches at Daniel, he instructs the young man to remember to "Wax on, wax off." When Daniel executes the waxing motions, he discovers that he has all along been learning the correct movements for deflecting karate punches. In this case, learning waxing skills readily transferred to karate blocking skills. Daniel had received his first lesson in positive transfer.

The results of near transfer studies support two different approaches to the design of practice experiences. These are the approaches we identified in Chapter 4 as the specificity and variability of practice hypotheses. We will leave the discussion of how these approaches might provide insights into the design of effective practice schedules for Chapter 11. For now, our purposes have been served by better understanding the influences among various skills that can facilitate (or hinder) learning.

LEARNING FROM PLAY TO DELIBERATE PRACTICE

Our discussion of learning has left largely unanswered one especially important question. That is, does the quality of skill performance, its intent and organization, affect the principles of learning we have considered? Do the patterns of learning as described by the law of practice, or the principles of transfer, for example, apply equally to the highly structured practice of athletes as they do to the play activities of children?

In a comprehensive review of the literature on learning and motor skills, Ericsson, Krampe, and Tesch-Romer (1993) concluded that the most effective learning situations are those that are highly structured and in which learners engage in activities with the express purpose of developing specific skills. The most beneficial performance environments for learning they termed as **deliberate practice**. Deliberate practice is defined as practice that is (1) effortful, (2) closely monitored and instructed, (3) directed toward the attainment of future goals rather than immediate rewards, and (4) motivated by the desire to improve skill performance. Deliberate practice, as defined, obviously covers many skill-learning situations. The practice sessions of athletic teams, patients working to regain functional abilities in therapy sessions, workers training for new job skills, and musicians practicing under the guidance of an instructor are all examples of deliberate practice.

deliberate practice: Practice that is effortful, highly structured and organized, and directed toward extrinsic goals and rewards.

If we were to form a continuum of performance conditions with deliberate practice at one end, then at the other end of the continuum we would place **play**, the immediately intuitive opposite of deliberate practice. There have been many definitions offered for play over the years, ranging from those based on scientific observation and description to the highly speculative and philosophical. Although a precise and consensually agreed upon definition remains elusive, a good working definition has been offered by Smith et al. (1986). Based upon their review of the literature, they identified five critical aspects delineating play from other forms of behavior. According to their definition, play (1) is intrinsically motivated, engaged in for its own sake rather than for bodily, social, or external reasons; (2) has a positive affect, being pleasurable and enjoyable; (3) is nonliteral, not carried out seriously but having an "as if" or pretend quality; (4) has a means rather than ends orientation, with participation in the activity itself of more interest than the outcome or result of participation, and (5) possesses the quality of flexibility, showing variation in form and content from one play experience to the next.

play: Activity which is spontaneous, intrinsically motivated, enjoyable and imaginative, and not pursued for any external rewards or goals.

The demarcation between play and deliberate practice is not a clear one, as the perceptive reader may already have recognized. What about organized sports for children, where even though the rules and structure of games apply, children may still engage in such activities largely for their intrinsic value and enjoyment? Is the weekend golfer out to enjoy a sunny day, a break from household chores, and hitting a bucket of balls on the driving range being more playful or deliberate about practice? What about the athlete practicing to improve his or her skills apart from the organized setting of practice and the presence of an instructor or coach?

Recently, Cote and Hay (2002) have proposed a useful classification of activities viewed on a continuum ranging from play to deliberate practice. They identify four broad types of activity based upon considerations of participant perspective, performance goals, monitoring during activity, corrections made during activity, source of enjoyment, and immediacy of gratification. Based upon these criteria, they identify four distinct categories of activity ranging from free play, to deliberate play, to structured practice, to deliberate practice. These are described in Table 5.2.

To date, researchers have not specifically investigated the interaction between activity types of the kind suggested here, and the principles of learning as described in this chapter. Perhaps this is because learning is a primary goal for skills practiced in a structured performance context, especially when the practice is accompanied by instruction, but viewed as being relatively less important in the play experiences. There is also a more obvious problem in conducting research on play, which is that the very act of doing research, of observing and collecting data, changes the circumstances surrounding the play experience, often such that the play experience itself is altered or even destroyed. Whatever the reasons for this lack of research, until further research is directed toward exploring the generalizability of learning principles across the entire spectrum of activity types, some questions concerning the extent of learning will remain speculative, at best.

In regard to the principles of learning presented in this chapter, as well as others discussed in other chapters of this book, the reader should feel confident in assuming that the information presented can be reliably applied to the learning of skills performed in the context of structured practice and deliberate practice, as they are defined here. This conclusion is supported by considerable research (Ericsson, Krampe, and Tesch-Romer, 1993). It is also reasonable to assume that the same principles as apply to structured and deliberate practice apply to the learning of skills performed in the context of deliberate play, at least to some extent, as well, though further research is needed to establish this with certainty. It may yet be found, for example, that some reconsideration of the strength and effect of many learning principles will need to be made when applying them to deliberate play conditions. It is in the area of skill performance classified here as free play that the most questions remain. Is learning of movement patterns and skills significantly improved as a result of play, even when time devoted to play is extensive? Do play experiences transfer to other contexts or skills (this is one of the reasons often advanced as a benefit of play)? Does the law of practice apply to play activities? For the present, these and many other questions about play and learning remain unanswered or speculative at best.

TABLE **5.2**

Comparison of Free Play, Structured Play, Structured Practice, and Deliberate Practice

Orientation of activity	Free play	Deliberate play	Structured practice	Deliberate practice
Perspective	Immediate "lived" experience of participation	Experience of participation, including movement experimentation	Improvement of performance, though other factors may also contribute to participation	Improvement of performance; other reasons subjugated to skill improvement
Goal	Fun, enjoyment, make-believe (process oriented)	Fun, intrinsic interest in exploring bodily capabilities (process oriented)	Improvement of skills, especially short-term improvement goals (outcome oriented)	Improvement of skills, with both short-term and long-term goals directed toward high levels of accomplishment (outcome oriented)
Instructional monitoring	None	Little or none	Instruction and monitoring of performance; may be directed toward group rather than individual	Carefully monitored and expertly instructed; extensive individual instruction
Correction and evaluation	None	Little or none; when provided is informative rather than corrective	Correction provided by instructor or through self-discovery learning methods	Immediate correction of errors; instructor source of evaluation and correction
Source of enjoyment	Inherent in participation	Inherent in participation and self-discovery	Predominantly extrinsic and based on improvement	Extrinsic and based on improvement
Gratification	Immediate	Immediate	Immediate and delayed	Delayed

SUMMARY

Learning may seem as simple as what happens as a result of practice. Upon further reflection, however, the processes involved in learning new skills are varied and complex. The acquisition of all motor skills, however, shares many fundamental processes revealed through research and experimentation.

- It is critical to distinguish between learning and performance, because the level of a person's performance is not always an accurate indicator of learning.

Because learning cannot be observed directly, it must be inferred from observations of performance. Three measurements of performance are typically assessed in order to accurately determine degree of learning: acquisition, retention, and transfer.

Performance curves illustrate the generalized pattern of improvement in performance of skills during acquisition. Four types of performance curves have been identified: Linear, negatively accelerating, positively accelerating, and S-shaped.

A number of fundamental laws and principles of learning observed during the practice of motor skills have been identified.

- According to the law of practice, learning occurs as a function of practice and continues as long as practice continues, though improvements in performance becomes progressively and predictably less over time.
- Learning approaches an upper limit called an *asymptote*, which differs among individuals.

Overlearning refers to practice beyond the attainment of a mastery level. The primary goal of overlearning is to enhance long-term retention of skills.

- Overlearning schedules of between 50 and 200 percent have been demonstrated as optimal in maintaining retention.

It has long been established that the learning of one skill often has an effect on the learning of other skills, a phenomenon called *transfer*. Transfer can be either positive or negative, or no transfer may occur.

Motor skills may be performed in a wide variety of contexts and conditions ranging from highly spontaneous and playful expressions, to highly structured and organized practice experiences.

LEARNING EXERCISES

1. Using three tennis balls, beanbags, or rolled-up socks, practice juggling for 10 minutes each day for 10 days. Begin by juggling one item, and then progressively add the remaining two items as you are able. After each 10-minute practice session, wait 5 minutes and then perform a retention test using all three items. Your performance score for the retention test is the time, in seconds, that you can keep all three items in motion without dropping any of them (your score may be zero seconds on the first and second days' trials). Record your retention data for all 10 days. After the

10th day, prepare a performance graph of your retention results. What kind of performance curve is best represented by your graph (draw in the best-fitting performance curve)? What does this performance curve tell you about the rate and pattern of your learning for this juggling skill?

2. Prepare a table of overlearning schedules including four columns labeled "50%," "100%," "150%," and "200%" overlearning. Based upon what is known about the amount of overlearning optimally required for promoting the long-term retention of different skills (e.g., Driskell, Willis, and Copper, 1992), list seven skills in each column for which that column's overlearning percentage would be appropriate.

3. Select two different skills between which you believe positive transfer may occur, but you are uncertain. Design an experiment for assessing whether there are transfer effects between the two skills. Describe and illustrate your experiment, including the groups used, which skills and how many trials each group performs, the order in which skills are performed, and when and how performance is measured. For the purposes of this exercise, make up performance data for each group in a way that seems most realistic to you. Using your data, calculate the percentage transfer between the two groups, showing the formula used and your calculations. What conclusion could you draw from these data?

4. Select a skill in which you have an interest and then, using Table 5.2 as a guide, describe under the appropriate columns the various dimensions (perspective, goal, monitoring, corrections, source of enjoyment, and gratification) for each of the four types of movement activity (i.e., free play, deliberate play, structured practice, and deliberate practice). Your descriptions should be specific examples for the skill you selected.

FOR FURTHER STUDY

HOW MUCH DO YOU KNOW?

For each of the following, select the letter that best answers the question.

1. Which of the following terms, in reference to motor learning research, refers to "observable behavior"?
   a. Practice
   b. Learning
   c. Performance
   d. Skill

2. Of the four types of performance curves typically observed when learning motor skills, the one that is consider "normal" or "standard" is the
   a. linear performance curve.
   b. positively accelerating performance curve.
   c. S-shaped performance curve.
   d. negatively accelerating performance curve.

3. If subjects in a motor learning experiment practice a task for 100 acquisition trials and then are tested on their learning by how well they perform five additional trials after a 30-minute rest period, the type of test is called a
   a. transfer test.
   b. retention test.
   c. acquisition test.
   d. learning test.

4. In one of the most important experiments in the history of motor learning research, the predictions of the law of practice were demonstrated by Crossman using the task of
   a. radio assembly.
   b. anti-aircraft gunnery.
   c. cigar assembly.
   d. rotary pursuit tracking.

5. Overlearning is measured as a percentage of
   a. original learning.
   b. original skill level.
   c. absolute skill level.
   d. target skill level.
6. When learning skill A enhances the learning of skill B, what kind of transfer is said to have taken place from skill A to skill B?
   a. Near transfer
   b. Positive transfer
   c. Neutral transfer
   d. Common transfer

Answer the following with the word or words which best complete each sentence.

7. According to the law of practice, the _____ represents an upper limit of learning.
8. In their review of research on overlearning, Driskell, Willis, and Copper (1992) found that a minimum of _____ percent overlearning was required before effects on retention enhancement became significant.
9. Implicit in the law of practice is the assumption that learning never completely stops as long as practice continues. What is the name given this assumption?
10. A theory of transfer stating that transfer between two skills is facilitated to the degree that both skills share common cognitive processing elements is called _____ theory.
11. When graphing performance curves, what is measured on the ordinate (i.e., vertical or Y-axis)?
12. As opposed to play, _____ entails practice that is highly structured, effortful, closely instructed, goal-directed, and motivated by a desire to improve.

Answers are provided at the end of this review section.

STUDY QUESTIONS

1. What is meant by the "learning–performance distinction?" Provide five examples of performance variables responsible for learning–performance distinctions.
2. When conducting motor learning experiments, why are three types of tests necessary for the accurate assessment of learning? What, specifically, do acquisition, retention, and transfer tests measure?
3. Describe each of the four performance curves typically observed in motor learning research. What does each type of curve suggest about the rate of learning as practice progresses?
4. Define the law of practice. Why might the predictions of the law of practice not always be observed through actual performance measures?
5. If people continue to learn as long as they continue to practice a skill as specified by the law of practice, then why do performance levels for sports skills ultimately wane and fade over time? What factors contribute to the eventual fading, as well as persistence, of performance capabilities in sports?
6. Discuss reasons for considering the use of overlearning schedules, providing five examples of when overlearning might be especially desirable.
7. Compare and contrast identical elements and transfer-appropriate processing theories as explanations of transfer of learning effects.
8. Define *deliberate practice* and contrast it with *play*.

ADDITIONAL READING

Christina, RW. (1997). "Concerns and issues in studying and assessing motor learning." *Measurement in Physical Education and Exercise Science, 1,* 19–38.

Lane, NE. (1987). *Skill acquisition rates and patterns: Issues and training implications.* New York: Springer-Verlag.

Lee, TD, and Swinnen, SP. (1993). "Three legacies of Bryan and Harter: Automaticity, variability, and change in skilled performance." In JL Starkes and F Allard (eds.), *Cognitive issues in motor expertise* (pp. 295–315). Amsterdam: Elsevier.

Memmert, D, Raab, A, and Baner, P. (2006). "Laws of practice and performance plateaus concerning complex motor skills." *Journal of Human Movement Studies, 51,* 239–255.

Newell, A, and Rosenbloom, PS. (1981). "Mechanisms of skill acquisition and the law of practice." In JR Anderson (ed.), *Cognitive skills and their acquisition.* Hillsdale, NJ: Lawrence Erlbaum.

Schmidt, RA, and Young, DE. (1987). "Transfer of movement control in motor skill learning." In SM Cormier and JD Hagman (eds.), *Transfer of learning.* Orlando, FL: Academic Press.

Welford, AT (1987). "On rates of improvement with practice." *Journal of Motor Behavior, 19*(3), 401–415.

REFERENCES

Adams, JA. (1977). "Motor learning and retention." In MH Marx and ME Bunch, *Fundamentals and applications of learning.* New York: Macmillan Publishing Company.

Anderson, JR (ed.) (1981). *Cognitive skills and their acquisition.* Hillsdale, NJ: Lawrence Erlbaum.

Bransford, JD, Franks, JJ, Morris, CD, and Stein, BS. (1979). "Some general constraints on learning and memory research." In LS Cermak and FIM Craik (eds.), *Levels of processing in human memory* (pp. 331–354). Hillsdale, NJ: Lawrence Erlbaum.

Cote, J, Baker, J, and Abernethy, B. (2003). "From play to practice: A developmental framework for the acquisition of expertise in team sports." In JL Starkes and KA Ericsson (eds.), *Expert Performance in Sports: Advances in Research on Sport Expertise* (pp. 89–114). Champaign, IL: Human Kinetics.

Crossman, ERFW. (1959). "A theory of the acquisition of a speed skill." *Ergonomics, 2,* 153–166.

Driskell, JE, Copper, C, and Moran, A. (1994). "Does mental practice enhance performance?" *Journal of Applied Psychology, 79,* 481–491.

Driskell, JE, Willis, RP, and Copper, C. (1992). Effect of overlearning on retention. *Journal of Applied Psychology, 77,* 615–622.

Druckman, D, and Bjork, RA. (1991). "Optimizing long-term retention and transfer." In D Druckman and RA Bjork (eds.), *In the mind's eye: Enhancing human performance.* Washington, DC: National Academy Press.

Ellis, HC. (1965). *The transfer of learning.* New York: Macmillan.

Ericsson, KA, Krampe, RT, and Tesch-Romer, C. (1993). "The role of deliberate practice in the acquisition of expert performance." *Psychological Review, 100*(3), 363–406.

Haskell, RE. (2001). *Transfer of learning: Cognition, instruction, and reasoning.* San Diego, CA: Academic Press.

Lane, NE. (1987). *Skill acquisition rates and patterns: Issues and training implications.* New York: Springer-Verlag.

Lee, TD, and Swinnen, SP. (1993). "Three legacies of Bryan and Harter: Automaticity, variability, and change in skilled performance." In JL Starkes and F Allard (eds.), *Cognitive issues in motor expertise* (pp. 295–315). Amsterdam: Elsevier.

Logan, GD. (1985). "Skill and automaticity: Relations, implications, and future directions." *Canadian Journal of Psychology, 39,* 367–386. Proctor, RW, and Dutta, A. (1995). *Skill acquisition and human performance.* Thousand Oaks, CA: Sage Publications.

Rosenbaum, DA, Carlson, RA, and Gilmore, RO. (2001). "Acquisition of intellectual and perceptual-motor skills." *Annual Review of Psychology*, 453–470.

Rudisill, ME, and Jackson, AS. (1992). *Lab manual: Theory and application of motor learning.* Onalaska, TX: MacJ-R.

Schendel, JD, and Hagman, JD. (1982). "On sustaining procedural skills over a prolonged retention interval." *Journal of Applied Psychology*, 67, 605–610.

Schmidt, RA, and Wrisberg, CA. (2008). *Motor learning and performance: A problem-based learning approach*, 4th ed. Champaign, IL: Human Kinetics.

Schmidt, RA, and Young, DE. (1987). "Transfer of movement control in motor skill learning." In SM Cormier and JD Hagman (eds.), *Transfer of learning*. Orlando, FL: Academic Press.

Shea, JB, and Morgan, RL. (1979). "Contextual interference effects on the acquisition, retention, and transfer of a motor skill." *Journal of Experimental Psychology*, 5(2), 179–187.

Shea, JB and Kohl, RM. (1991). "Composition of practice: Influence on the retention of motor skills." *Research Quarterly for Exercise and Sport*, 62, 187–195.

Smeeton, NJ, Ward, P, and Williams, AM. (2004). "Do pattern recognition skills transfer across sports? A preliminary analysis." *Journal of Sport Sciences*, 22, 205–214.

Smith, PK, Takhvar, M, Gore, N, and Vollstedt, R. (1986). "Play in young children: Problems of definition, categorization and measurement." In PK Smith (ed.), *Children's play: Research, developments, and practical applications* (pp. 37–54). New York: Gordon and Breach.

Snoddy, GS. (1926). "Learning and stability: A psychophysical analysis of a case of motor learning and clinical applications." *Journal of Applied Psychology*, 10, 1–36.

Thorndike, EL, and Woodworth, RS. (1901). "The influence of improvement in one mental function upon the efficiency of other functions." *Psychological Review*, 39, 212–222.

Answers to How Much Do You Know questions: (1) C, (2) D, (3) B, (4) C, (5) A, (6) B, (7) asymptote, (8) 50, (9) monotonic benefits assumption, (10) transfer-appropriate processing, (11) performance, (12) deliberate practice.

CHAPTER **6**

Memory and Learning

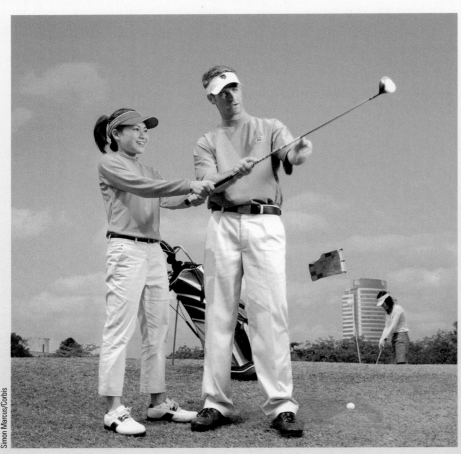

Simon Marcus/Corbis

"It's a poor sort of memory that only works backwards,"
said the Queen.
—Lewis Carroll (1832–1898)
Alice in Wonderland

KEY QUESTIONS

- What is memory?
- What different memory systems underlie the learning and performance of motor skills?
- How do beginners and experts differ in their use of memory?
- How does memory explain "choking" during the performance of motor skills?
- Why can you perform well-learned skills without remembering doing so—like driving a car for many miles?
- Why do people forget well-learned skills?
- How can skills be practiced in ways that they will be better remembered?

CHAPTER OVERVIEW

Learn new skills twice as fast and with half the effort through scientifically proven memory enhancement techniques. . . . Yes, you can develop a super memory that will give you that edge over all opponents. Learn to remember like the champions do, using. . . .

We need not complete the sentence identifying the product promoted in this advertisement. Advertisements like this one promise to help athletes and recreational enthusiasts develop super memories for their activities, ease the effort of learning, and make one a more highly skilled performer by unlocking the secrets of memory.

If this advertisement seems too good to be true, that is because it is. There are no shortcuts to developing the memories underlying skill learning. Just because there are no shortcuts, however, does not mean that there are not better, as well as worse, ways of working with memory. In fact, no one really needs to worry about developing a super memory—everyone already has one. Memory is one of the most amazing capabilities humans possess; it is, in fact, arguably the most amazing. The many billions of neural circuits that form your memories are already capable of super feats. Your memory is able to store and to calculate more information than the most powerful computer. The secret, if there is one, is not to develop additional memory capacities, but simply to learn to take advantage of those you already possess. In this chapter, we will learn how memory works and how, when learning new motor skills, we can best take advantage of the remarkable natural capacities inherent within memory.

In the previous chapter, we defined learning as a set of unobservable processes developed as a result of practice that must be inferred from relatively stable changes in performance observed over time. Those processes underlying learning are, to a large extent, functions of memory. As stated in the words of an old phrase, "Memory is learning that sticks." Jack Adams, one of the prominent founders of the academic study of motor learning, stated that learning and memory are "just different sides of the same coin" (Adams, 1976, p. 87). The study of memory is therefore essential to our understanding of how skills are acquired and how practitioners can design better practice experiences for learners. Understanding how to work with memory, rather than against it, is a hallmark of the knowledgeable and effective instructor of motor skills.

WHAT IS MEMORY?

memory: The processes enabling humans to retain information over time.

An obvious fact is that we learn from experience. Something about our experiences changes our capacity to perform practiced skills in the future. The mechanism responsible for this change, for learning, is called **memory**. Simply stated, memory is the persistence of information over time, the capacity to learn from our experiences.

BOX **6.1**   Ten Myths about Memory

In his book *Your Memory: How It Works and How to Improve It*, Kennett Higbee, a researcher specializing in the factors underlying memory, cites the following 10 myths that people commonly hold concerning memory (2001):

Myth 1: Memory is a thing.
Myth 2: There is a secret to a good memory.
Myth 3: There is an easy way to memorize.
Myth 4: Some people are stuck with bad memories.

Myth 5: Some people are blessed with photographic memories.
Myth 6: Some people are too old/young to improve their memories.
Myth 7: Memory, like a muscle, benefits from exercise.
Myth 8: A trained memory never forgets.
Myth 9: Remembering too much can clutter your mind.
Myth 10: People only use 10 percent of their mental potential.

memory trace: A network of neuronal brain cells encoded to store a specific memory.

Whatever else memory might be, its basic physical structure is housed in the brain through networks of neurons (referred to as a **memory trace**). These neural nets, comprised of thousands and even hundreds of thousands of individual neurons, are joined through millions of synaptic connections forming vast highways of electrochemical patterns representing specific memories—how to ride a bicycle, a favorite poem, where one attended first grade, how to best defend against a switch in a soccer game.

In the not too recent past, it was believed that neural networks were static, fixed structures located in specific brain centers and immutable to change. Modern instruments for studying memory, like PET scanners that provide a close-up of which parts of the brain are active during the formation and later recall of memories, are painting an entirely new picture of how and where memories are formed in the human brain, however. It is now clear that there is no single center for a memory (Baddeley, Eysenck, and Anderson, 2009; Johnson, 2004; Kandel, 2006; and Ratey, 2001). Rather, a memory is compartmentalized into various brain regions—hippocampus, frontal lobes, motor cortex, and so on—from which it can later be retrieved and reassembled when needed. Memories are like puzzle pieces spread out across the brain, which we bring together as a whole only when we retrieve them.

The question naturally arising is whether a memory is located someplace or is a process that occurs only when the memory is retrieved. Endel Tulving, one of the best known memory researchers in the world, after a lifetime studying memory confessed that he did not know if memory was "a storage space, or the act and strategy of retrieval" (quoted in Ratey, 2001, p. 185). We might best think of memory as a coin, with one side being storage and the other side process. When we take the coin out to use, we can focus our attention on whichever side is most beneficial at the time for providing the answers we seek (see Box 6.2).

BOX **6.2** The Vocabulary of Memory

Any memory system, regardless of the system in question, requires three things—the capacity to encode, store, and retrieve information. These form the primary processes describing memory. Definitions for these terms are provided below:

encoding The processes involved in originally registering information from the environment into memory.

storage The capacity to retain encoded information in both active and nonactive forms until needed.

retrieval The ability to locate and recall information stored within memory systems.

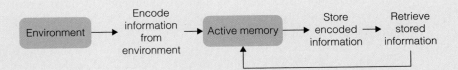

Theoretical Perspectives on Memory

Although modern brain research is adding to our understanding of memory, theoretical consensus remains elusive. A theoretical gap exists between those theorists, on the one hand, who view new memory findings in ways supporting cognitive-based theories, and those on the other hand who interpret new evidence as supporting dynamical systems theories.

Cognitive-Based Theories of Memory

Cognitive-based theorists have focused attention on the brain structures responsible for storing individual memory components. They can rightly point to the fact that memory (at least in its pre-retrieved form) is located in specific brain regions on which specific neurological processes act. A widely accepted theory among cognitive-based scientists is that the individual components of memory, when retrieved, come together in **convergence centers** (Damasio, 1994; Ratey, 2001).

convergence center: A theory that memories are stored in parts across the brain and only brought together through retrieval processes near the sites where they were initially perceived.

In this view, when a memory is retrieved, its individual components are assembled near the sensory neurons where the events forming the memory were initially registered, with this specific location being called a *convergence center*.

The notion of convergence centers carries an even greater appeal for cognitive-based theories than merely the hierarchical location of control centers in the brain. Advocates of this approach posit that convergence centers are hierarchical. That is, convergence centers range from low-level centers for general memory features, to high-level centers for specific memory features. In theory, there could be (as a hypothetical illustration) a lower-level center for all striking skills, a somewhat higher-level center for striking skills using a tennis racquet, an even higher-level center for returning balls using a backhand striking movement, and finally a highest-level center for shot placement in a specific situation using a backhanded return. Instead of having to store many individual memory elements, such hierarchical arrangement makes both storage space and retrieval processes manageable. If this idea looks familiar, that is because it reflects the ideas underlying schema theory presented in Chapter 4 (see Box 6.3). Memory, in this view, is seen as a top-down, hierarchical arrangement in which higher brain centers, those associated with managing the organization and retrieval of memories, are the essential features underlying the control of actions.

Dynamical Systems Theories of Memory

Just as cognitive-based theorists find much to support their ideas in contemporary views of memory, dynamical systems theorists also find much to support their major theoretical positions. Certainly, the neural structures underlying memory fit the definition of complex, adapting systems. Most critical to these theorists is that newly developing views of memory appear to highlight processes of self-organization, adapting networks, and emergence. Inherent in the modern science of memory is the concept, which we have only briefly sketched, that neural networks adapt to their environments (through sensory inputs to the system) and organize into larger collectives, with a specific memory being the final emergent property.

Dynamical systems theorists also point to the fact that memory appears conditioned by specific environmental features both at the time of formation and later during recall, and by an individual's previous knowledge, perceptual capabilities, and psychological state. That is why two people can experience exactly the same event yet have very different memories of it. The point is, though, that many aspects of the original event ultimately encoded within memory must be taken into account. Neural processes alone are not sufficient to explain memory. Thus, memory is viewed as a bottom-up process in which many systems and subsystems interact and have equally important roles to play in memory and the learning of movement skills (see Box 6.4).

The Current Theoretical Landscape

We should not proceed before noting that most of the research directed toward the effects of memory on the learning of motor skills has been conducted from cognitive-based theoretical perspectives. Although dynamical systems theorists have focused considerable attention on how neural networks are formed and how they behave, they have to date focused less attention on memory and even less on memory for motor skills (an exception is the study of perception and memory from an ecological perspective). This lack of systems-based approaches is probably due more to the relative newness of dynamical systems theory compared to cognitive-based approaches and to the greater focus therefore paid to basic questions of theory rather than more applied areas such as learning theory. Most of the research studies reviewed

---

BOX **6.3** Memory of Motor Skills as Schema

According to schema theory, memories for movement skills are stored in hierarchical arrangements. The details for controlling skills in specific ways are embedded within larger, all-encompassing memories for entire classes of action (see Chapter 4). Memories for executing skills in specific ways are retrieved by first accessing a higher-order, generalized memory structure, from which lower-order details for executing the skill in specific ways can then be retrieved. An interesting experiment illustrating how schema theory works was reported in the cognitive domain of learning by Bransford and Johnson (1972).

In this experiment, subjects were asked to read the following passage, after which they were tested for their recall and understanding:

The procedure is quite simple. First, you arrange items into different groups. Of course, one pile may be sufficient depending on how much there is to do. If you have to go somewhere else due to lack of facilities that is the next

step; otherwise, you are pretty well set. It is important not to overdo things. That is, it is better to do too few things at once than too many. In the short run this may not seem important but complications can easily arise.

Subjects read the passage either with or without reading a title beforehand. Those who read the passage without first reading its title remembered very few details and were unable to provide any meaningful context for the described procedures. Those who were first presented with the title of the passage displayed good recall of described procedures, and were able to place those procedures perfectly into their proper context. The title of the passage was "Washing Clothes." The schema for movement skills works in the same way. First accessing higher-order memory for an entire class of movement skills allows much easier retrieval of the details for specific actions, simplifying the entire memory storage and retrieval process.

in this chapter necessarily represent cognitive-based approaches, though their descriptive findings should prove acceptable to those representing either theoretical approach.

MEMORY SYSTEMS

If asked the seemingly odd question "How many different memory systems are there?" most people would probably reply that everyone has just one system for memory—the one he or she is consciously aware of and thinks with. Memory, however, is actually composed of two independent systems, one of which is then further made up of two subsystems, so that three distinct memory systems comprise human memory (Baddeley, 2004; Baddeley, Eysenck, and Anderson, 2009). These three memory systems include the declarative system, comprised of semantic and episodic subsystems, and the procedural system. We will examine each of these memory systems.

BOX 6.4   The Rhythms of Memory

In the view of dynamical systems theorists, memories emerge as the result of the self-organizing activities of networks of neurons within the brain. One result of self-organization of neuronal collectives is that all of the neurons within the network synchronize their activity so that rather than random firing patterns among many individual neurons, a single pattern of activity emerges. In 2001, Fell and colleagues (cited in Strogatz, 2003) offered the first experimental evidence for the synchronization of neurons as a prerequisite for memory.

In their study, Fell and associates asked subjects to memorize a list of words one at a time. Later, after engaging in distracting activities, subjects were tested on their recall of the list. During the original learning period as subjects were attempting to memorize the list of words, the researchers measured the firing patterns of neurons in two different areas of the brain known to be associated with memory—the hippocampus and rhinal cortex. (This was possible because subjects were epileptics who had electrodes implanted in these brain regions in preparation for neurosurgical procedures, which allowed for direct monitoring of neural activity during memorization.)

As would be expected, subjects remembered some words, but not others. What was amazing, though, was that when subjects were attempting to learn the word list, during their memorization activities, for some of the words the firing patterns of neurons in both brain regions would spontaneously shift into a perfectly synchronized pattern of firing, with rates of firing varying rhythmically, as in an orchestrated symphony of electrical impulses, between 30 and 50 cycles per second. While attempting to memorize other words, however, firing patterns remained random and displayed no degree of synchronization indicative of self-organization. What was truly amazing came when the researchers compared the words for which synchronous firing patterns were evident in both brain regions, to those words that were later remembered in the recall test. There was a perfect correlation. Those words that were remembered were the ones in which synchronized firing patterns occurred during learning. Subjects were unable to remember, however, those words for which random firing patterns only were observed. Although much more research is needed in this area, studies such as this one (there have been others since as well) offer strong evidence supporting the dynamical systems approach to the conceptualization of memory.

Declarative Memory System

declarative memory:
A memory system specialized for holding and operating on information concerning objective facts and events.

Declarative memory is a system containing our memories concerning facts and events, both those of a personal nature as well as those about the world around us. Declarative knowledge is knowledge that we can "declare," that is, which we can articulate and tell others about. The declarative memory system contains the knowledge of which we are consciously aware; when we think about our memories, we are really thinking about declarative memories. Declarative memories are further divided into two subsystems called the semantic and episodic systems (note that some theorists consider these two systems as merely different aspects of declarative memory, whereas others view them as entirely distinct and separate systems) (Tulving, 1972).

Semantic Memory

semantic memory:
A memory system specialized for holding and operating on information of a generalized factual nature.

Semantic memory includes generalized knowledge about the world: the capital of North Dakota, who wrote *The Iliad* and *The Odyssey*, the distance to the moon, how to tell time, the rules of baseball, and which club to use for a chip shot, for example. Semantic memory allows us to make sense of the world; it provides the knowledge necessary to organize, interpret, and give meaning to ongoing events. Semantic memory is also independent of the sequence and context in which information occurs; that is, semantic memories are stored independently from where and when they were originally acquired. You know that you should not cross a street on a red light, for example, but have probably long forgotten the specific time and place where you originally acquired this fact.

Episodic Memory

episodic memory:
A memory system specialized for holding and operating on information of a personal nature and specifying the time and place that events occurred.

Episodic memory stores information concering specific events as related to an individual where and when you attended grammar school, your favorite movie, your least favorite food, a remembered smile from a friend, or knowledge that you left the TV on when leaving home this morning. Episodic memory is autobiographical. It is also context and sequence related; it tells us when and where events occurred and provides the basis for organizing events into a meaningful time frame (i.e., putting events in temporal order—which came first).

Procedural Memory System

For a considerable time, psychologists and others studying memory believed that only declarative memories—those that could be articulated—underlay all human behaviors, including skilled motor behaviors. This notion was shattered in the 1950s when scientific reports first appeared concerning a young amnesic patient anonymously referred to simply as H.M. (see Squire and Kandel, 2000, pp. 11–16). As a boy of 9, H.M. suffered head injuries in a bicycle accident that ultimately led to epilepsy. Over the years, H.M.'s condition grew worse, and by the time he was 27 in 1953, he was severely impaired. Because at that time epilepsy was believed centered in the hippocampus of the brain, doctors decided on radically experimental surgery to remove this structure. The surgery proved a success in alleviating H.M.'s epilepsy. Unfortunately, there were unforeseen consequences. From the time of his surgery, H.M. appeared no longer able to form new memories (at least ones of which he was conscious). He could retain information for a few minutes but then forgot what had just happened. His recall of events that had occurred prior to his surgery, even those from earliest childhood, remained intact throughout the rest of his life, however. Over a long life that followed, he believed, whenever asked about current events, that Dwight Eisenhower had just been elected president; the song currently topping the music charts was "How Much Is That Doggie in the Window?" and that the New York Yankees had recently beaten the Brooklyn Dodgers four games to two in the World Series. The events proceeding his surgery became his current reality for the remainder of his life.

What had not been realized prior to his surgery was that the hippocampus, which was removed from H.M., was critical to the formation of declarative memories, at that time the only type of memory believed to exist. But then one of the most remarkable experiments in memory research was conducted (Scoville and Milner, 1957). Based more on intuition than on either theory or evidence, a researcher by the name of Brenda Milner decided to test whether H.M. could learn new motor skills. The motor skill that Milner selected for her research was star-mirror tracing, a frequently used task among motor learning researchers. In this task, subjects are required to perform fine hand–arm movements by quickly guiding a stylus over a narrow line shaped in the pattern of a star while viewing their hand and the star pattern in a mirror reversing the normal image. The results of H.M.'s learning of this skill stunned memory experts. Not only did H.M. improve his skill level, he improved at a rate as great as that observed within the normal population. Even so, each time he was presented with the tracing task, H.M. believed that he was experiencing it for the first time.

At first, many researchers were prone to interpret these astonishing findings as evidence that motor skills must be stored in some special and separate memory system apart from other memories. It soon became apparent, however, that not only motor skills, but also the entire range of behaviors that could be classified as skills were also controlled by a memory system that had to be different from the one used to store declarative memories. What the story of H.M. revealed was not that a specialized memory system exists for motor skills, but that a separate memory system exists that underlies all skill learning. Because this system stored information relative to the procedures for accomplishing skills, regardless of the particular type of skill, it was called the **procedural memory** system.

procedural memory:
A memory system specialized for holding and operating on information pertaining to the execution of skilled behaviors and functioning at a nonconscious level.

The procedural memory system is specialized to store information for skills; it contains memories underlying skills in all three domains of skilled behavior—cognitive, perceptual, and motor. Procedural knowledge deals with "how to" perform various skills, rather than "knowing about" the skills; it is a rule-based system containing the procedures allowing for the expression of skilled action. You use procedural memory for hundreds of activities every day—to tie your shoelaces, ride a bicycle, catch a ball, type a letter, play a musical instrument, dance, and drive a car. If you stop to think about each of these activities for a moment, it becomes obvious that more than the knowledge

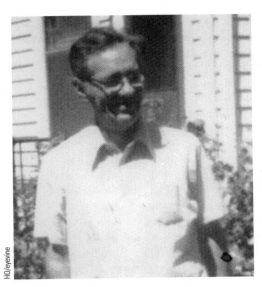

HO/eyevine

Henry Gustav Molaison, known worldwide as H.M. to protect his privacy, died at the age of 82 in 2008. From the time he received experimental brain surgery at age 27 in 1953, he could form no new memories, although his memory for events occurring prior to his surgery remained unimpaired. His intellect and personality also remained unimpaired— he was persistently happy and optimistic, and he was always eager to talk with the many memory researchers who came to study his case. He became the most widely studied patient in the field of memory research, and it is estimated that more is known about memory today because of him than any other source.

of each is necessary in actually accomplishing it. You can read hundreds of books about typing and "know" everything there is to understand about how to type, for example, and still not be able to type. Even though you may have an extensive declarative memory about typing, the actual steps for controlling the arm and hand movements, as well as the perceptual abilities necessary in finding the correct letters on a keyboard, are not encoded into memory along with merely learning the "facts" about typing. Memories governing the perceptual and motor components of typing must also be established in order for the declarative facts about typing to be actualized in the real world. So, procedural memories govern the "doing" of skilled behaviors (see Figure 6.1).

In the examples of procedural skills in the paragraph above, you might have noticed another important feature of each activity. That is, you perform them, at least when well learned, with little or no conscious thought. This distinction in cognitive awareness between declarative (conscious awareness) and procedural (nonconscious awareness) systems can easily be illustrated when considering any action in which you are highly skilled. To return to our typing example, for instance, as I type this page I have no difficulty in striking the correct letter keys to form the desired words on the page. In fact, I have been typing for so many years (since freshman year in high school) that my fingers

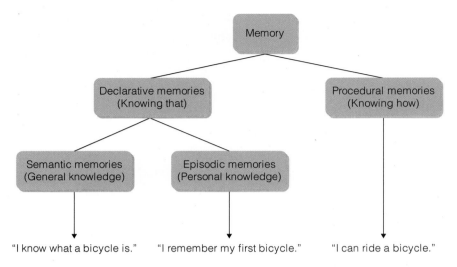

FIGURE **6.1** Memory Systems

Source: Created by author.

automatically go to the correct keys without "thinking" about how I do it—and without the need to look at the keyboard. That is, I have developed, over many years of typing, a rich procedural memory of rules for typing that underlies a fairly well-developed typing skill. I can type any letter needed to assemble the words I want on the page—as long as you do not ask me where the letter is on the keyboard or which finger (or even hand) I use to type it. If asked this question, I have to look on the keyboard and locate the respective letter key—I do not "know" where it is. What it means, in this case, to say, "I do not know where the letter is located," is really to say that I do not have access to my declarative memory for typing (the memory informing conscious awareness of where different keys are located). At some point in the past, when I was first learning to type, I obviously knew where the various letter keys were located on a standard keyboard. The information was in declarative memory but has long since been forgotten, and I can no longer retrieve it into conscious memory. Still, my procedural memory of typing—the one I use regularly and therefore frequently "refresh"—allows me to strike the correct keys accurately and to type even when I no longer remember "how" to type. The reader can no doubt think of many examples of skills contained in procedural memory that can be performed automatically and seemingly without thought, but if asked to elaborate upon the rules, one might have considerable difficulty articulating them.

Procedural memory has an advantage when performing skills that is so obvious that it may easily be initially overlooked. Procedural control of skills is carried out without the need for conscious attention, a capacity referred to as **automaticity**. This means that our conscious awareness, which is limited in its capacity, can be directed toward other activities while still performing skills

automaticity: The capacity of individuals to access and operate on procedural memory without the need for conscious attentional resources when executing well-learned skills.

effectively. Think, for example, of a basketball player dribbling a ball down-court during a game. If the player had to devote her limited attention to accomplishing the highly coordinated acts of running and dribbling, she would not have enough attentional resources remaining to think effectively about what to do in the game (i.e., whether to pass the ball to a teammate, how much time is remaining on the shot clock, what play to run, etc.). Procedural memory makes it possible for humans to carry out varied and highly complex skills while leaving cognitive resources available for other mental activities (planning ahead or carrying on a conversation, for instance), a capability sometimes called *dual tasking.*

Procedural knowledge does not appear to be stored directly into the procedural memory system, however, but is most frequently transferred from declarative memory (though there is still debate about this among experts). What, in effect, this means is that some degree of declarative knowledge must typically first be developed and is essential before procedural memory can be formed. You first have to learn the "facts" of the skill (i.e., the goals, rules, mechanics, what to pay attention to, etc.); that is, you first acquire some declarative knowledge of the skill. Early in learning a motor skill, for example, you "think" your way through performing the skill using the conscious facts you encode into declarative memory stores. Over time, this declarative knowledge fades and you begin to do more and more of the skill automatically, without "thinking" about it. This is an illustration that your knowledge of the procedures underlying the skill—the proceduralization of the skill—is being transferred from declarative memory to procedural memory. Over time, you may forget your original knowledge concerning how you perform a skill as declarative memory fades into a forgotten past, even though your capacity to perform continues to improve as procedural memories are used and reinforced (see Box 6.5 to test your ability to identify memory systems).

Novice and Expert Differences

The discovery of the procedural memory system answered many questions researchers had been asking about the acquisition of motor skills. Today, the

---

BOX **6.5**	**Can You Identify the Memory System?**

Three distinct types of memories have been identified and are believed to comprise three separate memory systems—the declarative system made up of semantic and episodic subsystems, and the procedural system. See whether you can identify the system—semantic, episodic, or procedural—of which each of the following memories would be a part.

- Being able to dribble a basketball
- Knowing the rules for playing tennis

- Remembering the score of the last game of tennis you played
- Being an excellent skateboarder
- The first time you played a Wii game
- The date of Columbus's first voyage to the Americas
- Your favorite musical group
- How you spell your name
- Signing your name

distinction between these systems continues to provide for meaningful analyses in many areas of inquiry. One area that has come under particular scrutiny is the differences between novice (i.e., beginner) and expert performers. Both cognitive-based and dynamical systems theorists have found the distinctions between these systems of memory useful in understanding the differences between individuals based upon skill level. Below we consider two studies designed to highlight differences between beginning and experienced performers based upon considerations of how each makes use of memory. One study, investigating the differences between novice and experienced golfers, was conducted under cognitive-based assumptions concerning memory. The other, examining differences in sport wall climbers of different skill levels, was completed using dynamical systems assumptions.

The Causes of "Choking"—When Declarative Memory Harms Performance

To test the roles played by declarative and procedural memories in acquiring motor skills, Beilock and Carr (2001) conducted an experiment comparing golf putting performance between expert and novice performers, subjects who could be expected to be differentially relying on declarative and procedural memory in their execution of golfing skills. Participants in the experiment were college students who were grouped as either expert or novice golf performers. Expert putters included subjects who had participated in at least two years of high school varsity golf and held a PGA (Professional Golf Association) certification; the novice group was comprised of students with no golfing experience. The task for both groups was the same and included putting a golf ball on a carpeted indoor green to a target on the floor from locations of various distances and angles. Scores were computed by averaging the distance off target for all putts for each of the conditions.

Following the 30-putt practice condition, each subject from both groups was asked to produce a "generic knowledge protocol" of how the golf putt should correctly be performed. Specifically, subjects were asked to respond to the question: "Certain steps are involved in executing a golf putt. Please list as many steps that you can think of, in the right order, which are involved in a typical golf putt." Answers were compared to a list of steps in executing a correct golf putt derived from interviews with professional golf instructors and an analysis of "how to" books on putting. Subjects were scored based upon the length, detail, and correctness of their answers as compared to this master list.

As might be expected, expert golfers were significantly better than novices at generating correct lists of steps for putting; their answers were longer, more detailed, and considerably more accurate. This is an indication that experts had superiorly developed semantic memories of putting compared to the less experienced novices. This is, not surprisingly, what one would expect to find.

The findings became more interesting when subjects were asked to describe in as much detail as possible their episodic memories of their putting performances. Specifically, they were asked: "Pretend that your friend walked into the room. Describe the last putt you took, in enough detail so that your friend could duplicate the last putt you just took in detail, doing it just like you did." When asked this question, the novices produced longer, more detailed, and more accurate descriptions of their performance than did the experts. Contrary to what might have been expected, novice performers displayed better episodic memory of their practice attempts than did experts. Beilock and Carr hypothesized that the experts' reliance on well developed, but automatic and nonconscious, procedural memories of putting actually blocked their recall of the performance events as they unfolded. That is, during the actual execution of a putt, experts controlled their actions through procedural memory structures that effectively blocked access to episodic monitoring of events as they occurred. Simply stated, the experts were less aware of their actions than were the novices, even though they were performing much better.

Surely, however, if experts knew in advance that they would be asked to recall their specific experiences, they would be able to apply their superior semantic knowledge to pay closer attention to a skilled performance and therefore be more proficient at analyzing their performances than would less experienced performers. To test this notion, Beilock and Carr repeated the same procedures on a second set of practice trials, but this time subjects were told before their last putt that they would be asked to describe it in detail just as they had after the first post-test. Although experts did somewhat better on this second recalling of their episodic memories, they still did not do as well as the novice group of subjects (see Figure 6.2). Surprisingly, experts, whose performances were much superior to novices largely because of their richer encoding of the skill requirements for putting into a procedural memory form, had less access to their declarative episodic memory of the skill than did novices (though not to their semantic memories of the skill). Highly skilled performances, it would appear, are controlled through automated procedural

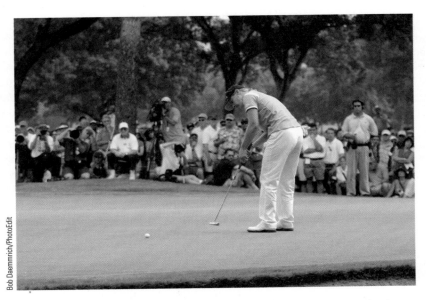

Overthinking when putting can block a skilled golfer's access to procedural memory, resulting in "choking" and degraded performance.

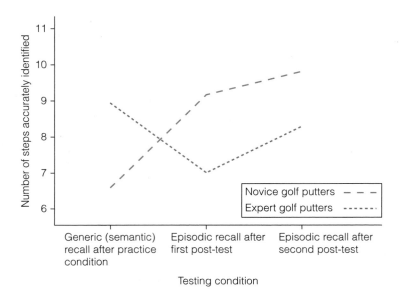

FIGURE **6.2** Results of Beilock and Carr Study

expert-induced amnesia: A term used to describe the tendency for highly skilled performers to exclude episodic monitoring during the execution of skills.

memory structures that operate outside of the scope of conscious attention and therefore remain substantially closed to explicit analysis and recall. Beilock and Carr called this phenomenon of experts' comparative impoverished episodic memories **expertise-induced amnesia.**

Based upon the findings of this research and several other supporting studies (e.g., Beilock et al., 2002; Beilock, Wierenga, and Carr, 2002; and Beilock et al., 2004), Beilock and Carr have argued that a primary cause of "choking" in athletic or other stressful situations in which highly skilled individuals perform (i.e., firefighters, police and military personnel, surgeons, heavy equipment operators, etc.) results when experts attempt to pay too much attention to their external environments (rather than too little, which has sometimes been argued as the cause of choking). That is, choking—performing worse than expected when under pressure—appears to be the result of attempts on the part of skilled performers to harness declarative memories in the execution of skills that have long since been encoded into procedural form. Accessing declarative memory structures during execution of these well-developed skills disrupts the normal functioning of procedural memories best operating in isolation from conscious semantic or episodic intervention, and which are capable of best guiding skilled action in automated and nonconscious fashion. These conclusions support a theory of choking called the *expert-monitoring hypothesis*, that paying too much attention to well-learned skills may prove detrimental to performance. Many current notions of high-level athletic performance also support this conclusion, such as the concepts of "flow" and "inner-game" theory (see, for example, Jackson and Csikszentmihalyi, 1999; and Kauss, 2000). An appreciation for the workings of memory, in this case, helps us to both understand and make practical instructional suggestions concerning a persistent, and still somewhat debated, aspect of highly skilled performances.

Attunement to Affordances

Before leaving our discussion of differences between beginning and experienced learners, we will consider an additional experiment, but this time, one from the perspective of dynamical systems theory. You may recall from Chapter 3 that dynamical systems theorists view memory as including the coupling of perceptual and action control systems, referred to as the perception of **affordances**. Memory means becoming more attuned to the possibilities available in the environment to accomplish skills effectively. Expert performers, in this view, are better able to perceive within the environment information maximizing their opportunities for successfully accomplishing the goals of a particular skill.

In a test of this theory of memory, researchers examined differences in memory use of expert and beginner sport wall climbers (Boschker, Bakker, and Michaels, 2002). Highly experienced wall climbers were compared to beginners with some experience, but who were still in the early stages of learning. Both groups were exposed to a climbing wall that they could study for several minutes. They were then asked to record on a model their recollections of the wall surface (hand- and footholds, overhangs, etc.). Beginners displayed a rich semantic memory of wall features, but those features they recalled were random structural features bearing no relationship to how they might actually climb the wall (that is, they afforded a low opportunity for climbing the wall successfully). Experienced climbers, on the other hand, did not recall nearly as much detail concerning the specific location of wall features, but they did recall available pathways for climbing the wall that would afford the best opportunities for achieving success. This is another example of how highly skilled performers appear to rely upon procedural memory to the exclusion of declarative memory structures, and indicated that such a prioritizing of memory resources provides many distinct advantages for highly skilled performers.

affordances: The properties of an object or of the environment that offer opportunities for action.

THE STAGES OF MEMORY

If individuals are to be aware of their environment and to respond effectively to it, three essential things must happen. Each of these three things in turn requires specialized functions of memory. First, as obvious as it seems, we must be aware of what is in the environment; more to the point, we must focus our limited attentional resources on the most critical and important aspects of our perceived environment. Once we focus on important environmental information, we must next decide what to do in response, as well as how to do it. Finally, if learning is to occur, we must be able to retain the lessons of past experiences for use in the future. These three functions are made possible through human memory. Because each of these three essential functions is accomplished by separate memory structures and processes, it is typical to consider memory as involving three separate stages. These stages are labeled

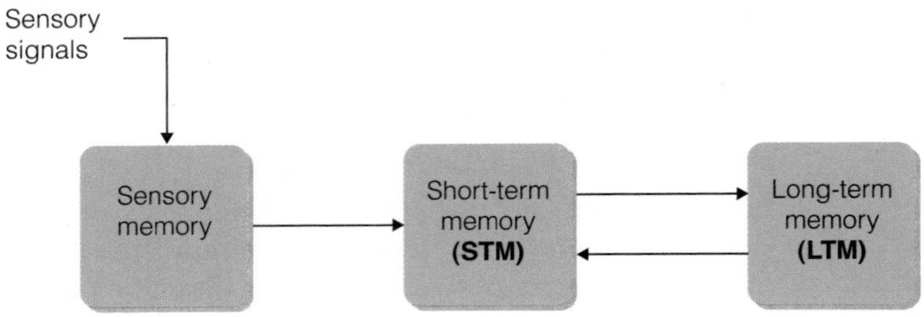

Sensory
signals

FIGURE **6.3** Stages of Memory

Source: Created by author.

sensory memory, short-term memory, and long-term memory (Figure 6.3). An early influential model of these stages was reported by Atkinson and Shiffrin (1968, 1971), so it is often referred to as the Atkinson and Shiffrin model of memory (for fuller and good discussions of this model, see Baddeley, 2004; Klatzky, 1980; and Smith, 1998).

Sensory Memory

sensory memory:
A memory system specialized for encoding all incoming sensory signals and transferring relevant information to short-term memory for attention and possible action.

Sensory memory is the first stage in the process of memory. Information from the environment first enters memory through this stage. This stage of memory takes in virtually everything registered by the body's various sensory receptors and holds it for a brief period during which it can be organized, prioritized, and encoded in transferable form for transfer to following stages in the chain of memory formation. In this capacity, sensory memory acts as a kind of filter or clearinghouse, sorting through the cacophony of mostly extraneous incoming information continuously bombarding our senses and channeling only what is important forward for further attention and possible action.

Sensory memory can be demonstrated in a number of ways. If you move your finger back and forth quickly in front of your eyes, you will observe that the image of your finger appears to be in more than one place at a time (a physical impossibility). This is because the visual image of your finger in each location it traverses is held for a brief period within sensory memory after the stimulus (your finger) is no longer there. This persistence of information, albeit brief, makes it available for further processing even after the stimulus has moved or terminated. The brain seems to possess separate sensory memory stores (called *registers*) for each of the sensory modalities—i.e., vision, hearing, touch, smell, and taste. The most extensively studied registers for motor behavior have been those for vision and touch—these are called *iconic* and *haptic* registers, respectively. Visual information is held for about one-half of a second in sensory memory, whereas auditory information is held for a second or longer (some researchers believe for up to about five seconds). However long, this is a brief storage sufficient only long enough for sensory information to be acted upon and either discarded or transferred on for further processing. Most information entering sensory memory (99% or more) is never further acted upon and is lost to the system (i.e., is forgotten) before being transferred for additional processing.

Short-Term Memory

short-term memory: A memory system that holds and operates on information transferred from sensory memory or retrieved from long-term memory; it is under conscious control and capable of operating on only a limited amount of information at a single point in time.

Information that is transferred from sensory for further processing goes to **short-term memory** (abbreviated STM). STM can hold only a limited amount of information, and then only temporarily. When we think about memory, we are usually thinking about STM because it is the only memory system of which we are consciously aware. Whether we are daydreaming, listening to music, solving a mathematics problem, or performing a motor skill, our awareness of our actions is part of STM.

When Atkinson and Shiffrin proposed their three-stage system of memory, they described STM as a "working memory" that was flexible and could be used in many ways in meeting environmental demands. Over the years, this capacity of STM has come to play a central role in the study of learning and cognition among modern theorists, especially those working from a cognitive-based, information processing perspective. STM is viewed today as much more than a passive memory storage system. It is seen as including a temporary workspace in which long-term memories can be retrieved and coupled with current sensory inputs as part of decision-making processes. In modern cognitive-based views, STM is an essential part of conscious awareness, attention, mental activity, and motor control. The coupling of current sensory inputs into STM, attentional processes, and relevant information from long-term memory stores is referred to as **working memory**. Alan Baddeley (2004), describing the functions of working memory as an integral part of STM, has characterized STM as a multicomponent system comprised of an attentional system, a central executive system responsible for cognitive processing of information, and separate subsystems for storage of sensory information. (Although some theorists prefer to view working memory as a separate stage apart from STM, we will follow the more common approach of viewing working memory as a part of STM and shall often use the terms more or less interchangeably.)

working memory: A temporary work space within short-term memory combining incoming perceptions with information from long-term memory.

magic number 7+/−2: The number of chunks, or bits, of information that short-term memory is capable of holding and operating on at any one time.

chunk: A singularly coherent and meaningful unit of information within short-term memory.

Because STM is so cognitively intensive, being both responsible for decision making and commanding the musculature to carry out those decisions, it has a limited capacity in terms of the amount of information that can be processed and acted upon at any one time. For many years, scientists studying memory have recognized that there is a fixed, seemingly universal amount of information that can be processed as a single unit of action. This fixed limit on the processing capabilities of STM is known as the **magic number 7+/−2**, and represents the number of **chunks,** or bits of information, that STM is capable of handling in a single process. That is, STM can hold no more than 5 to 9 chunks of information at any point in time; this number establishes a limit to the amount of information that can be acted on as a single unit for purposes of decision making and response. This limit represents the "memory span" of STM.

The attentive reader has properly already asked, "What is a chunk?" Unfortunately, there is no clear-cut or agreed-upon definition, and answers tend to fall quickly into the quagmire of circular reasoning (i.e., a chunk is what STM

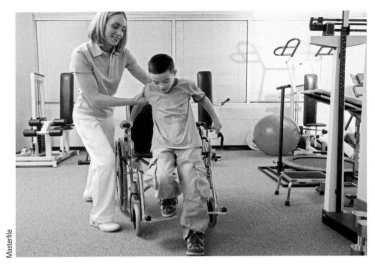

Masterfile

Effective skills instructors understand that beginners have a limited capacity for the number of task-items that they can remember and, therefore, learn during a single practice experience.

can hold about 7 of; STM is the system that can hold 7 chunks). Still, the concept of a chunk, if not the actual definition of it, is fairly well agreed upon. Conceptually, a chunk is a coherent, meaningful amount of information that can be processed as a single unit in memory. A chunk can be a relatively small amount of information, or relatively large, depending on whether the information contained in the chunk can be associated as a single meaningful item for recognition and processing. For example, the letters n, a, l, t, o, p, e, c, a, and u probably represent 10 chunks of information for most people, because there appears to be no logical connection among these letters. In this case, each letter would be encoded, remembered, and processed as a single chunk of information in STM, and because there are 10 letters, this would present a daunting task as it is beyond the memory span of STM (5–9 chunks). However, if one learns to associate all 10 letters in a meaningful way (or recognizes that they already are associated), then the 10 individual chunks can be held and processed in STM as the single chunk *cantaloupe*. The point is that large amounts of information can be handled by STM, as long as it is meaningfully associated into no more than 7+/−2 chunks of information, a technique when used in teaching called **chunking**. Early in learning, before associations among informational units have been made, the capacity of STM for working on information is small; as learning proceeds and associations among informational components are recognized and encoded into memory, more and more information can be held and acted upon at any one time (see Figure 6.4). In a literal sense, learning is about forming associations so that greater amounts of information can be processed in short-term, working memory at a single time.

Just as there is an item limit to the amount of information that STM can process at any single time, there is also a temporal limit to the operations of this

chunking: The process of grouping skill elements into meaningful units for purposes of instruction.

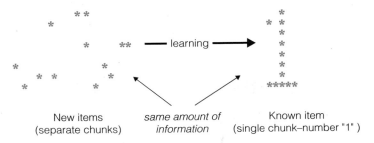

New items   *same amount of*   Known item
(separate chunks)   *information*   (single chunk–number "1")

FIGURE **6.4** Effects of "Chunking" New Items into a Single Known Item

Source: Created by author.

stage. Once information enters STM, it can be held—if not acted upon—for only about 20–30 seconds before it dissipates and fades from memory. Information not acted on within this time frame is quickly lost, and cannot be retrieved for further processing or action. With rehearsal (thinking about it, attending to it), however, information can be maintained in STM for a theoretically indefinite period, although most people find it difficult to maintain information for longer than about 8–10 minutes (it is so difficult, in fact, that this figure can be considered an upper limit for STM). As with sensory memory, most information (99% or more) encoded into STM will be permanently lost (forgotten) before being transferred to the next stage of memory—long-term memory.

Long-Term Memory

long-term memory:
A memory system that permanently stores all information encoded from short-term memory; responsible for learning.

Long-term memories are those responsible for learning. Once information enters **long-term memory** (abbreviated LTM), it is more or less permanent (there is some debate about this among experts, but certainly the vast majority of LTMs are stored permanently). LTM contains our memories of past experiences and forms the basis for learning. In fact, by definition, learning means getting things into LTM. Not only is the duration of LTM permanent, but its capacity appears unlimited as well. That is, it is capable of storing an entire lifetime of experiences. Table 6.1 compares the capacity and duration capabilities of long-term memory with the two previous memory stages that we have discussed.

TABLE **6.1**
Characteristics of the Three Stages of Memory

	Sensory Memory	STM	LTM
Capacity	Unlimited	7+/–2 items	Unlimited
Duration	1/10–1 sec.	20–30 sec. or 8–10 min. with rehearsal	Permanent

Long-term memory includes procedural, semantic, and episodic information encoding in a way that allows for retrieval. The process of encoding information from active, working memory (i.e., STM) into permanent LTM is highly dependent upon rehearsal (amount of time or number of trials practiced), attention, and motivation (interest). That is, encoding is a function of these three variables. Simply stated, the more times you practice something, the greater your attention to it during practice, and the greater your motivation or interest in it, the greater the probability that it will be encoded into LTM and learned. In fact, although the role of rehearsal and attention may appear obvious, in regard to motivation it appears to be nearly impossible to form LTMs for something in which a person has absolutely no interest or motivation (which is what typically occurs when people say that they have a learning "phobia" such as math phobia—it is probably not intellectual capability that is lacking, but sufficient interest and motivation to learn). Whether they realize it or not, instructors of motor skills are concerned with the factors responsible for encoding information into LTM when they focus their instructional methods on increasing learners' attention, motivation, and practice time, or with fostering the indestructible vestiges of skill, to echo James (Box 6.6). We will discuss specific instructional methods for facilitating memory for motor skills in Chapters 9 through 11.

Practice Considerations for Enhancing Long-Term Consolidation

An obvious fact concerning the three stages of memory is that the ultimate goal of practice is almost always to encode practiced skills into long-term memory before they are forgotten. The processes by which memories become permanent—that is, transferred into long-term memory structures—is called **consolidation**. According to current thinking, the imprint of experiences takes time to solidify because it requires structural changes in the synaptic connections between neurons, and those changes require time, usually between 24 and 72 hours, to reach fruition (Baddeley, Eysenck, and Anderson, 2009). Over the period of consolidation, the new memory trace is gradually woven into the fabric of long-term memory.

A number of practice variables have been identified that facilitate the process of consolidation. Besides the factors of amount of practice, attention, and motivation, which have already been mentioned and will be given special consideration in later chapters, a number of factors related to the scheduling and

consolidation: The process by which a new memory trace is gradually transferred to long-term memory.

BOX 6.6 William James on the Stages of Memory

The stream of thought flows on; but most of its segments fall into the bottomless abyss of oblivion. Of some, no memory survives the instant of their passage. Of others, it is confined to a few moments, hours or days. Others again leave vestiges which are indestructible, and by means of which they may be recalled as long as life endures.

—William James (1842–1910)
nineteenth-century American
philosopher/psychologist

presentation of practice can play important roles in enhancing the prospects for effective consolidation of practiced skills. We consider several of these next.

Primacy-Recency Effects   An important factor in whether new information will "stick" in LTM (i.e., will consolidate) has to do with the order in which it is originally presented. An obvious factor in learning any skill or activity is that some parts of the skill are practiced first, some in the middle, and others last within a practice session. This may seem of no real significance until one considers that the positioning of information during practice has a significant influence on what will be remembered. In fact, the effect on learning of positioning during a practice session is well established across all domains of learning and is called the **primacy-recency effect** (or, perhaps as frequently, the *serial-order effect*).

primacy-recency effect: The phenomenon that information presented at the beginning and ending of a practice session is more readily learned, all other factors being equal, than is information presented in the middle of practice.

The primacy-recency effect is the observation that in any sequencing of things to be learned, those practiced in the beginning (primacy) and ending (recency) of practice will be best recalled. In the practice of motor skills, this means that those activities or components of a skill instructed early and late in practice are the ones most likely to be remembered (i.e., learned), and those in the middle part of the practice session, the least likely to be remembered (i.e., are relatively more difficult to learn). Figure 6.5 illustrates the effects of primacy-recency positioning on remembering and learning.

As can be observed in Figure 6.5, those skill activities or components in the primacy and recency positions of a practice session are most easily consolidated within LTM. That is, all other things being equal, they are most easily remembered and, therefore, the best learned. So instructors of motor skills do well to consider the relative positioning of skills or skill components when instructing new or more difficult skills or activities within practice sessions. Unless there is good reason for doing otherwise, new or more difficult items to be learned should be presented in the beginning and/or ending of practice sessions while reserving middle portions of practice for easier task components or for reviewing previously learned activities.

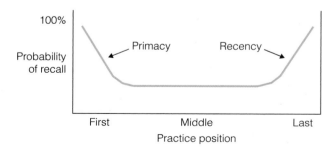

FIGURE **6.5** Primacy-Recency Effects

Source: Created by author.

The Von Restorft Effect

An interesting exception to the primacy-recency effect is that some information presented in the middle parts of practice can be encoded into memory as well as, and perhaps even better than, information presented at either the beginning or ending of practice. This occurs whenever information is given a special meaning, or stands out in some way from other information being presented. An instructor who presents information in an especially dramatic and "unforgettable" way, or who gives special meaning to information or an activity, is relying on the **von Restorft effect** (also called the *outstanding item effect*) to make that information more meaningful and easily remembered by learners (see Figure 6.6).

von Restorft effect: An exception to the primacy-recency effect in that information presented during the middle of a practice session in a particularly meaningful or dramatic fashion increases the likelihood that it will be learned.

Practice Distribution Effects

Considerable research across all domains of learning has cogently demonstrated that distributing practice over a longer period punctuated by rest breaks significantly enhances the retention and recall of information (Dail and Christina, 2004). For most cognitively demanding learning situations, which could include preparing for a school examination or practicing a new motor skill, 45 minutes to an hour seems to be an upper limit to the amount of practice time that is effective for learning (Baddeley, 2004). In many situations, even shorter practice periods are recommended. Regardless of the activity, shorter practice sessions distributed across longer periods of time typically result in significant increases in learning (see Figure 6.7).

In practice, the amount of time that motor skill instructors have to work with is often limited by the length of a class, therapy session, or training session. Whenever possible and practical, however, instructors should weigh the benefits to memory of spreading practice out and including more short breaks between practice experiences in order to enhance learning. (The application of this principle should be carefully weighed against other factors, however, and a more extensive discussion of these ideas is presented in Chapter 11.)

priming: The brief introduction of new information prior to the time when it is actually practiced; increases the likelihood that the information will be learned when it is later practiced.

Priming Effects

Increasing the likelihood that learners will remember information is significantly enhanced through the use of a technique called **priming**. Priming means the brief introduction of new information or a new skill prior to actually practicing it; priming is presented to help learners "get the idea" of what it is they are going to practice.

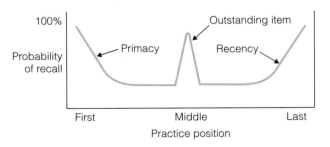

FIGURE **6.6** The Von Restorft (or Outstanding Item) Effect

Source: Created by author.

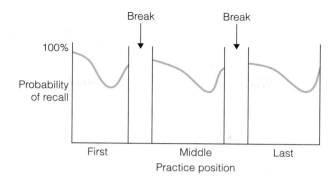

FIGURE **6.7** Effect of Practice Breaks on Recall

Source: Created by author.

Priming can be especially helpful in reducing some retention disadvantages associated with activities practiced in the middle parts of a practice session by briefly introducing the activities at the beginning of practice. Priming activities do not need to be extensive in order to be effective, and in fact probably work best when brief. An instructor who visually demonstrates a new skill at the beginning of practice, for example, even though not instructing it until later in practice, is using priming. Later, when learners practice the skill, the initial priming will enhance the likelihood that they will remember and learn the skill. Priming might also occur at the completion of one practice session for a skill to be instructed on a following day. An important point here is that priming is a brief demonstration designed to help learners get the basic idea of what is to come and is not meant as instruction or practice.

Emphasizing Location Cues When learning a motor skill, any one of many characteristics of movement could be encoded into memory. For example, we could store the location of points along the path of limb movements, the distance of limb movements, the velocity of movements, the force of muscular contractions producing movements, or some abstract representation of spatial-temporal patterning concerning movements.

Although all of the above features of movements for skill are probably stored in memory, a considerable amount of research has demonstrated that various locations along the path of a movement, and particularly movement endpoint locations, are given priority in the encoding activities of memory—at least in the early stages of learning (Chieffi, Allport, and Woodfin, 1999; Diewert, 1975; and Hagman, 1978). That is, location points of limb and body movements, and especially limb endpoint location, are remembered before distance, velocity, force, or other features of the movements' underlying skill.

Understanding how memory works in this respect can aid the instructor of motor skills. Because memory processes function to encode important location points, an instructor can enhance the learning capabilities of individuals by pointing out critical position points in skills being practiced—and this is especially true of the final endpoints of limb movements. For example, when providing instructions for the tennis serve to a beginning learner, a knowledgeable instructor should focus sufficient attention on body and limb locations associated with critical points in the serve; these could include the beginning position of body and arms, arm position at the top of the backswing, and arm and body position at the point the racquet strikes the ball. The position of the striking arm at the point the racquet contacts the ball would be especially critical and should be emphasized. As another example, a therapist working with a patient to regain gait control might point out important hip and leg positions during walking, particularly the positions associated with extreme flexion and extension during the gait cycle. In this regard, just as in the others seen in this chapter, knowledgeable motor skill instructors learn to work with, rather than against, memory.

Sleeping on It   The importance of getting a good night's sleep following motor skill practice has been offered as advice by motor skill instructors for as long as anyone can remember. Considerable research in recent years has supported this observation. Sleep following motor skill practice has repeatedly been demonstrated to enhance the learning of motor skills, and even to play an essential role in skill learning (Brashers-Krug, Shadmehr, and Bizzi, 1996; Walker et al., 2002; Walker, Brakefield, and Stickgold, 2003). Although the neural mechanisms connecting sleep and consolidation are still debated, mounting evidence suggests that sleep plays an essential role in the consolidation of memories, and especially in the consolidation of procedural memories.

Although restive sleep is important for optimal skill learning, this should not be interpreted as meaning the more sleep, the better. Sleep representative of a person's normal nightly sleep cycle, which is restful in nature, is sufficient in maximizing consolidation effects. Sleep beyond the normal range appears to have no additional benefits. What is apparent, though, is that a lack of sufficient sleep, or sleep that is interrupted and nonrestful, has detrimental effects on memory consolidation and resultant learning.

More work still is needed to fully understand both the mechanisms through which sleep enhances memory consolidation, as well as the types of skills and individual characteristics which may be most impacted by sleep. Evidence to date would suggest, for example, that younger persons may benefit more from sleep than older individuals, although this is still debatable. Recent evidence also is leading to a conclusion supporting the significant benefits of sufficient sleep in regaining skills lost to injury or neurological impairments (Siengsukon and Boyd, 2009). Other research has shown that the benefits of sleep can be enhanced by short daily naps (Sheth, Janvelyan, and Khan, 2009). Whatever the continuing research in this area ultimately reveals, it is now evident that coaches, teachers, and therapists have been correct all along in encouraging their charges to "get a good night's sleep."

WHY DO WE FORGET LEARNED SKILLS?

In the previous section, we stated that considerable information held in both sensory memory and STM stores is permanently lost, either because it is not needed or because it is insufficiently attended to or practiced. We also noted that most theorists believe that information encoded into LTM is permanently stored. The question then becomes, why is this information lost, or in the case of LTM, why can it not be retrieved and used? The answer in both cases is that the memories are forgotten.

forgetting: The loss of, or failure to retrieve, information from memory.

Forgetting is the loss of or inability to retrieve information from memory. Forgetting does not necessarily mean that previously learned information is no longer in the memory system, only that it is no longer accessible. Forgetting of information occurs for one of two reasons: trace decay or interference. These two reasons imply different processes involved with forgetting and underlie different reasons for forgetting from the three stages of memory. We will examine both reasons for forgetting as well as the implications for motor skill practice.

Trace-Decay Theory

trace decay: A theory of forgetting that the memory trace fades over time and reverts to its original state; an explanation of forgetting from sensory memory and short-term memory.

Trace-decay theory is probably what most people think about when they think about forgetting. Trace decay means that the original memory trace stored in one of the memory systems decays before being permanently encoded in LTM. The original excitation of neurons in the brain (the memory trace) caused by electrochemical activity transmitted from sensory receptors diminishes over time as energy is dissipated. Once the original trace is gone, it can no longer be retrieved (because it is no longer anywhere in memory). The process of decay may take only a fraction of a second in sensory memory, or between seconds

---

BOX 6.7   A Hierarchy of Memory Difficulty

Things are difficult or easier to remember based upon a number of factors. Donald Norman (1988), a noted cognitive scientist, summarizes the ease with which things are remembered as falling into the following three categories.

1. **Memory for arbitrary things.** The items or information to be retained seem arbitrary, with no meaning and no particular relationship to one another or to things already known. This represents the category of things that are the most difficult to remember.

   Example: Teaching the serve in tennis by presenting the individual components of the swing in isolation (i.e., rotate at the hips, lead with the elbow of the striking arm, snap the wrist at contact, etc.).

2. **Memory for meaningful relationships.** The items or information to be retained form meaningful relationships with themselves or with other things already known. This category represents only moderate difficulty of remembering.

   Example: Illustrate how the tennis serve uses the same movement pattern as throwing a ball.

3. **Memory through explanation.** The material does not have to be remembered, but rather can be derived from some explanatory mechanism. This represents the easiest category of remembering.

   Example: Build upon the illustration of throwing a ball by explaining the biomechanical principles involved (i.e., rotating the hips and leading with the elbow increases the distance the racquet head travels prior to contacting the ball, thus increasing speed and force at contact).

and minutes in STM. In either case, information that is not transferred to the next stage of memory vanishes due to trace decay and are eliminated from the system and further processing activities. Trace decay is the explanation for forgetting from both sensory and STM. Some information that originally enters LTM may also be lost to trace decay if it is not made permanent through sufficient rehearsal and attention, though this conjecture remains debatable. Once the memory trace is encoded in LTM, its structure and function are immutable to decay, and so trace decay is no longer an explanation for forgetting. If the trace is impervious to decay, though, why do people forget information stored in LTM? The answer is not that the trace decays, but that interference prevents retrieval of the memory.

Interference Theory

interference: A theory of forgetting that memories encoded into long-term storage may fail to be retrieved into short-term memory because other memories stored in the long-term system block retrieval processes.

Interference theory is the notion that memories in LTM interfere with, or get in the way of, one another (Baddeley, Eysenck, and Anderson, 2009; Del Ray, Liu, and Simpson, 1994; Keppel and Underwood, 1962; and Underwood, 1957). The problem is not that memories stored in LTM diminish in strength in any way, but that they cannot be effectively retrieved. Because LTM is such a vast store of memories, those covering a lifetime of experiences, it should not be surprising that memories can interfere with one another. Put simply, given the vast number of memories stored in LTM, so many are similar in some respect that finding the correct one becomes a challenge to memory's retrieval capabilities.

Not all memories have the same potential to interfere with one another, however. Two factors seem especially important in determining the strength of interference between any two memories; these are their similarity and their temporal closeness. That is, the more two memories are similar—the more they are about the same thing—and the closer together in time they were originally registered in LTM, the greater the potential for interference between them to occur.

The storage of information with respect to the comparative time in which memories are placed into LTM has an effect on the strength of interference, and further denotes two types of interference effects called *retroactive inhibition* and *proactive inhibition* (which are also termed *retroactive interference* and *proactive interference*).

Retroactive Inhibition

retroactive inhibition: The interference of newer memories with retrieval of older memories.

Retroactive inhibition (see Figure 6.8) refers to the interference of new memories with the retrieval of older memories. (Another way of saying the same thing is that new learning interferes with old learning.) We have all experienced that as things we once learned and knew well recede in time without being practiced, we tend to forget them. This is because the things we have subsequently learned affect our ability to recall previous memories. It is, of course, to our benefit that memory is structured in a way making what we are currently experiencing more readily accessible to recall and use (think what it would be like if you could remember everything you did a year ago, but had trouble remembering what you did earlier in the day). Still, retroactive inhibition can become problematic relative to skilled performance, especially when skills are not continuously practiced.

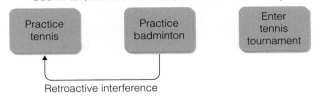

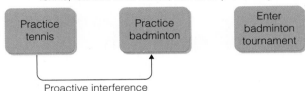

FIGURE **6.8** Retroactive and Proactive Inhibition

Source: Created by author.

Skills that are learned and then not used for long periods of time are susceptible to retroactive inhibition. Since the time of the first scientific studies on forgetting by the German psychologist Hermann Ebbinghaus (1885, 1913) in the late nineteenth century, it has been known that the rate at which newly presented information is forgotten is steep. Although many factors affect the rate of forgetting, a generalized finding is that about 70 percent of the information originally recalled in a practice session is forgotten within the first 24 hours after practice, and that figure quickly increases to about 80 percent after 48 hours. After that, the rate of forgetting gradually diminishes over longer periods of time, with perhaps no more than 5 or 10 percent of the originally learned information ultimately retained (or, at least, accessible). The effects of retroactive inhibition can be significantly decreased in several ways, however. These include following overlearning practice schedules, as discussed earlier, in Chapter 5, providing for periodic refresher practice of skills, and using mental rehearsal of skills during periods of nonuse. The type of skill also interacts significantly with rates of forgetting, with continuous motor skills considerably more resistant to forgetting than are discrete motor skills.

Proactive Inhhibition

proactive inhibition:
The interference of older memories with the learning and retrieval of newer memories.

Proactive inhibition (see Figure 6.8) refers to the interference of old memories with the retrieval of newer memories. (Again, another way of saying the same thing is that old learning interferes with new learning.) A common example of proactive inhibition is seen when experienced racquetball players attempt to learn tennis; their previous learning of racquetball interferes with their initial ability to learn tennis.

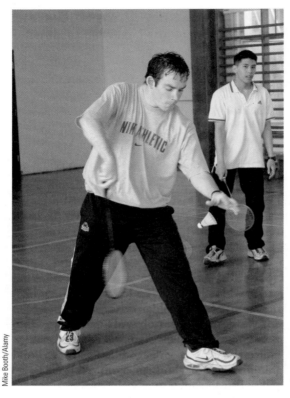

Mike Booth/Alamy

Individuals who take up the skill of badminton after having learned tennis, often experience an initial period of difficulty acquiring the correct racquet techniques for badminton because the differences in racquet techniques between tennis and badminton are a source of proactive interference.

Of the two types of inhibition, though, retroactive inhibition causes considerably more problems during learning and is the stronger of the two types relative to interference effects.

Strategies for Reducing Interference (and Forgetting)

Based on an understanding of interference and the effects it has on memory and learning, the motor skill instructor can apply several principles to the design of practice experiences that will increase the likelihood learners will successfully remember what they practice. These principles inform the following two guidelines, which would be well considered in the teaching of any motor skill.

1. *Separate similar skills within a practice schedule as far apart as "practically" possible in order to reduce the effects of interference.* For example, a dance instructor teaching several different steps to a class

might determine which of the steps are most alike and then separate them so that instruction initially occurs on different days. (Note that this goes against much commonly heard advice about teaching similar skills together, which can be effective but only once some initial degree of learning has occurred making memories more resistant to interference.)

2. *Prefer proactive rather than retroactive inhibition when presenting a new skill.*

   When instructing a skill for the first time, presenting it late in practice (or even at the end) has a considerable effect on reducing interference and gives learners the best chance of encoding the skill and getting it into memory while it is still "fragile" and susceptible to interference. Practice does not need to be extensive at this stage, although somewhat more than an introduction is probably desirable. (The reader will note that this consideration based upon reducing interference effects also takes advantage of primacy-recency effects.)

Putting together the several principles discussed in this section on forgetting, the motor skill instructor should be able to design effective practice schedules giving learners the best chance of retaining information and acquiring desired motor skills.

The secret of a good memory is attention, and attention to a subject depends upon our interest in it. We rarely forget that which has made a deep impression on our minds.

—Tryon Edwards (1809–1894)

MEMORY AND PLACE: ENCODING SPECIFICITY PRINCIPLES

By now, the reader will hopefully recognize that memory impinges upon nearly every aspect concerned with the learning of motor skills. Because of this, most practice considerations are based at least to some extent, and often to a great extent, upon memory principles. In focusing on memory, however, it is easy to consider only those aspects of practice of which we are consciously aware and which seem directly related to skill performance. After all, it is what we attend to, what we are consciously aware of wanting to learn, that is encoding into memory. Or is it?

When we learn a motor skill, we consciously practice and hopefully encode into long-term memory the important aspects of bodily movements required for executing a skill properly. We also remember, again hopefully, strategies for executing the skill under various conditions. Such information forms what is called **explicit memory**. These are memories of the things we consciously intend to learn, and of which we are consciously aware when we retrieve them. But there are also other facets of learning environments that are encoded and stored along with explicit memory, those of which we are unaware and which we do not intend to remember. We might think of these features as a backdrop of the practice environment, something like the canvas of a painting. When we look at a painting, we are aware of the various images portrayed, the colors, the background on which the figures are displayed, indeed all of the visual elements and details the artist placed upon the canvas. We probably do not think about the canvas itself, however. Yet it forms the supporting surface making the painting possible.

explicit memory: Memory that is open to intentional retrieval (synonymous with declarative memory).

When we learn a new skill, many features of the practice environment form the supporting background of practice; they are like the canvas on which an artist paints. We may not be aware of them, but they provide the context in which those aspects of practice of which we are aware are embedded, and much of this background context is stored in memory along with the explicit memories we intend to learn. These memories are called **implicit memories**, and they are entwined with our explicit memories of a skill so that memories are really compositions of both consciously and unconsciously learned elements of the practice environment.

In learning a motor skill, we store in memory information pertaining to movement patterns, the goals and rules of the skill, and perceptual cues related to the performance of the skill—all things we intentionally practice and of which we are aware. These are all explicit memories. But we also encode into memory many aspects related to the conditions of learning of which we are not consciously aware—or at least which we do not intentionally practice and intend to remember. These implicit memories may include aspects of the place in which we practice the skill such as specific spatial dimensions related to performance (extent and distances of the practice space), lighting conditions, patterns of color and texture, temperature, time of day, verbal feedback, the order in which skill events are typically sequenced during practice, the way in which skills are practiced (active vs. passive, or slow vs. fast, for example), social conditions (how we relate to those with whom we practice), and even mood (our level of arousal, attention, motivation, etc.). None of these aspects of practice are things we specifically pay attention to with the intention of remembering them as they relate to learning a skill; nonetheless, they are (or many such aspects are) encoding into memory along with the more obviously practiced elements of a skill.

Researchers have observed for many years that when the original conditions of practice change, people have some increased difficulty in recalling learned information. This is true for both declarative and procedural memories, including memories for motor skills (see Tulving and Thomson, 1973). Scientists call the conditions of learning in which memories are originally formed the **encoding condition**. The conditions existing later, when a person attempts to perform the skill, are called the **recall condition**. The closer the encoding and recall conditions resemble one another (the more similar they are), the easier it will be to retrieve the memory of a skill and perform it well (Magill and Lee, 1987; Thompson and Madigan, 2005). The observation that retrieval and performance of learned skills are facilitated to the degree that encoding and recall conditions are similar is known as the **encoding specificity principle**.

A Classic Demonstration of the Encoding Specificity Principle

Godden and Baddeley demonstrated the encoding specificity principle in a landmark experiment in 1975. Their experiment consisted of training 60 experienced scuba divers to recall a list of 36 nonassociated words practiced under one of two conditions. Half of the divers practiced learning the list on the dock next to the water, while the other half practiced for the same amount of time

implicit memory: Retrieval of information from long-term memory through performance rather than conscious recall; nondeclarative memory.

encoding condition: The context in which a skill is practiced and learned.

recall condition: The context in which a skill is performed as a result of practice.

encoding specificity principle: The principle that skills executed in situations similar to those in which they are learned will be better remembered and performed.

but 15 feet underwater a few feet away from the dock. On the following day, all divers were asked to recall as many of the words on the list as they could. During the recall test, however, half of each group was asked to recall the list of words in the same setting as they were originally learned, and the other half of the group was asked to recall the list in the opposite setting. That is, half of the divers who practiced on the dock performed the recall test on the dock, while the other half performed the test underwater. Likewise, half of the group who practiced underwater performed the recall test underwater, while the remaining half performed the test on the dock (see Figure 6.9).

Results of the experiment revealed that both groups remembered best when they were tested in their original learning condition. On the other hand, attempting to recall the list of words in the opposite condition resulted in considerably less proficiency for both groups. The group that learned on the dock correctly recalled 37 percent of the words on the list when tested on the dock, but only 23 percent when tested underwater. The group that learned the list underwater successfully recalled 32 percent of the words when tested underwater, but only 24 percent when tested on the dock (see Figure 6.10). Godden and Baddeley concluded that the similarity of contexts between learning and recall conditions provided retrieval cues, whereas the greater forgetting in the dissimilar contexts was due to the absence of context-dependent retrieval cues encoded along with the original learning.

Encoding Specificity and Practice Guidelines

Since Godden and Baddeley's original study, many other experimental investigations have established the principle of encoding specificity (e.g., Lee and Hirota, 1980; Magill and Lee, 1987; Smith, Glenberg, and Bjork, 1987; Smith and Vela, 2001; and Vaidya et al., 2002). What this principle means for instructors of motor skills is that the closer practice conditions (i.e., encoding

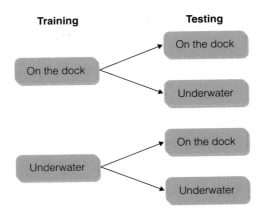

FIGURE **6.9** Experimental Design of Godden and Baddeley Study

Source: Created by author.

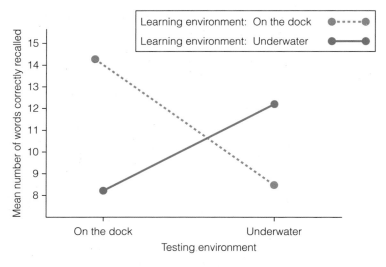

conditions) are matched to those conditions in which a learner is ultimately expected to perform (i.e., recall conditions), the more effective practice will become. Examples include matching practice conditions as closely as possible to game conditions in the practice of athletics, clinical conditions to home or work conditions in therapy settings, training conditions to work conditions in industrial training programs, and training conditions to expected combat conditions in military training programs.

To some extent, of course, practice conditions are seldom able to mimic expected recall conditions precisely. The application of encoding specificity principles can prove especially effective, though, when both the practice context and skill remain highly constant from practice to recall conditions. This situation is most relevant when closed motor skills are being instructed. With closed skills, the anticipated performance conditions are typically stable and predictable so that practice conditions can be established to closely mirror the expected performance conditions. Practice conditions that are designed to conform as closely as practically possible to expected performance conditions in these cases represent sound application of encoding specificity principles to the instructional setting.

Consider, for example, a field-goal kicker in football practicing for an upcoming game. In order to maximize the number of kicks practiced, he will kick many balls. Most of these will be kicked in isolation from his teammates, under nonpressured conditions, while setting his own pace concerning when to kick the ball. None of these conditions will exist in the actual game, however, in which he will be called upon to perform quickly when the ball is snapped and with the sights and sounds of opposing players closing in on him. In this case, it is particularly important that as many kicking attempts as possible during practice be accomplished under more authentically game-like situations as part of practice with the entire team during game-simulated conditions.

As another example, it is interesting to observe the efforts made to provide realistic skill performance situations in professional police and military training programs. Once basic skills have been acquired, both military and police personnel are put through training that is as close to the expected actual conditions of policing and combat as possible, including environmental considerations such as location, time of day, lighting, weather, ambient noise (sirens, explosions, shouting, etc.), and obstacles—all of this while wearing their service uniforms complete with webbing, utility belts, and backpacks.

SUMMARY

Learning is made possible by memory, which most simply defined is the capacity to maintain some aspects of previous experiences in order to guide current behaviors. The mechanisms responsible for memory are viewed differently within cognitive-based and dynamical systems theories.

Memory is comprised of the declarative and procedural memory systems, with the declarative system further subdivided into semantic and episodic subsystems.

- The semantic memory system stores generalized knowledge about the world; it includes memories about objective and nonpersonal facts and events.
- The episodic memory system stores information about personal events; it includes the what, where, and when of personal experience.
- Procedural memory contains the rules governing skills, including but not limited to motor skills.

There are three distinct stages of memory, each devoted to specific functions involved in the processing and storage of information.

- Sensory memory processes all available sensory information from a person's environment and body; it acts as a filter, eliminating unnecessary information from further consideration and transferring relevant information to the next stage for further processing.
- Short-term memory (STM) holds essential information for a brief period of time (a few seconds to minutes) so that it can be consciously worked on, decisions made, and actions carried out.
- Long-term memory contains those memories that have been permanently stored in memory, and it is the system ultimately responsible for learning (i.e., learning occurs when what has been practiced gets into long-term memory).

The consolidation of long-term memories (learning) can be significantly enhanced through instructional techniques based upon memory considerations including chunking, primacy-recency effects, the Von Restorft effect, practice distribution, priming effects, and the emphasizing of location cues.

Forgetting is the loss of or inability to retrieve and use information stored in memory. An important goal of practice is the presentation of information in ways that learners are less likely to forget it. Two theories, trace-decay theory and interference theory, explain why people forget.

- Trace decay occurs when the original neural trace associated with an event or practice experience decays or dissipates before becoming permanently encoded into LTM.
- Interference occurs when a memory has been encoded permanently into LTM, but other memories interfere with a person's ability to retrieve and use the memory. Interference can occur through either retroactive or proactive inhibition.

When practicing skills, both explicit and implicit aspects of the practice context are encoded into long-term memory.

- Retrieval of the memory for a skill is facilitated to the degree that the encoding and retrieval conditions are similar.

The study of how memories for motor skills are formed provides many important guidelines for the provision of practice experiences and instructions. Knowledgeable practitioners learn to work with, rather than against, memory.

LEARNING EXERCISES

1. For this exercise, identify a setting of interest to you in which you can observe an instructor teaching a motor skill to either an individual or small group of individuals in the initial or early stages of learning for at least 30 minutes (larger groups may be used if you are still able to closely observe the instructor). Describe the setting, including the methods you used for observing and collecting data.

   Prior to making your observations, discuss with the instructor his or her goals for the practice session, a description of previous practice activities if any, and whether the instructor uses any specific teaching methods based upon memory considerations. Once observing the practice, your goal is to analyze the effectiveness of the instructional setting in relation to considerations concerning memory. Make a list of memory considerations you think relevant to the situation and for which you will make observations (e.g., are primacy-recency considerations observed, are chunking methods employed, are important location cues pointed out, etc.? Many more items can be included). As you observe practice, keep notes on your observations.

   After your practice observations have been completed, prepare a written evaluation of your experiences and conclusions. Discuss those aspects of instruction that reflected good techniques for facilitating the memory of learners, as well as ways in which practice could have been instructed to produce greater memory consolidation and later recall of skills. How would you have instructed practice differently based upon your understanding of memory?

2. Design a practice schedule for instructing a motor skill in which you are both interested and knowledgeable to an individual having no previous experience with the skill. Describe the basic activities in which this learner will engage for a period covering the initial 10 practice periods. Describe in general terms your instructional goals for each of the practice sessions. Describe for each practice session how memory considerations will help you achieve your practice goals, including specific techniques you will use in providing instructions.

3. For this exercise, describe a motor skill in which you are experienced and believe yourself highly proficient and one in which you are inexperienced and would like to become better. Provide a detailed description of how you believe you use your memory when performing both of these skills. Specifically, how do both declarative and procedural memories help you describe and understand your performance characteristics for both skills?

FOR FURTHER STUDY

HOW MUCH DO YOU KNOW?

For each of the following, select the letter that best answers the question.

1. The process by which information in the environment is translated into a form that can be registered by a memory system is called
   a. storage.
   b. consolidation.
   c. retrieval.
   d. encoding.

2. Studies in the 1950s with a young man identified only as "H.M." resulted in the discovery of
   a. the memory trace.
   b. the procedural memory system.
   c. episodic memory.
   d. convergence centers.

3. In a series of items practiced in the order A, B, C, D, E, F, G, H, I, and J, assuming all items are of equal difficulty and new to the learner, which items would most likely be the easiest to remember and therefore the most likely to be learned?
   a. A, B, C, and D

   b. G, H, I, and J
   c. A, B, I, and J
   d. D, E, F, and G

4. Forgetting from short-term memory is explained by ___(1)___, while forgetting from long-term memory is explained by ___(2)___.
   a. (1) trace decay, (2) interference
   b. (1) proactive inhibition, (2) retroactive inhibition
   c. (1) interference, (2) trace decay
   d. (1) retroactive inhibition, (2) proactive inhibition

5. Which of the following is a characteristic of short-term memory?
   a. Is capable of storing an unlimited amount of information
   b. Has a duration capacity of one second or less
   c. Has an item capacity of five to nine chunks or bits of information
   d. Stores information in the form of schema

6. Which memory system would store knowledge of the rule "Three strikes and you are out?"
   a. Semantic system
   b. Procedural system
   c. Episodic system
   d. Working system

Answer the following with the word or words which best complete each sentence.

7. What is the term for the type of forgetting illustrated in the figure below?
   Learn Skill A → Learn Skill B → Difficulty recalling Skill A
8. The encoding of implicit details along with the explicit memory of a skill illustrates a principle called _____.
9. In the experiment by Beilock and Carr described in this chapter, expert golfers were less able to recall their actual putting experience than were beginner golfers. What did these researchers term the observation that attempts by experts to access declarative memory during skill execution, can hinder access to procedural memory causing experts to choke in their performances of well-learned skills?
10. When an instructor briefly presents new information at the end of one practice session that she intends to teach in the following practice session, the memory principle she is using is called _____.
11. Theorists working within the dynamical systems perspective focus considerable attention on the role played by memory in attuning individuals to the meaning of perceptual information from the environment. Such information, called _____, conveys information concerning opportunities for action manifest in the learner's environment.
12. An instructor who presents new information to be learned in the middle of a practice session in a particularly dramatic and meaningful way is likely depending on the _____ effect to promote memory and learning.

Answers are provided at the end of this review section.

STUDY QUESTIONS

1. What are the major differences between cognitive-based theories and dynamical systems theories in their view of memory?
2. What is memory? Offer a working definition.
3. Discuss what it means to say that memory is both the storage of information located in a specific place in the brain, and a retrieval process? How can these two claims be reconciled?
4. Describe the differences between declarative and procedural memory. How is each related to the learning of motor skills?
5. What are the advantages of procedural memory as a system for housing the memories of motor skills?
6. Describe Beilock and Carr's concept of expert-induced amnesia? Based upon this concept, what suggestions would you make to experts when performing motor skills?
7. Describe the major function of each of the three stages in the Atkinson and Shiffrin model of memory. What are the characteristics of each stage (consider both capacity and duration)?
8. What factors relevant to the practice of motor skills can be suggested to increase the likelihood that practiced skills will be consolidated into long-term memory?
9. Why are practice skills forgotten, even when they are originally well learned? What practice considerations can be suggested to enhance the long-term memory of skills?
10. Explain why performing a skill in either the same or a similar context to that in which it was practiced can enhance performance.

ADDITIONAL READING

Baddeley, A, Eysenck, MW, and Anderson, MC. (2009). *Memory*. New York: Psychology Press.

Beilock, SL, and Carr, TH. (1994). "From novice to expert performance: Memory, attention and the control of complex sensorimotor skills." In AM Williams and NJ Hodges (ed.), *Skill acquisition in sport: Research, theory and practice*. New York: Routledge.

Dail, TK, and Christina, RW. (2004). "Distribution of practice and metacognition in learning and long-term retention of a discrete motor skill." *Research Quarterly for Exercise and Sport, 75*(2), 148–155.

Higbee, KL. (2001). *Your memory: How it works and how to improve it*. New York: Da Capo Press.

Imanake, K, and Abernethy, B. (1992). "Interference between location and distance information in motor short-term memory: The respective roles of direct kinesthetic signals and abstract codes." *Journal of Motor Behavior, 24*, 274–290.

Magill, RA. (1998). "Knowledge is more than we can talk about: Implicit learning in motor skill acquisition." *Research Quarterly for Exercise and Sport, 69*, 104–110.

Sohn, YW and Doan, SM. (2003). "Roles of working memory capacity and long-term working memory skill in complex task performance." *Memory & Cognition, 31*, 458-466.

REFERENCES

Adams, JA. (1976). *Learning and memory: An introduction*. Homewood, IL: Dorsey.

Atkinson, RC, and Shiffrin, RM. (1968). "Human memory: A proposed system and its control processes." In KW Spence and JT Spence (eds.), *The psychology of learning and motivation: Advances in research and theory*, vol. 2. New York: Academic Press.

Atkinson, RC, and Shiffrin, RM. (1971). "The control of short-term memory." *Scientific American, 225*, 82–90.

Baddeley, A. (2004). *Your memory: A user's guide*. Buffalo, NY: Firefly Books.

Baddeley, A, Eysenck, MW, and Anderson, MC. (2009). *Memory*. New York: Psychology Press.

Baumeister, RF. (1984). "Choking under pressure: Self-consciousness and paradoxical effects of incentives on skillful performance." *Journal of Personality and Social Psychology, 46*, 610–620.

Beilock, SL, Bennett, LB, McCoy, AM, and Carr, TH. (2004). "Haste does not always make waste: Expertise, direction of attention, and speed versus accuracy in performing sensorimotor skills." *Psychonomic Bulletin and Review, 11*(2), 373–379.

Beilock, SL, and Carr, TH. (2001). "On the fragility of skilled performance: What governs choking under pressure?" *Journal of Experimental Psychology: General, 130*(4), 701–725.

Beilock, SL, Carr, TH, MacMahon, C, and Starkes, JL. (2002). "When paying attention becomes counterproductive: Impact of divided versus skill-focused attention on novice and experienced performance of sensorimotor skills." *Journal of Experimental Psychology: Applied, 8*, 6–16.

Beilock, SL, Wierenga, SA, and Carr, TH. (2002). "Expertise, attention, and memory in sensorimotor skill execution: Impact of novel task constraints on dual-task performance and episodic memory." *The Quarterly Journal of Experimental Psychology: Human Experimental Psychology, 55*, 1211–1240.

Boschker, SJ, Bakker, FC, and Michaels, CF. (2002). "Memory for the functional characteristics of climbing walls: Perceived affordances." *Journal of Motor Behavior, 34*(11), 25–37.

Bransford, JD, and Johnson, MK. (1972). "Contextual prerequisites for understanding." *Journal of Verbal Learning and Verbal Behavior, 11*, 717–726.

Brashers-Krug, T, Shadmehr, R, and Bizzi, E. (1996). "Consolidation in human motor memory." *Nature, 382*, 252–255.

Chieffi, S, Allport, DA, and Woodfin, M. (1999). "Hand-centered coding of target location in visuo-spatial working memory." *Neuropsychologia, 37,* 495–502.

Dail, TK, and Christina, RW. (2004). "Distribution of practice and metacognition in learning and long-term retention of a discrete motor skill." *Research Quarterly for Exercise and Sport, 75*(2), 148–155.

Damasio, AR. (1994). *Descartes' error: Emotion, reason, and the human brain.* New York: Grosset/Putnam.

Del Ray, P, Liu, X, and Simpson, KJ. (1994). "Does retroactive inhibition influence contextual interference effects?" *Research Quarterly for Exercise and Sport, 65*(2), 120–126.

Diewert, GL. (1975). "Retention and coding in motor short-term memory: A comparison of storage codes for distance and location information." *Journal of Motor Behavior, 7,* 183–190.

Ebbinghaus, H. (1885, 1913). *Memory.* New York: Columbia University Press.

Godden, DR, and Baddeley, AD. (1975). "Context-dependent memory in two natural environments: On land and underwater." *British Journal of Psychology, 71,* 99–104.

Hagman, JD. (1978). "Specific-cue effects of interpolated movements on distance and location retention in short-term motor memory." *Memory and Cognition, 21,* 432–437.

Higbee, KL. (2001). *Your memory: How it works and how to improve it.* New York: Da Capo Press.

Imanake, K, and Abernethy, B. (1992). "Interference between location and distance information in motor short-term memory: The respective roles of direct kinesthetic signals and abstract codes." *Journal of Motor Behavior, 24,* 274–290.

Jackson, SA, and Csikszentmihalyi, M. (1999). *Flow in sports: The key to optimal experiences and performances.* Champaign, IL: Human Kinetics.

Kauss, DR. (2000). *Mastering your inner game.* Champaign, IL: Human Kinetics.

Keppel, G, and Underwood, BJ. (1962). "Proactive inhibition in short-term retention of single items." *Journal of Verbal Learning and Verbal Behavior, 1,* 153–161.

Klatzky, RL. (1980). *Human memory: Structures and processes,* 2nd ed. New York: W. H. Freeman.

Lee, TD, and Hirota, TT. (1980). "Encoding specificity principles in motor short-term memory for movement extent." *Journal of Motor Behavior, 12,* 63–67.

Magill, RA, and Lee, TD. (1987). "Verbal label effects on response accuracy and organization for learning limb positioning movements." *Journal of Human Movement Studies, 13,* 285–308.

Norman, DA. (1988). *The design of everyday things.* New York: Currency/Doubleday.

Scoville, WB, and Milner, B. (1957). "Loss of recent memory after bilateral hippocampal lesions." *Journal of Neurology, Neurosurgery and Psychiatry, 20,* 11–21.

Siengsukon, CF, and Boyd, LA. (2009). "Does sleep promote motor learning?" *Implications for physical rehabilitation. Physical Therapy, 89*(4), 370–383.

Smith, F. (1998). *The book of learning and forgetting.* New York: Teachers College Press.

Smith, SM, Glenberg, AM, and Bjork, RA. (1978). "Environmental context and human memory." *Memory and Cognition, 6,* 342–353.

Smith, SM, and Vela, E. (2001). "Environmental context-dependent memory: A review and meta-analysis." *Psychonomic Bulletin and Review, 8*(2), 203–220.

Squire, LR, and Kandel, ER. (2000). *Memory: From mind to molecules.* New York, NY.

Strogatz, S. (2003). *Sync: The emerging science of spontaneous order.* Hyperion, New York: W. H. Freeman.

Thompson, RF, and Madigan, SA. (2005). *Memory: The key to consciousness.* Princeton, NJ: Princeton University Press.

Tulving, E. (1972). "Episodic and semantic memory." In E Tulving and W Donaldson (eds.), *Organization of memory* (pp. 381–403). New York: Academic Press.

Tulving, MT, and Thomson, DM. (1973). "Encoding specificity and retrieval processes in episodic memory." *Psychological Review, 80,* 352–373.

Underwood, BJ. (1957). "Interference and forgetting." *Psychological Review, 64,* 49–60.

Vaidya, CJ, Zhao, M, Desmond, JE, and Gabrieli, JD. (2002). "Evidence for cortical encoding specificity in episodic memory: Memory-induced re-activation of picture processing." *Neuropsychologia, 40,* 2136–2143.

Walker, MP, Brakefield, T, Morgan, A, Hobson, JA, and Stickgold, R. (2002). "Practice with sleep makes perfect: Sleep-dependent motor skill learning." *Neuron, 35,* 205–211.

Walker, MP, Brakefield, T, and Stickgold, R. (2003). "The time course of sleep-dependent motor-skill learning." *Sleep, 26,* A441–A442.

Answers to How Much Do You Know questions: (1) D, (2) B, (3) C, (4) A, (5) C, (6) A, (7) retroactive inhibition, (8) encoding specificity, (9) expert-induced amnesia, (10) priming, (11) affordances, (12) Von Restorft or outstanding item.

CHAPTER 7

Stages of Learning

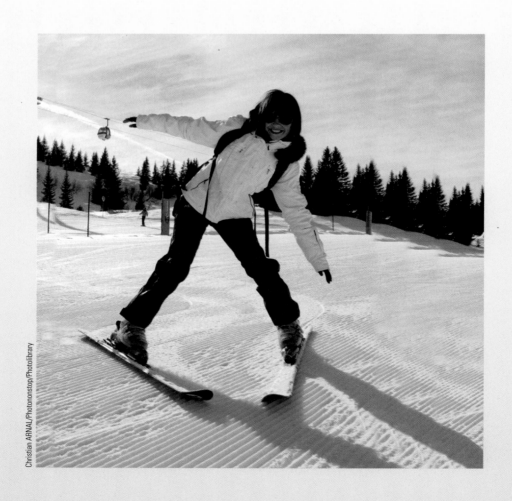

Christian ARNAL/Photononstop/Photolibrary

If learning weren't so hard, everyone would be an expert at everything.
—**former motor learning student**

KEY QUESTIONS

- Are there identifiable stages of learning that people pass through when acquiring motor skills?

- Does everyone go through the same stages of learning when acquiring motor skills?

- How do cognitive-based and dynamical systems theories differ in their conceptualizations of stages of learning in the acquisition of motor skills?

- What is expertise, and how does someone become an expert at a motor skill?

- Given sufficient motivation and practice, is everyone capable of becoming an expert?

- Is initial performance when first learning a motor skill a good indicator of a person's ultimate potential for learning the skill?

CHAPTER OVERVIEW

Everyone has experienced learning a challenging new movement skill. We all know the frustration attending the first, clumsy adventures in learning. In the beginning, we struggle just to understand what to do. How do we coordinate the movements of our limbs? How far? How fast? How much force? How do we respond to this situation or to that one? How do we begin? When?

Too frequently in our attempts to find movement solutions to these questions, our bodies resist our efforts. We move awkwardly and are confused about what to do. Our joints stiffen, our muscles tighten, we forget what comes next, and our performance misses the mark. As practice continues, however, our bodies do eventually begin to respond to our desires with greater loyalty. Our movements become smoother. We have some small successes. With continued practice come even more successes. We experience a growing sense of confidence as our movements become more consistent and accurate.

The experience of acquiring a new motor skill may be common to everyone, but are there commonalities shared equally by everyone regardless of the relative ease, or difficulty, with which learning is experienced? Are there stages in the learning process that we can identify, and if there are, does everyone pass through the same stages in the same way?

In this chapter, we will look at the stages of learning people go through in acquiring motor skills. The ability to identify various stages of learning is far from a mere intellectual exercise. Effective instructors of motor skills are capable of identifying the stages of skill attainment and of tailoring instructional and practice experiences to best match the needs of learners in each stage. Indeed, the ability to distinguish among the stages through which people progress in acquiring motor skills is a prerequisite to effective instruction and is one of the hallmarks of the effective motor skills instructor in whatever setting he or she may be found.

When mastering new skills, the learner typically advances through a predictable series of learning stages. At the start, a learner is usually halting and uncertain as he or she tries to use the target skill. With instruction and lots of practice, the learner becomes more fluent, accurate, and confident in using the skill.

—Haring et al. (1978)

stage of learning: Phase in the learning process exhibiting distinct behavioral characteristics; Fitts and Posner have identified three such stages: the cognitive, associative, and autonomous.

Although to the casual observer it might appear as though people learn motor skills in different ways, some acquiring them relatively quickly and easily while others struggle to make even slight progress, movement scientists and thoughtful instructors have known for many years that there are identifiable behavioral stages that all learners experience in their acquisition of motor skills. These stages may be experienced at different rates, sometimes markedly different, but passage through each stage, even if briefly for some, seems a prerequisite for all learners.

Over the years, a number of different models have been proposed for identifying the various stages people experience when acquiring motor skills (Adams, 1971; Bandura, 1986; Fitts and Posner, 1967; Gentile, 1972, 2000; Marteniuk, 1976; Newell and van Emmerik, 1989; Southard and Higgins, 1887; Vereijken, 1991; and Vereijken, Whiting, and Beek, 1992). Although each model describes the same movement characteristics, each categorizes them somewhat differently—some authors preferring to compress performance changes into two stages, some into three, and still others into four **stages of learning.** Regardless of how many stages are identified, though, each model describes the same progression of learner characteristics and adaptation to practice (although perhaps interpreting these from differing theoretical perspectives).

THE FITTS AND POSNER THREE-STAGE MODEL OF MOTOR LEARNING

As is often the case, the first model became the most widely accepted. In 1967, two psychologists, Paul Fitts and Michael Posner, proposed a three-stage model of motor skill learning (Fitts and Posner, 1967). Since that time, their model has become the most widely accepted and used in fields concerned with the learning and teaching of motor skills. It has become the standard model for describing the learning of motor skills (Belka, 2002).

Based upon observations that different cognitive, perceptual, and motor processes are involved at different points in the learning process, the Fitts and

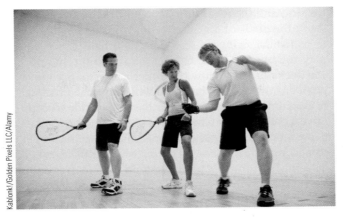

Kablonk!/Golden Pixels LLC/Alamy

The experience of acquiring motor skills can be classified into various stages of learning common to all skills and individuals.

Posner model identifies three stages in the acquisition of motor skills: cognitive, associative, and autonomous (see Figure 7.1). The model represents a cognitive theoretical approach to classifying learning stages, with the progression from declarative to procedural memory serving to explain changes in observable behaviors in each stage. Each stage presents the learner with a unique set of problems, and the role of memory and cognition is seen as key in solving those problems.

The Cognitive Stage of Learning

cognitive stage of learning: The initial stage of learning in Fitts and Posner's three-stage model of learning.

In the Fitts and Posner model, the first stage is called the **cognitive stage of learning**. Fitts and Posner referred to this stage as cognitive because conscious mental processes dominate early in learning. In this stage, learners are almost totally dependent on declarative memory, and information is consciously manipulated and rehearsed in formulating motor commands. Learners quite literally attempt to "think" their way through the performance of skills in this stage.

The primary problem confronted by learners in this stage of learning is attempting to grasp the basic idea of the skill. This includes both the goals of

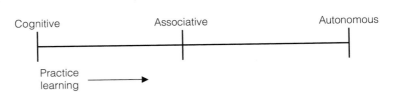

FIGURE **7.1** Fitts and Posner Model of the Stages of Learning

Source: Created by author.

the skill and the means for achieving them. Even when learners initially understand the goals of a skill, they may not understand the correct movement patterns for achieving those goals. A softball player learning to bat, for instance, may fully understand that her goal is to hit an approaching pitched ball, but she does not know how to properly control her movements to accomplish this goal, or how to tell where and when a pitched ball will cross the plate and then to coordinate the swing of her bat to coincide with its arrival. She has a declarative knowledge of what to do—hit the ball over the outfield wall and win the game—but has not yet developed the procedural rule-based knowledge needed to accomplish this goal. The major need of learners in the cognitive stage of learning, therefore, is to understand *how* to accomplish the outcome goals of a skill. Learners need especially to understand the correct movement mechanics of a skill, and how information from both the environment and bodily sources should be interpreted and applied to producing correct movements.

Because learners in this stage lack the prerequisite knowledge needed to interpret their movement environment, produce correct movement patterns, and evaluate the results of their movement attempts, they are highly dependent upon outside sources of information. Learners, in fact, are so dependent on outside sources of information at this stage that they will disregard their own intrinsic knowledge and instead rely almost entirely on the instructions and feedback provided by an outside source. Indeed, so inadequate is learners' knowledge at this stage, and so great their need for information, that studies have shown that even when information provided by an instructor is clearly wrong and contrary to learners' own perceptions, they will nonetheless disregard their own correct sources of information (visual, auditory, kinesthetic, etc.) and rely instead on that provided by an instructor (e.g., Buekers, Magill, and Hall, 1992). (This fact should make motor skills instructors especially sensitive to the importance of providing clear and accurate information to beginning learners.)

In their attempts to compensate for their lack of knowledge, learners engage in a somewhat experimental approach to practice in this stage of skill acquisition. At least in formal instructional situations, learners will conform their movement attempts almost exclusively to information provided by instructors. Such information may include verbal instructions, visual demonstrations, physical guidance, video displays, and verbal feedback. Based on these sources of information, learners will generate an attempt to accomplish the goals of a skill. They will then evaluate the success of their experimental attempt through information provided from their own sensory sources as well as the feedback provided by the instructor (and as just mentioned, will rely mostly on the instructor's feedback). Learners then engage in a process of evaluation and correction, comparing the instructor's feedback to their own sources of sensory feedback and making adjustments before next attempting the skill. Finally, in their endeavor to correct and update movement commands, learners will attempt to connect their current movement needs with existing sources of information in long-term memory. That is, they will attempt to "transfer" old, previously learned information that is applicable to their current needs in performing the new skill. An example of this might be seen among beginning racquetball players who gradually, over practice attempts, become sensitive to ways in which accomplishing novel racquetball skills can be made easier by applying their existing knowledge of tennis skills.

Characteristics of Learners in the Cognitive Stage

The observable results of these experimental attempts by learners in the initial, cognitive stage of learning are all too familiar to us. A learner's performance is highly inconsistent; there are frequent errors, and errors are significantly large in magnitude. Moreover, the errors that are observed tend to vary widely in both type and extent. Many inappropriate movement attempts are made in this stage, as learners are experimenting, as it were, with various movement strategies in their attempts to find solutions for achieving movement goals. Because cognitive processes are primarily used in seeking solutions to movement problems in this stage, learners direct conscious attention to finding such solutions and may engage in "self-talk" and subverbalization activities; learners can almost be seen as trying to "talk" their way through performance attempts. Learners may, in this stage, sense that their movements do not meet the goals of the skill, but they do not know how to correct them. This may lead to behaviors indicating confusion, frustration, and even the waning of interest and motivation on the part of learners.

Progression through the Cognitive Stage

How long learners will remain in the cognitive stage of learning depends on a number of factors. Learners may pass through this stage after completing only a few practice attempts or a few minutes of practice when learning fairly simple skills, especially if they are adults and experienced with similar skills. Practice in the cognitive stage may, however, take considerably longer for complex skills; this is true for experienced adult learners but especially true for younger, less experienced, or physically challenged learners. With effective practice, however, almost everyone is capable of passing through this stage of learning for most motor skills. In fact, with rare exception, anyone is capable of reaching the next, or associative, stage of learning.

The Associative Stage of Learning

In Fitts and Posner's associative stage of learning, learners are no longer wholly dependent on declarative memory. Some elements of skill have been encoded into procedural memory form, even though others remain under the control of declarative memory. As practice progresses, however, more and more movement-related elements become procedurally encoded. The need for every aspect of movement to be controlled consciously is therefore gradually attenuated throughout the **associative stage of learning**.

Characteristics of Learners in the Associative Stage

In the associative stage, learners have come to understand the basic goals of a skill. As a result, a number of behavioral changes are observed. Errors become less frequent, and the variability among errors—both in their type and magnitude—decreases. One of the keys to identifying behaviors indicating

associative stage of learning: The intermediate stage of learning in Fitts and Posner's three-stage model of learning.

the associative stage of learning, in fact, is that the variability among errors decreases and remaining errors begin to show a distinct bias. In previously discussing the cognitive stage of learning, we used the example of a softball player learning to bat a ball. In the cognitive stage of learning, her errors were gross and widely varied. Specifically, she may have swung her bat too late on one pitch and then too early on the next. Her swing may also have been too high on one pitch and then too low on the next pitch. Errors appeared random, ranging from those that were small to those that were large, and from one type of error to another. As our player moves into the associative stage of learning, however, noticeable changes will occur in the type and extent of her errors. Rather than making large errors, in both timing and magnitude errors will be expected to become smaller; the variability of those errors will also significantly abate and a particular bias will increasingly become more evident. For instance, most of our player's errors in the associative stage might entail swinging her bat slightly too early and a little too high. Or they might be mostly late and low. The point is that an increased tendency toward one type of error becomes more pronounced in the associative stage, with the extent of these errors decreasing as practice continues.

Also, in the associative stage of learning, movements become quicker and smoother. Much of the jerkiness seen in earlier learning disappears as various component parts of a skill become more effectively integrated and linked together. Some components of the skill are controlled more or less automatically and with little need for conscious attention; others still require cognitive processing and appear attention demanding. As a consequence, the need for "self-talk" or subverbalization decreases throughout this stage, as procedural memory comes to dominate the control of action.

In this stage too, learners are beginning to understand and to integrate relevant features of the environment into their performance. In the cognitive stage of learning, performance is often abstracted from the context in which it is accomplished. That is, learners seemingly perform movements in a stereotypical fashion disregarding changes that may occur in the environment (almost as though performing in isolation from the environment). In the associative stage of learning, however, performers begin to integrate aspects of the environment into their performance. They begin to link sensory input with appropriate movement responses. That is, they can make changes to movement patterns based on changes in the environment. For example, learners develop the ability to speed up or slow down the movements of a skill as changes in environmental conditions dictate. Consider again the example of our softball player as she now learns to catch a pop-up fly ball. In the cognitive stage of learning, she is concerned mainly with performing the movement mechanics of the skill correctly, not having yet developed the ability to integrate her movements to changing patterns of the ball's flight. The pattern of performance that she will adopt, and which is typical of beginners, is to focus on the mechanics of performing the skill correctly while all but disregarding the particular characteristics of the ball's flight. Most likely, she will run to the spot where she anticipates the ball will come down, and while doing so extend her gloved hand above her head with her other hand positioned below in a catching position.

She will then wait for the ball to come down, as though performing the movement mechanics for catching were independent of what was environmentally taking place regarding the actually flight of the ball. Once in the associative stage, however, our player's arm movements will be timed to coincide exactly with the arrival of the ball, her gloved hand extended to catch the ball just an instant before it arrives overhead.

Progression through the Associative Stage

The amount of time a learner will remain in the associative stage of learning is highly variable, depending on a number of factors such as skill complexity, underlying abilities of the learner, and quality of instruction. Learning simple skills may require only a few hours of practice in the associative stage before progressing to the next stage. Highly complex skills, however, may require many weeks or months of practice before leaving the associative stage. In fact, many learners will attain the associative stage of learning rather quickly but fail to advance to the next stage of learning. For complex motor skills, attaining the final, autonomous stage of learning will most likely require skill-specific abilities on the part of the learner, as well as adequate motivation and effective instruction.

The Autonomous Stage of Learning

autonomous stage of learning: The third and final stage of learning in Fitts and Posner's three-stage model of learning.

The transition from the associative stage to the **autonomous stage of learning** is marked by the ability to perform skills more or less automatically with little, if any, conscious attention paid to the actual mechanics of the skill. In this stage, the underlying knowledge needed to perform skills has been entirely transferred from declarative memory into procedural memory. Learners no longer need to think about *how* to perform a skill. In fact, over time, learners may even forget exactly how they perform a skill, even though they can do it proficiently. (This has been suggested as one reason that highly skilled performers do not always make the best instructors. Those in the autonomous stage of learning, having encoded the knowledge of a skill entirely in nonconscious procedural memory form, simply forget, over time, their conscious declarative knowledge of the skill.)

Characteristics of Learners in the Autonomous Stage

Because movement at this stage is controlled by the procedural memory system, learners do not need to focus on actual movement mechanics involved in a skill but can direct their attention to other areas of concern. A clear indication of having reached the autonomous stage of learning is the ability to perform a skill well while thinking about something else. The worker using machinery while thinking about his upcoming vacation, the basketball player dribbling downcourt while observing opposing players and planning her next move, or the driver of an automobile daydreaming about winning the next lottery are all in the autonomous stage of learning. They are clearly in the autonomous stage because they can perform their respective skills well, even though paying little or no attention to how they are actually performing them—and in fact have the ability to concomitantly attend to other, even unrelated, thoughts.

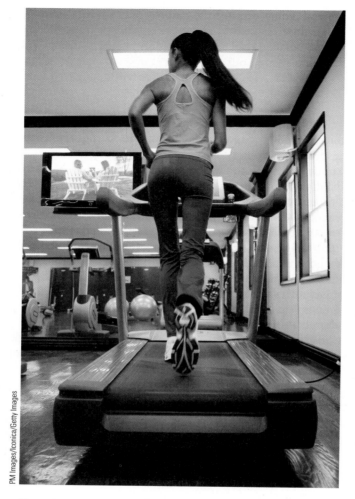

PM Images/Iconica/Getty Images

The autonomous stage of learning is marked by the ability to attend to other activities without compromising the performance of a motor skill.

Improved performance levels become obvious once the autonomous stage of learning is reached. Learners are able to adjust their movements to a wide range of environmental situations. Skills become highly accurate, quicker, and require less effort. Learners appear to move automatically, and indeed automaticity of performance in a variety of environmental settings is an indicator of the autonomous stage. In this stage, learners are also able to draw fairly good conclusions about their errors, including how to correct them. Because of this ability, reliance on instructional feedback becomes markedly less important. Performance characteristics for the three stages of learning are summarized in Table 7.1 (and see Box 7.1 to test your knowledge of these.)

TABLE **7.1**

Performance Characteristics across the Three Stages of Learning

Cognitive Stage

- Many errors
- Wide variability in errors
- Jerkiness of movement patterns
- Limbs remain "stiff" in complex movements
- Slow response time
- Conscious attention needed for all, or most, skill elements
- Subverbalization ("self-talk") evident
- Stereotypical movements regardless of environmental changes
- Inability to articulate appropriate movement mechanics

Associative Stage

- Decreased frequency of errors
- Errors are less gross
- Errors show particular outcome bias
- Basic skill requirements are understood
- Smoother movements (jerkiness mostly disappears)
- Quicker movements
- Some movement segments appear automatic
- Beginning to match movement parameters to environmental changes

Autonomous State of Learning

- Few errors
- Little variability among errors
- Smooth, coordinated action of limbs
- Quick response in executing skill
- Automaticity of performance
- All components of skill well integrated
- Ability to attend to extraneous information while still performing skill well
- Ability to perform well in a variety of environmental contexts
- Little need for augmented feedback in correcting errors
- Decreased reaction time associated with decision-making
- Minimum expenditure of energy

Reaching the Autonomous Stage

Not everyone who practices a skill reaches the autonomous stage. As previously stated, reaching the autonomous stage of learning typically requires considerable practice, effective instruction, high motivation, and some prerequisite motor capabilities. Although simple tasks, such as those often employed in laboratory research, may require relatively few practice attempts (e.g., 500–600 trials), more complex skills may require many thousands of practice attempts before automatic processes fully develop.

Instructional Priorities in the Fitts and Posner Stages of the Learning Model

As individuals progress through the stages of learning, their needs for instruction change. Instructors, therefore, need also to consider the stage of learning when designing and delivering instructions to learners. Instructions that may be most helpful in one stage of learning may actually hinder learning in another stage. In prioritizing the instructional needs of learners, Fitts and Posner paid special attention to the changes in memory structure that evolve over the course of learning, with learners first needing to develop a cognitive understanding of a skill within declarative memory and then progressively transferring that learning to the control of automatic, procedural memory.

Instruction in the Cognitive Stage

Fitts and Posner preface their suggestions concerning the provision of instructions in the cognitive stage of learning in the following way:

> Whether left to his own devices or tutored by an experienced instructor, the beginner in most adult skill-learning situations tries to "understand" the task and what it demands. A good instructor will call his attention to important perceptual cues and response characteristics and give diagnostic knowledge of results.
> He may also shape behavior by calling "good" any sequence of acts that at all resembles the correct one. (Fitts and Posner, 1967, p. 13)

Based on an understanding of the problems confronting learners in the cognitive stage of learning, knowledgeable motor skill instructors will do several things to help promote learning in the most effective manner. Although we will discuss these in greater detail in following chapters, we can briefly mention the more pertinent ones here. In providing the most effective instruction to learners who can be classified into the cognitive stage of learning, instructors will (1) use verbal instructions and demonstrations to help learners grasp the goals of the skill and the correct mechanics for accomplishing them, (2) help learners identify and differentiate between appropriate and irrelevant sources of environmental information, (3) identify and point out to learners how their previously acquired skills and knowledge can be transferred to the new learning situation, (4) provide frequent verbal feedback concerning learners' major errors, and (5) help learners maintain a sufficient level of motivation and interest. The use of simplification techniques, such as part-practice scheduling, may at times be warranted in this stage as well. Of special concern in this stage of learning is the potential for visual information to dominate other sources of sensory input and to impede learning, the phenomenon called **visual dominance** discussed in Chapter 3.

visual dominance:
The tendency for vision to dominate in the processing of sensory information during the initial stage of learning.

Instruction in the Associative Stage

It is tempting to conclude that the associative stage of learning is merely a half-way mark between the earlier cognitive stage and the final autonomous stage of learning, a blending of the two as it were. But such a premise would lead to false conclusions on several points and, most importantly, would lead to ineffective instructional decisions regarding learner needs in the associative stage of learning.

The associative stage has its own unique characteristics and learner needs, and the effective motor skills instructor will come to appreciate them. As with our discussion of instructional priorities in the cognitive stage of learning, a detailed presentation of effective practices in the associative stage is left for following chapters, but we can again briefly point out some of the more crucial things instructors should be aware of in planning instructional strategies for learners in this middle stage of learning.

It is particularly important in this stage that instructors begin helping learners to identify and respond to changes in environmental conditions as opposed to focusing instruction primarily on movement mechanics, as is the case in the cognitive stage of learning (though this also remains important). For example, when instructing a patient who is regaining the skill of walking after a knee replacement, a therapist may begin in the cognitive stage of learning by focusing exclusively on basic movement goals, helping the patient relearn the proper mechanics of gait on a consistently flat, smooth, and unimpeded surface. Once the basic mechanics of the skill are mastered, however, and the learner judged to have progressed to the associative stage of learning, the therapist will begin helping the patient learn to respond to different—and real-life—environmental situations by altering the features of the walking surface. These alternations could include walking on carpeted surfaces, up and down inclines, on

BOX **7.1**	**Identifying Characteristics in Fitts and Posner's Stages of Learning**

For the following skills, think about the observable characteristics specific to the particular skill that can tell you whether a person performing the skill is most likely in the cognitive, associative, or autonomous stage of learning. What characteristics can you think of for each stage of learning in each of these skills? (See whether you can think of at least five for each stage.)

- Taping an athlete's injured ankle
- Driving a golf ball
- Driving an automobile
- Typing
- Line dancing
- Riding a bicycle

undulating surfaces, and with obstacles placed in the patient's path. Instruction would focus on how to alter basic movement mechanics to respond to such environmental changes (e.g., shorten one's gait stride and contract the gluteal muscles more on inclined surfaces).

It is also critical in this stage that instructors begin to reduce the amount of feedback, as well as the type of feedback, provided to learners. Because learners are beginning to develop the ability to make sense of some of their own sensory-produced sources of feedback, the effective instructor will gradually withdraw the amount of feedback that he or she provides, thus requiring learners to gradually gain the capacity for evaluating and correcting errors on their own. Because errors are significantly fewer in the associative stage, feedback should also be directed more at reinforcing correct movement behaviors, as well as changing incorrect ones (we will discuss the role of feedback in greater detail in Chapter 12). Other instructional priorities include the elimination of part-practice scheduling if it was used in the cognitive stage, instructing learners on methods for appropriately redirecting visual and attentional resources, and the continued need for maintaining appropriate levels of motivation.

Instruction in the Autonomous Stage

Because learners have reached advanced levels of performance, obvious improvements in performance become less noticeable. For those in the latter phases of autonomous learning, even minute improvements in performance may require long periods of time. As improvements in performance become less obvious and take longer to recognize, learners may become frustrated with what appears as their lack of progress. The perception that improvement is not occurring can sometimes prove problematic for learners, resulting in a dwindling of motivation. Given that even slight changes in motivation can affect performance, coupled with the fact that considerable time and effort must be devoted to practice even to maintain current levels of performance, maintaining learner motivation becomes a main goal of instruction in the autonomous stage of learning. Learners need to be assured that improvement is still occurring, even when it might not seem that it is.

Because basic movement mechanics are well encoded into procedural memory at this stage, instruction is best focused on refining movements and adapting them to varying situations. In sport settings, learning to couple variations of skill to changing game situations (i.e., the development of strategy) replaces instruction of basic skill mechanics. The effective instructor will engage in a thorough analysis of the various situational conditions in which a skill may be performed, and assist learners in refining and adapting the skill to meet these changing conditions. Helping learners to adapt well-learned skills to the various environmental situations in which they will be called on to act, as well as maintaining high levels of motivation, are the principal instructional priorities in the autonomous stage of learning.

Progression through the Stages of Learning

Even though Fitts and Posner's three-stage model distinguishes unique stages of skill through which learners advance, progression through these stages is best regarded as continuous rather than discontinuous. As Fitts and Posner state, "one phase merges gradually into another, so that no definite transition between them is apparent" (1967, p. 11). Transition from one stage to the next is gradual and seldom marked by abrupt performance shifts. In fact, transition from one stage to the next is frequently ambivalent, exhibiting behaviors representing both stages (in such cases, it is usually best to assume that the higher stage has been reached and provide instructions accordingly). Moreover, as previously stated, a learner may not make the transition to later stages. Skill learning can therefore be conceived of as occurring on a continuum (Figure 7.1), with progression advancing over practice from the cognitive to autonomous stages.

THE STAGES OF LEARNING FROM A DYNAMICAL SYSTEMS PERSPECTIVE

Viewed from the perspective of dynamical systems theory, the stages of learning take on a different interpretation than that offered by Fitts and Posner. Dynamical systems theorists recognize the same behavioral characteristics manifested by learners as they acquire motor skills, but interpret them in a different way. Based upon their interpretation of the stages of learning, dynamical systems theorists also focus on a different set of priorities for the instruction of motor skills.

Learning theories within the dynamical systems perspective are still in the early stages of development, though a number of models have been advanced and there is general consensus concerning the primary features involved in the learning of motor skills. Much of the work in identifying stages in the learning process from a dynamical systems perspective is grounded in the contributions of Bernstein (1967); Gibson (1979); Kugler, Kelso, and Turvey (1982); and Newell (1986). According to these theorists, coordinated patterns of movement (i.e., motor skills) arise as a result of the constraints imposed upon learners. Constraints, recall from Chapter 4, are those factors that provide the boundaries on movement possibilities. They set the limits within which movement patterns are possible, and they guide patterns of movement toward preferred states called *attractors*. Taken together, various attractors spread across the bodily systems shape movement into preferred patterns. Constraints do not impose particular movement patterns, but they make it more likely that certain patterns, those resulting in the greatest degree of stability, will emerge. Newell (1986) has identified three basic types of constraints: organismic, task, and environmental (see Chapter 4).

Coordination emerges as learners adapt their movement behaviors to the constraints imposed upon them and learn to exploit their movement environment in ways to take greater advantage of those constraints. To do this, learners must be able to control the many different ways that the various bodily components contributing to movement are capable of functioning. Again, as we saw in Chapter 4, Bernstein was the first to point out that the various systems and components of the body operate independently, each being free to assume many different states or values. That is, human movement systems contain an extremely large reservoir of degrees of freedom, reaching at the cellular level well into the many millions. The fundamental challenge faced by learners is how to control such a vast number of movement possibilities. According to Bernstein, coordination (i.e., skill learning) is the process of learning to control the many redundant degrees of freedom available within the human movement apparatus.

Based upon Bernstein's observations concerning the degrees of freedom problem, Vereijken (Vereijken, 1991; Vereijken, van Emmerik, Whiting, and Newall, 1992; and Vereijken, Whiting, and Beek, 1992) has offered a three-stage model of motor learning. In her model, these three stages are called *novice*, *advanced*, and *expert* (see Figure 7.2). We will turn next to a description and consideration of each of these three stages. (Although not a description of the specific stages, a discussion of the general features of this model was presented in Chapter 4).

The Novice Stage of Learning

novice stage of learning: The initial stage of learning in Vereijken's dynamical systems model of the stages of learning.

When first learning a motor skill, which Vereijken refers to as the **novice stage of learning**, the major challenge facing the learner is how to control the many muscles and joints involved in the movement. Not only must each joint be controlled, but it must also be coordinated with the movements of other joints. This requires the control of many independent degrees of freedom within the muscles involved in controlling joint actions underlying movement. Faced with what would be an overwhelming task for cognitive processes alone, the learner simplifies the control problem by reducing the number of individual elements that must be controlled. In the terms of dynamical theorists, the learner "solves" the movement "problem" by manipulating the "dynamics" of the movement task. This is accomplished by **freezing the degrees of freedom** within the movement systems involved in producing the skill, as we saw earlier in Chapter 4.

freezing the degrees of freedom: Limiting the movement of limbs and joints.

The strategy of freezing degrees of freedom was first proposed by Bernstein. This involves locking some joints within limbs so that the limb moves as a single unit, in a sticklike fashion, rather than as a multijoint system with each joint free to move independently. In similar fashion, the body is kept relatively rigid ("frozen"), with only limited movement allowed of the most essential limbs and bodily components. For example, consider a beginner faced with

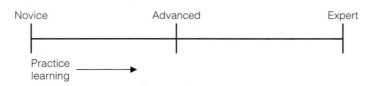

FIGURE **7.2** Dynamical Systems Model of the Stages of Learning as Proposed by Vereijken

Source: Created by author.

the challenge of controlling the many body segments involved in kicking a soccer ball (see Savelsbergh et al., 2007, for a complete description). When first learning to kick a soccer ball, beginners typically keep their bodies relatively rigid and involve only their lower body in the kicking action. The upper body and arms remain fixed, the arms perhaps stretched out to help maintain balance, but not allowed to swing freely. Movement of the lower body is also constrained, with the movements of some joints coupled. The hip and knee of the kicking leg, for example, are coupled in their actions. As the hip begins to flex in the kicking motion, the knee synchronously begins to extend. Flexion and extension at the hip and knee are locked into a single reciprocal pattern of motion (with the ankle remaining fixed). For those relatively few joints that are not frozen, coupling their actions makes the control problem much easier

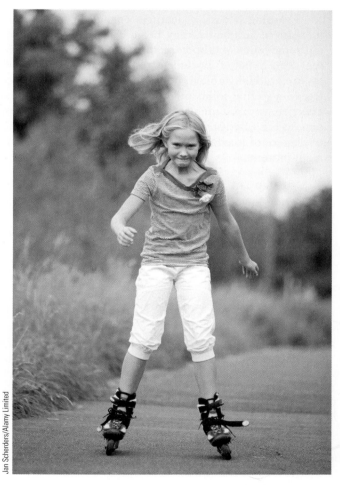

Jan Scherders/Alamy Limited

When initially learning a new motor skill, people reduce the degrees of freedom they must control by "freezing" movement in various joints and limbs.

to solve. Savelsbergh et al. (2007) have described this strategy as analogous to controlling the wheels of an automobile. If all four wheels were controlled independently, you would need four different steering wheels to control the car's movements. By coupling the wheels so that they act as a single unit, only one steering wheel is required to control all four wheels, significantly reducing the control problem.

By freezing some degrees of freedom through holding various limbs and body regions rigid and fixed, and coupling the actions of joints of other limbs, the number of degrees of freedom that must be controlled by the novice learner are reduced to a manageable number (see Box 7.2). This approach to simplifying the control problem, however, is insufficient to allow for coordinated and effective movement control. Improvement in performance is possible only as some of the degrees of freedom (i.e., movement possibilities) are freed to assume values independently of the actions of other body components.

Learning occurs as learners engage in a type of trial-and-error experimentation. Gradually, they begin releasing some degrees of freedom, allowing some joints and body segments to move more freely, and explore how this may lead to better movement results. Through this exploratory process, learners are gradually able to unfreeze, or to use the preferred term, *free*, degrees of freedom so that joints might be controlled in more flexible, independent, and effective ways. Gradually this process leads to conversion to a controllable system, to echo Bernstein's definition of a skill, a system in which a large number of degrees of freedom across the body can be coordinated into effective movement patterns.

The Advanced Stage of Learning

Over the course of learning, those in the novice stage explore movement possibilities and learn to free more and more degrees of freedom. The eventual result is the freeing of degrees of freedom so that optimal coordination patterns

---

BOX **7.2**   **Freezing Degrees of Freedom**

For the activities listed below, imagine a novice performing the skills for the first time. Think about the minimum movements that would be required to roughly accomplish the skill. For each skill, consider the body's movement components that you could constrain (joints, limbs, body segments) and still perform the skill. Which joints and limbs could you freeze, and which joints could you couple into a single action unit? Which regions of the body could you keep rigid? What are the minimum bodily components that you would need to allow to freely move?

Experiment by attempting various movement patterns (you need not actually perform the skills,

but just go through the bodily motions as though you were performing them). Determine which movement patterns are essential and which can be eliminated (i.e., frozen). How does your experience with this exercise help you better understand the awkward movements beginners often exhibit?

- Throwing a baseball or softball
- Driving a golf ball
- Downhill skiing
- Jumping rope
- Hula Hoop twirling

advanced stage of learning: The intermediate stage of learning in Vereijken's dynamical systems model of the stages of learning.

freeing the degrees of freedom: Releasing frozen limbs and joints to move freely.

are achieved. When this occurs, the learner has, in Vereijken's dynamical systems model of learning, moved into the **advanced stage of learning**. If the novice stage is marked by freezing movement possibilities (degrees of freedom), the advanced stage is marked by the freeing of movement possibilities (**freeing the degrees of freedom**).

In the advanced stage, previously frozen joints can be incorporated into larger and more sophisticated units of action. In dynamical systems terminology, these larger action units are called *coordinated structures*, or *synergies*.

Synergies

Referring to the process of exploration during the novice stage that leads into the advanced stage of learning, we said that this occurs as learners acquire the ability to control increasingly greater numbers of degrees of freedom. That is, learners acquire the ability to control many more independent movements of joints and muscles over the course of learning, resulting in the ability to coordinate complex movements often involving whole body patterns of movement. The thoughtful reader may have wondered how this is possible. If the novice can control only a limited number of movement components initially, how is it that the learner in the advanced stage can control so many more? After all, the original problem is in the novice's inability to control a large number of individual movement components, because doing so imposes too large of a cognitive load (according to dynamical systems theory) on the central nervous system. It should be clear that practice of a motor skill does not enhance cognitive abilities sufficiently to be able to manipulate such large increases in movement demands. This was the problem that Bernstein grappled with, and his solution was the synergy. The primary mechanism responsible for reducing computational demands on the central nervous system and for facilitating coordination, according to Bernstein, is the development of synergies over the course of practice. A **synergy**, recalling Chapter 4, is a group of muscles, often extending over several joints, which are linked together and act as a single unit when activated. Such linkage occurs over practice as neurological connections among muscles are recruited to take advantages of naturally existing neural pathways and reflexes. The development of a synergy does not inhibit other movements involving the linked muscles, but when activated, the muscles comprising the synergy temporarily act as a single unit, orchestrating a symphony of effectively timed contractions among the many muscles comprising it. This results in greater coordination among limb segments and between limbs.

synergy: A grouping of joints, muscles, and cells that temporarily cooperate in acting together as a single collective action unit; can be assembled and unassembled as the need arises; also called a *coordinative structure*.

As an analogy to help visualize how synergies work, think about a puppet on strings (Shea, Shebilske, and Worchel, 1993). Typically, there are eight strings controlling the various segments of the puppet's arms and legs. To make the puppet perform a complex, multilimb movement, like walking, for example, requires that the strings controlling each arm and leg segment be pulled or released at the correct time. In this case, that would mean that eight strings must all be individually controlled (which is a difficult challenge using two hands). Experienced puppeteers, however, know that they can temporarily hold groups of strings together (link them) in such a way that the puppet can be made to walk by manipulating only two groups of strings. In this case, instead of eight individual puppet body segments that must be controlled, only two linked segments must be controlled to make the puppet walk. Synergies work in the same way so that rather than controlling individual muscles, groups of muscles can be controlled as single units, requiring less mental effort and resulting in effectively coordinated limb movements.

The advanced stage of learning, in summary, results from freeing the many degrees of freedom needed to fully coordinate actions required for accomplishing the movement patterns of a skill. This freeing and expansion of movement possibilities is made possible through the development of muscle synergies. Movements in this stage are fluid, smoothly coordinated, and relatively effective.

The Expert Stage of Learning

expert stage of learning: The third and final stage of learning in Vereijken's dynamical systems model of the stages of learning.

The final stage of learning in Vereijken's three stages model is the **expert stage of learning**. Although movement coordination is achieved in the advanced stage, the most effective coordination of movements, especially in complex skills, typically requires the exploitation of passive and reactive forces in various body systems as well as the environment. If "freezing" is a key descriptor of the novice stage of learning, and "freeing" of the advanced stage, then "exploitation" is the best descriptor of the expert stage of learning (see Table 7.2). In the expert stage, the learner continues to release degrees of freedom, and reorganize others in order to achieve the most energetically efficient movement patterns. The primary focus in this stage, though, is on the exploitation of internal and external forces, which can contribute in significant ways to movement effectiveness.

TABLE **7.2**

Manipulation of Degrees of Freedom across the Stages of Learning in the Dynamical Systems Model as Proposed by Vereijken

Stage of Learning	Degrees of Freedom (DF)	How Accomplished
Novice	Freezing DF	Lock some joints while coupling others; maintain body rigidity; limit movement of joints, limbs, and bodily components.
Advanced	Freeing DF	Release frozen joints and limbs as synergies develop, freeing more degrees of freedom to increase control and flexibility of bodily movements.
Expert	Exploiting DF	Use passive and reactive forces inherent in bodily systems, as well as those in external environment, to contribute to movement dynamics.

In the example of learning to kick a soccer ball mentioned earlier, for example, we saw that learners originally freeze out most movements of the body and rigidly move the kicking leg as a single action unit. Gradually, over the course of learning leading to the advanced stage of learning, learners release degrees of freedom and begin moving the hip and knee independently. Through exploring various combinations of hip and knee (and ankle) actions, learners come to recognize that some are more effective than others. In the expert stage, once basic movement patterns have been developed, this exploration involves learning to exploit the passive and reactive forces generated by the kinetic actions of the hip-knee-ankle system (**exploiting the degrees of freedom**). The three joints of the leg act as a kinetic chain such that the timing among them can result in the maximal production of force at the end of the chain (i.e., the ankle). The greatest force is transferred to the foot, and in turn the soccer ball, when the hip is flexed at maximum velocity, adding its force to the knee at the same time as the knee is extended at its maximum velocity, resulting in maximum velocity of the foot at the instant it strikes the ball. Through continued exploration of movement possibilities, learners learn to exploit such biomechanical forces, as well as other forces such as the buildup of forces in muscle due to their elastic properties, and harness these as part of movement solutions adding to improved coordination, energy conservation, and performance effectiveness.

In addition to forces within bodily systems, learners also benefit from exploiting features of the environment. This often involves learning to make adjustments in the use of equipment. Shifting one's grip slightly toward the handle of a golf club, as well as learning to take a greater backswing before hitting the ball, both contribute to greater force being transferred to the club head at impact with the ball. Learners also acquire the ability to exploit physical properties within the environment such as inertia, friction, and gravity that are inherent in the environmental context. In this latter sense, the learner's perception of the interaction of environment and task is redefined, allowing for greater performance proficiency and movement flexibility.

Perceptual Degrees of Freedom and Learning: Attunement to Affordances

In addition to the bodily dynamics involved in coordinated movement, dynamical systems theorists have focused considerable attention on the role of perception during learning. We saw this in both Chapters 4 and 6 in discussing the concept of affordances. You will recall that an affordance is a property of an object or of the environment that offers ("affords") the opportunity for an action. According to the dynamical systems perspective, affordances are developed as individuals learn to couple perceptions to certain actions; that is, as they learn the various possibilities for moving given specific sensory information. Learning to expand the degree of perceptual-action coupling so that one can take advantage of greater opportunities for movements is viewed as analogous to the sequence of freezing, freeing, and exploiting degrees of freedom of bodily components (Savelsbergh and van der Kamp, 2000). This has been referred to as the *perceptual degrees of freedom*. In an initial stage, learners focus on specific sensory information to control their movements, freezing out all other perceptual informational sources. This often involves allowing visual

exploiting the degrees of freedom: Using passive and reactive forces inherent in bodily systems and in the environment to assist in producing bodily movements.

information to dominate attempts at movement control, because it is the most readily accessible and understood, even when it may prove a relatively ineffective source of information. Analogous to the advanced stage of learning, learners explore additional informational sources, developing a rich repertoire of possible perceptual-action couplings, enhancing their flexibility for selecting among different movement patterns to meet changing conditions and goals. Finally, as in the expert stage of learning, learners gain the ability to exploit the movement environment. That is, they learn to use different perceptual sources to accomplish the same movement goals, making them more able to continue moving skillfully when environmental and perceptual conditions change.

In the dynamical systems theory, an essential key to learning involves the development of the learner's ability to couple perceptual information with appropriate actions, a process called *attunement*. We saw how attunement to affordances is developed over practice when discussing memory in Chapter 6. To dynamical systems theorists, memory is too indirectly connected to perception, and the retrieval of memories too slow and uncertain for it to play a critical role in learning. Rather, it is the direct linkage between perception and movement that is critical to learning. As perception and movement are coupled, the perception of affordances in a given situation will become automatic. Once the individual has decided on a goal to be achieved (and this is a function of memory), he or she will explore the perceptual landscape in order to find its affordances. Over time, through the natural processes of trial and error, attunement to the affordances offered in various situations will develop. When this happens, the learner will respond automatically. If he or she has also developed the underlying synergistic structures required for coordinated actions, the result will be a highly skilled action.

Instructional Priorities in the Dynamical Systems Model of Learning

From a dynamical systems perspective, the learner is an active seeker of information. This has led those espousing a dynamical systems approach to learning to the advocacy of **discovery learning** methods (van Emmerik et al., 1989; Vereijken, Whiting, and Beek, 1992). In discovery learning, the learner attempts to solve the movement problem (to "discover" a solution) through exploration of various task solutions. The role of the instructor is to facilitate such discovery through the manipulation of task requirements. The instructor introduces the movement problem and the goal to be achieved to the learner, and then facilitates and encourages the learner's attempt to discover movement solutions. Rather than beginning by providing specific instructions, the instructor provides a general overview of movement possibilities that the learner then uses as a framework for exploration and discovery of what works best. Instructors can assist the learner's self-discovery by asking questions directing the learner's attention to relevant cues and perceptual information, as well as by providing feedback. Once the learner acquires an effective movement pattern, the instructor can then use verbal instructions and demonstrations to help refine the learner's movements.

In traditional instructional settings, instructors tend to rely on preconceived idealizations of correct techniques and movement patterns. Research

discovery learning: Practice based upon the theory that learners learn best when they discover through exploratory methods the most effective ways of accomplishing motor skills.

has revealed, however, that even for highly stable closed skills such as golf and rifle shooting, optimal movement patterns do not exist (Davids, Button, and Bennett, 2008). This is because both initial body conditions (body sway, physiological conditions, psychological factors, etc.) and environmental conditions (light, wind, surface conditions, equipment, etc.) change every time a skill is performed. Given that the constraints shaping movement change constantly, practice should encourage adaptation to changing situations rather than consistency to hypothetically optimal, and unchanging, patterns of movement.

Because, from a dynamical systems perspective, self-discovery of what works best is the key to the most effective learning, then the learner's engagement in the learning process is critical. This means that a major instructional goal during practice is the maintenance of a high degree of motivation on the part of the learner. In selecting instructional strategies and creating learning environments, movement skill instructors need to facilitate high levels of motivation on the part of learners, leading to the learners' full engagement in the learning process.

Benefits of Considering Two Approaches to the Stages of Learning

It might at first appear as though the two models of the stages of learning that we have considered contradict one another. A closer examination, however, will reveal more similarities than differences. Both recognize the same observable changes in performance as individuals acquire motor skills. The difference is in the theoretical constructs used to interpret and explain these observable changes over the course of learning.

Although the theoretical differences between the two models may be at odds, the insights provided by both models may be harmonized into effective instructional practices. Fitts and Posner help us understand the cognitive demand faced by learners and increase our sensitivity to the limits of human processing capabilities and the need to provide instructional resources in ways matching learners' developing processing capabilities. Vereijken's dynamical systems perspective turns our attention to the interaction of learners with changing characteristics of the environment and task, and to a consideration

---

BOX **7.3**   **Getting to the Expert Stage of Learning**

For a skill at which you consider yourself to be in the expert stage of learning, compare your present performance of the skill with your performance when you were in the novice and advanced stages of learning. How did you perform differently in each stage? How did your performance in each stage relate to the degrees of freedom?

Using degrees of freedom as a concept to better understand your acquisition patterns in acquiring

the skill at which you are now expert, consider how you would explain your performance of the skill in the novice, advanced, and expert stages of learning. As an extension of this exercise, explain your performance across the stages of learning as related to degrees of freedom to someone who you believe will find it interesting.

of the unique characteristics of each learner. It also focuses attention on the need to orient learners to important perceptual cues in the practice environment. An understanding of both models can facilitate recognition of specific needs of learners in various situations. Some individuals may, in a given situation, benefit from developing a better cognitive grasp of the mechanics of a skill, whereas others, given the same conditions, may be better served by allowing more automatic processes to act as they are encouraged to explore various movement options.

THE ACQUISITION OF EXPERTISE IN A MOTOR SKILL

Our civilization has always recognized exceptional individuals, whose performance in sports, the arts, and science is vastly superior to that of the rest of the population.

—Ericsson, Kramps, and Tesch-Romer (1993, p. 363)

Both Fitts and Posner's and Vereijken's three-stage models of learning encompass the entire range of human motor skill learning. It becomes obvious upon reflection, however, that those individuals in the autonomous or expert stage of learning, depending on the model considered, may exhibit a considerably wide range of different skill levels. Although most people would easily be classified as being in the third stage of both models for driving an automobile, few would be capable of earning a spot on the NASCAR racing circuit, for instance. Other examples can easily be added. Would we conclude that there are few significant differences between a low-handicap weekend golfer and the current Masters champion, for example? What about the intramural tennis champion of her high school and the most recent winner of the Women's Singles at Wimbledon? Do high school basketball players differ significantly in their abilities compared to NBA or WNBA players?

Obviously, there exist significant performance differences among those cited in the examples above. Yet, all are in the third stage of learning (autonomous or expert) for their respective skills. Unfortunately, perhaps, neither Fitts and Posner, nor Vereijken, considered this extreme range of performance that can be exhibited by those in the respective third stages of their models. This should not be considered a failing or neglect on their part, however. Their interest, in the case of both models, was not on extremely talented individuals, but rather on the vast majority of people learning jobs, playing sports, pursuing recreational activities, regaining skills lost to injury or disease, or any of the other myriad of movement skills that make daily life possible and meaningful. These researchers, rightly for their purposes, eschewed elitism in developing their respective models.

In recent years, however, there has been an increased interest concerning those relatively few individuals who reach the extreme limits of learning and performance (Ericsson, 1996). If people practice a skill long enough and well enough, they may ultimately reach a level of learning called *expert*. It must quickly be pointed out that in this context, "expert" does not denote the same level of learning as the term does when used in the dynamical systems model of learning. Being an expert or acquiring expertise means something different from the stage of learning called expert by Vereijken in her conceptualization of the stages of learning. On the learning stages continuum represented by both three-stage models presented here, the level of learning we are referring to as

expertise: The attainment of superior levels of performance and knowledge related to a specific skill, reached only by those experts at the highest levels of achievement.

expert, or **expertise**, represents the area all the way to the extreme right of the continuums, at the end of the third stage (refer to Figures 7.1 and 7.2). Because of the large commitment of time and energy required to attain **expertise** in a particular skill, most experts are professionally involved in the performance of their respective skill.

A burgeoning field of scholarship and research now exists concerning the stage of learning called expertise (for good reviews of this research, see Ericsson, Krampe, and Tesch-Romer, 1993; and Starkes and Ericsson, 2003). This growing scholarly interest has mirrored the study of expertise in a wide variety of other human endeavors. Although movement skills, especially sports skills, would seem a logical area for the study of expertise, motor learning theorists, in comparison to those in other areas of academic and scholarly study, were somewhat late in beginning to apply concepts of expertise to the study of motor skills. Perhaps this is because the study of expertise as a concept places such a great emphasis on the development of cognitive and perceptual elements of skill that motor behavior researchers either failed to recognize its importance to motor expertise early on or failed to recognize the importance of cognition and perception to highly developed levels of performance for motor skills. But whatever the reason, this early neglect has given way to a robust research agenda in the motor behavior domain concerning the development of expertise, and recognition—even if somewhat late—of the importance of cognitive and perceptual aspects of motor skill performance, especially at the extreme upper limits of performance.

As a consequence of this recent interest in motor expertise, a fairly extensive literature now exists informing our understanding of how experts differ from beginners or indeed even the highly skilled. In the field of motor expertise, this literature is almost entirely to this point concerned with sport and athletic skills. In this regard, strong evidence suggests that motor expertise is both sport and context specific; that is, experts are only experts in their specific sports or areas of expertise (Ericsson and Smith, 1991). Experts are not only better than others at the actual movement patterns of a skill, but also better in their ability to perceive, understand, and respond to the various environments and situations in which the skill is performed. (Consequently, therefore, expertise cannot be measured simply through measures of skilled performance alone, but involves assessing cognitive and perceptual aspects of skill as well.)

An exact definition of expertise is somewhat difficult to arrive at, and scholars differ on some issues. However, a consensus of scholarly opinion would probably agree with the description offered by Abernethy, Burgess-Limerick, and Park (1994) that motor skill experts, when compared to others in their particular domain of skill, are known to (a) be faster and more accurate in recognizing patterns; (b) have superior knowledge of both factual (declarative) and procedural matters; (c) possess knowledge organized in a deeper, more structured form; (d) have superior knowledge of situational probabilities; (e) be better able to plan their own actions in advance; (f) be superior in anticipating the actions of an opponent; (g) be superior perceivers of essential kinematic information; (h) perform in a less effortful, more automatic fashion; (i) produce movement patterns of greater consistency and adaptability; and (j) possess superior self-monitoring skills. Many of these distinguishing characteristics separating motor experts from others in the motor domain, it should be noted, entail the cognitive and perceptual aspects of skilled performance. Indeed, the finding that experts in a particular sport are better than others not only at physical skills, but also at the underlying cognitive and perceptual components of a sport, is strongly supported in both laboratory and field research.

How Long Does It Take to Become an Expert?

How long does it take to become an expert? Research in sport, as well as other domains, has repeatedly demonstrated that somewhere on the order of 10 years experience (or 10,000 hours) of practice is needed to reach the expert stage of performance. This 10-year criterion has been observed for skills as diverse as chess, music, air-traffic control, teaching, medicine, dance, science, experimental research, piloting an airplane, soccer, field hockey, baseball, quarterbacking, figure skating, and coaching (Starkes, Helsen, and Jack, 2001).

10-year rule: A rule derived from observation across several skill domains that it generally requires a minimum of 10 years of deliberate practice to attain expertise in a skill.

Research in a number of skill domains has supported the consistency of a "**10-year rule.**" This is, indeed, one of the most ubiquitous findings in the literature concerning expertise. There are, however, limitations to this 10-year rule. Though somewhere on the order of 10 years of practice may be required to reach the expert level, any coach or teacher can attest to the fact that as important as the amount of time committed to practice may be, the quality of that practice is just as important. This observation has led to the notion of **deliberate practice** (see Table 5.2).

deliberate practice: Practice that is effortful, highly structured and organized, and directed toward extrinsic goals and rewards.

In perhaps the most extensive review of deliberate practice, Ericsson, Krampe, and Tesch-Romer (1993) identified several factors as defining the concept. Deliberate practice is highly structured and (1) requires effort and worklike intensity, (2) is engaged in for hours a day, (3) generates no immediate rewards, and (4) is motivated by the goal of improvement rather than inherent enjoyment. As already mentioned, deliberate practice also assumes the provision of optimal, often personalized, instruction for a minimum of 10 years. Of course, simple tasks are acquired in less than 10 years. For example, we would not expect someone to take 10 years to learn how to ride a bicycle expertly or to dribble a basketball (although we should still expect it to take 10 years to become a champion mountain biker or a professional basketball player). For complex skills, however, those most representative of sports

| BOX **7.4** | **Do You Know Any Experts?** |

Experts are found in many domains—among athletes, musicians, dancers, pilots, air traffic control operators, chess masters, surgeons, automotive repair specialists, typists, writers, and card players, among others. Do you personally know any experts? What makes them experts?

activities, the assumption is made and supported by research that the 10-year rule, entailing 10 years of deliberate practice, applies.

In the first investigation of the amount of deliberate practice required for attaining expertise, Starkes et al. (1996) reported that athletes participating in individual sports spent at least 10 years in practice before reaching the international level in competition. International level wrestlers reported reaching their peak levels of performance at an average age of 25 or, on average, 12 years after beginning their competitive wrestling training. International level wrestlers also reported spending considerably more time in practice (an average of 38.7 hours per week by the sixth year of training) compared to a similar group of wrestlers who did not attain international competitive levels (20.9 hours per week at year six of training).

Extending this early work on individual sports, Helsen, Starkes, and Hodges (1998) studied the practice histories of provincial (i.e., local), national, and international soccer players from Belgium. On average, the soccer players studied began systematic practice on local youth soccer teams by age 7 and reached their peak levels of performance at an average age of 22, 15 years into their careers. Those players reaching the national and international levels of team competition spent 9.9 and 13.3 hours per week on practice, respectively, over their playing careers, compared to 6.9 hours for the provincial team members. Interestingly, the percentage of time spent in team practice, compared to practicing skills individually, was highest for the international group at each year, and increased each year over the international players' athletic careers. This finding suggests that deliberate "team" practice may be especially important for the development of expertise in team sports.

One reason that team practice may prove significantly more beneficial than the individual practice of skills, at least for team sports, is that team

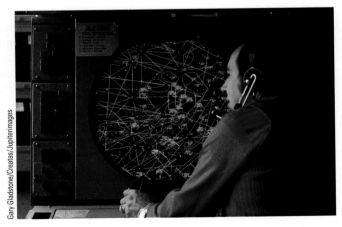

The ten-year or ten-thousand hour rule for attaining expertise in a skill applies across skill domains (represented here is air-traffic control).

practice is more likely to be instructed by a coach. The presence of a coach, it can be argued, makes it more likely that practice will include training in the cognitive and perceptual elements of a skill, in addition to practice of the motor patterns involved in performance. A strong conclusion reached from the literature on expertise recall is that practice of the perceptual and cognitive elements of a motor skill appear just as important, and perhaps even more important, than the actual execution of a skill's movement patterns in attaining high levels of skill. It is becoming more clear from recent research concerning expert performance that even beginning learners may benefit significantly by increasing the quality and amount of practice attention devoted to the perceptual and cognitive elements of a skill (Abernethy, Burgess-Limerick, and Park, 1997, p. 345).

The 10-year rule provides a guideline indicating the amount of practice necessary for reaching the highest levels of performance in athletic and other motor skills. Just as important as the amount of practice, however, is the quality of the practice. Deliberate practice under the guidance of a knowledgeable and effective instructor is necessary to turn years of practice into expert levels of performance. Although recent research on expertise has expanded our understanding of the quality of instruction and amount of practice needed for attaining high levels of motor performance, a number of questions still remain. There is debate, for instance, over the original proposals by researchers in the field that the type of practice necessary is not inherently enjoyable. Evidence to the contrary, although mostly anecdotal, suggests that in the realm of sports, practice may frequently be experienced as enjoyable. Considerable debate remains, also, concerning the relative importance of practice and inherited abilities individuals bring to practice. Although Ericsson and other original developers of the expertise approach have suggested that intensive, deliberate practice for a sufficient period of time can reshape underlying genetic factors toward skill-specific attributes, others reject this premise. Singer and Janelle (1999) join a chorus of voices from within the research community in suggesting that it would be a mistake to ignore the influence of genetic predispositions on the acquisition of motor skills, especially in the sports domain where cognitive and perceptual components are a critical part of achieving high levels of performance. Sternberg (1996), perhaps the most vocal critic of the expertise approach, has even suggested that the tendency to practice in the intense fashion described by the concept of deliberate practice may itself be genetically determined.

Whatever the underlying factors responsible for the achievement of exceptionally high levels of athletic or other forms of motor performance, there is no question that considerable amounts of practice are required for its attainment. Although many variables interact in the attainment of sport expertise, and no exact amount of practice experience can be identified for its attainment, an interesting analysis of the amount of practice necessary to attain high levels of success in a sample of elite performers in differing domains was reported a number of years ago by Ericsson (1990) and can serve here to stimulate further thought on the question of the amount of practice necessary to achieve expertise (see Table 7.3).

TABLE **7.3**

Years of Deliberate Practice to Achieve World-Class Performance

Domain	Starting Age	Years to International Performance	Age at Peak Performance
Tennis	6.5	10+	18 to 20
Swimming	4.5	10	18 to 20
Piano	6	17	NA
Chess	10	14	30 to 40

Source: Adapted from Ericsson, KA. (1990). "Theoretical issues in the study of exceptional performance." In KJ Gilhooly, MTG Keane, RH Logic, and C Erdos (eds.), *Lines of thinking: Reflections on the psychology of thought* (vol. 2). Mahwah, NJ: Lawrence Erlbaum.

PREDICTING INDIVIDUAL SUCCESS ACROSS THE STAGES OF LEARNING

One of the more interesting questions arising from a study of the stages of motor learning is, How predictive of the later stages of learning is performance in earlier stages of learning? That is, are observations of performers' initial experience with a skill a good indication of how well they might ultimately learn to perform the skill? Put more technically, what is the correlation among performance measures across the stages of motor learning?

Many variations of this basic question can be posed. By watching a group of performers in the early stages of learning, can you accurately predict who might ultimately be the best performer? Are those who perform best when first learning a skill more likely to remain comparatively best at the skill throughout the stages of learning? Are those who start poorly, on the other hand, destined to always lag behind? Such questions have considerable theoretical and practical importance. Should a coach select players for an athletic team, for instance, based on performance by young players still new to a sport? Is performance in a job-training program a good predictor of who will become the best workers? Is early difficulty in relearning a skill lost to injury a precursor of ultimate failure? A commonly held notion, including among many professionals in motor skill instruction, is that initial performance of a skill in the early stages of learning is a good indicator of one's ability to ultimately learn the skill. Is this assumption true?

There is a large body of research answering this question, and it is one of the oldest areas of investigation in skill learning, going back to the early part of the last century. Although an analysis of the literature is beyond the scope of this chapter, the research findings in this area have yielded consistent results over the years, and there is a well-established answer to such questions as posed above. (The interested reader will find good reviews of the research in this area in Ackerman, 1988, 1992; Day, Arthur, and Shebilske, 1997; and Henry and Hulin, 1987.)

Correlational Analysis and the Predictive Strength of Learning Potential at Various Stages of Learning

Research investigating the relationship of skill performance between early and later stages of learning typically involves the correlation of some performance measure over time (i.e., as an individual progresses through the stages of learning). For example, if 100 people were measured on the performance of a skill in the initial stage of learning and then ranked by their relative performance ability from 1 to 100, how consistent would this ranking remain as practice proceeded? Would those initially ranking high (say in the 1–10 positions) continue to be ranked high (1 to 10) over all stages of practice? Would they, just as likely, be ranked in a lower grouping of learners at some point as practice progressed (say in the 31–40 positions, or even the 91–100 positions)?

To answer this question, a correlational analysis is conducted. Correlation, in this case, tells us the degree of likelihood that individuals will remain in the same relative ranked positions as practice progresses. If the correlation is high, learners stay in the same relative ranked position on performance scores as they progress through the stages of learning, making prediction of relative skill level across learning reliable (i.e., those who perform the best initially also perform the best in the middle and later stages of learning—indeed, at any stage of learning they are among the best performers). If the correlation is low, however, individuals change in their ranked positions as they progress through the stages of learning, and prediction of later performance level based upon early performance ranking is unreliable (i.e., the worst performers initially may be among the best performers in the middle or later stages of learning).

Such correlational analyses have yielded consistent findings and inform a well-established relationship between skill level and stage of learning. Generally, for most types of skills, the correlation between initial performance and later performance is low. As one progresses through the stages of learning, however, the correlation between current performance and later performance gradually increases and becomes more predictive. Simply put, early performance is an unreliable predictor of later performance, at least in the initial stages of learning. As one progresses through the stages of motor skill learning, however, performance becomes more and more reliable as a predictor of ultimate performance abilities. In a perhaps helpful but admittedly simplistic way of stating the case, performance in the early stages of learning is not predictive of ultimate levels of skill learning; prediction in intermediate stages of learning is somewhat predictive of ultimate skill achievement; and prediction in later stages of learning is highly predictive of ultimate skill level achievement. A more technically sound way of stating this finding has been made by Henry and Hulin (1987) in their excellent review of the literature on the stability of skilled performance across the stages of learning. They state that:

> A ubiquitous finding in the study of relations of ability and performance is the decreasing predictive validity that occurs as a function of time and interpolated practice. Correlations between ability measures, assessed at Time i, and performance, assessed successively at Times $i + 1, i + 2, ..., i + k$, decrease regularly as a function of the ordinal position of the performance assessment. Studies done longitudinally with constant samples of subjects, almost without exception, display this general trend. (p. 457)

Figure 7.3 illustrates the general findings concerning the relationship between early and later performance measures as people progress through the stages of learning a motor skill. In this figure, a common technique of interpreting correlation has been used by squaring the correlation coefficient (R^2) to obtain a percentage; this number indicates the percentage of times a prediction of future performance level based on current level of performance would be accurate.

As Figure 7.3 illustrates, accuracy of prediction increases in a rather linear fashion with progression through the stages of learning. In the figure, for example, the predictive power of observations in the initial phase of learning is

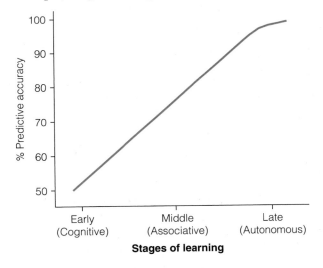

FIGURE **7.3** Prediction of Final Level of Skill Performance Based Upon Earlier Stage of Learning Observations

Source: Copyright © 1992 by the American Psychological Association. Reproduced with permission. Ackerman, PL (1992). "Predicting individual differences in complex skill acquisition: Dynamics of ability determinants." *Journal of Applied Psychology, 77,* 598–614. The use of APA information does not imply endorsement by APA.

only about 50 percent, meaning that only half of the time that one attempted to predict later skill-learning levels from early observations would the prediction be accurate (and the other half of the time, one would be incorrect). As learning progresses, say to the middle stages of learning in the figure, accuracy in predicting future performance levels increases to the 65 to 80 percent level. Finally, when entering the later stages of learning, prediction becomes reliable (90 percent or greater). Note, however, that the tail end of the prediction line is curved as it approaches the 100 percent prediction accuracy level, never reaching that asymptote (that is, even at high levels of skill, absolute prediction accuracy is not possible— there can still be surprises).

A consistent research finding is that an early level of success in a motor skill is not a reliable predictor of one's ultimate potential to learn the skill. Prediction becomes more reliable, however, as individuals progress through the stages of learning, though even in the intermediate stages of learning prediction remains somewhat tentative at best. This finding should be of considerable practical importance to practitioners responsible for making assessments of ultimate skill learning based on early observations of novice learners or even, for that matter, of more experienced learners.

Ackerman's Theoretical Explanation of Learning Effects across the Stages of Learning

Although the relationship between skill level and stage of learning is well established in the literature, the reasons for it remained unclear until Ackerman (1988, 1992), an experimental psychologist, proposed an explanation that has received considerable research support (Matthews, Jones, and Chamberlain, 1992). Ackerman proposed that different types of abilities are primarily responsible for performance in each of the three stages of learning proposed by Fitts and Posner and that there is a weak correlation among these ability types. Figure 7.4 illustrates Ackerman's model of abilities and skill level.

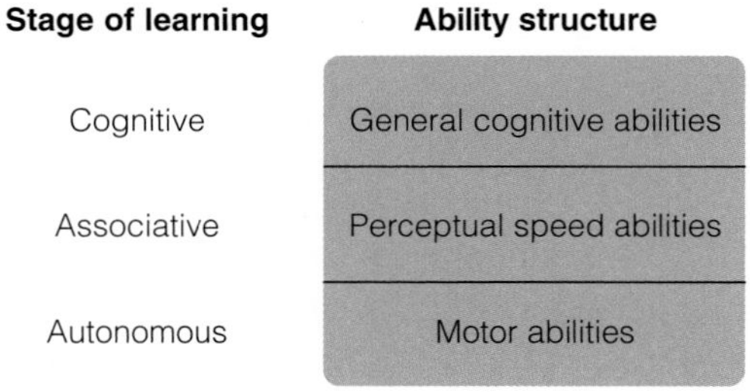

Stage of learning	Ability structure
Cognitive	General cognitive abilities
Associative	Perceptual speed abilities
Autonomous	Motor abilities

FIGURE **7.4** Ackerman's Model of Relationship Between Critical Learning Abilities and the Fitts and Posner Stages of Learning

Source: Copyright © 1992 by the American Psychological Association. Reproduced with permission. Ackerman, PL (1992). "Predicting individual differences in complex skill acquisition: Dynamics of ability determinants." *Journal of Applied Psychology, 77,* 598–614. The use of APA information does not imply endorsement by APA.

As Fitts and Posner posited, in the cognitive stage of learning, individuals must acquire knowledge about the goals, rules, movement characteristics, and important perceptual cues involved with skill production—i.e., they must understand the task and how to perform it. As Ackerman (1992) states, this stage of learning is "characterized by a high cognitive load on the learner in the context of understanding task instructions, general familiarization with task goals, and formulating strategies for task accomplishment" (p. 599). Ackerman goes on to state that in this stage of learning "general cognitive" and "broad-content" abilities predominate. **General cognitive abilities** include reasoning, problem solving, and verbal abilities, among others; broad-content abilities include spatial orientation, attentional control, and so on.

general cognitive abilities: A generalized abilities pattern broadly encompassing such cognitive traits as reasoning, problem solving, and verbal abilities.

perceptual speed ability: The ability to assess environmental stimuli and respond quickly.

As individuals progress to the associative stage of learning, cognitive abilities become less important and **perceptual speed ability** becomes more dominant in accounting for performance success. Again as stated by Ackerman (1992), the associative stage "involves the proceduralization of task strategies in a manner that makes performance quicker and less error prone. In Fitts and Posner's terms, this phase is characterized by strengthening associations between stimulus and response" (p. 599). The perceptual abilities most important in this stage of learning include the ability to assess environmental factors and respond to them quickly. This ability especially relates to visual search and memory (i.e., how quickly one can locate and attend to correct cues in the environment and then correctly retrieve the associated memory and make accurate stimulus–response connections). At this stage, the learner's problem is not knowing what to do, but in being able to do it quickly. In the associative stage of learning, perceptual abilities are of the greatest importance for performance and continued improvement in learning.

BOX 7.5   Predicting Success for Michael Jordan?

From the time he was a young child, Michael Jordan loved sports. He played organized youth baseball and football, and loved playing basketball in the backyard against his older brother. So, when in his sophomore year he tried out for the Laney High School basketball team in his hometown of Wilmington, North Carolina, it was not a surprise. What was a surprise, perhaps, was that at the end of tryouts Jordan was cut from the team as having insufficient skills to develop into a good basketball player.

Instead of giving up on basketball, though, Jordan began practicing for many hours each day on the court in preparation for tryouts the following year. Of that time, he has said, "Whenever I was working out and got tired and figured I ought to stop, I'd close my eyes and see that list in the locker room without my name on it, and that usually got me going again."

Of course, Jordan did get going again. He went on to be a college All-American leading his team to a national championship, won an Olympic gold medal, and as a professional led his Chicago Bulls team to three straight NBA championships. Today, he is almost universally regarded as the best basketball player of all time. All of this from an athlete who was considered insufficiently skilled to be a member of his high school team.

Why do you think that Jordan may have failed to perform well enough in his early attempts at basketball to make his high school team? How might Ackerman's model help explain Jordan's initial performance difficulties? How does Jordan's response help us better understand why he eventually went on to such great success?

motor abilities: Stable, inherited traits that underlie the execution of movements and skills (i.e., reaction time, rate control, dynamic strength, etc.).

When an individual moves into the autonomous stage of learning, cognitive and perceptual abilities have become well encoded into memory and no longer limit further progress. At this stage, the demand on **motor abilities** increases so that these become the abilities most highly correlated with performance success. Motor abilities are unchanging, genetically determined traits that underlie and support movement skills. At this stage of learning, the individual has acquired a cognitive (declarative) understanding of the skill as well as memory structures informing appropriate stimulus–response associations. What is essential for further performance improvement is the individual's underlying motor abilities as related to specific skill requirements. These include such abilities as reaction time, manual dexterity, balance, multilimb coordination, dynamic strength, flexibility, and so forth (these abilities are described in more detail in Chapter 8). Until an individual understands skill requirements, and has formed appropriate stimulus–response connections to allow for rapid perceptual decision making, the motor abilities underlying a skill are relatively less important in performance achievement. Once the task is well understood and perceptual speed in decision making achieved, however, motor abilities become the dominant factor in the further development of skill.

The relative importance of each of these ability types is represented in Figure 7.5. This figure illustrates the importance of each of the three ability types at the various stages of motor skill learning. Because there is a weak correlation among the three types of ability (perhaps even a zero correlation), prediction becomes unreliable. A person possessing high general cognitive abilities, for example, would perform well relative to others in the early stages of learning most motor skills. However, if this same person has rather weak motor abilities relative to the skill, then performance in the later stages of learning will be marked by relatively weak performance measures compared to others. Because there is little predictive association among the three ability types, it is impossible to accurately predict an individual's performance across the stages of learning since the requisite abilities most importantly underlying performance (and learning) at each stage change in a highly uncorrelated (nonpredictive) fashion.

One caveat must be stated before drawing any final conclusions concerning these three categories of abilities and predictive decisions about skill learning. The Ackerman model should be viewed as a general description of how abilities inform progression across the stages of learning. This is because, for some skills, abilities that account for a person's performance success may not change as drastically across the stages of learning as indicated in the model. That is, for some skills, cognitive abilities may remain dominant across all the stages of learning (billiards and watch repair, for example), whereas for others, perceptual abilities dominate in all stages (Game Boy and driving). Still, for most motor skills (though not all) the progression of learning is most dependent on underlying ability structures as suggested in Ackerman's model, making prediction of future successes based upon earlier stages of performance tentative, at best.

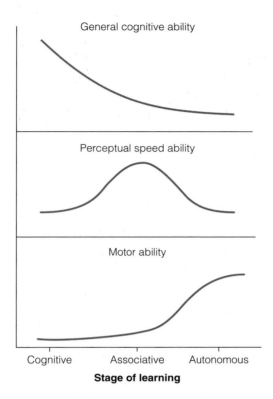

FIGURE **7.5** Ackerman's Hypothetical Skill-Ability Relationship Across the Stages of Learning

Source: Copyright © 1992 by the American Psychological Association. Reproduced with permission. Ackerman, PL (1992). "Predicting individual differences in complex skill acquisition: Dynamics of ability determinants." *Journal of Applied Psychology, 77,* 598–614. The use of APA information does not imply endorsement by APA.

SUMMARY

- As people learn motor skills, they exhibit similar behavioral characteristics that can be grouped to identify distinct stages of learning.
- In 1967, Fitts and Posner proposed a three-stage model of learning that has become the most widely accepted and used model of learning.
  - In the initial cognitive stage of learning, individuals attempt to understand the goals and proper movement mechanics of a skill. Skills are controlled through declarative memory structures.
  - The associative stage is an intermediate stage of learning in which individuals begin to put longer and longer sequences of skill components together.
  - The final stage of learning is the autonomous stage, in which learners perform most or all components of a skill automatically without the need of attentional resources. Skills are encoded into procedural memory.

- Dynamical systems theorists have proposed their own three-stage model of learning based upon notions of constraints, degrees of freedom, and affordances.
  - In the novice stage of learning, learners freeze the degrees of freedom in limbs and joints as they attempt to solve movement problems by exploring the movement landscape.
  - The advanced stage is marked by the freeing of degrees of freedom and the development of synergies.
  - In the expert stage of learning, learners exploit features of bodily systems and the environment in order to facilitate greater coordination, reduce energy demands, and optimize performance levels.
- In recent years, considerable research attention has been focused on the acquisition of expertise. Experts perform at the extreme limits of human performance in a specific skill.
  - Expertise is domain and skill specific.
  - The acquisition of expertise requires a minimum of 10 years of deliberate practice.
  - Experts in motor skills possess optimally developed movement patterns as well as highly developed cognitive and perceptual resources relative to the skill in which they are expert.
- Prediction of performance potential across the stages of learning is fairly unreliable; there is little correlation of comparative performance proficiency between earlier and later stages of learning among people.
  - Ackerman proposed that the low correlation observed between performance and amount of practice as people progress through the stages of learning is explained by different sets of unrelated ability types playing a prominent role in each stage of learning.

LEARNING EXERCISES

1. Locate a setting where you can observe people performing the same or similar motor skills representing all three stages of learning (i.e., a recreational setting; physical education class; dance, martial arts, or gymnastics studio; workplace; clinic setting; etc.). For each of the three stages of learning, identify and observe one person you judge to be in that stage. Observe each of these people for at least 10 minutes, taking notes on the behaviors that you judge as revealing his or her stage of learning. Prepare a written report discussing your findings and explaining why you categorized your subjects into the three stages of learning. *Note:* For this exercise you may use either the three-stage model of Fitts and Posner or the dynamical systems model proposed by Vereijken.

2. For this exercise, observe an individual who is in the early or intermediate stage of learning (either the first or second stage in one of the two models presented in this chapter) practicing a motor skill. For this individual, what specific instructional suggestions do you think most appropriate?

If you were the person's instructor, what would be your focus, and what specific instructions and practice manipulations would you provide? Prepare a written discussion of your answers, including your analysis of your subject's performance and stage of learning. Your suggestions should be specific to the individual learner, task, and situation. *Note:* You may use either the three-stage model of Fitts and Posner or Vereijken's dynamical systems model as the bases of your analysis and instructional suggestions.

3. Select a motor skill of interest to you for completing this exercise. For the skill you select, describe, in detail specific to the skill, the characteristics and behaviors that would indicate an individual who was in each of the stages of learning for both Fitts and Posner's model and Vereijken's dynamical systems model of the stages of learning. Prepare a written report of your analysis for each stage, and include a summary statement comparing and contrasting your observations relative to the two learning stage models.

4. Think of a skill (it can be from any skill domain) at which you would most like to be an expert. Prepare a written plan detailing how you can give yourself the best chance for achieving expertise in this skill.

5. Think about a skill in which you are proficient (in the third stage of learning relative to the models we discussed in this chapter) and which you remember originally learning. Using Ackerman's model of stage-specific abilities, analyze and discuss in a written report the specific abilities you deem most important to performance and learning of this skill in each stage of learning. Recalling your learning of the skill, was there a stage you had more difficulty with than the others? Do you feel you were equally proficient in all stages of learning, or did you notice a difference in your learning experiences as you progressed in learning the skill? How would you evaluate your abilities in each of the three stages of learning, and what effect did this have on the rate and relative ease with which you learned the skill?

FOR FURTHER STUDY

HOW MUCH DO YOU KNOW?

For each of the following, select the letter that best answers the question.

1. In Fitts and Posner's three-stage model of learning, the stage in which sub-verbalization is most evident is the _____ stage.
   a. cognitive
   b. perceptual
   c. associative
   d. autonomous

2. In which stage of Fitts and Posner's stages of learning model are skills controlled primarily by procedural memory?
   a. Cognitive
   b. Perceptual
   c. Associative
   d. Autonomous

3. Which word best describes the functions of the second stage of learning in Vereijken's dynamical systems model of the stages of learning?
   a. Freezing
   b. Freeing
   c. Elaborating
   d. Exploiting

4. According to the dynamical systems theory of learning, learners can best be thought of as
   a. passive receivers of information.
   b. cognitive processors of instructions.
   c. active problem solvers.
   d. duplicators of visually modeled activities.

5. In order for the practice of a motor skill to be deliberate, which of the following characteristics need *not* be true?
   a. Motivated by the goal of improvement
   b. Requires effort and work-like intensity
   c. Engaged in for hours on most days
   d. Experienced as being enjoyable
6. As a general rule, achieving expertise in a sport (or other skill) requires a commitment to deliberate practice for a minimum of
   a. 5 years.
   b. 10 years.
   c. 15 years.
   d. one-half the number of years as a person's age.

Answer the following with the word or words that best complete each sentence.

7. Which stage of learning in Vereijken's dynamical systems model of learning stages is analogous to the cognitive stage of learning in the Fitts and Posner model?

8. According to the dynamical systems theory of learning, in what stage of learning have synergies been mostly developed?
9. The elastic properties of muscles are a type of _____ constraint that individuals can learn to exploit in solving movement problems.
10. _____ to affordances is the process by which individuals develop their abilities to recognize perceptual cues and couple them with appropriate movement responses.
11. Bernstein labeled the strategy adopted by beginners of locking some joints and coupling others in order to reduce the cognitive demands on motor control as _____ the degrees of freedom.
12. What kind of abilities are the most essential in the associative stage of learning according to Ackerman?

Answers are provided at the end of this review section.

STUDY QUESTIONS

1. What are the stages of learning according to Fitts and Posner? Name and describe each stage.
2. What are the stages of learning from a dynamical systems perspective as described by Vereijken? Name and describe each stage.
3. What are the instructional priorities, and how do they change over the stages of learning according to the Fitts and Posner model of the stages of learning?
4. How do the memory structures controlling movement change over the stages of learning according to the Fitts and Posner model of learning?
5. What are the instructional priorities, and how do they change over the stages of learning according to Vereijken's dynamical systems model of the stages of learning?

6. What are constraints, and how do they influence the learning of motor skills?
7. What is meant by attunement to affordances? How does it facilitate learning?
8. In what ways can individuals learn to exploit the properties of bodily systems and movement environments? How is this beneficial to learning?
9. What is expertise? How is an expert different from somebody who is highly skilled, but not an expert?
10. How is expertise developed?
11. How predictive of a person's potential for future learning is his or her level of learning within each stage of learning?
12. Describe Ackerman's model for explaining differential learning potential within the three stages of learning described by Fitts and Posner.

ADDITIONAL READING

Ackerman, PL. (1992). "Predicting individual differences in complex skill acquisition: Dynamics of ability determinants." *Journal of Applied Psychology, 77,* 598–614.

Darden, GF. (1999). "Videotape feedback for student learning and performance: A learning stages approach." *Journal of Physical Education, Recreation and Dance, 70*(9), 40–44.

Ericsson, KA, Krampe, RT, and Tesch-Romer, C. (1993). "The role of deliberate practice in the acquisition of expert performance." *Psychological Review, 100,* 363–406.

Fitts, PM, and Posner, MI. (1967). *Human performance.* Belmont, CA: Brooks/Cole.

Savelsbergh, G, Verheal, M, van der Kamp, J, and Marple-Horvat, D. (2007). "Visuomotor control of movement acquisition." In J Liukkonen, Y Vander Auweele, B Vereijken, D Alfermann, and Y Theodorakis (eds.), *Psychology for physical educators: Student in Focus,* 2nd ed., Champaign, IL: Human Kinetics.

Starkes, JL, Helsen, W, and Jack, R. (2001). "Expert performance in sport and dance." In RN Singer, HA Hausenblas, and CM Janelle (eds.), *Handbook of sport psychology,* 2nd ed. New York: John Wiley & Sons.

Verejiken, B, van Emmerik, REA, Whiting, HTA, and Newall, KM. (1992). "Free(z)ing the degrees of freedom in skill acquisition." *Journal of Motor Behavior, 24,* 133–142.

REFERENCES

Abernethy, B, Burgess-Limerick, R, and Park, S. (1994). "Contrasting approaches to the study of motor expertise." *Quest, 14,* 186–198.

Ackerman, PL. (1988). "Determinants of individual differences during skill acquisition: Cognitive abilities and information processing." *Journal of Experimental Psychology: General, 117,* 288–318.

Ackerman, PL. (1992). "Predicting individual differences in complex skill acquisition: Dynamics of ability determinants." *Journal of Applied Psychology, 77,* 598–614.

Adams, JA. (1971). "A closed-loop theory of motor learning." *Journal of Motor Behavior, 3,* 111–150.

Bandura, A. (1986). *Social foundations of thought and action: A social cognitive theory.* Englewood Cliffs, NJ: Prentice Hall.

Belka, DA. (2002). "A strategy for the improvement of learning task-specific presentations." *Journal of Physical Education, Recreation, and Dance,* August.

Bernstein, N. (1967). *The co-ordinary and regulation of movement.* Oxford: Pergamon Press.

Buekers, MJA, Magill, RA, and Hall, KG. (1992). "The effects of erroneous knowledge of results on skill acquisition when augmented feedback is redundant." *Quarterly Journal of Experimental Psychology, 44A,* 105–112.

Darden, GF. (1999). "Videotape feedback for student learning and performance: A learning stages approach." *Journal of Physical Education, Recreation and Dance, 70*(9), 40–44.

Davids, K, Button, C, and Bennett, S. (2008). *Dynamics of skill acquisition: A constraints-led approach.* Champaign, IL: Human Kinetics.

Day, EA, Arthur Jr., W, and Shebilske, WL. (1997). "Ability determinants of complex skill acquisition: Effects of training protocol." *Acta Psychologica, 97,* 145–165.

Ericsson, KA. (1990). "Theoretical issues in the study of exceptional performance." In KJ Gilhooly, MTG Keane, RH Logic, and C Erdos (eds.), *Lines of Thinking: Reflections on the Psychology of Thought,* vol. 2. Mahwah, NJ: Lawrence Erlbaum.

Ericsson, KA. (1996). *The road to excellence: The acquisition of expert performance in the arts and sciences, sports, and games.* Mahwah, NJ: Lawrence Erlbaum.

Ericsson, KA, Krampe, RT, and Tesch-Romer, C. (1993). "The role of deliberate practice in the acquisition of expert performance." *Psychological Review, 100,* 363–406.

Ericsson, KA, and Smith, J. (1991). "Prospects and limits of the empirical study of expertise: An introduction." In KA Ericsson and J Smith (eds.), *Toward a General Theory of Expertise: Prospects and Limits* (pp. 1–38). Cambridge, England: Cambridge University Press.

Fitts, PM, and Posner, MI. (1967). *Human performance*. Belmont, CA: Brooks/Cole.

Gentile, AM. (1972). "A working model of skill acquisition with application to teaching." *Quest*, 17, 3–32.

Gentile, AM. (2000). "Skill acquisition: Action, movement, and neuromotor processes." In JH Carr, RB Shepherd, J Gordon, AM Gentile, and JM Hands (eds.), *Movement science: Foundations for physical therapy in rehabilitation*, 2nd ed. Gaithersberg, MD: Aspen Publishers.

Gibson, JJ. (1979). *The ecological approach to visual perception*. Hillsdale, NJ: Erlbaum.

Haring, NG, Lovitt, TC, Eaton, MD, and Hansen, CL. (1978). *The fourth R: Research in the classroom*. Columbus, OH: Charles Merrill Publishing.

Helsen, WF, Starkes, JL, and Hodges, NJ. (1998). "Team sports and the theory of deliberate practice." *Journal of Sport and Exercise Psychology*, 20, 12–34.

Henry, RA, and Hulin, CL. (1987). "Stability of skilled performance across time: Some generalizations and limitations on utilities." *Journal of Applied Psychology*, 72, 457–462.

Kugler, PN, Kelso, JAS, and Turvey, MT. (1992). "On the control and coordination of naturally developing systems." In JAS Kelso and JE Clark (eds.), *The development of movement control and co-ordination* (pp. 5–78). New York: Wiley.

Marteniuk, RG. (1976). *Information processing in motor skills*. Dubuque, IA: Wm. C. Brown.

Matthews, G, Jones, DM, and Chamberlain, AG. (1992). "Predictions of individual differences in mail-sorting skills and their variation with ability level." *Journal of Applied Psychology*, 77, 406–418.

Newell, KM. (1986). "Constraints on the development of coordination." In MG Wade and HTA Whiting (eds.), *Motor development in children: Aspects of coordination and control* (pp. 341–360). Dordrecht, Germany: Martinus Nighoff.

Newell, KM, and van Emmerik, REA. (1989). "The acquisition of coordination: Preliminary analysis of learning to write." *Human Movement Science*, 8, 17–32.

Savelsbergh, GJP, and van der Kamp, J. (2000). "Information in learning to co-ordinate and control movements: Is there a need for specificity of practice?" *International Journal of Sport Psychology*, 31, 467–484.

Savelsbergh, G, Verheal, M, van der Kamp, J, and Marple-Horvat, D. (2007). "Visuomotor control of movement acquisition." In J Liukkonen, Y Vander Auweele, B Vereijken, D Alfermann, and Y Theodorakis (eds.), *Psychology for physical educators: Student in focus*, 2nd ed., Champaign, IL: Human Kinetics.

Shea, CH, Shebilske, WL, and Worchel, S. (1993). *Motor learning and control*. Englewood Cliffs, NJ: Prentice Hall.

Singer, RN, and Janelle, CM. (1999). "Determining sport expertise." *International Journal of Sport Psychology*, 30, 117–150.

Southard, D, and Higgins, T. (1987). "Changing movement patterns: Effects of demonstrations and practice." *Research Quarterly for Exercise and Sport*, 58, 77–80.

Starkes, JL, Deakin, J, Allard, F, Hodges, NJ, and Hayes, A. (1996). "Deliberate practice in sports: What is it anyway?" In KA Ericsson (ed.), *The road to excellence: The acquisition of expert performance in the arts and sciences, sports, and games* (pp. 81–106). Mahwah, NJ: Lawrence Erlbaum.

Starkes, JL, and Erricsson, KA. (2003). *Expert performance in sports: Advances in research on sport expertise*. Champaign, IL: Human Kinetics.

Starkes, JL, Helsen, W, and Jack, R. (2001). "Expert performance in sport and dance." In RN Singer, HA Hausenblas, and CM Janelle (eds.), *Handbook of sport psychology*, 2nd ed. New York: John Wiley & Sons.

Sternberg, RJ. (1996). "Attention and consciousness." In *Cognitive Psychology*, New York: Harcourt Brace.

van Emmerik, REA, den Brinker, BPLM, Vereijken, B, and Whiting, HTA. (1989). "Preferred tempo in the learning of a cyclical action." *The Quarterly Journal of Experimental Psychology*, 41, 251–262.

Verejiken, B. (1991). *The dynamics of skill acquisition*. Unpublished dissertation, Free University, Netherlands.

Verejiken, B, van Emmerik, REA, Whiting, HTA, and Newall, KM. (1992). "Free(z)ing the degrees of freedom in skill acquisition." *Journal of Motor Behavior*, 24, 133–142.

Verejiken, B, Whiting, HTA, and Beek, WJ. (1992). "A dynamical systems approach towards skill acquisition." *Quarterly Journal of Experimental Psychology*, 45A, 323–344.

Answers to How Much Do You Know questions: (1) A, (2) D, (3) B, (4) C, (5) D, (6) B, (7) novice, (8) advanced stage, (9) organismic, (10) attunement, (11) freezing, (12) perceptual-speed abilities.

CHAPTER 8

Individual Differences

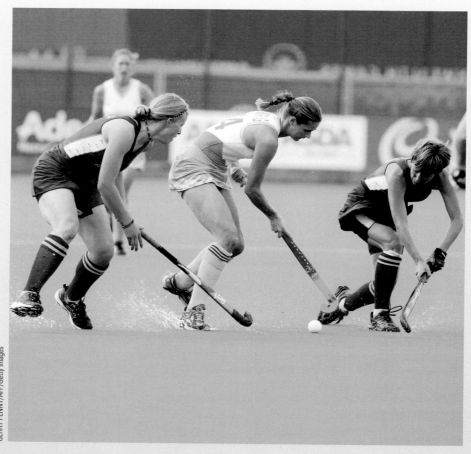

GERRY PENNY/AFP/Getty Images

Nobody has things just as he would like them. The thing to do is to make a success with what material I have.
—Dr. Frank Crane (1861–1928)

KEY QUESTIONS

- Why do people differ in their capacities for learning motor skills?

- Are some people genetically endowed to be better than others at learning and performing motor skills?

- Which influences a person's potential for learning motor skills more—genetics or experience?

- What are motor abilities?

- Are there limits to how accomplished people can become in specific motor skills?

- Is there such a person as an "all-around athlete"?

CHAPTER OVERVIEW

Outstanding athletic performance by an individual is as breathtaking as it is rare. That is probably why we marvel when we observe siblings excel in athletics. Consider brothers Peyton and Eli Manning, for example. Both excelled as college quarterbacks and were the first professional football players selected in their respective draft classes. Both have also gone on to outstanding professional careers, and in fact, each has led his team to a Super Bowl victory, Peyton for the Indianapolis Colts and Eli for the New York Giants. Their story is even more intriguing because their father, Archie, was also an outstanding collegiate quarterback, and the second player selected in his draft class, going on to an All-Pro career quarterbacking the New Orleans Saints.

The probability that two siblings, let alone a parent and siblings, would achieve such elite performances in the same sport (and position within the sport) seems to defy odds. The example of the Manning family offers a unique challenge for those interested in explaining why some people excel at given motor skills, while others do not. Did Peyton and Eli benefit from some genetic factor they inherited from their father, or was it the environment of their father's role modeling, encouragement, and coaching that was the decisive factor in the sons' development? Or, perhaps, was it some combination of both? Nature or nurture?

In this chapter, we will look at some of the approaches movement scientists use to disentangle the influences of genetic and environmental factors in the development of motor behavior. By the completion of the chapter, you should be able to provide a reasoned and compelling explanation of the Manning family's athletic success.

———————

People vary widely in their individual characteristics and capabilities. This is one of the most obvious facts of human life. Some people are tall, and others are short, for instance. Some people can sing better than others or are more artistic or are better at solving mathematical problems. Some people are fast and others strong—some are both.

People differ from one another on virtually every identifiable human characteristic and dimension of observed behavior (but see Box 8.1). Sometimes the differences are only slight, sometimes extensive. Individual differences may be attributable to either heredity or to environmental experience or to some combination of both. Although both genetic and environmental factors are important in understanding individual differences, inherited factors establish the basic structures upon which experience builds, and they are particularly important to our understanding of individual differences in skilled motor behaviors.

Questions concerning individual differences in motor learning and performance have been scientifically studied and debated since the latter part of the nineteenth century. Edward Thorndike (1874–1949) was the first to extensively investigate individual differences. He asked whether people became more alike or less alike in their performance characteristics as they practiced a skill, and he carried out the first experiments to investigate individual differences (Thorndike, 1908). Since Thorndike's initial inquiries, the study of individual differences in skill acquisition, and particularly in motor skill acquisition, has waxed and waned with various theoretical movements and changing scholarly interests among researchers (see Boyle and Ackerman, 2004, for a review of this research). Although many questions of interest still remain, research has established solid approaches to the study of why people differ in the learning and performance of motor skills.

BOX **8.1**   Individual Differences Depend on Where You Are Looking

Similarity is the shadow of difference. A short man is different from a tall man, but two men seem similar if contrasted with a woman. A man and a woman may be very different, but by comparison with a chimpanzee, it is their similarities that strike the eye. A chimpanzee, in turn, is similar to a human being when contrasted with a dog: the face, the hands, the 32 teeth, and so on. And a dog is like a person to the extent that both are unlike a fish. Difference is the shadow of similarity.

(Matt Ridley, 2001, p. 7)

THE CONCEPT OF INDIVIDUAL DIFFERENCES AND TRAITS

traits: Inherited factors that are stable and enduring and that underlie and support activity across the entire spectrum of human behaviors.

The study of individual differences is grounded in the study of **traits** (Buss and Poley, 1976; Cooper, 1999; Minton and Schneider, 1980). Traits are genetically inherited factors that underlie behavior; they are stable and enduring, and cannot be changed. Traits make people different and predispose them to being relatively better or worse on the entire spectrum of human behaviors.

Some traits underlie intellectual capabilities like mathematical reasoning, language skills, artistic expression, musical abilities, and creativity; other traits form the character of our personality, like interpersonal skills, self-awareness, motivation, behavioral control, and aggression. Other traits underlie our emotions and include, as examples, feelings, interests, curiosity, empathy, and attachment. Still other traits underlie the entire array of skilled human movement behaviors. Together, the various kinds of traits responsible for human behavior, and which differentiate people from one another, can be classified as cognitive, personality, emotional, and physical traits, as illustrated in Figure 8.1. It is important to remember, however, that traits overlap and interact with one another, forming the rich tapestry of individual differences making up diversity. Only when taken together are traits fully responsible for the complexities of motor skill behaviors observed among people.

You will notice from Figure 8.1, that everyone possesses the same traits. That is, traits are nomothetic—they are shared by all members of a population,

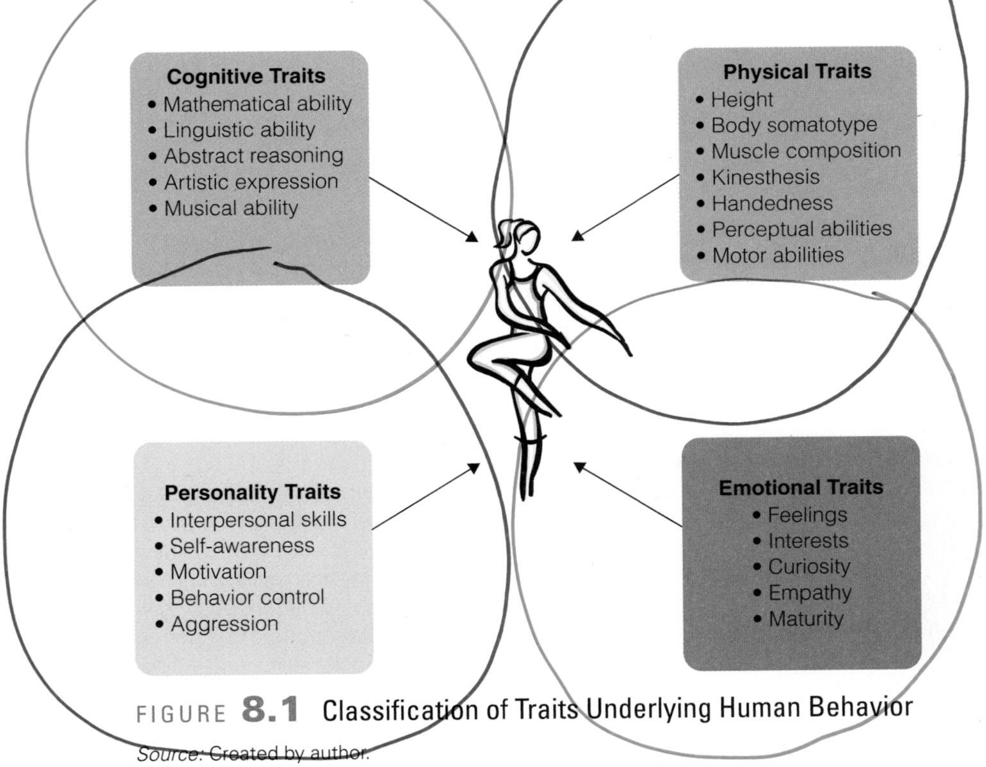

Cognitive Traits
• Mathematical ability
• Linguistic ability
• Abstract reasoning
• Artistic expression
• Musical ability

Physical Traits
• Height
• Body somatotype
• Muscle composition
• Kinesthesis
• Handedness
• Perceptual abilities
• Motor abilities

Personality Traits
• Interpersonal skills
• Self-awareness
• Motivation
• Behavior control
• Aggression

Emotional Traits
• Feelings
• Interests
• Curiosity
• Empathy
• Maturity

FIGURE **8.1** Classification of Traits Underlying Human Behavior

Source: Created by author.

in this case, by all humans. Everyone possesses every trait. But you probably also recognize that some people are better at (we might say "have more of") some of these traits than others. Some people who are good at mathematical reasoning, for example, possess poor language skills. Other people are proficient at language but lack musical skills. An important feature to note is that although everyone is able to improve their performance in each of these areas—become better at math or language or playing a musical instrument—they nevertheless have limits in each area. Some people will struggle with mathematical concepts and eventually become competent mathematicians, whereas others will achieve genius status as mathematicians with seemingly little effort. We often refer to people as *naturals* if they possess great amounts of some particular trait—a natural scientist, a natural musician, a natural artist, a natural writer, a natural athlete, and so on. (This is, of course, an old idea in philosophy and religion—i.e., that people have different capabilities or talents and that it is not their differences but how people use their differences that is important. See Box 8.2.)

This brings us to another important feature of traits: they are unipolar. That is, their value increases in one direction only. It is typical to specify the quality of (the amount of) any specific trait for an individual by noting the individual's **percentile rank** for the given trait as compared to the general population. Percentile rank is the position or relative strength of a trait within a given population. Percentage rank is typically specified for all people, although it can also be specified for people within specific groups (i.e., all adults living in North America, all females, all males living in North America of Asian heritage, all college athletes, etc.). For example, if an individual's percentile rank were 65

percentile rank: A ranking indicating a person's position relative to trait strength among the general population of people and being equal to the percentage of persons below him or her in strength of the trait.

BOX **8.2** **What Are Your Strongest Traits?**

The relative strength of an individual's various traits is genetically determined. The strength of any trait is also due to random genetic variation. Every person has traits that are strong, average, and weak relative to the general population. For the list of traits below, rank them from 1 though 7, with 1 being the trait for which you consider yourself the strongest, 2 the next strongest, and so on. Do not worry about your current skill levels, but rank these traits according to where you think your greatest potential lies given sufficient practice. After ranking the traits, ask yourself whether you believe that you are definitely stronger in some traits than in others or whether you believe you possess the same potential in all of them. What is your conclusion?

- Artistic expression (painting, drawing, sculpture, interior decorating, etc.)
- Language skills (writing, speaking, debating, verbal imitation, etc.)
- Logical reasoning (seeing the "big picture," reflective, rational, curious about "why" questions, enjoy thinking things through, etc.)
- Mathematical reasoning (good at numbers, can do mathematical calculations such as adding and dividing in your head, understand how mathematical formulas relate to real world situations, can remember numbers and equations, etc.)
- Musical skills (sing, play a musical instrument, remember the words to songs, sing to yourself when doing other things, etc.)
- Physical skills (good body awareness, coordination, enjoy games and sports, proficient at learning most new physical skills, etc.)
- Social skills (enjoy socializing, get along with people from many walks of life, are often the leader in groups, look forward to social events, etc.)

for a specific trait, that would mean that he or she was better at (or had more of) the trait than 65 percent of the general population (i.e., all other people). It would mean as well, though, that 35 percent of the population possessed greater amounts of the trait. Percentile rank is a measure of the strength of a particular trait when compared to all other people (or to a particular group so specified). Remember that traits are genetically determined and do not change (think of height or eye color, for example). An individual's percentage rank, or place in the general population, for a given trait is unaffected by experience (i.e., practice) and remains stable.

Though people differ in the relative strength of their traits, it is also important to note that within the entire population of people, traits exhibit a **normal distribution**. This means that most people will tend toward average (normal) strength for any given trait, with progressively fewer people exhibiting extremes in either comparative weakness or strength of traits. If we represent the percentage of persons possessing any trait graphically, the result will be a normal distribution in the form of a bell-shaped curve, with most people tending toward a central average value, and fewer and fewer persons exhibiting extreme scores in either direction. The relative strength of the trait within the population, however, will increase in one direction (be unipolar) as a function of percentile rank (see Figure 8.2).

As illustrated in Figure 8.2, the relative strength for any trait increases in one direction from weak to strong. People are not, however, equally distributed

normal distribution: The tendency for individuals within a population to cluster about the average value on any given measurement of trait strength, and for progressively fewer individuals to exhibit measurements of either high or low trait strength as distance increases from the norm.

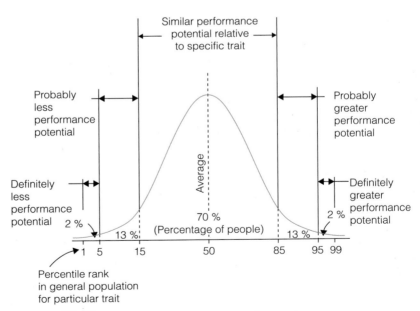

FIGURE **8.2** **Distribution and Relative Strength of Traits in the General Population**

Source: Created by author.

along the continuum from weak to strong. Most people cluster around average, with the number (percentage) of persons who are relatively weak or strong on a given trait decreasing progressively as extremes of either weakness or strength are approached. Most people, for example, tend toward average height. We would not expect to see the same numbers of either very tall or very short persons as of persons of normal or near normal height. In a sense, through random genetic processes, nature attempts to maintain equality and balance while avoiding extremes within the human population. The large majority of people will be average or relatively close to average for any particular trait, with a smaller percentage being either relatively strong or weak and only an exceptional few individuals at the extremes of strong or weak for a specific trait. As shown in Figure 8.2, approximately 70 percent of people cluster closely around an average or central value of strength measurement for a specific trait. These people would also be expected to perform more or less similarly on skills where the trait in question played a critical role in performance. Extreme percentile rank scores predisposing individuals to perform particularly well or poorly in skills critically relying on the specific trait are relatively few. For an illustration of how people are normally distributed on virtually every expression of human behavior, attempt the exercise shown in Box 8.3.

INDIVIDUAL DIFFERENCES AND MOTOR SKILLS

Individuals differ significantly in their capacity to perform and to learn motor skills. Some people seem good at almost every new motor skill they attempt; others experience difficulty when first attempting new physical skills. Most people appear average at the majority of skills. Still others are good at one or a few skills but frustratingly unskilled at others.

Why do people differ so widely in their capacities to perform motor skills? The answer to this question, at least in large part, entails a study of the underlying traits responsible for skilled motor performance. In the study of motor skills, the traits most essential to learning and performance are called *motor abilities*.

BOX **8.3** **Most Human Behaviors Are Normally Distributed**

Explain how each of the phenomena listed below are normally distributed. Think of specific values you might obtain if you observed many examples of each item, including an average value, the total range of values, and how the range of values would be clustered or dispersed about the average. Do the values you chose support the assumptions of a normal distribution?

- Intelligence as measured by IQ for all adults
- Average game score for recreational bowlers

- Hours per week spent doing homework by college students
- Average daily temperature during summer months in your hometown
- Average score on the Scholastic Aptitude Test (SAT) for all exam takers
- Time in the 100-yard dash for female college students
- Number of words typed per minute by all college students

Motor Abilities

Most people are already familiar with a few motor abilities, such as reaction time, manual dexterity, depth perception, and balance, for example. **Motor abilities** are defined as genetically determined traits that are stable and enduring and that underlie or support the performance of motor skills. There are four features of this definition that are important to note. First, motor abilities are genetically determined. Like hair color or sex or height, motor abilities are determined at conception. They are not developed or acquired after birth. A person is born with all of the motor abilities (and all of each of their abilities) that they will ever possess. Everyone is also born with the same motor abilities—people do not have different ones or a different number of abilities. People do, however, differ in the relative strength of their inherited motor abilities. Just as with intellectual traits, so also people possess motor abilities on a range from weak to average to strong relative to the population as a whole (i.e., they are normally distributed).

Second, motor abilities are stable and enduring. They do not change over the course of a person's lifetime, and they cannot be improved with practice (or lost from nonuse). Motor abilities may vary as a result of developmental factors, of course. An infant does not possess as fast a reaction time as an adult, for example, and most adults will experience some reduction in reaction time as they age beyond a certain point. But these changes represent developmental processes rather than underlying alterations to motor ability structures. This might be observed, for instance, if reaction time were measured for 100 young children who were then ranked from best to worst (1–100) on reaction time. Should reaction time again be measured at any point during the lifespan of these 100 individuals, their relative ranking would not change (assuming the absence of disease or injury). Those ranked in the top positions as children would remain in the top positions at whatever age they were comparatively ranked throughout their lifespan; those with average reaction time would likewise remain average compared to their peers at every age; and those exhibiting the slowest reaction times as children would always fall among the slowest at every age. In this case, as for all motor abilities, the underlying physical and neurological structures responsible for reaction time do not change over the course of the person's lifespan, even if developmental and aging processes have an effect on the overall expression of reaction time.

Third, motor abilities underlie or support the performance of motor skills. Motor abilities are considered the building blocks of motor skills. It is important to distinguish here between abilities and skills. Skills, as we saw in Chapter 2, are acquired—we are not born with them. We learn skills through practice, and they are directed toward the accomplishment of specific environmental goals. Motor abilities are the "basic equipment" that people are born with and from which they draw in order to learn and to perform skills. (See Table 8.1 for some of the distinctions between abilities and skills.)

Fourth, motor abilities are trans-situational. That is to say, a given motor ability may be manifested in a wide variety of skill situations. Any given motor ability may be an essential building block for a large number—and variety—of different skills. Motor abilities are not specific to any particular class or type of

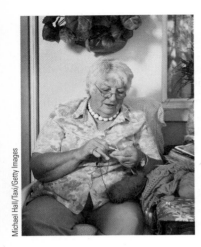 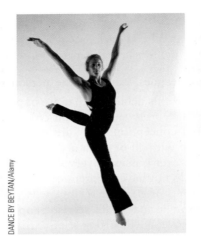 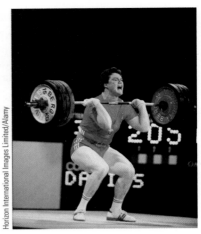

Different skills rely on different combinations of motor abilities for their performance.

motor skill, but the same motor ability may cross many classification lines in contributing to a large variety of actions. Conversely, a motor ability may also play little or no role in the performance of other motor skills.

Motor Abilities as a Limiting Factor for Skills

As just noted in the last sentence of the previous section, in the process of building up motor skills by drawing on the resources of one's underlying motor abilities, not all motor abilities are important, or at least as equally important, for all skills. Every skill is dependent upon a combination of some collection of specific motor abilities. Think about the contributions to various skilled performances of a motor ability like reaction time, for instance. It would obviously be

TABLE 8.1
Some Differences Between Motor Abilities and Motor Skills

Abilities	Skills
Stable, cannot be changed	Changeable, can be improved with practice
Inherited, genetically determined	Acquired through practice or experience
Relatively few (40–50?)	Many (1,000s)
People possess all abilities	People possess relatively few of the many skills available
Support the performance of skills	Depend on differing subsets of abilities
Not directly observable or manifested as behaviors	Observable and manifested as behaviors
Do not act directly on environment	Act directly on environment

important that a person have a good reaction time (be ranked relatively high among the general population) to be a successful fastball hitter in baseball. But is reaction time important for success in bowling? In this example, having a relatively fast reaction time would be important for a successful career in the major leagues, but even the person with a slow reaction time could have the potential for a career on the professional bowling circuit. As another example, manual dexterity—the ability to make quick and precise movements using the fingers and wrist—is important in carving a turkey on Thanksgiving or casting a line in fly-fishing but would be of no real benefit in performing a long jump (in fact, a handless person could still be a good long jumper). Contrarily, though, success in the long jump depends on explosive strength, which is hardly needed for fly fishing and could result in a badly butchered turkey.

The point here is that motor abilities are the requirements for performing skills, as well as the determinants for how well one can perform and learn particular skills, but not all motor abilities are important, or as equally important, to all skills. In fact, most motor skills probably depend on no more than a few motor abilities for their performance, with three to five motor abilities most likely accounting for most of the variance in skill observed between individual performers (Chaiken, Kyllonen, and Tirre, 2000; Fleishman, 1972). Depending on the particular cluster of motor abilities necessary for successful performance in any given skill, people will be predisposed to certain limits on their performance and ultimate learning of a skill based on the strength of their relevant motor abilities. Motor abilities inform a ceiling or limit on both the performance and learning of motor skills, with people manifesting differing limits based upon their individual pattern and relative strength of motor abilities.

As an example of the ceiling effect imposed by an individual's specific motor abilities profile, consider the limits in performance attainable in the skills of Olympic weight lifting and distance running based upon traits related to strength and endurance. At first, it may seem that strength and endurance are poor choices to be classified as traits because both can be considerably improved by practice. But consider that both traits are largely conditioned by the muscle composition of an individual. Muscle fibers are comprised of both fast-twitch (types II and III) and slow-twitch (type I) fiber types (see discussion in Chapter 3). Fast-twitch fibers are specialized to act quickly and exert maximal contractile force in the absence of oxygen—they are specialized for strength and explosive power (referred to as anaerobic work). Slow-twitch muscle fibers, on the other hand, are specialized for lesser force production but for sustained contraction over longer periods of time and work in the presence of oxygen (referred to as aerobic work). Most people have a fairly equal percentage of both fiber types as part of their inherited body makeup. Some individuals, however, possess significantly greater amounts of one fiber type than of the other—perhaps as much as 90 percent fast-twitch or slow-twitch fiber. This composition of muscle fiber type is an inherited trait that cannot be altered. An individual's muscle composition will act to either predispose or limit potential attainment in skills dependent on strength and endurance requirements. The individual with a high percentage of fast-twitch muscle fibers will have much greater potential in skills requiring strength like weight lifting than will the person with high quantities of slow-twitch muscle fibers. The inverse is also true; the individual with a significantly high composition of slow-twitch fibers will have greater potential in endurance activities like distance running than either the average person or the person with a high composition of fast-twitch muscle fiber. In this case, the motor traits related to strength and endurance are determined to a significant degree by inherited muscle composition patterns that cannot be altered through environmental experiences. These traits in turn establish limits on performance, and these limits are most greatly manifested as the extremes of performance are approached. In our example, everyone probably has the potential for meaningful performance in both weight lifting and distance running. However, only those with the most advantageous motor abilities relative to strength and endurance, as conditioned by inherited muscle composition patterns of fast and slow-twitch muscle fibers, will have the potential of attaining elite performance in these disparate motor skills.

Motor Abilities Establish Upper Limits on Skills

The debate over the relative effects of heredity and environment in explaining human behaviors is a long and still contentious one. Our argument here is not that environmental factors do not play a significant role in the acquisition of motor skills, but that genetic factors (i.e., motor abilities) establish the limits within which environmental factors are free to operate. Although little empirical research has addressed this contention directly, mounting evidence from twin studies has offered strong support for the primary role played by genetics in establishing upper limits on an individual's potential in given motor skills.

The Evidence from Twin Studies

Twin studies are an especially good method for studying the relative effects of genetic and environmental influences because both influences can be isolated within various research designs (Segal, 1999). This advantage of twin studies arises from the fact that twins may be one of two distinct types. Monozygotic, or identical, twins develop from a single fertilized egg and therefore share all of their genes (i.e., they are 100% genetically similar). Dizygotic, or fraternal, twins develop from two fertilized eggs and share, on average, 50 percent of their genes, or the same genetic similarity as found in non-twin siblings.

An especially powerful research approach to studying genetic and environmental influences is a design that identifies both fraternal and identical twins reared apart. Twins raised apart do not share a common environmental background influencing their behaviors. This allows for the influence of genetic factors to be isolated because identical twins share exactly the same genetics, which fraternal twins do not. Studies of twins raised apart have revealed a number of interesting patterns relative to physical activity levels and choices. Although specific motor ability levels have received little research attention as yet, behavioral preferences have been well established. These studies most typically are conducted through survey and case study methodologies. Generally, fraternal twins raised apart are somewhat more likely to exhibit similarities in activity levels and choices relative to motor skills than would be expected by chance. On the other hand, for identical twins raised apart studies show highly similar patterns in their activity choices, often including engaging in the same sports, playing the same positions, and attaining the same levels of skill proficiency (Ridley, 2003; Segal, 1999). The only factor explaining these marked patterns of similar activity choices and attained proficiency levels in identical twins is genetic determinism. Because behavior choices do, at least to some extent, reflect an individual's behavioral strengths more than weaknesses, an argument can be sustained that the similarity in genetic traits related to motor skill potential appears a likely candidate for explaining similarity patterns in motor skill selection among twins. Genetic predisposition to engage in and succeed at specific motor skills depends on an individual's underlying pattern of motor abilities.

In contrast to twin studies identifying interest and participation patterns, relatively few studies have investigated physical and motor traits among twin samples. A number of suggestive studies have been completed in recent years, however (Dowling, 2004; Segal, 1999). These studies involve actually bringing twins into laboratories and measuring various physical and motor traits. Although research in this area remains scant, some interesting conclusions are beginning to emerge (Segal, 1999, p. 213). A general finding is that twins show considerable similarities in some areas, but little similarity in others. Specifically, twin studies have reported that twin pairs are extremely similar in reaction time and in measures of agility and coordination, suggesting genetic influences on these measures. They are no more similar than would be expected of non-twins in the various physical measures of strength and endurance, however. (An interesting note is that similarities are observed in those traits classified as perceptual-motor abilities in Fleishman's Taxonomy, while those traits classified as physical proficiency abilities show little or no genetic link among twin pairs—see Table 8.2 for the distinction between these ability types.)

Results of twin studies suggest that a strong link exists between genetic influences and a person's choices and proficiency relative to sports and physical activity, and that some combination of genetically determined underlying motor traits plays an important role in personal choice and proficiency. Considerably more research is still needed to, however, fully disentangle the relative influences of genetic and environmental factors.

HOW MANY MOTOR ABILITIES ARE THERE?

Most theorists believe that about 40 to 50 motor abilities underlie all human motor skill behavior, though not all have been identified and there remains debate about the exact number (Boyle and Ackerman, 2004). In fact, some theorists, with Franklin Henry being the most prominent, have even proposed the existence of thousands of motor abilities! This latter number seems unlikely for several theoretical reasons, however, and the more conservative estimate of 40 to 50 seems much more likely and is accepted by broad consensus today. (Before reading further, you are encouraged to see how many different motor abilities you can think of and list; we have already mentioned some examples including reaction time and balance, as examples).

Of the 40 to 50 motor abilities believed to exist, not all have been identified (this figure is an estimate based on statistical modeling of how many

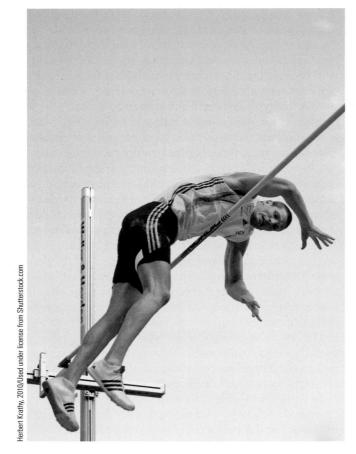

Herbert Krathy, 2010/Used under license from Shutterstock.com

Motor abilities may be conceived as establishing an upper limit to a person's potential in a specific skill, while factors such as practice, motivation, previous experience, and opportunity determine the degree to which that potential is achieved.

Fleishman's taxonomy of motor abilities: A widely used classification of motor abilities identifying 21 separate abilities.

abilities would be required to produce the various basic movement patterns observed in a wide variety of skills). The most complete system for identifying and classifying motor abilities is one developed in the mid-1960s by ergonomics engineer Edwin Fleishman (see Fleishman and Bartlett, 1969, for an overview of this research). **Fleishman's taxonomy of motor abilities** is based on a tremendous amount of research and resulted in the identification of 21 separate motor abilities (see Table 8.2).

In his classification system, Fleishman identified two broad categories of motor abilities (Fleishman, 1967; Fleishman, 1972; Fleishman and Quaintance, 1984). He labeled these categories *perceptual-motor* and *physical proficiency* abilities (Table 8.2). The first, perceptual-motor abilities, is comprised of motor abilities for which the central nervous system is the primary determinant of the ability's relative strength (percentile ranking in the general population). The second, physical proficiency motor abilities, depends upon, in addition to neurological factors, such underlying physiological factors as muscle composition (as we have already seen), the mechanical properties of muscle based on length and origin and insertion locations, the efficiency of sensory receptors associated with movement, and other physiological factors such as lung volume and body somatotype. The first category—perceptual-motor abilities—includes motor abilities such as reaction time, manual dexterity, and multilimb coordination that are fully realized through normal developmental processes. That is, one does not have to do anything to maximize perceptual-motor abilities such as reaction time. In this case, reaction time is realized to its full potential simply through normal interaction with one's environment (i.e., as part of the maturation process). Physical proficiency abilities such as static strength, extent flexibility, and stamina, on the other hand, require some degree of use and training to be fully realized. Static strength, for example, is not maximized without considerable training relative to muscular development. Still, as we have already observed, there is an upper limit to the amount of static strength people can possess relative to their unique muscle properties and biomechanical features.

[handwritten margin note: Perceptual motor abilities → normal development; physical proficiency abilities → use & training]

TABLE **8.2**
Fleishman's Taxonomy of Motor Abilities*

Perceptual-Motor Abilities

multilimb coordination—Ability to coordinate the movement of a number of limbs simultaneously. A high level of this ability is probably important when serving a tennis ball or playing the piano.

control precision—Ability to make highly controlled movement adjustments, particularly when large muscle groups are involved. An example is operating a bulldozer or other type of earth-moving equipment that requires careful positioning of the arms and feet.

response orientation—Ability to make quick choices among numerous alternative actions, often measured as choice reaction time. An example is the task of a goalie in hockey, where the type of shot on goal is often uncertain.

rate control—Ability to produce continuous anticipatory movement adjustments in response to changes in the speed of a continuously moving target or object. Examples include the tasks of high-speed auto racing and white-water canoeing.

manual dexterity—Ability to manipulate relatively large objects with the hands and arms. An example is package handling at the post office.

finger dexterity—Ability to manipulate small objects. Examples include threading a needle and eating spaghetti with a fork and spoon.

arm–hand steadiness—Ability to make precise arm and hand positioning movements where strength and speed are not required. A waiter who carries trays of food and dispenses the contents without incident has a high level of this ability.

(Continued)

TABLE **8.2** *(Continued)*

wrist–finger speed—Ability to rapidly move the wrist and fingers with little or no accuracy demands. An example is playing the bongo drums or keyboard entry tasks.

aiming—A highly restricted type of ability that requires the production of accurate hand movements to targets under speeded conditions. An example is the task of hitting a target with a rapid throw of a dart.

Physical Proficiency Abilities

---

explosive strength—Ability to expend a maximum of energy in one explosive act. Advantageous in activities requiring a person to project his or her body or some object as high or far as possible. Also important for mobilizing force against the ground. Examples of tasks requiring high levels of explosive strength include the shot putt, javelin, long jump, high jump, and 100 m dash in track and field.

static strength—Ability to exert force against a relatively heavy weight or some fairly immovable object. Tasks requiring high levels of static strength include near maximum leg and arm presses in weightlifting, as well as moving a piano.

dynamic strength—Ability to repeatedly or continuously move or support the weight of the body. Examples include climbing a rope and performing on the still rings in gymnastics.

trunk strength—Dynamic strength that is particular to the truck and abdominal muscles. Tasks requiring high levels of trunk strength include leg lifts and performing on the pommel horse in gymnastics.

extent flexibility—Ability to extend or stretch the body as far as possible in various directions. An example of a task requiring high levels of extent flexibility is yoga.

dynamic flexibility—Ability to make repeated, rapid movements requiring muscle flexibility. Ballet dancers and gymnasts need high levels of dynamic flexibility.

gross body equilibrium—Ability to maintain total body balance in the absence of vision. Circus performers who attempt to walk across a tightrope while blindfolded require high levels of this ability.

balance with visual cues—Ability to maintain total body balance when visual cues are available. This ability is important for gymnasts who perform on the balance beam.

speed of limb movement—Ability to move the arms or legs quickly, but without a reaction-time stimulus, to minimize movement time. Examples include throwing a fast pitch in baseball or cricket or rapidly moving the legs when tap dancing or clogging.

gross body coordination—Ability to perform a number of complex movements simultaneously. Individuals needing high levels of this ability include ice hockey players who must skate and stick-handle at the same time or circus performers who try to juggle duckpins while riding a unicycle across a tightrope.

stamina—Ability to exert the entire body for a prolonged period of time; a kind of cardiovascular endurance. Individuals requiring high levels of stamina include distance runners and cyclists.

---

*Adapted from Fleishman (1964) as reported by Schmidt and Wrisberg (2008).

Since Fleishman's original research in the 1960s, several additional motor abilities have been either identified or proposed. Magill (2007), for example, has pointed out that Fleishman's original analysis, though extensive, did not include a sufficient breadth of skills to reveal the important motor abilities of static balance, dynamic balance, visual acuity, visual tracking, and eye–hand or eye–foot coordination. Additionally, Scott Keele, a productive researcher in the area of motor learning, and his colleagues have identified four motor abilities related to the timing of movement skills as identified in Table 8.3 (see Keele and Hawkins, 1982; Keele, Ivry, and Pokorny, 1987; and Keele et al., 1985). These include movement rate (the ability to make a series of movements rapidly), motor timing (accuracy of timed movements), perceptual timing (ability to accurately judge the timing of movements), and force control (ability to make changes in force production during movements). An important finding of Keele's work is the discovery that each of the timing abilities appears to correlate highly within individuals (i.e., a person manifests the same general level of proficiency among all of the timing abilities). This suggests that there may be a general timekeeping ability that underlies the performance of a variety of timing skills.

Although Keele's observations are intriguing and bode the need of further research, Fleishman's system remains the accepted standard in the field and is widely used in developmental, industrial, ergonomic design, therapy, educational, and physical education settings. Importantly, though, neither Fleishman's nor Keele's models of motor ability were produced through research involving

TABLE **8.3**
Motor Abilities Identified by Keele and Colleagues*

movement rate—Similar to Fleishman's speed of limb movement, this ability applies more to situations in which a series of movements must be made at a maximum speed. Examples include typing or keyboarding.

motor timing—Ability to perform tasks in which accurately timed movements are essential. Examples include most open sport skills as well as driving an automobile in traffic, stepping on a moving escalator, and playing drums in a band.

perceptual timing—Ability to perform tasks in which accurate judgments about the time course of perceptual events are required. Examples include making judgments about the timing of a musical score by a ballet dancer or a vocalist, timing a partner's movements in pairs dancing or a horse's movements in equestrian competition, or estimating the speed of a moving object such as a ball in tennis, cricket, or soccer.

force control—Ability to perform tasks in which forces of varying degrees are needed to achieve the desired outcome. Examples include changing mood or emphasis when playing a musical instrument such as the piano or violin and performing sport tasks such as billiards, figure skating, and floor exercise in gymnastics.

*Reported by Keele et al. (1982, 1985, and 1987) as presented by Schmidt and Wrisberg (2008).

gross motor skills similar to those displayed in most sports. Until further research includes this important classification of skills, how long the final list of motor abilities will be remains elusive. The 40 to 50 figure remains a sound guess, but a guess nonetheless.

THE MYTH (?) OF THE "ALL-AROUND ATHLETE"

all-around athlete: Description of an individual who appears to excel at most motor activities he or she attempts.

Most people know somebody who seems to excel at every motor skill he or she attempts. Such people are often star athletes and typically excel in a variety of sports. The temptation is to say that such people are naturally born to succeed at all sports—that they are destined by birth to be "all-around athletes" (see Box 8.6 on p. 306). Saying that someone is born an all-around athlete is really saying that he or she is born to perform proficiently at any motor skill, whether a sports skill or any other kind of movement skill. Parenthetically, the opposite conclusion would also hold, that some people are born predisposed to poor performance in all sport and movement skills. If this assumption is correct, then there must be some sort of trait for general motor proficiency, and some people must be fortunate enough to be strongly endowed with it, whereas others are as equally unendowed.

The idea of a genetic trait predisposing some people to superior performance in any motor skill goes back to at least the 1880s, when scientists first begin to identify links between neurological factors and motor performance. This was the notion that a singular, global motor factor underlies all motor behavior. That is, a single factor (some sort of inherited neurological mechanism) was believed responsible for all of the separate motor abilities with which a person is endowed. If that single factor—typically referred to as a **global motor ability**—is superior relative to the general population, then all of the specific measures of separately identified motor abilities will also be superior. On the other hand, if the global motor ability is inferior or weak, then all individual motor abilities will likewise be inferior or weak. Extending this notion, most people are believed to have an average global ability, making them average at all individual motor abilities (as well as the skills built up from motor abilities).

global motor ability: The notion that a single global factor is responsible for the relative strength of all motor abilities.

This idea that motor abilities are generalized across the motor system is a compelling one, as it would appear to explain why some people are proficient

---

BOX 8.4 | **Can You Tell Which Motor Abilities Underlie the Performance of Specific Skills?**

For each of the following skills, see whether you can identify two or three motor abilities from those listed in Table 8.2 that underlie performance of the skill.

- Jumping rope
- Hammering a nail
- Driving a golf ball
- Performing a spike in volleyball
- Walking on crutches
- Standing from a chair
- Springboard diving
- Bouncing on a trampoline
- Typing

at so many motor skills (i.e., all-around athletes) and why a few others appear clumsy at most motor skills. It would also explain why most people seem average at most skills, because any such global ability would tend to be normally distributed in the population.

The idea that a global motor ability exists—a genetic endowment that a person is born with—is analogous to the notion of a single trait underlying all intellectual abilities. It is interesting that the concept of a generalized motor ability was developed at about the same time as the concept of a single intellectual ability (IQ) was developed. Because this notion is a rather old one, it has been thoroughly tested, and a conclusion concerning it is firmly established in the research literature to which we will turn next.

TWO COMPETING HYPOTHESES CONCERNING THE ALL-AROUND ATHLETE

generalized motor abilities hypothesis (GMA): The notion that motor abilities are positively correlated, and that a person's percentile rank in one motor ability is fairly similar to his or her comparative ranking in all other motor abilities.

specificity of motor abilities hypothesis (SMA): The notion that motor abilities are not significantly correlated and that a person's percentile rank in one motor ability does not predict his or her ranking for any other motor ability.

In explaining the phenomenon of the all-around athlete, perhaps someone like Babe Didrikson Zaharias (Box 8.6) or simply the individual good at many sports and physical activities, two hypotheses are tenable. The first is that people are good at many different skills because some singular underlying factor (i.e., global motor ability) is responsible for the strength of all individual motor abilities, and these people possess this factor at a high level relative to the general population. Remember that motor skills are comprised of subsets of various combinations of motor abilities. In this view, because the underlying general factor is strong, all individual motor abilities will also be strong. It then follows that any motor skill, regardless of the specific combination of motor abilities drawn upon in its production, will result in superior performance. This notion is referred to as the **generalized motor abilities hypothesis**, or the GMA hypothesis for short.

The alternative position to the GMA hypothesis is that no singular global motor ability exists but that motor abilities are independent of one another. This notion, referred to as the **specificity of motor abilities hypothesis**, or the SMA hypothesis, holds that motor abilities are randomly spread throughout the motor system and have no positional relationship to one another. That is, a person's relative strength (as measured by his or her percentile rank) on one motor ability has no influence or relationship to his or her strength on any

BOX **8.5**   **What Are Your Strongest Motor Abilities?**

Think of the movement skills at which you are the most highly proficient. What commonalities do you recognize among them? Can you identify any specific motor abilities common to these skills? Based upon your analysis, what other skills in which you do not currently engage do you think you might learn to perform well?

BOX **8.6**   Who Was the Greatest All-Around Athlete?

Babe Didrikson Zaharias, the daughter of immigrant parents from Norway, was born in Port Arthur, Texas, in 1911. She was exuberant about sports almost from the time she could walk, and over her athletic career became highly accomplished in many different sports—basketball, track, golf, baseball, tennis, swimming, diving, boxing, volleyball, handball, bowling, billiards, skating, and cycling. As a teenager, she wrote in a school paper that "My goal is to be the greatest athlete who ever lived." A survey of sports experts and writers conducted by the Associated Press resulted in her being named the "greatest female athlete of the twentieth century," and many would argue that she was simply the greatest athlete period.

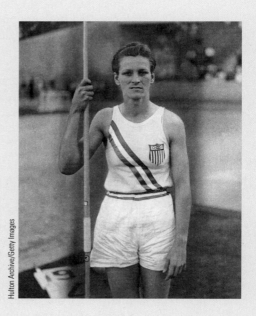

Hulton Archive/Getty Images

After starring in nearly every sport during her high school years, Babe was recruited by the Employers Casualty Insurance Company of Dallas to play on their athletic teams (the primary sports governing organization of the time was the Amateur Athletic Union, and company teams competed equally alongside college teams). In her first year of competition, Babe led the company women's basketball team to the national championship and was named All-American. The following year, she competed in track and field in preparation for the Olympics to be held in Los Angeles. She represented her company in the national track and field team championships as its only athlete. Competing in all 10 women's events, she placed first in 6 and second or third in each of the remaining events to win the overall team championship. In the 1932 Olympic Games that summer, she was limited to participation in only three events by the rules, but still won two gold medals and a silver (and would have won all gold if her final world-record high jump had not been discounted because she went over the bar head-first, which was not allowed at the time).

After the Olympics, Babe formed a traveling team in basketball and toured the country playing against the best competition of her day. She also competed professionally in pool and pitched in exhibition games against professional baseball teams (until her success in striking out professional players led to teams refusing to participate against her).

At the age of 25, Babe took up golf for the first time and quickly mastered the game. Denied status as an amateur, she competed successfully on the men's professional circuit because there was no professional golf association for women. Recognizing the need for a women's professional organization, Babe spearheaded the creation of the Women's Professional Golf Association (WPGA) and became the first female golf celebrity and the leading player of the 1940s and early 1950s.

In her personal life, Babe was married to George Zaharias, a star of the professional wrestling circuit of the time. She died in 1955 at the age of 45. Today, the Babe Didrikson Zaharias Trophy is awarded annually to the best female athlete in America. Clearly, Babe fit the description of an All-Around Athlete.

other motor ability—no global factor connects motor abilities. Box 8.7 summarizes the distinctions between the GMA and SMA hypotheses.

Research investigating the GMA and SMA hypotheses involves an analysis of the correlation among motor abilities. To grasp the research conclusions concerning these two hypotheses, we will first need to turn to a consideration of the statistical concept of correlational analysis. More than simply a mathematical tool, correlational analysis provides a strong intellectual basis for understanding the relationships among variables and for drawing meaningful explanatory conclusions about those relationships. In this case, correlational analysis provides both the means for testing the two alternative hypotheses possible, and the bases for constructing a deeper understanding of those factors influencing skilled motor performance.

Understanding the Language of Correlational Analysis

correlation: The degree of association between two things, or the percentage of component parts the two things have in common; the strength of a correlation is mathematically expressed as a number ranging from −1.00 to +1.00.

Correlation refers to the degree of association between two things. For instance, we would say that there is a high correlation between amount of time a student studies and his or her grades in school. Generally, the more hours of study, the better will be one's grades. Would there be a correlation between hair color and grades, though? In this case, the answer is obvious—hair color and grades do not correlate (referred to as a **zero correlation**). You could not predict by a person's hair color anything about what kind of grades he or she might earn.

zero correlation: A complete lack of association between two things, such that changes in the value of the first are not accompanied by any predictable changes in the value of the second.

More technically, correlation is the degree to which two things vary together. In the example of time devoted to studying and grades earned, we would recognize that there is a high correlation between the two, but not a perfect one. That is, there is certainly a tendency for students who study more to get the best grades and for grades to vary (go up or down) proportionally to the amount of time spent in study. But other things besides time preparing for an exam also influence grades—like intelligence, motivation, previous

---

BOX **8.7**	**Two Views Concerning the Relationship among Motor Abilities**

Generalized Motor Abilities Hypothesis	Specificity of Motor Abilities Hypothesis
• All individual motor are highly related to one another.	• All motor abilities are relatively independent.
• A singular global ability is responsible for determining the strength of each individual ability.	• The relative strength of a person's individual motor abilities varies unpredictably and can range widely.
• People are generally capable of performing all motor skills at similar levels of proficiency.	• People will typically possess different capabilities relative to the potential for proficiency in different motor skills.

knowledge, emotional state, and quality of teaching, for example. The best that we can say is that there is a tendency for study time and grades to go together, but that that tendency is not perfectly predictable.

Correlations are specified in numerical terms ranging from -1.00 to $+1.00$. A perfect **positive correlation** of $+1.00$ means that two things vary together exactly. As the value of one changes, so does the value of the other, and it changes in the same direction and to the same degree. We would say that there is a perfect positive correlation between the length of a person's foot and shoe size, for example. For every one-half inch a person's foot length increases, shoe size increases by one-half inch. An equal change in one thing (foot length) is matched every time by an equal change in the other thing (shoe size).

positive correlation: A correlation between two things such that increases in the value of the first are accompanied by increases in the value of the second.

Similarly, a perfect **negative correlation** (-1.00) means that two things vary equally, but in opposite directions. Consider the correlation between altitude and percent of atmospheric oxygen, for example. Every equal increase in altitude is matched by an equal decrease in oxygen. The higher up you go, the less oxygen there is, and the change in the amount of oxygen remains proportional to the change in altitude.

negative correlation: A correlation between two things such that increases in the value of the first are accompanied by decreases in the value of the second.

Most correlations are not perfect ones, of course, as with the example of study time and grades. Consider another example: Is there a correlation between body weight and strength? Most of us would recognize that larger people tend to be stronger than lighter people, but that you cannot always tell this with certainty. Some lighter people are stronger than those larger than them. Still, if you picked a hundred people at random (let's say all males to avoid the complication of sex-related strength differences), there would be a strong tendency—though not a perfect one—for the larger people to be the strongest. Hypothetically, suppose you further grouped these 100 people into the 50 largest and the 50 smallest; from which group do you suspect that most of the strongest people would be found? Obviously, you would expect significantly more of the stronger people in the larger group (though you still might find some in the smaller group who ranked among the strongest—as well as a few in the larger group who were among the weakest of the groups). In this case, we would say that there was a high positive correlation (strength goes up as body weight goes up), but not a perfect one. The strength of the correlation is measured as a number somewhere between 0.00 (no correlation) and 1.00 (a perfect correlation).

The actual degree of correlation (its strength) is computed by a statistic called the *Pearson product moment,* and is expressed by a correlation coefficient (labeled as the Greek letter ρ, pronounced "rho"). Without going into these statistical calculations, we can state that the strength of association (the correlation) between any two variables can be determined through research and a correlation coefficient calculated. These values can be expressed in words, as illustrated in Table 8.4. Remember that a correlation can be either positive or negative, depending on the direction in which two things vary together. Also, remember that a zero (0.00) correlation coefficient means that there is no relationship between two variables.

TABLE **8.4**
Strength of Correlation between Two Variables

Correlation Coefficient (rho)	Word Description of the Strength of Correlation
0.01–0.20 =	negligible relationship
0.21–0.40 =	low relationship
0.41–0.70 =	moderate relationship
0.71–0.90 =	marked relationship
0.91–0.99 =	very strong relationship
1.00 =	perfect relationship

Note 1: A minimum correlation coefficient allowing valid predictability is 0.85.

Note 2: For negative correlation coefficients, the same relationships exist but are inverse.

The Correlation among Motor Abilities: Testing the GMA and SMA Hypotheses

The search to confirm the GMA hypothesis was extensive in the 1950s and 1960s. Typically, researchers would test individuals on different types of motor ability tests or actual motor skills (often ones that were similar) and determine the correlation between the various pairs of abilities or skills. It soon became apparent, however, that even similar skills (or motor ability tests) typically exhibited low correlations between groups of subjects performing both skills (or motor ability tests). In fact, the correlation coefficients observed in the many research investigations completed typically ranged in the very low numbers (typically -0.20 to $+0.20$). Eventually, the inability to confirm the GMA hypothesis resulted in accepting its logical alternative: the SMA hypothesis. A classic example is a study conducted by Drowatzky and Zuccato in 1967. Using a large sample of Air Force recruits, they examined scores on six different balance tests, three static balance tests, and three dynamic balance tests. The assumption was that the same subset of motor abilities would underlie all three tests for static balance and that a closely similar subset of abilities would underlie performance for the dynamic balance tests. The researchers expected to discover how similar the two groupings of abilities were that were responsible for static and dynamic balance. Surprisingly, the correlations among all six tests were very low, with none of the performance scores within either the static or dynamic grouping of balance tests significantly correlated. As can been seen in Table 8.5, the correlations between balance tests varied from -0.12 and 0.31, which indicates a negligible to low relationship among pairs of balance tests. These results indicate that even for similar skills such as different tests of balance, different subsets of highly independent motor abilities are responsible for performance proficiency.

In fact, after literally hundreds of research studies, a correlation of +0.04 is generally accepted among researchers as the average correlation among motor abilities. A correlation coefficient of this value can be interpreted as meaning that any two motor abilities typically have less than 1 percent of their variance in common (this figure is arrived at by squaring 0.04 and multiplying by 100 to equal 0.16%). Another way of saying this is that whatever causes one motor ability to vary (change) accounts for less than 1 percent (i.e., 0.16%) of the variance (change) in another motor ability. This correlation coefficient is so small as to be negligible, and it certainly does not establish predictive power (i.e., you could not predict a person's strength in one motor ability from knowing his or her strength in any other motor ability).

As a result of these many research investigations into the correlation among skills and motor abilities, the validity of the SMA hypothesis has become one of the most strongly accepted concepts in the field of skill acquisition. This acceptance leads to several important conclusions about making predictions relative to skill level in one skill by making observations of another skill (even a similar one) as well as predicting future success in a skill by observing early performance when learning the skill.

TABLE **8.5**

Correlations Among Tests of Static and Dynamic Balance
Reported by Drowatzky and Zucato (1967)

Test	Static Balance Tests			Dynamic Balance Tests		
	Stock Stand	Diver's Stand	Stick Stand	Sideward Leap	Stepping Stone Test	Balance Beam Test
Stock Stand	—	0.14	−0.12	0.26	0.20	0.03
Diver's Stand		—	−0.12	−0.03	−0.07	−0.14
Stick Stand			—	−0.04	0.22	−0.19
Sideward Leap				—	0.31	0.19
Stepping Stone Test					—	0.18
Balance Beam Test						—

PREDICTING MOTOR PROFICIENCY BETWEEN SKILLS

If motor abilities are randomly distributed throughout the motor system and independent of one another as suggested by the SMA hypothesis, then this has important implications when predicting success in one skill from observations made of another skill. Most people, without knowing it, intuitively accept the GMA hypothesis, however.

We saw in Chapter 7 that early performance is not a reliable indicator of athletic potential. Remember that we highlighted this by recounting the story of how Michael Jordan, considered by most experts as the best basketball player of his day, was cut from his high school freshman team. Michael Jordan comes to our assistance again in making the point that skill in one motor activity, even if one is the best at that activity, is not a predictor of success in any other motor activity. The story in this instance begins when Jordan retired from the Chicago Bulls basketball team and signed to play professional baseball with the Chicago White Sox. The White Sox assigned him to their minor league team in Port Charlotte, Florida, to learn the game. There was a great deal said and written at the time about Jordan's potential as a baseball player. Most sports commentators, as well as most sports fans, believed that it was just a manner of time until Jordan became a good professional baseball player. After all, he possessed so many natural athletic gifts that he could certainly learn to transfer them to the game of baseball. Basketball and baseball had much in common—they both required good body coordination, quick movements, timing skills, team play, and general athletic ability. Without knowing it, such prognosticators had accepted the GMA hypothesis as correct. It seemed reasonable, to them, to predict that if someone was good at one skill, they would also be good at another skill, particularly one seemingly having many things in common.

What was the outcome of Jordan's foray into baseball? As one sports writer phrases it in the pages of *Sports Illustrated* magazine (Wulf, 1994):

> Granted, he looks good in a baseball uniform. Granted, he is the best basketball player who has ever lived. Granted, a few weeks of batting practice, an intrasquad game and two exhibitions against the Texas Rangers are not a lot to go on. But this much is clear: Michael Jordan has no more business patrolling right field in Comiskey Park than Minnie Minoso has bringing the ball upcourt for the Chicago Bulls.

With all of his abilities to play basketball, Jordan was unable to transfer these abilities successfully to the game of baseball. This was because the abilities allowing him to play basketball so well were not the same ones required to be a baseball player. There is, as we have seen, no general athletic ability (i.e., no global motor ability) that is transferable from one skill to another. Jordan was so good at basketball because (among other factors) he possessed strong motor abilities underlying the skill of basketball. As soon as he moved to baseball, however, he was required to harness a different set of motor abilities, and there was no relationship in the strength of these motor abilities compared to the ones underlying his basketball skills (a conclusion supported by acceptance of the SMA hypothesis).

In fact, as we first saw in the Drowatzky and Zuccato study mentioned earlier in this chapter, skills appear to be highly specific in relation to underlying motor abilities. Even skills that appear very similar and could be expected to rely on many of the same traits (e.g., basketball and baseball, tennis and racquetball, gymnastics and springboard diving) draw on substantially different clusters of motor abilities for their execution. This fact is illustrated in Figure 8.3, which shows the motor abilities supporting two different skills, A and B. As can be observed, skill A draws from a strong set of motor abilities. Skill B, however, even though it has something in common with skill A and relies equally on motor ability D, nevertheless draws from a substantially different set of motor abilities. In the case of the underlying motor abilities needed for skill B, D is strong, N is moderately strong, but U and W are weak. The result is that skill B will never be performed at the same high level as is possible with skill A. Other factors may contribute to the performance and learning of both skills, but the underlying building blocks of skill B limit the level of skill that can be attained (and this is regardless of practice or motivation). (This should not, however, be taken as meaning that the person who has weak motor abilities for a particular skill cannot obtain meaningful and satisfactory performance levels, only that he or she is limited in his or her ultimate level of performance. Michael Jordan could learn to be a good baseball player, just not a professional leaguer.)

The implications of the SMA hypothesis, parenthetically, correlate well with what is known about transfer between different skills (remember from Chapter 5 that transfer refers to the degree to which experience in one skill "transfers" to a different skill; i.e., learning one skill improves performance in another skill). There is an extensive literature concerning transfer, and it has generally been found that transfer between any two complex skills (even those appearing similar) is weak.

A good example of weak transfer between similar skills is a study on the relation of perceptual abilities to performance in basketball conducted by Beats and his associates (Beats et al., 1971). These researchers obtained the field goal and free-throw shooting averages for an entire season of one college basketball

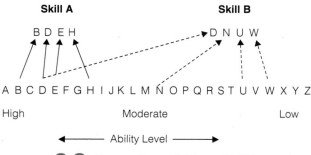

FIGURE **8.3** Comparison of Motor Abilities Underlying Two Different Skills

Source: Created by the author.

team. They then measured each player on four visual abilities; these were static visual acuity (the perception of fixed objects), dynamic visual acuity (the perception of moving objects), size consistency (the perception of objects of different size), and depth perception. Correlational analysis revealed that dynamic visual acuity was the only visual trait contributing significantly to field-goal shooting performance and that static visual acuity was the only visual trait related to free-throw accuracy. These results suggested that even within a single sensory modality (vision), differing abilities are required for the performance of even similar skills (e.g., field-goal and free-throw shooting). Research support for the SMA hypothesis strongly supports the conclusion that predicting level of success in one motor skill by observing success achieved in a second motor skill (even one very similar) is unreliable.

THE MYTH OF THE "ALL-AROUND ATHLETE" RECONSIDERED

motor educability:
The concept that a single factor underlies all motor skills and that an individual possesses the same performance potential in all skills.

Earlier in this chapter, we discussed the myth of the all-around athlete, that is, the person who seems to be naturally good at all (or at least many) motor skills. A tendency concerning such individuals, as we stated, is to assume that they possess some genetic factor supporting performance in a wide variety of (even all) motor skills (i.e., a "global motor ability" as proposed by the GMA hypothesis). This notion actually has a long history in the scientific study of skill. A concept called **motor educability**, first proposed in the 1920s, argues that a single factor is responsible for all motor abilities and that individuals can be determined to possess some general ability (ranging from weak to strong) underlying their capacity to learn any motor skill. As already stated, this concept of a single factor underlying motor performance is similar to the notion of IQ as a single factor responsible for all intellectual abilities. As should be clear to the reader of this chapter by now, however, no such single factor exists. That is, motor educability is a myth, although one that is still heard in many circles.

If motor educability is a myth, what are we to make of the all-around athlete? Does such a person exist? At one level, the answer is obvious: Yes, all-around athletes do exist. There are individuals who are good at a wide variety of motor skills, as is apparent to anyone who has spent much time involved in sports. The more important question, however, concerns why these relative few individuals (e.g., Babe Didrikson Zaharias) are good at so many motor skills.

There are two possibilities in answering this question. The first is that there is some genetic factor predisposing individuals to be good at all motor skills, and some people are lucky enough to be born possessing it. We might say that they have a high motor educability quotient. As we have seen based upon extensive correlational research studies, however, this is not the case. The GMA hypothesis, which expresses this notion in a scientifically testable way, has not been supported. (Indeed, tests of motor educability have proven particularly unsuccessful, also—even though they are still used in many schools today!)

If the alternative SMA hypothesis is true, then how are all-around athletes explained? The answer is so obvious as to be elusive; they are lucky! As a thought experiment, suppose that you had 100 people randomly draw playing cards. Would you expect everyone to draw a good card hand? Obviously not, but you might reasonably expect one or two individuals would be lucky enough to do so. In an analogous fashion, some people are lucky at the genetic draw of motor abilities, just as some people are lucky at the drawing of playing cards in our example. The odds are, though, that most people will be average—they will get a few good cards and a few bad ones, just as people get a few strong motor abilities and a few weak motor abilities, with most tending somewhere toward average. So people who are all-around athletes have been lucky at the genetic draw of motor abilities—nature did not specifically design them to be all-around athletes, but random genetic factors worked to their advantage.

This last point is important. Nature (i.e., the biology of genetics in this case) produces variety, but always tends toward the average. There is no known genetic mechanism designed to differentiate people into categories of low and high on any biologically determined characteristic. Human differentiation—individual differences—results from the processes of random distribution of genetic factors. This accounts for an important observation in human differentiation called **regression toward the mean.** What this means is that biologically determined characteristics—like height, intelligence, and motor abilities—tend toward intergenerational regression toward an average level. Tall parents may produce tall children but, on average, their children will be shorter than they are and "regress" back toward the average height of the entire population. Likewise, shorter parents are, on average, more likely to have children taller than are they. If nature did not function in this fashion, then given the way in which people select mates, after a few generations there would probably be only two classes of people—tall, smart, athletic people; and short, dull, clumsy people.

regression toward the mean: The intergenerational tendency for individuals, regardless of their parents' trait characteristics, to move toward the 50th percentile rank on specific motor abilities.

What about Motor Skill Similarities within Families?

If it is chance rather than biology that is responsible for the all-around athlete, how do we explain the fact that all-around athletes often appear to run in families? At the start of this chapter (Chapter Overview), we presented the example of the Manning family in professional football. Recall that Peyton Manning is the all-star quarterback of the Indianapolis Colts, while his younger brother Eli stars at quarterback for the New York Giants. Their father, Archie Manning, was an outstanding professional quarterback for the New Orleans Saints. Surely this family has great quarterback genes—something making them good at all the requisite skills needed to successfully play quarterback. There is too much coincidence to be explained by genetic luck.

Everything that research has revealed about motor abilities, including the acceptance of the SMA hypothesis, argues against this conclusion, however. So, how do we explain the Manning family? The answer is found in a psychological fallacy that we can call, for our purposes, the **fallacy of observed correlation.** This fallacy refers to people's psychological tendency to draw conclusions based upon what they see rather than what they do not see. A more technical way of expressing this idea is that epistemologically humans are disposed to infer facts based upon the presentation of sensory data, and when relevant data are missing, it is disregarded in decision making.

fallacy of observed correlation: The tendency to draw conclusions based only upon relationships that can be readily observed.

As an illustration, consider Figure 8.4. If asked "Are A and B related?" our immediate response would be "yes," because the only thing that we have to infer from is that A and B are correlated in the only instance we can observe. But what we do not consider in arriving at a conclusion are all the instances that we do not see where there is no correlation between A and B, as all the other pairings (the "unseen" ones in the figure) demonstrate. So rather than saying that A and B go together 1 out of every 100 pairings, our tendency is to infer a perfect correlation (because all we see is A and B together) and say that every time we see A, we also see B, and that there must therefore be a connection between the two. Had we considered all the pairings we did not see but which existed nonetheless, we would probably be inclined to say that a 1 in 100 correlation was most likely due to random chance, and that A and B really are not significantly related.

The same kind of reasoning holds true in our example of the Manning family. For every professional quarterback who has a son playing in the big leagues, there are many more former quarterbacks whose sons are not professional quarterbacks (and maybe not even childhood league quarterbacks). Yet we draw inferences and come to conclusions based upon the single datum that we have before us, disregarding the many more data that are not obviously presented for our consideration. In this case, we allow an exceptional case resulting from purely random factors (the Manning family) to generalize to a much larger population, even when the evidence, if considered, would invalidate such a conclusion. A better conclusion is that both of Archie Manning's sons benefited from random genetic factors that predisposed them to gain maximally from advantageous environmental factors related to the family into which they were born. (Although we have considered only one family in our example,

AB (A and B appear strongly correlated)

Seen
- -
Not seen

AD	AR	AT	AW	AV	AH	AO	AJ	AK	AZ	AM	AN
AS	AP	AR	AH	AT	AU	AV	AW	AX	AY	AM	AP
AD	AZ	AA	AH	AJ	AX	AT	AO	AK	AM	AK	AR
AK	AT	AJ	AN	AC	AR	AY	AV	AS	AD	AX	AW
AN	AZ	AM	AH	AT	AR	AD	AC	AJ	AK	AU	AP
AK	AQ	AC	AD	AV	AO	AJ	AM	AP	AT	AS	AY
AR	AD	AT	AW	AV	AH	AO	AJ	AK	AZ	AM	AN
AP	AS	AR	AH	AT	AU	AV	AW	AX	AY	AM	AP

(A and B are not significantly correlated)

FIGURE **8.4** "What is the correlation between A and B?"

Source: Created by author.

conclusions are most typically drawn by pointing to many such examples of athletic families. What must be recognized, though, is that these still represent a relatively small number of the total families that would need to be considered in sustaining such a conclusion of familial genetic superiority relative to motor abilities and athletic performance).

SOME OTHER FACTORS CONTRIBUTING TO MOTOR SKILL ACHIEVEMENT

In the example of the Manning family discussed above, we alluded to the fact that advantageous environmental factors in addition to genetic endowment most likely also influenced the two sons' skill levels. It should indeed be noted that many other factors besides underlying motor abilities contribute to performance potential and individual differences in motor skill learning.

In the case of the Manning family, one would suspect that parental encouragement and instruction played a significant role in developing the quarterbacking skills displayed by Archie's two sons. Psychological factors like the interest and motivation manifested in sons of a famous athlete could also play a significant role, as might social and emotional factors transmitted through family dynamics. What is important to recognize, however, is that without the underlying motor abilities, these other factors would not in and of themselves be sufficient to produce such high degrees of skill. When the required motor abilities are present at a sufficient level of strength, though, other factors come into play and are important in promoting athletic success. That is, the underlying motor abilities remain the fundamental building blocks of skill, and without sufficient strength in the subset of motor abilities underlying a particular skill, individuals will not be able to learn or perform past a certain level. Given the requisite strength of essential motor abilities, however, a wide variety of other factors can interact with the supporting abilities to produce a champion athlete (or, perhaps, a star musician or chess master). Motor abilities establish a ceiling of performance potential, but many other factors influence how closely a person will come to reaching it. A summary of some of the other factors important in explaining the individual differences observed among people in relation to motor skill learning and performance is presented in Table 8.6.

Given the large number of factors that influence motor performance and learning, it may be tempting to think of motor abilities as only one part of the equation specifying why people differ in such pronounced ways in the acquisition and execution of skills. Other factors, such as those identified in Table 8.6, surely play an important role also. Although this is certainly true, we must state again as cogently as possible that underlying patterns of motor abilities are the single most essential factor in explaining individual differences among people in terms of their performance and learning of motor skills. As we have previously observed, motor abilities are the basic building blocks of skills, establishing an asymptotic upper limit to performance that other factors—regardless of their influence—cannot bridge.

TABLE **8.6**

Factors That Can Contribute to Differences in Movement Skill Proficiency

Factor	Example
Abilities	Reaction time, finger dexterity, stamina
Attitudes	Open, closed, or neutral to new experiences
Body type	Stocky, tall, lean, muscular, round
Cultural background	Ethnicity, race, religion, socioeconomic status
Emotional makeup	Boredom, excitement, fear, joy
Fitness level	Low, moderate, high
Learning style	Visual, verbal, kinesthetic
Maturational level	Immature, intermediate, mature
Motivational level	Low, moderate, high
Previous social experience	One-on-one, small group, large group
Prior movement experience	Recreational, instructional, competitive
Social reference group	Nonathletic, moderately athletic, athletic
Parental encouragement	Low, moderate, high
Parental instruction	None, moderate, extensive

The Challenge Raised by the Study of Expertise

In the last chapter, we presented the concept of motor expertise. Recall that advocates of this approach suggest that a minimum of 10 years (or 10,000 hours) of deliberate practice is required to obtain the expert level of performance. In recent years, a number of proponents of this approach have challenged the underlying assumptions concerning the deterministic qualities of inherited factors in the learning and ultimate levels of one's performance potential in a motor skill. Ericsson, in particular, has argued that the extensive levels of practice required to obtain expertise can reshape the underlying structures of individual motor abilities (see Ericsson, Krampe, and Tesch-Romer, 1993). Although Ericsson's critique has elicited new lines of debate concerning the relative contributions of nature and nurture in the area of motor skill development, it has also been open to considerable criticism. Singer and Janelle (1999), for instance, have pointed out that it would be mistaken to ignore genetic factors, because cognitive abilities play a strong role in development of motor expertise, and such abilities are firmly held to be genetically determined. Sternberg (1996, 1998), perhaps the biggest critic of the expertise approach, notes that the tendency to practice may itself be an inherited trait. Most damaging to the expertise critique, though, is the observation that the correlation between motor expertise and the underlying motor abilities deemed most critical to the performance of a particular skill increase, rather than decrease, over prolonged periods of practice (Ward, Williams, and Starkes, 2004). That is, those individuals initiating practice of a particular skill are more likely to possess the requisite motor abilities for the skill, and more likely to continue practicing and developing expert levels of achievement than are those whose underlying abilities are not as strong initially. This would suggest that the initial strength of one's requisite subset of abilities is critical to obtaining expertise in a particular motor skill (the conclusion could also be drawn that those who do not perform as well as practice progresses are more likely to disengage from further practice).

Any final conclusion regarding the role of deliberate practice in mediating the influences of genetic factors awaits further research (in itself problematic because subjects willing to practice skills deliberately for 10 years in controlled experiments are difficult to locate). A more practical conclusion can currently be arrived at, however. Few people will ever engage in the amounts of intense practice required to reach, or even closely approach, expert levels of performance in a motor skill. For the vast majority of individuals learning sport, recreational, occupational, or rehabilitative skills, the influence of genetic factors continues to shape patterns of achievement, which effective practice experiences can then optimize.

EVERYONE IS GOOD AT SOMETHING!

It might be tempting to conclude that because some individuals are lucky at the genetic draw of motor abilities, then some people are also unlucky and destined—not by nature but by chance—to be poor at every motor skill. The truth concerning this observation is not so simplistic, however. People who appear good at everything are really only good at many things—at least the things they attempt (and they are probably not interested in attempting skills in which they would not prove successful). The opposite is also true—nobody is poor at every motor skill. In fact, given the number of motor abilities and all the possible combinations available to support various skills, it is nearly impossible (mathematically) for any person not to possess the requisite strength in subsets of motor abilities informing the potential for highly skilled performance at a number of different motor skills and sports activities. That is, assuming 40 to 50 motor abilities to exist—and there may be more—and clusters of no more than 3 to 5 of these abilities as deterministic of performance in any given skill, there are so many possible combinations of 3 to 5 motor ability subsets that it is statistically unlikely for there not to be at least a few motor skills in which every individual has the potential to excel.

We must look to other factors—things such as poor motivation, lack of encouragement, poor instruction—to account for the reasons some people perform poorly at the motor skills they do attempt. Everyone, unless profoundly physically or neurologically impaired, possesses the "basic equipment" to be good at a number of different motor skills. Indeed, it is probably not an exaggeration to suggest that every individual is a potential champion at some sports activity. This should motivate those responsible for the teaching of motor skills to people (and perhaps especially to children) to steadfastly encourage every learner until they find an enjoyable skill at which they might succeed. This is one reason that children should be exposed to a broad range of movement activities and sports skills during their school years. Such exposure can help them discover those activities that they enjoy and at which they can excel. It can also provide movement skill professionals opportunities for observing and identifying dominant patterns of motor abilities in children and then encouraging activity in the direction of skills most dependent upon those motor abilities in which a child is most likely to succeed.

SUMMARY

- Individuals differ across the entire spectrum of human behaviors, with both hereditary and environmental factors contributing to these differences.
- Although both genetic and environmental factors contribute to differences in motor skill proficiency among individuals, genetic factors establish upper boundaries to the performance of motor skills.
- Motor abilities are genetically determined traits underlying all skilled motor actions; they are the building blocks of motor skills.
  - Approximately, 40 to 50 motor abilities are believed to exist and underlie all human motor skill behavior.
  - Most skills depend on no more than a few (three to five) motor abilities.
- Based upon random differentiation, some individuals will possess more, perhaps many more, relatively strong motor abilities compared to others in the general population, increasing the probability that they will be advantaged in learning and performing a significantly larger number and variety of motor skills. Such individuals are frequently credited as being "all-around athletes."
  - Those individuals designated as being "all-around athletes" have been lucky at the "genetic draw" of motor abilities; there is no mechanism or global genetic factor through which nature predisposes some individuals to be superior to others in motor skill learning or performance.
- Because the motor abilities underlying skills change quickly from skill to skill, drawing conclusions about a person's potential in one skill from observations of his or her capabilities in another skill is misleading.
- Given the diversity of motor abilities and motor skills, the probability is extremely high that every individual possesses the potential to become highly proficient in a number of different motor skill activities.

LEARNING EXERCISES

1. Identify someone who reasonably could be considered an all-around athlete (he or she might be a family member, classmate, acquaintance or friend, or a person recommended by someone you know). Interview the person and obtain answers to the following questions: At what five sports or recreational activities are you the best? What sports or other movement skills have you experienced the greatest difficulty in learning? Do sports skills often seem to come naturally to you, or do they take a lot of practice before you feel comfortable performing them? Based upon answers to these questions (and any others you might think warranted), prepare an analysis and discussion of the person's specific strengths (and perhaps weaknesses) relative to the motor abilities underlying sports skills, as well as the role "natural" as compared to practice "experiences" play in influencing his or her skill development. Draw a conclusion as to whether the person is indeed an all-around athlete, and support your position based upon the information presented in this chapter and the data you collected from your interview.

2. Prepare a simple questionnaire asking people to rate their general interest in participating in sports activities as well as the extent of their participation (i.e., occasional informal participation, belonging to school teams, etc.). Ask subjects to provide the same information concerning any siblings they have. Your questionnaire need not be extensive and should take only a minute or less to complete. Include at least 20 subjects in your survey (your instructor may decide to make this a class project and have all class members complete the same questionnaire). Based upon the results of your survey, discuss the likelihood of sports interests and capabilities running in families, including the relative roles played by genetics and experience.

3. For a sport or other movement skill of interest to you, perform an analysis of the factors most essential to success in the skill.

FOR FURTHER STUDY

HOW MUCH DO YOU KNOW?

For each of the following, select the letter that best answers the question.

1. Traits
   a. can be improved with practice.
   b. include only physical capacities.
   c. vary in number from one person to another.
   d. are genetically inherited.

2. Although not all motor abilities have been identified, the number believed to exist by most experts is
   a. between 20 and 30.
   b. between 40 and 50.
   c. between 100 and 200.
   d. in the thousands.

3. Any person's potential for performance success in a particular motor skill is
   a. a combination of genetics and experience.
   b. determined entirely by inherited factors.
   c. determined entirely by experience.
   d. directed by inherited interests but determined by experience.

4. Compared to fraternal twins raised apart, identical twins raised apart are _____

to have similar patterns of interest and performance in sports and physical activities.
   a. less likely
   b. more likely
   c. no more or less likely
   d. The evidence is unclear and still debated.
5. Keele and colleagues have identified several highly correlated motor abilities, leading them to suggest the existence of a general _____ ability.
   a. balancing
   b. force production
   c. timing
   d. locomotive
6. The best conclusion regarding all-around athletes is that they
   a. are genetically predetermined to excel at all motor skills.
   b. possess a strong global motor ability.
   c. have benefited from richer environmental experiences than others.
   d. are lucky at the genetic draw.

Answer the following with the word or words that best complete each sentence.

7. How many motor abilities are identified within Fleishman's taxonomy?
8. What is the correlation coefficient for a perfect positive correlation?
9. Parents who are exceptionally tall are most likely to have children who are shorter than they are, just as parents who are significantly shorter than normal are most likely to have children taller than they are. This phenomenon is called_____.
10. The testable hypothesis that motor abilities are independent and not related in strength by any global factor is called the _____ hypothesis.
11. The ability to make quick choices from among many alternative movement possibilities is called _____ (i.e., name the motor ability).
12. The pattern of motor abilities in the general population can be represented by a curve known as a _____ distribution.

STUDY QUESTIONS

1. How are motor abilities defined and in what ways do they differ from motor skills?
2. Explain what is meant by referring to motor abilities as the "building blocks" of skills.
3. How many motor abilities are there? Describe the two categories of abilities in Fleishman's taxonomy and the four related abilities identified by Keele and colleagues.
4. Which is most critical in establishing a person's performance potential within a particular motor skill, inherited motor abilities or experience?
5. Explain how motor abilities establish an upper limit or ceiling to skilled performance.
6. How does the study of twins help us understand the relative influences of genetics and experience in people's interests and performance of motor skills?
7. Define the GMA and SMA hypotheses and explain how they are evaluated. Which has been supported by research evidence?

8. Explain whether an individual's performance in one skill or sport is a reliable predictor of his or her potential in another skill or sport, especially if the two activities are similar in some way.
9. Why are some people much better than average at many different motor skills (i.e., all-around athletes)?
10. Does athleticism run in families? If so, is there a genetic explanation for it?
11. Based upon an analysis of the distribution of motor abilities within the general population, defend the position that "Everyone has the potential to excel in the performance of a motor skill."
12. Based upon a consideration of motor abilities, why is it important that children and adolescents be exposed to a broad educational program of movement activities?

ADDITIONAL READING

Ackerman, PL. (1992). "Predicting individual differences in complex skill acquisition: Dynamics of ability determinants." *Journal of Applied Psychology, 77,* 598–614.

Campbell, LS and Catano, VM. (2004). Using measures of specific abilities to predict training performance in Canadian forces operator occupations. *Military Psychology, 16,* 183-2-1.

Fleishman, EA, and Reilly, ME. (1992). *Handbook of human abilities: Definitions, measurements, and task requirements.* Potomac, MD: Management Research Institute.

Johnson, PJ. (2002). "Psychomotor abilities tests as predictors of training performance."

Canadian Journal of Behavioral Science, 34, 75–83.

Klawans, H. (1996). *Why Michael couldn't hit: And other tales of the neurology of sports.* New York: W. H. Freeman.

Segal, NL. (1999). Entwined lives: Twins and what they tell us about human behavior (Chapter 11— Two Base Hits and Triple Toe Loops: Physical Growth and Athletic Prowess (pp. 208–229). New York: Plume Publishers.

Vescovi, JD and McGuigan, MR. (2008). Relationship between sprinting, agility, and jump ability in female athletes. *Journal of Sport Science, 25,* 97–107.

REFERENCES

Ackerman, PL. (1992). "Predicting individual differences in complex skill acquisition: Dynamics of ability determinants." *Journal of Applied Psychology, 77,* 598–614.

Beats, RP, Mavyasi, AM, Templeton, AE, and Johnston, WI. (1971). "The relationship between basketball-shooting performance and certain visual attributes." *American Journal of Optometry, 48,* 585–590.

Boyle, MO, and Ackerman, PL. (2004). "Individual differences in skill acquisition," In AM Williams and NJ Hodges (eds.), *Skill acquisition in sport: Research, theory, and practice.* London: Routledge.

Buss, AR, and Poley, W. (1976). *Individual differences: Traits and factors.* New York: Gardner Press.

Chaiken, SR, Kyllonen, PC, and Tirre, WC. (2000). "Organization and components of psychomotor abilities." *Cognitive Psychology, 40,* 198–226.

Cooper, C. (1999). *Intelligence and abilities.* London: Routledge.

Dowling, JE. (2004). *The great brain debate: Nature or nurture?* Washington, DC: Joseph Henry Press.

Drowatzky, JN, and Zuccato, FC. (1967). Inter-relationships between selected measures of static and dynamic balance. *Research Quarterly, 38,* 509–510.

Ericsson, KA, Krampe, RT, and Tesch-Romer, C. (1993). "The role of deliberate practice in the acquisition of expert performance." *Psychological Review, 100,* 363–406.

Fleishman, EA. (1967). Performance assessment based on an empirically derived task taxonomy. *Human Factors, 9,* 349–366.

Fleishman, EA. (1972). "On the relationship between abilities, learning, and human performance." *American Psychologist, 27,* 1017–1032.

Fleishman, EA, and Bartlett, CJ. (1969). "Human abilities." *Annual Review of Psychology, 20,* 349–380.

Fleishman, EA, and Quaintance, MD. (1984). *Taxonomies of human performance.* Orlando, FL: Academic Press.

Fleishman, EA, and Reilly, ME. (1992). *Handbook of human abilities: Definitions, measurements, and task requirements.* Potomac, MD: Management Research Institute.

Johnson, PJ. (2002). "Psychomotor abilities tests as predictors of training performance." *Canadian Journal of Behavioral Science, 34,* 75–83.

Keele, SW, and Hawkins, HI. (1982). "Explorations of individual differences relevant to high level skill." *Journal of Motor Behavior, 14,* 3–23.

Keele, SW, Ivry RI, and Pokomy, RA. (1987). Force control and its relation to timing. *Journal of Motor Behavior, 19,* 96–114.

Keele, SW, Pokomy, RA, Corcos, DM, and Ivry, RI. (1985). "Do perception and motor production share common timing mechanisms: A correlational analysis." *Acta Psychologica, 60,* 173–191.

Klawans, H. (1996). *Why Michael couldn't hit: And other tales of the neurology of sports.* New York: W. H. Freeman.

Minton, HL, and Schneider, FW. (1980). *Differential psychology,* Monterey, CA: Brooks/Cole.

Ridley, M. (2003). *Nature via nurture: Genes, experience, and what makes us human.* New York: Harper Collins.

Segal, NL. (1999). *Entwined lives: Twins and what they tell us about human behavior.* New York: Plume.

Singer, RN, and Janelle, CM. (1999), "Determining sport expertise: From genes to supremes." *International Journal of Sport Psychology, 30,* 117–150.

Sternberg, RJ. (1996). "Costs of expertise." In KA Ericsson (ed.), *The road to excellence: The acquisition of expert performance in the arts and sciences, sports, and games* (pp. 347–354). New York: Lawrence Erlbaum.

Sternberg, RJ. (1998). "If the key's not there, the light won't help." *Behavioral and Brain Science, 21,* 425–426.

Thorndike, EL. (1908). "The effect of practice in the case of a purely intellectual function." *American Journal of Psychology, 19,* 174–184.

Ward, P, Hodges, NJ, Williams, AM, and Starkes, JL. (2004). "Deliberate practice and expert performance: Defining the path to excellence." In AM Williams and NJ Hodges (eds.), *Skill acquisition in sport: Research, theory and practice.* New York: Routledge.

Wright, L. (1997). *Twins: And what they tell us about who we are.* New York: John Wiley and Sons.

Wulf, S. (1994). "Try as he might, Michael Jordan has found baseball beyond his grasp." *Sports Illustrated,* March 14.

Answers to How Much Do You Know questions: (1) D, (2) B, (3) A, (4) B, (5) C, (6) D, (7) 21, (8) 1.00, (9) regression toward the mean, (10) specificity of motor abilities, (11) response orientation, (12) normal.

CHAPTER 9

Preparing Learners for Practice: Motivation and Attention

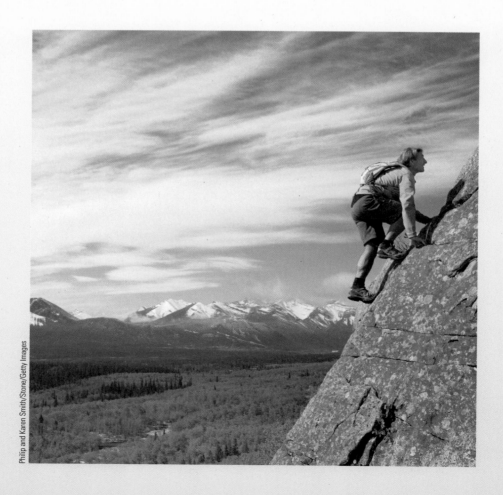

Philip and Karen Smith/Stone/Getty Images

To be prepared is half the victory.
Miguel de Cervantes (1547–1616)

KEY QUESTIONS

- How is motivation defined? How important is motivation to the learning of motor skills?

- What factors influence motivation?

- Why is setting goals important to learning?

- How should goals be set? What different types of goals should be established for practice?

- How is attention conceptualized? On what should learners concentrate during the performance of motor skills?

- How can attention be improved and directed most effectively?

- How does a performer's visual gaze influence attention and performance? What is the "quiet eye"?

CHAPTER OVERVIEW

Two students, Mary and Martha, are both enrolled in a high school physical education class in beginning golf. Three days a week they attend the same class sessions, are taught by the same highly capable instructor, and use identical equipment. Let us assume for the purposes of this illustration that we can know that both young women possess identical physical and mental abilities, are equally industrious in their various scholastic pursuits, and that neither has previous experience in golf or any other skill that might effectively transfer to learning golf. They are beginning at exactly the same point and with the same capacity for learning golf.

Now assume for the purposes of our hypothetical example that Mary sees no reason for learning golf and finds the entire class experience meaningless and boring. She is constantly distracted during class, fails to concentrate either on the teacher's instructions or her practice attempts, and as a result finds performing required practice skills both confusing and difficult.

In contrast to Mary, Martha is excited about going to class, looks forward to the experience, and anticipates being able to join the local recreational golf league once she completes the class. She listens attentively during class instructions and concentrates on what the teacher tells her during her practice attempts.

Which student, Mary or Martha, do you think will acquire the greatest golf skills during the class?

The answer, and our point in this illustration, may seem obvious. In actual practice, though, instructors too frequently fail to recognize the obvious fact that unless learners are properly motivated and unless they focus their attention on the proper cues during practice, optimal learning will not occur regardless of how well all the other aspects of practice may be planned and executed. In this chapter, you will learn the fundamental concepts of how to effectively motivate learners and focus their practice attempts in optimal ways.

Before the first ball is thrown out in practice, before the first dance rehearsal, or before a patient begins on the road to recovering impaired skills, experienced motor skills instructors have already begun preparing learners for the practice experience. To gain the most from practice, effective instructors know that learners must be sufficiently motivated, have identified realistic yet challenging goals they want to achieve as a result of practice, and have begun receiving guidance concerning focusing their attention on the most essential aspects of their practice attempts. Preparing the learner for practice is, in many ways, the most critical aspect of motor skills learning. Without such preparation, learners too often become confused and frustrated, and either fail to learn skills effectively or, worse, disengage from practice altogether, feeling as though they have failed. When motivation and attention are properly considered, practice is much more likely to lead to enjoyable practice experiences, good learning outcomes, and the attainment of desired practice goals.

MOTIVATION

Teachers, therapists, and coaches frequently point to motivation as the key to success. "She was too motivated not to succeed." "They were not the most talented team but won anyway because they were highly motivated." "He had all the necessary abilities but lacked the needed motivation to succeed."

Highly motivated individuals often achieve performance goals in spite of challenging situations and physical limitations. People who are motivated work harder, persevere longer, and are more focused on achieving their goals than are those who are less motivated. It is not surprising that motivation plays an essential role in the learning of motor skills. Indeed, insufficient levels of motivation may be the main reason that most people fail to achieve their goals relative to the acquisition of movement skills.

Although motivation plays a central role in learning, its definition remains debated by experts and is somewhat elusive. Kleinginna and Kleinginna (1981), after reviewing 102 definitions of motivation from a variety of textbooks on the subject, defined motivation as "an internal state or condition that serves to activate or energize behavior toward a goal" (p. 363). Petri (2003), in his highly regarded textbook on motivation, defines it as "the concept we use when we describe the forces acting on or within an organism to initiate and direct behavior." "We also use the concept of motivation," Petri adds, "to explain differences in the intensity of behavior" (p. 3). Weinberg and Gould (2007), in their text on sport psychology, define motivation simply as "the direction and intensity of one's effort (p. 52)." Many theorists also accept a role for motivation in maintaining the persistence of behavior over time, although it remains unclear as to whether the factors that energize and direct behavior are the same as those that provide for its persistence (Franken, 2001). Based upon the available literature, we will conceive of **motivation** as describing a state or condition of an individual that is (1) internal (i.e., a need, desire, want, or other state), (2) directed toward the accomplishment of some general or specific goal (i.e., initiates and directs behavior toward accomplishment of some goal), (3) energizing (i.e., promotes the intensity of behavior), and (4) involved in maintaining persistence of the motivated behavior.

motivation: An internal state or condition directing and energizing behavior.

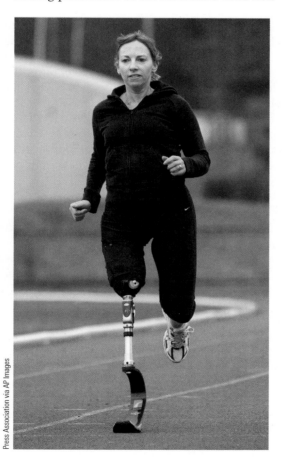

Press Association via AP Images

Many obstacles and limitations on performance can be overcome when a person is highly motivated.

The importance that motivation plays in the learning of motor skills is obvious. Unless they are sufficiently motivated, people will neither have the interest nor maintain the effort needed to persevere toward motor learning goals. Unfortunately, adequate levels of motivation on the part of learners cannot be assumed. High school students required to take physical education, for instance, too often fail to see the relevance of these classes to their lives and therefore lack sufficient interest and motivation to improve their skills in the instructed activities. Patients in physical therapy settings may become easily discouraged by their physical limitations and become unmotivated, thereby hindering their progress toward recovery. Even competitive athletes, usually considered highly motivated in their sporting pursuits, may become discouraged in the face of competition for team positions, or from defeat in competitive contests, with the result being a decline in levels of both motivation and performance. No matter how much potential a person possesses for a given activity or sport, that potential will remain untapped without sufficient levels of motivation to achieve it. Helping individuals to achieve and maintain the high levels of motivation required to realize their movement potential is therefore a requisite ability of the successful motor skills instructor. To effectively motivate individuals, though, practitioners must first understand and appreciate those factors influencing a person's level of motivation. Instructors need to be able to answer questions such as these: What factors motivate people? Under what conditions is motivation increased or decreased? How do people differ in the things that motivate them? How can motivation be maintained? What aspects of motivation can and cannot be changed? Understanding the answers to such questions can help motor skill instructors choose and apply the most effective motivational techniques in various practice and performance contests.

Most of the important things in the world have been accomplished by people who have kept on trying when there seemed to be no hope at all.

—Dale Carnegie
(1888–1955)

Characteristics of Motivation

Even though an exact and exhaustive definition of motivation may remain elusive, most of us, experts and nonexperts alike, have some intuitive feeling for what constitutes motivation. However specifically defined, there are two essential characteristics of motivation agreed upon by virtually all observers; these are most typically labeled as *activation* and *direction* (Petri, 2003).

Activation

activation: The persistence and energy level of behavior indicating motivation.

Activation is the easiest characteristic of motivation to observe. Activation is observed in the production of behavior within individuals. Is a person behaving in some way? If some degree of behavior is present, even if minimally so, then a person is assumed to be motivated. That is, it is assumed that motivation initiates and is manifested through some form of overt behavior, some action that can be observed. (In this sense, all behavior is viewed as a product of motivation.) Although overt behavior clearly indicates the presence of motivation, the absence of behavior does not necessarily mean, however, that motivation is absent. An individual's level of motivation may simply be too insufficient to trigger an overt expression of behavior. At other times, the individual might be highly motivated in a way that is expressed through the suppression of overt behaviors. Consider, for example, a photographer who waits silently and motionlessly for long hours hidden among the thickets next to a mountain lake in anticipation of wild animals arriving to quench their thirst, so that he can photograph them. Even in this example, though, we would still expect a behavioral response indicating a somewhat elevated level of motivation. No doubt, the photographer's anticipation would be accompanied by some increase in heart rate, adrenaline output, and other physiological measures. So even though behavioral indices are considered necessary expressions of motivation, the behavior need not always be overt. Fortunately, however, for both researchers and movement skill instructors, motivation is typically expressed through observable actions and changes in behavior, especially in the context of motivation eliciting movement responses.

A second characteristic of motivation expressed through activation is persistence. The persistence of behavior is one of the primary characteristics indicating both the presence and strength of motivation. People typically do not persist in activities for which they have little motivation. If two people begin a 12-week aerobics program, and one person drops out after only a few sessions while the other person perseveres for the entire 12 weeks, we assume that the person completing the program was more motivated than the person who dropped out. Of course, there could be other reasons than lack of motivation behind why the one person dropped out of training, and these would have to be investigated before any definitive conclusion regarding the influence of motivation could be determined. But other factors being equal and accounted for, it is assumed that persistence is a reliable indicator of motivational strength.

A third characteristic of motivation based upon activation is energy or vigor. Both laboratory and casual observations suggest that highly energetic behavior is more motivated than is less energetic behavior. The person who visually exerts greater effort during a practice session is most likely more motivated than the person lethargically going though the motions. The person who stays after an athletic practice to continue rehearsing new skills is probably more motivated than the person who does not. Again, factors other than motivation could account for observed levels of energetic expression, which should always be considered when assessing the motivational intensity of individuals. But again, assuming that other factors can be ruled out, the level of energetic expression in the practice and performance of a skill is most typically a good indicator of motivation.

Directionality

As we have just seen, overt behavioral responses, persistence, and energy level are considered properties indicating the presence and intensity of motivation. Activation, however, is only one of two major characteristics of motivation. This is because, as a number of researchers have pointed out, activation alone does not adequately account for the fact that humans are more or less continuously active. This has led researchers to propose a second characteristic, **directionality**, when analyzing motivation. How do we decide to direct our behavior toward accomplishing one thing rather than another? Why do we change our behaviors from performing one task to performing another having

directionality: The specific behaviors indicating a person's level of motivation.

a different goal? Although the mechanisms responsible for how we direct our attention are debated, scientists who study motivation hold that it plays an essential role in directing human behavior. Directionality is considered a primary indicator of motivation and of motivational strength.

Suppose that college students enrolled in a physical education weight training class were offered the option of completing a specified number of supervised additional training hours each week outside of class. The students who chose the additional hours could select between receiving either a small cash reward or a personalized trophy recognizing their additional efforts. Which would the most students choose? Another way of posing this question is to ask whether these students would be more motivated by extrinsic (money) or intrinsic (personal recognition of accomplishment) rewards. The change in behavioral direction would allow us to evaluate the effects and relative strengths of both types of reward systems in promoting individuals' motivation to exercise. Therefore, directionality is an indicator not only of the presence of motivation, but also of the strength of factors influencing motivation.

What Causes Motivation?

What causes people to be motivated? What specific factors best motivate people? Are there even "best" motives? Why do two people perform exactly the same behaviors, yet they are motivated by different reasons? One of the perplexing problems confronting scientists attempting to understand motivation, as well as practitioners attempting to motivate behaviors in those whom they instruct, is that people are motivated by a wide variety of situational factors and personal goals. Before examining the underlying causes of motivation, consider just some of the many everyday reasons motivating people to engage in exercise behaviors, for example. A number of different reasons people exercise are shown in Table 9.1.

TABLE **9.1**
Motivational Reasons to Exercise

Why Exercise?	Illustration
Fun, enjoyment	Children exercise spontaneously—they run and jump and chase, and they do so simply for the sheer fun of it.
Personal challenge	Athletes get "in the zone" when their sport optimally challenges their skills.
Forced to do it	Students exercise because their coach tells them to do so.
Paid to do it	A coach or instructor is paid to exercise and to help others exercise.
Accomplish a goal	Runners see whether they can run a mile in 6 minutes or less.

(Continued)

TABLE **9.1** *(Continued)*

Health benefits	People exercise to lose weight or to strengthen their heart.
Inspired to do so	People watch others exercise and become inspired to do the same.
A standard of excellence	Snow skiers race to the bottom of the mountain trying to beat their previous best time.
Satisfaction from a job well done	As exercisers make progress, they feel more competent, more effective.
An emotional kick	Vigorous jogging can produce a runner's high (a rebound to the pain).
Good mood	Beautiful weather can pick up exercisers' moods and invigorate exercise spontaneously as they skip along without knowing why.
Alleviate guilt	People exercise because they think that is what they should, ought, or have to do to feel good about themselves.
Relieve stress, silence depression	After a stressful day, people go to the gym, which they see as a structured and controllable environment.
Hang out with friends	Exercise is often a social event, a time simply to enjoy hanging out with friends.

Source: J. Reeve (2008), p. 4.

As illustrated in Table 9.1, people are motivated for many different reasons. But what do these many reasons have in common? What is the underlying cause of motivation? Is there some root cause, regardless of specific situational factors, from which all motivation springs? In the study of motivation, at least three different points of view have been identified as explanations of the factors responsible for motivation, although most researchers also assume some overlap among all of these factors (Petri, 2003).

Innate Factors

Scientists across many scholarly fields of study have debated the relative contributions to human behavior of innate versus acquired tendencies for over 100 years (i.e., of genetics versus experience as discussed in chapter 8). Early theorists saw motivation as controlled by innate factors they labeled *instincts*. These early views did not last, but today many theorists still believe that genetic factors are the primary determinants of motivation. This perspective is called the **trait-centered view of motivation** and holds that motivated behaviors are primarily the products of individual characteristics that are genetically determined. In this view, personality, needs, and attitudes are studied as the prime motives shaping motivation in sport, exercise, and movement-based performance.

trait-centered view of motivation: The theory that a person's motivational proclivities and tendencies are the result of genetic factors.

Acquired Factors

In contrast to the trait-centered view is the contention that motivations are primarily acquired through experience. In this view, individuals learn the motives guiding their behaviors from the accumulation of experiences, and learning plays the central role in the development of a person's motivations. Early childhood experiences are believed to form the strongest motivations, but even such early acquired motive states can be reshaped through adult learning. The most important instructional principle to emerge from this view is probably the concept of **incentive motivation**. This is the notion that individuals learn that some behaviors result in greater rewards than do others, and they seek out the greatest rewards when deciding among alternative behavioral choices. For example, a college student planning to try out for the college's dance company knows from previous experience that she can work herself into acceptable physical condition for tryouts with a minimum of time and effort devoted to training. She also has learning from previous experiences that if she begins training sooner and devotes considerably more time and effort to training, her chances of making the dance company will improve. She is confronted with

incentive motivation:
The idea that people have greater incentive to behave situationally in ways that have previously been rewarded.

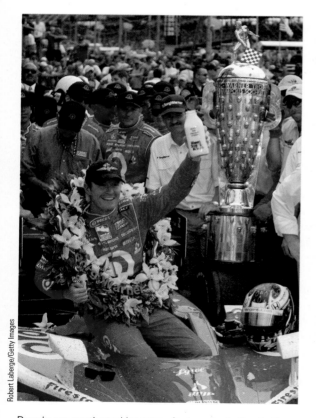

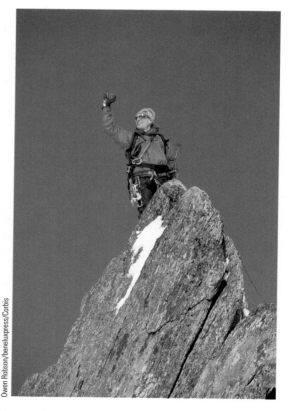

People are motivated by many factors, including both external factors (trophies, praise and adulation, monetary rewards) and internal factors (overcoming obstacles, personal achievement).

two different incentives. There is an incentive to increase her chances of making the dance company, as well as the incentive to experience greater comfort and freedom for other activities during the period prior to tryouts (and to avoid the discomfort of extensive training). In this example, there are two competing motivational states. Based upon previous learning, our aspiring dancer will weigh the alternatives and choose the one having the greatest incentive for her. The decision concerning how to train is not hard-wired genetically, but is the product of previous learning.

From an instructional standpoint, this view of acquired motivational states leads to a focus on situational factors. Unlike a trait-centered view, where instructors attempt to identify underlying personality traits and devise individualized approaches to motivate behavior, the opposing view that motivations are learned leads to a focus on situational factors and how they are rewarded. From this view, instructors will look for the most effective ways of changing learning experiences and then provide rewards and punishments to reinforce desired actions, which in turn presumably will shape the individual learner's motivations in desired ways.

A Combination of Innate and Acquired Factors

In recent years, an increasing number of researchers and practitioners have come to view motivation as a function of both innate and acquired factors. In this view, innate characteristics are held to impose certain predispositions for motives, though with room also remaining for the learning of new motive states within established personality structures. Researchers promoting this view hold that personality has genetically defined parameters but that it is also much more flexible and adaptable than previously conceived. Even within fixed general personality frameworks, there remains ample opportunity for significant reshaping of motivated behaviors. What most motivates you (see Box 9.1)?

Factors Influencing Motivation

Having considered the underlying causes of motivation, we turn next to a consideration of situational factors influencing motivation. Although the situational factors motivating people's behavior are complex and multidimensional, four factors are especially important in understanding those motives underlying the performance and learning of motor skills. These include (1) the relevance of the task to the learner, (2) the level of task difficulty, (3) the learner's perception of control, and (4) feelings of progress and success in meeting task goals.

BOX **9.1**   **What Motivates You?**

For a skill in which you regularly participate (preferably a motor skill), think of the five reasons most motivating your participation. Do these reasons share anything in common? Why do you think these reasons motivate you more than others?

Relevance of Task

We can begin by noting the obvious fact that people will seldom engage, at least with any enthusiasm, in activities that they do not see as relevant to their interests, needs, or desires. When introducing a unit on volleyball, as an example, an elementary physical education specialist may find that her students—especially the boys—show little motivation for learning this skill because they probably have not seen it on television, at least not to the same extent as they have football and basketball, and so do not think of it as a "real" sport. In this case, the teacher, having been properly trained in motor learning theory, might begin the unit with a video of competitive Olympic volleyball, thereby increasing her students' interest and motivating them to learn how to play the sport. Even when the relevance of a skill to an individual may seem obvious, such as an athlete working to regain full function of an injured limb or a worker training for a new job skill, an experienced instructor can usually point out potential results of skill enhancement that the learner has not considered (review the many options available for exercising shown in Table 9.1, for instance). Matching the outcomes of learning a new skill to the motives and needs of individuals can be a challenging task for instructors, but it is an essential one if practice is to be the most productive and meaningful. Fortunately, there are many techniques and strategies for helping people appreciate the relevance of acquiring skills in various settings (e.g., videos, demonstrations by experts, group discussions, prizes and awards, certificates of recognition, tournaments, etc.).

Level of Task Difficulty

The level of task difficulty also plays a major role in shaping an individual's motivation. Tasks that are presented at too high a level of difficulty given a performer's abilities or stage of learning will result in frustration and anxiety, quickly extinguishing any motivation there might have originally been for the task. Likewise, tasks that are too easy can lead to boredom and decrease motivation just as much as tasks that are too difficult. It is critical, therefore, that motor skill instructors determine learners' initial levels of skill proficiency and provide practice that is sufficiently challenging, but not so much so as to dampen enthusiasm and motivation. Depending upon the nature of a skill and the goals of learning, this may be accomplished by simply observing a learner's initial skill level, but may also require the administration of appropriate skills tests or other evaluation techniques in order to be determined. The results of such initial assessments may lead to the necessity of providing modified or other developmentally appropriate forms of skill practice before moving on to practice skills in the manner in which they are eventually intended to be performed. Or such assessment could also result in directing a learner to a class or training situation that is more challenging, but better suited given his or her capabilities.

Perception of Control

Another reason that tasks must be presented at appropriate levels of difficulty is to help facilitate the learner's perception of control over his or her own learning. Considerable research supports the observation that those who believe that they have control over whether they will learn are more likely to exhibit higher levels of motivation than are those who believe that they have little control over their learning outcomes (these findings are formally expressed through attribution theory). The effective instructor can do much to help enhance learners' sense of control, however. Besides assuring that the activities practiced match learners' skill levels, instructors should provide feedback and encouragement pointing out learners' successes and progress. Keeping practice experiences enjoyable and fun can help to reduce learners' anxiety and enhance motivation. When instructing groups of learners, maximizing the involvement of each group member is important for maintaining each learner's sense of control and motivation. Perhaps the key to helping learners develop their perceptions of personal control, however, is through **empowerment**. Learners can be empowered in their practice experiences in many ways. Allowing learners to choose the order in which they practice skills, what equipment to use, with whom they will team during practice, when to request feedback, and, most especially, to set their own goals for practice are all effective methods of empowering learners and heightening their levels of motivation. Of course, not all such methods will fit every circumstance, and instructors must be aware of individual differences in people's needs for direction and guidance. Where appropriate, however, methods designed to empower the learner by enhancing his or her sense of self-control over learning experiences can be very effective.

empowerment: The degree to which a person feels in control of his or her own learning.

Success in Meeting Task Goals

Generally, the more successful an individual is in a given situation, the more he or she will be motivated. Those who experience little success in their practice or performance attempts become discouraged and less motivated. A major reason that low-skilled performers so often exhibit little motivation for an activity is because they have experienced little success in it. A person's perception of success can be dramatically influenced by the way task goals are presented. In establishing the criteria against which instructors will make evaluations and learners will judge the success of their actions, instructors can focus attention either on how an individual's performance compares to others (called **peer-referenced judgments**) or on how it compares to the learner's previous performances (called **self-referenced judgments**). In a peer-referenced judgment situation, performance is competitive and the individual learner has little control over his or her own success. Instead, it is the quality of others' performances that determines how learners will be judged, and how they will judge themselves, as being successful or not. In self-referenced judgment situations, however, learners judge the results of their practice experiences against their own previous levels of performance. ("See whether you can bend your knee three degrees more today." "See if you can hit the ball farther today than yesterday." "See whether you can beat your time from the last race today.") Establishing self-referenced norms and goals for individuals can increase their experiences of success, maintain high levels of motivation, and enhance learning. Some learning situations will, of course, require that individuals attempt to meet peer-referenced standards (i.e., athletic and rehabilitative goals, for example), but even then the provision of a combination of peer- and self-referenced standards can be effectively established as guides for practice, as we will see in this chapter's section on goal setting.

peer-referenced judgments: Evaluation of skill performance in comparison to the performance of others.

self-referenced judgments: Evaluation of skill performance in comparison to one's previous performance levels.

Guidelines for Promoting Motivation

To summarize the factors important in promoting and maintaining high levels of motivation in learners, motor skill instructors should keep the following guidelines in mind when planning practice experiences:

1. Devise methods to help individuals understand and appreciate the ways in which the tasks to be learned are relevant to their needs, desires, and interests.
2. Evaluate an individual's abilities and readiness to learn in order to determine the most appropriate skill level for practice, being sure that practice requirements are challenging but attainable.
3. Provide opportunities empowering individuals to determine their own practice goals and practice experiences where appropriate.
4. Provide ample opportunities for individuals to experience success in their practice attempts, focusing at least some practice goals on increasing personal performance levels rather than on absolute performance measures or comparisons to performances of others.

Shaping the Motivational Climate

motivational climate:
The curricular and instructional factors influencing performers' motivation in structured performance environments.

Although learners may come to skills practice situations already sufficiently motivated, how the motor skills instructor structures and instructs learning experiences will typically play the most significant role in learners' continued levels of motivation. By considering the four factors shaping motivation presented above, motor skills instructors can create a supportive **motivational climate**. Motivational climate consists of instructional and design factors that combine to motivate the behaviors of participants in a practice or performance context, and is typically conceived of as enhancing motivation in appropriate ways. A widely used model for enhancing motivation among students enrolled in physical education classes, for example, is the TARGET model developed by Ames (1992). TARGET is an acronym standing for the main factors instructors of motor skills should consider in order to provide a highly motivational climate in a physical education setting: tasks, authority, rewards, grouping, evaluation, time. (It should be noted that the model is also applicable in other settings as well, such as those found in clinical, recreational, and training environments.) An illustration of the model is presented in Table 9.2.

Though there are many aspects of motivation, and therefore many guidelines that can be established to effectively enhance motivation, all of these guidelines have one thing in common—each is, to some degree, conditioned by the goals established for practice. How relevant a task is for an individual, the appropriate entry point for practice, the individual's feelings of self-confidence in achieving the goals of practice, and an individual's judgments of success in meeting task goals are all determined by what goals for practice have been established. Hence, an especially critical factor in maintaining adequate motivational levels and in achieving performance and learning success involves the process of goal setting, to which we next turn our attention.

TABLE **9.2**
TARGET Principles for Enhancing Motivation in Physical Education

TARGET Principles	How to Promote a Positive Motivational Climate	What Should Be Avoided
Tasks	Include variety, challenge and purpose for each activity. Give students the opportunity to choose from a variety of tasks. Encourage students to set their own goals.	Basing task goals on who will be first or who will score the most points, and so on
Authority	Foster active participation and a sense of autonomy. Use questioning skills. Give students the opportunity to choose (within the assigned content framework). Involve students in decision making during teaching (e.g., how to complete tasks, what materials to use, and so on).	Assuming all the responsibility as the teacher. Giving students orders and no choices
Rewards	Focus on individual progress and improvement. Recognition of students' accomplishments is kept private, and rewards are given for improvement.	Recognition of students' accomplishments is public, and rewards are given in comparison with others.
Grouping	Use individual and cooperative learning. Students work on individual tasks, in dyads or in small cooperative groups. Grouping is flexible and heterogeneous.	Grouping is based on ability.
Evaluation	Evaluation is self-referenced and private. Give opportunities to improve. Use diverse methods. Progress is judged on the basis of individual objectives, participation, effort, and improvement. Students are encouraged to evaluate their own performances.	Evaluation is based on norms and on comparing with others.
Time	Allow students to participate in scheduling. Time limits for task completion are flexible. Students help schedule timelines for improvements.	Time is not flexible.

Source: Liukkonen et al. (2007), p. 5.

Goal Setting

Virtually everyone comes to a skill-learning situation with some goal or goals in mind. "I want to beat my sister in tennis." "I want to learn to tango." "I want to regain the full use of my knee that was operated on." "I want to bat 300 next season." A common feature of skill learning is that it is goal directed; people engage in practice, often long and laboriously so, because they have some goal that they want to achieve. Locke et al. (1981) have defined a goal, simply, as "What an individual is trying to accomplish; it is the object or aim of an action" (p. 126).

Although nearly everyone has a goal or goals that he or she wants to achieve as a result of practice, not all goals are equally beneficial in promoting learning. Setting goals for practice may be a natural human propensity, but to be effective, goals must be specified and implemented correctly. Goals that are either too challenging or insufficiently challenging, unattainable given a person's physical abilities or limitations, unrealistic based on previous experiences, or too vaguely specified can lead to frustration and feelings of failure, typically resulting in a loss of motivation, diminished learning, and often withdrawal from further practice altogether. To be effective, goals must be challenging, attainable, realistic, and specific. These qualities of effective goals can be remembered by the acronym CARS.

Challenging
    Attainable
        Realistic
            Specific

To promote adherence to practice and optimize learning, goals should be set that sufficiently challenge an individual to improve; are attainable given the conditions of practice (i.e., there is adequate time, equipment, and instructional support to achieve goals); are realistic based upon a person's previous learning and innate abilities; and are specific and measurable, which allows for the assessment of progress in obtaining the goals.

Types of Goals

goal setting: The process of establishing targets for skill improvement as a result of practice.

In the study of **goal setting**, three types of goals have been identified as important in promoting effective practice. These are outcome goals, performance goals, and process goals (Burton, Naylor, and Holliday, 2001; Hardy, Jones, and Gould, 1996; Weinberg and Gould, 2007).

Outcome Goals

outcome goals: Targets for skill improvement focusing on the results of performance and often involving comparison to others.

Outcome goals focus upon the desired results or end product of practice in comparison to others. Beating your school's record in the 100-yard dash, making an athletic team, consistently striking out batters, and winning a league championship are examples of outcome goals. Outcome goals are objectively specified measures of performance that involve comparisons with the performance of others. Thus, although such goals provide challenging incentives, a person could still experience significant improvement in skill level but fail to meet the goal of practice. A competitive swimmer, for instance, might dramatically improve her time in the 100-meter free-style, but still fail to meet her goal of winning a particular race by losing to a faster opponent. On the other hand, she might not improve her performance at all and still meet the goal of winning a race because the other contestants performed worse than she did. Outcome goals are not under the control of the individual attempting to obtain the goal. For this reason, it is important also to prioritize performance and process goals.

Performance Goals

performance goals: Targets for skill improvements in comparison to a person's previous skill level.

In contrast to outcome goals, **performance goals** focus upon an individual's improvement relative to his or her previous performances and are therefore solely under the control of the individual. Performance goals, for this reason, are flexible—they are not conditioned by absolute standards or by the performances of others. Set realistically, performance goals should be challenging but attainable. Typing 60 words per minute, cutting 10 strokes off your average golf game, increasing your average bowling score from 180 to 200, and improving elbow flexion from 90 degrees to 100 degrees are examples of performance goals.

Process Goals

process goals: Targets for skill improvement that emphasize the quality of a movement.

To perform a skill at the level desired, as well as meet outcome goals, a person must be able to perform the skill sufficiently well. **Process goals focus on particular aspects of skill execution.** For example, a receiver in football may focus on watching the ball until it is in his hands, a stroke patient relearning to walk on rotating her hips as she steps forward, or a volleyball player on his follow-through after each serve. Process goals focus on the correct performance of movement patterns.

Goal-Setting Should Include All Three Types of Goals

All three types of goals—outcome, performance, and process—play a role in directing a learner's behavior and are important in motivating optimal achievement. Focusing on outcome goals helps keep learners motivated over the long run, keeping them excited and providing an eventual target that makes daily practice efforts more meaningful. Performance and process goals are important because they are entirely under the learners' control. They can be met by obtaining intermediate and attainable subgoals (i.e., rather than focusing on improving free throw average by 10%, subgoals of 1%, 2%, 3%, etc., can be more quickly and easily obtained). Process and performance goals can facilitate short-term motivational levels, keeping learners progressing toward their ultimate outcome goals. Examples of some outcome, performance, and process goals are illustrated in Table 9.3.

Given that each type of goal has a separate role in the learning process, it is important that all three types be part of an effective goal-setting program (Hardy, Jones, and Gould, 1996). A study by Filby, Maynard, and Graydon (1999) demonstrated that using a combination of all three goal types significantly enhanced learning when compared to the use of any single type of goal. Using beginning soccer players, the researchers randomly formed five groups based on the type of goal or goals provided to subjects. Three groups were provided with a single goal on which they were instructed to focus attention during practice, with the groups differentiated by whether they were provided with an outcome, performance, or process goal. A fourth group was given all three goal types and instructed to focus practice attention on meeting each of the three goals. An equal amount of prompting to attend to goals was provided to all four groups. Finally, a fifth group served as a control and received no practice goals. After five weeks of practice, all groups participated in a competitive

TABLE **9.3**

Examples of Outcome, Performance, and Process Goals

Task	Outcome Goal	Performance Goal	Process Goal
Typing	Be first in class to complete practice test with no errors.	Type 30 words per minute with no errors.	Maintain fingers on home row.
Baseball	Have highest batting average on team.	Keep majority of swings at balls in strike zone.	Keep eyes on pitched ball through strike zone.
Wrestling	Become league champion.	Add two new escape moves to match repertory.	Increase speed of escape moves.
100 Hurdles	Win 7 of 10 meets.	Complete all events clearing hurdles.	Fully extend leading leg and flex trailing leg parallel to ground.
Archery	Qualify for national regional meet.	Improve bull's-eye percentage from 20% to 30%.	Exhale slowly and maintain bow without motion before release.

soccer game. Results of the experiment clearly showed that goal setting provided both a practice and competitive advantage. The four groups given goals for practice improved more during practice sessions and also performed better in game competition than did the control group not provided goals for practice. The greatest improvement in learning, and best competitive performance, however, belonged to the group focused on multiple goal strategies involving outcome, performance, and process goals. You can evaluate your ability to set each of these three type of goals by completing the exercise in Box 9.2.

Why Does Goal Setting Work?

As we have just seen, goal setting facilitates learning and can have a pronounced effect on the quality of competitive sports performance. A basic question is, How do goals work? That is, what is it about goal setting that influences practice behavior and induces better learning outcomes? Theorists working in this area have identified four important functions that underlie the goal-setting process (Horn, 2002; Locke and Latham, 1990; Weinberg and Gould, 2007):

BOX **9.2**   **Setting Goals**

For each skill listed below, develop an outcome goal, performance goal, and process goal for a novice just beginning to learn the activity.

- Driving an automobile
- Playing golf
- Cooking
- Playing the piano
- Rehabilitating a sprained ankle
- Preparing for a motor learning exam
- A skill you desire to learn

1. Goals direct the learner's attention to important elements of the skill.
2. Goals increase the learner's effort and intensity.
3. Goals encourage persistence in the face of failure, adversity, or lack of immediate progress.
4. Goals promote the development of new learning strategies.

The first three of these functions of goal setting are fairly obvious. When learners set goals, their attention during practice is directed to important elements of the skill that they might otherwise neglect. Goals also motivate effort, as well as persistence, by providing incentives for performance.

In addition to these more obvious functions, goal setting has a hidden function, or at least a function not directly planned for. Goal setting encourages the development of new learning strategies. Assuming that goals are set at sufficiently challenging levels, performers may find that meeting them requires adjustments in their ordinary practice routines. A basketball player whose goal is to improve her free-throw average may find that she must increase the number of practice attempts that she takes daily or improve her form or perhaps both, to be more successful. The focus on goals, in this instance, can prompt a search for new practice strategies to help achieve those goals that would not otherwise occur. Goal setting in essence influences performance and learning indirectly by encouraging the search for task solutions, thereby empowering individuals as independent learners (the reader might recall this as a major instructional principle of dynamical systems theory).

Guidelines for Goal Setting

Helping individuals identify and set goals to meet their specific needs and desires requires sensitivity to individual differences, experience in the activity being practiced, and a good grasp of the principles of goal setting established in the scientific literature. The first two of these are beyond our scope here, but the third can be summarized fairly succinctly (but see Hall and Kerr, 2001, for a fuller discussion). Summarizing the research literature on goal setting, Weinberg and Gould (2007) have suggested a number of basic principles that should be considered when designing practice goals.

1. **Set specific goals.** Goals should be stated in specific, measurable terms. Many teachers, coaches, and therapists believe that it is best to provide goals in general terms such as "Do your best." Such goals, however, are too vague to be effective. Telling someone to do his or her best at lowering their golf handicap is not the same as telling them to strive to lower their handicap from 14 to 11 over par. To be most effective, goals must be stated in specific terms that specify the behaviors to be accomplished.
2. **Set moderately difficult but realistic goals.** Substantial research demonstrates that moderately difficult goals lead to the best performance and learning outcomes. Goals should challenge learners, though they should also be realistic and attainable. Goals that are too easy to achieve quickly result in learners losing interest and reducing effort. Goals that are too difficult to achieve, on the other hand, lead to frustration, loss of motivation, and poor performance. To be effective, goals must strike a balance between being too easy and too difficult.

3. **Set both long-term and short-term goals.** Both short-term and long-term goals are important if goal setting is to be effective (Kane, Baltes, and Moss, 2001). Long-term goals provide ultimate targets for learners and motivate adherence and sustained effort. If long-term goals alone are provided, however, learners can quickly become frustrated when they fail to see sufficient progress toward attaining the goal. Short-term, intermediate goals provide a sense of progress and encourage learners to continue working toward the long-term goals of practice. When designing goals, it is important that long-term and short-term goals be linked so that learners perceive the attainment of short-term goals as part of a progression leading to ultimate success in attaining long-term goals.

4. **Set outcome, performance, and process goals.** As we have already seen, pursuing a combination of outcome, performance, and process goals results in the most effective performance and learning outcomes. Too frequently, practitioners focus learners' attention on outcome goals alone (Steinberg and Marcy, 1999). Ironically, however, the best way of achieving outcome goals is to focus attention on performance and process goals. Though outcome goals are important in encouraging continued participation, especially in the face of difficulty periods of practice, placing too much emphasis on them creates anxiety and frustration, as well as diverts learners' attention from achieving essential progressive steps in the learning process.

5. **Record and display goals.** A number of studies have shown that to be most effective, learners must be frequently reminded of their performance goals. Recording goals and prominently displaying them in a manner that invites frequent review is an effective way of accomplishing this. Many techniques have been suggested, such as keeping goals on index cards and reviewing them prior to every practice session, displaying a listing of goals where they will be seen often, and listing goals in training logs and recording when specific short-term goals are met. No single method is optimal, and instructors and learners may express considerable creativity in finding methods that work best for specific individuals and in specific situations.

6. **Develop goal achievement strategies.** Establishing goals without consideration of the strategies that will be used in achieving those goals is like setting the goal of losing 10 pounds without considering the kind of eating or exercise program you will follow to accomplish such a weight loss. In establishing goals, one also must answer the question "How will I achieve this goal?" Strategies should be specific and quantifiable (What will you specifically do? How many times? For how long? Etc.). Strategies should also be flexible, so that learners can adapt to new situations as needed or as they discover better methods of promoting goal outcomes.

7. **Consider the learner's personality and motivation when setting goals.** In helping learners set and achieve goals, practitioners should take into consideration the unique characteristics of each learner and what things

motivate him or her the most (those things we reviewed in the previous section on learner characteristics). Is a learner a high achiever or low achiever, more motivated by the goal of success or the fear of failure, motivated more by personal or group goals, and so on? Consideration of previous experience, ability level, age, and any physical limitations may play a significant role in setting goals. Effective practitioners will be sensitive to individual needs and personalities, as well as learn about an individual's previous experiences and expectations of practice when establishing performance goals.

8. **Foster a learner's goal commitment.** Regardless of how well goals may be designed, learners will not benefit from them if they are not committed to achieving them. Practitioners should therefore involve learners fully in the goal-setting process, and then provide constant encouragement and feedback concerning the accomplishment of those goals.

9. **Provide evaluation and feedback about goals.** Once they have established the goals of practice for a learner, practitioners too often leave the specific evaluation of meeting those goals to the learner him- or herself. It is critical, however, that a regular and systematic method of evaluating and following progress in the attainment of goals be part of the overall goal-setting program. There are many ways of accomplishing this. Monitoring progress toward goals on charts or other records provided to a learner is one effective method, but many others can be effectively developed and implemented. The key is that learners are able to realize the accomplishment of intermediate short-term goals, as well as discern progress toward ultimate long-term goals.

10. **Limit the number of goals set, especially initially.** A common mistake beginners at goal setting often make is setting too many goals. In their desire to improve, both instructors and learners may set an unrealistically large number of goals to be achieved. Too many goals can easily distract the learner's attention, making the monitoring and attention devoted to specific goals almost impossible. It is recommended that one or two short-term goals initially be set and then others goals added gradually. Such a strategy makes it more likely that learners will initially acquire several short-term goals that will enhance enthusiasm and sustain optimal levels of motivation.

ATTENTION

attention: The direction of conscious mental resources toward specific sensory stimuli.

The study of **attention** and its relationship to motor performance and learning has both theoretical and practical importance. The theoretical importance lies in the fact that attention underlies the processes of memory and learning, central to an understanding of how motor skills are acquired from a cognitive theoretical perspective. From a practical perspective, attention plays a central role in nearly every facet of executing a motor skill. How many tasks can you perform at the same time? How rapidly can you switch attention from one task to another, or from one aspect of the performance environment to another? How broadly, or narrowly, should attention be focused? Can you learn to focus attention more effectively? The answers to such questions are critical to the performance and learning of movement skills.

Like motivation, attention is a concept readily recognized, but one not blessed with a consensually agreed-upon definition. The founder of American psychology, William James, is often quoted when defining attention. In his seminal text, *Principles of Psychology*, James (1890) wrote the following:

> Everyone knows what attention is. It is the taking possession by the mind, in clear and vivid form, of one out of what seem several simultaneously possible objects or trains of thought. Focalization, concentration, of consciousness are its essence. It implies withdrawal from some things in order to deal effectively with others. (pp. 403–404)

Although everyone may indeed know what attention is, theorists identify different characteristics of attention as being of central importance, and definitional issues are further compounded by the application of differing theoretical approaches.

Characteristics of Attention

Perhaps the major difficulty in arriving at a specific definition of attention, one enjoying broad consensus, results from the fact that a number of different characteristics are attributable to it (Schmidt and Lee, 2005).

Attention as Consciousness

The concept of attention as consciousness is the oldest view among scientists. Consciousness is defined as "awareness," which may refer both to one's awareness of internal psychological states and of those things making up the external environment. Although this original view is now considered overly simplistic, modern methods of brain research have led to a renewed interest in the aspects of consciousness associated with attentional states. Of particular interest has been the discovery that conscious and unconscious neural processes explain differences observed between automatic and controlled motor skills. For example, skills controlled by automatic (unconscious) processes have been found to be relatively resistant to forgetting as individuals age, often being retained well into old age. Controlled skills, on the other hand, which are processed using conscious attentional resources, are much more likely to decline as a result of aging.

Attention as Effort or Arousal

A feature of attention everyone has experienced is effort or arousal. Though most of the time the effort involved in attention is so small as to go unnoticed, we become aware, when focusing attention intently, that effort is a primary constituent of attention. Attention requires mental effort. Driving in heavy traffic, studying for an exam, and learning a complex motor skill are all accompanied by mental work that can leave participants feeling exhausted. In fact, the amount of mental work required of attentional processes is measured by increases in physiological measures of arousal such as respiration, heart rate, and galvanic skin resistance.

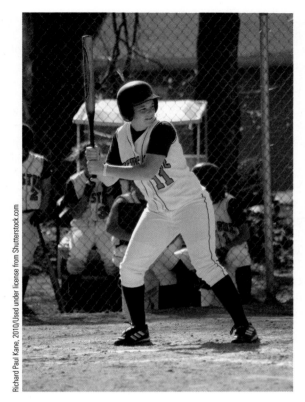

Richard Paul Kane, 2010/Used under license from Shutterstock.com

Success in many motor activities requires intense and highly focused attention directed toward a specific aspect of the performance environment.

Attention as a Limited Resource

The concept of attention as a limited resource is an essential feature of information processing models of motor control. According to this notion, people are limited in their capacity (i.e., their resources) for processing information from the environment at any one point in time. There are limits in how many things we can attend to at a time, for instance. Generally, we can consciously attend to only one thing at a time, although we may be able to switch quickly back and forth from one thing to another if the items we are attending to require relatively little attentional effort. We can perform two tasks at the same time only when one of the two is well learned and automatic, such as driving an automobile while carrying on a conversation with a passenger (see Box 9.3).

A corollary to the concept of attention as a limited capacity is the idea of selective attention. Selective attention is the concept that we can direct our limited attentional resources to specific tasks or environmental features among various alternatives with which we are presented. Listening to a friend's conversation when many other people are talking around you (called the *cocktail phenomenon*), following the movements of a puck in an ice hockey match, and watching a pitched ball in anticipation of whether to swing your bat are examples of selective attention. Each of these examples requires conscious effort to muster limited attentional resources that can be focused exclusively on the desired stimulus. We will examine the concept of selective attention in greater detail later in this chapter.

Theories of Attention

Given the breadth of the concept of attention, it should come as no surprise that several different theories and models of attention have been proposed. Many of these theories are concerned with explaining specific aspects of attention, such as how its capacity is determined or how selection among objects occurs. Other theories are concerned with explaining attention at different levels such as neurophysiological, cognitive, emergence, and mathematical levels of analysis. Although some recent theories have attempted to provide widely encompassing perspectives, as Styles (1997), in her text on attention, has written, "There is so much to explain that it seems unlikely that there could ever be a single unified theory of attention" (p. 109).

Although a single unified theory may remain elusive, existing theories can generally be classified into either of two broad theoretical approaches in explaining attention. These can be labeled as bottleneck theories and central-resource theories.

bottleneck theories:
The perspective that attention is limited to the processing of only one or two chunks of information at a time, which must be completed before additional sensory information can be processed.

Bottleneck Theory

A number of theories have been proposed over the years to explain the limitations of attention from an information processing perspective. These have typically been termed as filter or **bottleneck theories.** According to this theoretical

---

| BOX **9.3** | **Cell Phone Use while Driving** |

A long-held concern since the introduction of cell phones has been the effect that their use has on the attentional capacity of automobile drivers. Scientists from a number of fields of cognitive and neuromotor studies pointed to the attentional demands of driving and expressed concerns that limited human attentional capabilities made cell phone use and driving incompatible. Cell phone use, it was argued, would distract limited attentional resources away from essential driving requirements. Since the introduction of the cell phone and these original concerns, a growing body of research is confirming that the use of cell phones while driving increases a driver's chances of being involved in an accident by more than fourfold. Studies of actual accidents, as well as controlled laboratory studies using driving simulators, have consistently supported the finding of a fourfold increase in accident rates when driving using a cell phone. A review released by the American Automobile Association in 2008 of 84 separate investigations of cell phone use and accident rates confirmed a conclusion that cell phone use increased a driver's probability of being in an accident by a factor of more than four. The fourfold increase was observed with both handheld and hand-free phone use. Research has further revealed that cell phone use while operating an automobile impacts a number of performance variables, with the most critical being reaction time. Research from a number of laboratory studies has reported an average increase of more than 2/10 of a second in reaction time when responding to an emergency situation while using a cell phone. Recent research has also reported that cell phone use increases a driver's probability of being in an accident more than does being legally intoxicated.

approach, cognitive processes involved in information processing occur in serial order, and each stage of processing must be completed prior to the initiation of processing activities for additional stimuli entering the processing stage. Recall from Chapter 4 that the sequential stages of perception, decision making, and motor programming occur in a fixed, linear order. Because each of these stages has a limited capacity for processing information, once a chunk of specific stimuli enters any stage of the system, processing activities for that stimulus must be completed and either discarded or selected for further processing and forwarded before new stimuli can enter the stage for continued processing. Because only one piece of information can be processed at a time, if processing activities require too much time in any stage for a particular stimulus, following stimuli must wait their turn, as it were, before entering the processing stage. The analogy of informational chunks flowing through a bottle has been used to illustrate this process (see Figure 9.1). When informational chucks become too large (i.e., contain a complex array of stimuli), only one can get through the neck of the bottle at a time, with those chunks behind it having to wait their turn to be processed and pass through the bottle's neck to the next stage. Because processing activities take time, the buildup of processing delays can impede an individual's ability to attend to several items at a single point in time, and cause delays in shifting attentional focus when required.

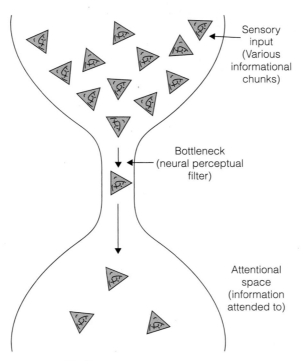

Sensory input (Various informational chunks)

Bottleneck (neural perceptual filter)

Attentional space (information attended to)

FIGURE **9.1** Bottleneck Theories of Attention

Source: Created by author.

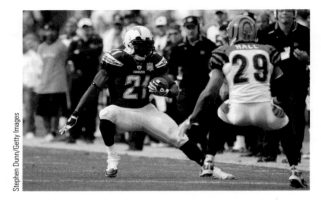

The Psychological Refractory Period offers an explanation for the effectiveness of the "fake" technique in sports.

psychological refractory period: Delay in responding to the second of two stimuli occurring closely in time.

Bottleneck theories offer an explanation for a number of perplexing features of attention, including the **psychological refractory period**. Everyone has experienced the state of seemingly being frozen for a brief time, usually only a fraction of a second, before responding to a stimulus. Whenever two stimuli occur closely in time, the first stimulus must be processed before the second, meaning that a response to the second stimulus will be delayed until the first stimulus is dealt with (either ignored or responded to). The time of this delay is the psychological refractory period. Many athletes are well versed in this theory. As one example (see Shea, Shebilske, and Worchel, 1993), a basketball player dribbling downcourt in a game may move to the right of the player guarding him and then, in the instant the defensive player moves to counter his movement to the right, quickly cut back to the left to pass the defender. The offensive player is counting on the psychological refractory period to give him enough time to get around the defender, who is delayed in responding to his cut to the left because he is still processing the original information about movement to the right. In sporting terminology, the defensive player "took the fake." The psychological refractory period is defined as the delay in responding to the second of two stimuli spaced closely in time.

Central-Resource Theories

Although bottleneck theories explain a number of characteristics of attention, they leave others unanswered. One of the main criticisms of such theories is their inability to offer an adequate explanation for how people are able to attend to more than one task at the same time. Bottleneck theories explain the simultaneous execution of two tasks by assuming that one of the tasks must be performed through unconscious automatic processes. But what about the situation in which two tasks are performed simultaneously and both require conscious attention? What if several tasks are performed simultaneously, and all must be consciously attended to?

To illustrate a situation requiring simultaneous attention to several aspects of the environment, consider a typical pass play by a quarterback in a football game. At the snap of the ball, the quarterback drops back to pass. In the next two or three seconds, he must attend to a number of things happening on the field at the same time and decide how best to respond. The quarterback must track the activities of two to three receivers running downfield, the movements of defenders guarding them, the location of defensive players rushing toward him, all the while moving to avoid being tackled by players from the opposing team. How can the quarterback focus his attention on all of these features of a single football play at the same time?

Bottleneck theories do not adequately explain situations like this quarterbacking example, never mind the many multiple tasks we all perform every day. For this reason, a number of newer theories have emerged that provide theoretical solutions to situations requiring attention to multiple tasks or situations at the same time. These theories can be grouped together as representing a basic theoretical approach called **central-resources theories.** Nobel laureate Daniel Kahneman (1973) was the first to propose this approach, and many newer theories have since advanced his basic theoretical premises. The basic assumption of all central-resource theories is that there is a central reserve of attentional resources available from which all activities requiring attention draw and compete. As an analogy, think about how a person must allocate his or her expenditure of money from a monthly paycheck. The check is of a fixed amount of money; there is a limited amount of dollars from which to draw, and when those are spent, there are no additional funds available. The person must decide how the fixed sum of money is to be spent. Rent and groceries will probably receive the highest priority, followed perhaps by laundry or gas money. If the entire check is allocated for these basic needs, there will be nothing left for the purchase of new clothes or dinners out or a new larger computer monitor. (Of course, resources could be allocated toward new clothes and the larger monitor, but then nothing would be left for rent and groceries.)

Central-resource theories assume that attention, like a monthly paycheck, is a fixed and limited amount of mental capital that is available to expend on attentional needs. Like the need to prioritize monthly expenditures, a person must decide which features of a situation most require attention, because the amount of attentional capital is limited. If we consider a person simultaneously performing two tasks, A and B, both of which require attention, and the attentional resources available for performing these two tasks as 100 percent of the total attentional capacity available from which the individual may draw, then the person may allocate attention to these two tasks in any way that does not exceed 100 percent. A person may, for example, draw 80 percent of the available resources for task A, leaving 20 percent for task B. However, the person could also use only 50 percent of the resources for task A, leaving 50 percent for task B. Some ways of allocating limited attentional resources will prove more effective than others, of course. One of the intended outcomes of skill practice is learning how to most effectively allocate limited attentional resources for different skills and situations. An example illustrating the allocation of attention to three tasks is presented in Figure 9.2.

In contrast to bottleneck theories, central-resources theories of attention hold that two or more tasks can be performed simultaneously as long as the

central-resource theories: The perspective that attention consists of a limited resources pool from which one must decide how much attention to allocate among competing needs.

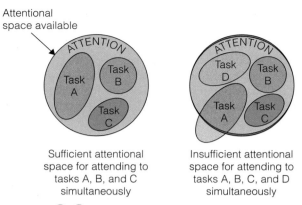

FIGURE **9.2** Central-Resource Theories of Attention

Source: Created by author.

combined attentional capacity does not exceed 100 percent of the total central resources available. As illustrated in Figure 9.2, the attentional requirements of the three tasks A, B, and C do not exceed the central resources available. The addition of a fourth task, D, however, exceeds available attentional resources. In this case, D must be ignored; resources must be reallocated to accommodate D, which will require ignoring at least one of the remaining tasks; or resources could be shared among all four tasks, resulting in inadequate attention to any of the tasks. In any of these cases, performance would be compromised.

Finally, the amount of attentional resources available for allocation is not considered fixed. Primary among the factors influencing the availability of attentional resources is an individual's state of arousal and anxiety. **Arousal** refers to a person's degree of physiological and psychological activity, which can range from a state of sound sleep to intense excitement. (Arousal also refers to the intensity dimension of motivation discussed earlier in this chapter.) As individuals become more aroused, they become more physically and mentally activated. Physically, physiological parameters including heart rate, respiration, adrenaline flow, and sweating increase. Mentally, one's focus narrows and becomes more intense; attentional resources are shifted from irrelevant environmental features to those that are more relevant. **Anxiety** refers to the experience of arousal as a negative emotional state. When a person experiences anxiety, feelings of nervousness, apprehension, and worry accompany increases in arousal.

Feelings of anxiety detract from attention. They compete with task-relevant stimuli for an individual's limited attentional resources. Arousal, on the other hand, typically has a positive effect in channeling one's attentional focus to relevant environmental cues, at least up to some optimal point. At a certain level of arousal, however, continued increases in one's arousal begin to detract from attentional capabilities. In his classic description of central-resource theory, Kahneman (1973) posits that the storage of attentional resources within the central nervous system (which he calls a "central pool" of resources) has a flexible capacity. This central capacity expands or contracts in attentional

arousal: General physiological and psychological activation of an individual; varies from a state of sleep to extreme excitement.

anxiety: Feelings of threat or apprehension in a given situation, accompanied by an increasing state of arousal.

resources available, depending on a number of factors, with the performer's level of arousal being a particularly critical factor. Managing a performer's degree of arousal to obtain the level that optimizes the attentional resources available is a critical instructional goal. Techniques designed to enhance motivation and establish attainable goals, particularly the attainment of process goals rather than outcome goals, as described earlier in the sections on motivation and goal setting, are particularly critical in promoting appropriate levels of arousal that provide for the greatest capacity in attentional resources.

Selective Attention

The performance environment is filled with a multitude of differing types of stimuli. Both internal and external sources of information compete for the performer's attention. To what should the performer pay attention? To what stimuli should the motor skill instructor direct the learner's attention? In the next chapter, we will discuss in considerable detail the important topic of focusing the learner's practice attempts on specific features of practiced skills through verbal instructions. For now, though, we will focus on the performer's general attentional orientation as it influences performance and learning in different types of motor skills.

Luckily, given the vast amount of sensory information from which learners must select in deciding how to allocate their limited attentional resources, humans are capable of selective attention. Everyone has experienced becoming suddenly aware of something obvious in their environment of which he or she had been completely unaware a second before, even though the thing suddenly noticed had been clearly present all along. This illustrates our tendency for **selective attention**. Because of our limited capacity to attend to things in our environment, we orient our attention toward a particular aspect of the environment to the exclusion of other aspects or parts. These selective tendencies are generally based upon our learning, interests, habits, and needs (see Box 9.4).

Selective attention can be either incidental or intentional. Incidental selective attention typically involves some feature of our external involvement suddenly capturing our attention, such as a loud noise, the face of a friend in a crowd, or being hit by an unexpected raindrop on a sunny day. Intentional selection occurs when we purposefully decide to attend to one thing rather than another (i.e., the exam we are taking in class, music playing on a radio, the movement patterns of players on an opposing team). Obviously, both intentional and incidental selective processes are responsible for the many shifts in attention people more or less continuously experience. An important role of the motor skill instructor is to help learners intentionally direct their selective attention resources to the most essential features of the performance environment while minimizing incidental distractions of attention through the management of the performer's motivation, goals, and arousal level.

Directing Attention

In helping learners direct their selective attentional resources to the most critical aspects of the practice environment, a number of models for directing attention have been proposed. The most widely used and intuitively appealing

selective attention: The human capacity for choosing among the many sources of sensory information to which one's attention could be directed.

is a model classifying attention into four categories developed by Nideffer (Nideffer, 1976a, 1976b, 1981, 1993; Nideffer and Segal, 2001).

Nideffer's view is that attention can be controlled by individuals along two dimensions of attentional focus, which he labels "width" and "direction" (see Figure 9.3). Width of focus varies on a continuum between a broad focus (attending to several stimuli at the same time; what is happening around you) and a narrow focus (limiting attention to one or two stimuli; focusing attention on some critical aspect of a task). Direction of focus varies between external focus (attending to the desired consequences of action, e.g., where you want a thrown ball to go) and internal focus (attending to the bodily movements that will produce the desired action, e.g., with how much force the ball should be thrown). Based upon a combination of these two dimensions, Nideffer identifies four distinct styles of attentional focus.

attentional focus: The allocation of attentional resources along dimensions of width of focus (broad to narrow) and direction of focus (external or internal).

- **Broad external attentional focus.** The performer must attend to and remain aware of several environmental cues at the same time, shifting focus constantly among changing aspects of the external environment. Constant awareness of what is happening around the performer is paramount in this style. Skills for which this attentional focus style is appropriate include many open skills requiring the ability to rapidly assess a situation and react quickly. Examples include a quarterback passing in a football game, driving bumper cars, playing musical chairs.
- **Narrow external attentional focus.** The performer attends to only one or two environmental cues, focusing attention exclusively on a limited scope of environmental possibilities. Concentrated attention focused upon a few aspects of one's performance environment is the essence of this style. Skills for which this style of attentional focus is appropriate include

---

BOX 9.4   Selective Attention: Would You Have Stopped to Listen?

An important capacity of attention is our ability to select those stimuli in our environment to which we will attend. Although this is an essential attentional capacity, it can also sometimes have unintended consequences. Consider the following example.

On a cold winter's day in early 2007, a man stood on the platform of Metro Station in Washington, DC, violin in hand, during rush hour as people scurried to catch the next train home after a day's work. For an hour, the man played six different Bach pieces. During the hour he played, six passersby stopped for between one-half to three minutes, but all quickly ran off to make their schedules. Only a few left money in the man's violin case, from which he collected $6.00 in earnings for the hour. When the man stopped playing and packed away his violin after the hour, no one noticed, no one applauded,

nor was there any recognition from any of the thousands of people who had passed by without acknowledging the man's playing.

No one who rushed past the man playing that afternoon knew that he was Joshua Bell, one of the greatest musicians in the world. He played one of the most intricate pieces ever written for the violin on one worth $3.5 million dollars. The evening before, he had played the same pieces, on the same violin, at a sold-out performance in Boston, where ticket prices averaged $100.

The performance had been arranged as part of a social experiment by a local newspaper. It was also a striking example of selective attention, especially how humans tend to divert their attention from current interests and things that do not fit in with their expectations.

open skills in which features of the environment change in regular ways representing a limited number of alternative situations, and closed skills in which the environment is stable. The environment may also be either moving or stationary, though a key for moving environments is that changes occur in a highly predictable way. Examples include putting in golf, batting in baseball and softball, and threading a needle.

- **Broad internal attentional focus.** This style involves focusing attention on a wide range of bodily sensations or mental processes and thoughts. Generally, the performer's focus is upon overall kinesthetic awareness of bodily movement rather than attention to a specific body part. Mental focus may include the focusing of thoughts and feelings in preparation for actual performance, or planning strategy related to performance. Whether attending to physical or mental activities, the key is that a wide range of sensations or thoughts are considered, typically encompassing the entire range of what is to be experienced in actual performance. Examples of motor skills in which a broad internal attentional focus style is appropriate include performing on a balance beam, ballet, and wrestling. Examples of mental preparations include "psyching up" prior to competition; deciding, when rock climbing, which of several paths on a mountain's rock face to follow; and planning goals for an exercise program.
- **Narrow internal attentional focus.** The performer focuses attention on a specific aspect of bodily movement when executing a skill, or on his or her thoughts concerning some specific mental aspect in preparation for practice or performance. This may include monitoring specific movement cues

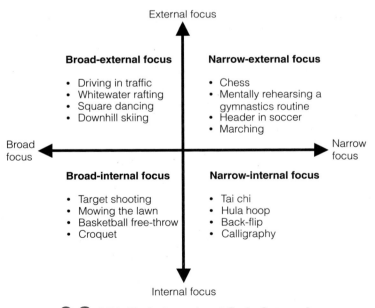

FIGURE **9.3** Nideffer's Attentional Style Categories

Source: Created by author.

when performing a skill, such as focusing on pointing one's elbow toward the intended target before extending the forearm when throwing a ball, or remembering the order of arm movements in an aerobics exercise routine. It can also include the mental rehearsal of a skill or the control of one's emotional state in preparation for performing a skill. Examples include a therapy patient focusing on achieving a certain degree of flexion during a knee extension exercise, a yoga student focusing on taking deeper and slower breaths during a routine, and a diver visualizing a dive prior to performance.

It cannot be assumed that learners will automatically adopt the correct attentional focus style when performing a skill, especially during early stages of learning. Learners experience considerable difficulty in harnessing and correctly focusing attentional resources (Wilson, Peper, and Schmid, 2001). An important instructional consideration involves promoting a learner's optimal attentional focus in various situations. By understanding attentional styles, instructors of motor skills can significantly enhance the learning and performance of skills. In fact, the available evidence suggests that with practice and instruction on focusing one's attention optimally, learners become more adept at allocating their attentional resources in the most efficient manner (Vickers, 2004; Weinberg and Gould, 2007). Although instructors must evaluate both task and learner needs in determining the optimal type of attentional focus for each given situation, some helpful guidelines can be offered. Research evidence suggests, for example, that an external attentional focus directing learners' attention to important environmental cues is generally preferred for open skills (Landin, 1994). A growing body of evidence has also supported the use of an external focus for closed skills, a topic to be considered in more detail in Chapter 10, which discusses verbal instructions. The combination of task requirements, environmental demands, and learner capabilities and needs must all be carefully evaluated in decisions concerning the allocation and proper focus of attentional resources (see Box 9.5).

Finally, Nideffer has suggested that people vary considerably in their attentional preferences and capabilities. He contends that most people are best suited to learn and perform motor skills requiring a dominant attentional focus style or a particular combination of styles (i.e., broad external, narrow external, broad internal, or narrow internal). By helping learners identify their preferred attentional style, Nideffer has suggested that opportunities for achieving athletic success might be significantly enhanced (Nideffer, 2007). An instrument he developed, *The Attentional and Interpersonal Style Inventory* (or TAIS), can be used for formally evaluating a person's dominant or preferred attentional style (Nideffer, 1976a).

Directing Attention Visually

Attention frequently follows vision. Research has supported the conclusion that a shift in visual gaze (i.e., where our vision is directed) to a new location is a reliable indicator of a shift in attention to that location (Henderson, 2003; Zelinsky et al., 1997). What we look at captures our attention; what we attend to directs what we look at. Vision and attention form a symbiotic dance, one leading and the other following, the next instant the other taking the lead, both reciprocally leading and following back and forth in the mutual search for the most relevant information to guide our actions.

Many movement skills, including most of those found in sports, involve either moving our bodies through space (tumbling), propelling some object through space (hitting a golf ball), or a combination of both (basketball lay up); other instances require the interaction of bodily movements with objects moving in space (hitting and catching a ball). Whichever the case, vision plays an essential role in our detection of environmental cues and in the direction of our attentional resources in response to those cues.

An important area of study for movement scientists is in understanding the relationship between vision and attention. Research by Vickers (2007) and her colleagues and graduate students at the University of Calgary has resulted in significant findings concerning visual search and attention. Vickers and her colleagues have shown in a number of studies that expert and novice performers in various sports skills use vision differently from one another. Specifically, expert performers engage in a period of eye fixation prior to and during the execution of a movement, which Vickers has called the **quiet eye** (Vickers, 1996, 2004). Four characteristics of visual gaze control characterize the quiet eye (Vickers, 2007, p. 77). First, the quiet eye is a fixation of the performer's gaze on a single critical location in the performance environment. Second, the onset of the visual fixation occurs prior to the beginning of the intended movement. Third, the duration of the performer's fixed gaze carries through and beyond the final movement. Fourth, a longer quiet eye period is characteristic of higher levels of both skill and accuracy. As an example of these four characteristics applied to a specific skill, Vickers offered the following description of the quiet eye as observed in elite golfers performing putting skills.

quiet eye: The fixation of one's visual gaze prior to and during the execution of an action.

> The Quiet Eye occurs when your gaze remains absolutely still on the ball just before and as the stroke is performed. There are two important aspects to this basic yet essential skill: location and duration. Our research has shown that golfers who putt well focus their gaze on either the back of the ball or the top of the ball, Which is better? Both locations are effective in improving accuracy, but a weight of evidence is beginning to favor the back of the ball.
>
> We've also studied the quiet eye duration. The expert putters had a Quiet Eye duration of two to three seconds on average, while the less skilled players held their gaze steady for one to two seconds. (Vickers, 2004, p. 96)

BOX 9.5   Which Attentional Style Should Performers Adopt?

For each of the activities listed, determine which attentional style (broad external, broad internal, narrow external, or narrow internal) should be recommended when performing the skill.

- Performing a yo-yo trick
- Learning to walk up a flight of stairs using crutches
- Painting a wall
- Canoeing in a lake
- Dribbling a soccer ball in a game
- Learning a dance step with a partner
- Skateboarding
- Bathing a dog in a tub

Research has also reported that the quiet eye characterizes elite performers in a wide variety of different sports skills, including golf, basketball, volleyball, darts, rifle shooting, billiards, table tennis, and ice hockey goaltending (Vickers, 2007, p. 11). It should be noted that most of the skills in this list involve aiming or tracking in one form or another. Other skill types have received less attention because of the difficulties involved in data collection when subjects are not relatively stationary (i.e., it is difficult to track eye movements of moving subjects). Until research can clarify the effects of gaze control in a wider range of activities, especially open skills with rapidly changing environments, it is prudent to limit quiet eye findings and techniques to the performance and instruction of skills in which such techniques are readily adaptable, with closed skills and open skills in which 2 or 3 seconds are available for initiating a response the most likely candidates.

To explain the beneficial effects of the quiet eye, Vickers has proposed the **location-suppression hypothesis** (Vickers, 1996). She suggest that visual fixations of relatively long durations (2–3 seconds) are required for the mental programming of parameters (recall from Chapter 4 that parameters are the features that vary each time a skill is executed). The timing and force of muscular contractions, timing and coordination of limb movements, and the direction and velocity of objects or implements propelled must be programmed. As Vickers points out, this programming entails the organization of billions of neurons in the human brain, a process that requires the stability of visual information from which the motor program is assembled and which therefore benefits from a "quiet" duration in which incoming sensory sources do not change. Once a movement is initiated, however, Vickers suggests that performers use suppression mechanisms to block out interfering visual information that may arise from the performer's movements (e.g., a golfer seeing his club and arms move as he is striking the ball). Expert performers, she has found, subvert their visual attention during the execution of a skill through such techniques as blinking or blocking out conscious thoughts. This supports the suggestion in using quiet eye techniques that performers maintain their gaze on the target beyond the actual execution of the skill, thus blocking a shift in their attentional focus caused by shifting their visual gaze. By maintaining a fixed visual gaze, the performer's gaze stays in exactly the same location relative to the performer's body, so that the programmed movements are executed from the same initial conditions in which they were planned. Vickers acknowledges that this maintenance of gaze throughout a movement is difficult, but she observes that expert performers do maintain such fixation of gaze and that it is an aspect of skilled performance that can be readily learned and lead to significant improvement in performance accuracy.

This last point is especially relevant for motor skill instructors. Although most research on the quiet eye has focused on describing differences between expert and novice performers, evidence from other studies, as well as considerable practical experience, supports the conclusion that the quiet eye technique can be learned and applied to many motor skills by novices and that the learning of such techniques significantly enhances skilled performance. By identifying critical locations on which learners should fixate their visual gaze for a

location-suppression hypothesis: The notion that fixation of one's visual gaze on a specific location before and during the execution of a skill enhances performance by stabilizing processing activities.

particular skill, and helping learners understand and achieve quiet eye proficiency, motor skills instructors can promote the learner's effective use of his or her limited attentional resources.

SUMMARY

If the practice of motor skills is to be optimally beneficial, learners must first be sufficiently motivated, have established effective goals for practice, and be guided in attending to the proper environmental cues and states of mental focus.

- Motivation is characterized by activation and directionality.
- Motivation to learn a motor skill is influenced by many factors, including task relevance, task difficulty, perception of control, and success in meeting task goals.
- An especially effective method of influencing motivation is goal setting. Goals should be challenging, attainable, realistic, and specific.
- Goals should include outcome goals, performance goals, and process goals.
- Attention is conceptualized as a state of psychological and physiological activation directed toward a specific stimulus or stimuli and characterized as a limited resource that must be allocated selectively.
- A number of different theories have been advanced to explain attention; these can be classified into two broad categories: bottleneck and central-resource theories.
- Attentional focus can be conceptualized in a number of ways. A widely accepted model developed by Nideffer classifies attention into four distinct styles, including broad external, narrow external, broad internal, and narrow internal.
- Compared to novices, experts in various sports activities exhibit visual gaze control characterized as the "quiet eye" phenomenon. The quiet eye facilitates greater attentional control and can be learned by beginning learners in many movement skills.
- Through education and guidance, individuals can learn to prioritize limited attentional resources in ways promoting the most effective performance of motor skills.

LEARNING EXERCISES

1. For this exercise, identify an instructional situation involving the practice of movement skills (e.g., physical education or recreational class, physical therapy clinic, athletic team, dance practice, etc.). Make arrangements to observe a practice session for at least 30 minutes. Your task is to observe, record, and analyze factors during practice that impact the motivation of participants. You should, therefore, be well prepared to identify relevant factors affecting motivation prior to making your observations, as well as having planned methods for recording your observations during practice. After completing your observations, prepare a written report

analyzing the motivational climate you observed. What specific things did you observe that you believe played a role in promoting the motivation of participants? What things did the instructor(s) do that might have enhanced, or detracted from, the motivation of participants? What was your overall impression of how motivational the practice situation was? What recommendations would you make for improving the motivational climate in this situation?

2. For this exercise, you will develop a set of practice goals for someone who is a novice or who is in the early stages of learning a motor skill. Skills may include, as examples, sports skills, recreational activities, dance or musical skills, driving, learning to type or use a computer, rehabilitating an injury, or any other complex skill involving a movement component. Interview the person for whom you will be developing goals to assess his or her current skill level, personal motivations, and goals for practice, and commitment of time and resources that can be expected. From this information, develop a set of immediate, intermediate, and long-term goals for the individual. Schedule at least one period of discussion to go over your planned goals with the individual, making any refinements or adjustments necessary before preparing the final goal plan. Provide a written statement of your goal plan to the individual for whom it was prepared, as well

as a final report of your activities and the goals developed for purposes of completing this exercise. (*Note:* This exercise could be used as a class or group assignment, and could use members of the class as subjects.)

3. For this exercise, select a skill that you can perform correctly but in which you are not overly proficient (technically, a skill in which you are in the early associative or early advanced stage of learning; good skill examples include a basketball free throw, putting in golf, throwing darts, billiards, or target shooting, although many other equally good examples could be added). For the skill you select, prepare a plan for how the quiet eye method can be used when performing it. Consider the location best suited for the point of your visual gaze and how you will assure good time delays in holding your gaze prior to and throughout the execution of the skill. Plan a time to practice the skill and to apply the quiet eye principles you have developed for this exercise. Attempt at least a dozen practice attempts in your normal fashion prior to using the quiet eye technique. When you are ready, continue practicing, employing the quiet eye for another two dozen practice attempts. Take your time and focus on developing your skill using the quiet eye. As a result of your practice experience, prepare a report of your thoughts, performance observations, and conclusions regarding the quiet eye method.

FOR FURTHER STUDY

HOW MUCH DO YOU KNOW?

For each of the following, select the letter that best answers the question.

1. Definitions of motivation almost always include the concept of
   a. recognition.
   b. intention.
   c. activation.
   d. variability.

2. Which of the following factors would be most likely to enhance an individual's motivation for performing a task?
   a. The task is easily performed.
   b. Task performance is evaluated in comparison to an absolute standard.

c. The task is difficult to perform correctly.

d. The performer feels in control of his or her resources for learning the skill.

3. In the TARGET model for promoting a positive motivation climate in physical education, the letter "G" stands for what?
   a. Grouping
   b. Goals
   c. Grounding
   d. Getting

4. In Kahneman's theory of attention, the amount of attentional space available from which individuals can draw is expanded or contracted by the individual's level of
   a. motivation.
   b. cognition.
   c. arousal.
   d. confidence.

5. Driving a race car during a race on a crowded track would require what type of attentional focus, as classified in Nideffer's attentional style inventory?
   a. Narrow external focus
   b. Broad external focus
   c. Narrow internal focus
   d. Broad internal focus

6. Which of the following is a feature of the quiet eye?
   a. Rapid shifts in visual focus
   b. Closing eyes for one or two seconds before initiating movement
   c. Closing nondominant eye during initial phase of movement
   d. Fixation of gaze prior to movement execution

Answer the following with the word or words that best complete each sentence.

7. _____ is the concept that learners have control over their learning of a skill and that they have the resources to accomplish their performance goals.

8. In the acronym CARS, used to guide goal-setting, the "R" stands for what?

9. _____ goals focus on improving some specific aspect of a skill over a person's previous levels of performance.

10. Theories of attention holding that humans have a pool of attentional resources from which to draw, and that they can attend to several things simultaneously as long as sufficient resources remain available in the pool, are called _____ theories.

11. Bottleneck theories of attention offer an explanation for the _____, which is the observation that when two stimuli are presented at the same time, there is often a delay in the time it takes to respond to one of the two stimuli.

12. The capacity of _____ attention enables humans to focus on stimuli of their choosing, as well as to shift attention at will from one stimulus to another.

STUDY QUESTIONS

1. Define motivation and explain why it is a critical variable in the learning and performance of motor skills.

2. Describe the activation and directionality characteristics of motivation. Provide examples of both in the context of motor skills performance.

3. What factors significantly influence a person's level of motivation when performing movement skills?

4. How might differences in the performance context (e.g., skills practice, exercise, rehabilitation, and competitive sports) have a role in which factors motivate one's performance?

5. What is meant by motivation climate, and what are some of the factors that influence it? (Consider the TARGET model in your answer.)

6. How does the setting of goals influence the performance and learning of skills? Why does goal setting work?

7. Define outcome, process, and performance goals. Explain how each differs and why all three are important.

8. For what does the acronym CARS stand? Explain how it establishes guidelines for the setting of performance goals.

9. Define attention and explain why it is critical to skill learning.

10. Define, compare, and contrast bottleneck and central-resource theories of attention.

11. Describe the psychological refractory period and provide a sports-related or other example. What is the theoretical explanation of this phenomenon?

12. Define and provide an example of selective attention in a sport or other movement-related context.

13. Define attentional focus and describe Nideffer's four attentional focus styles.

Provide examples of skill performance situations best served using each of these styles of focusing attention.

14. Describe differences in visual gaze between expert and novice athletes as revealed in research by Vickers and her colleagues. How have these differences led to the description of the quiet eye? What four features does Vickers posit as defining the quiet eye?

15. How can the concept of the quiet eye be applied to learning situations with novice learners in different sport and motor skill situations? How has Vickers described the benefits of the quiet eye through the development of the location-suppression hypothesis?

ADDITIONAL READING

Filby, W, Maynard, I, and Graydon, J. (1999). "The effects of multiple-goal strategies on performance outcome in training and competition." *Journal of Applied Sport Psychology, 11,* 230–246.

Hall, HK, and Kerr, AW. (2001). "Goal setting in sport and physical activity: Tracing empirical developments and establishing conceptual direction." In GC Roberts (ed.), *Advances in motivation in sport and exercise* (pp. 183–234). Champaign, IL: Human Kinetics.

Jaakkola, T, and Digelidis, N. (2007). "Establishing a positive motivational climate in physical education." In J Liukkonen, YV Auweele, B Vereijken, D Alfermann, and Y Theodorakis (eds.),

Psychology for physical educators: Student in focus (pp. 3–20). Champaign, IL: Human Kinetics.

Nideffer, RM, and Segal, M. (2001). "Concentration and attention control training." In JM Williams (ed.), *Applied sport psychology: Personal growth to peak performance,* 4th ed. (pp. 312–332). Mountain View, CA: Mayfield.

Vickers, JN. (2004). "The quiet eye: It's the difference between a good putter and a poor one." *Golf Digest,* January, 96–101.

Wilson, VE, Peper, E, and Schmid, A. (2001). "Strategies for training concentration." In J Williams (ed.), *Applied sport psychology,* 5th ed. (pp. 404–422). New York: McGraw-Hill.

REFERENCES

American Automobile Association. (2008). "Cell phones and driving: Research update." Washington, DC: AAA Foundation for Safety.

Ames, C (1992). "Classrooms: Goals, structures, and student motivation." *Journal of Educational Psychology, 84,* 261–271.

Burton, D, Naylor, S, and Holliday, B. (2001). "Goal setting in sport: Investigating the goal effectiveness paradigm." In R Singer, H Hausenblas, and C Janelle (eds.), *Handbook of sport psychology,* 2nd ed. (pp. 498–528). New York: Wiley.

Filby, W, Maynard, I, and Graydon, J. (1999). "The effects of multiple-goal strategies on performance outcome in training and competition." *Journal of Applied Sport Psychology, 11,* 230–246.

Franken, R. (2001). *Human motivation,* 5th ed. Pacific Grove, CA: Brooks/Cole.

Hall, HK, and Kerr, AW. (2001). "Goal setting in sport and physical activity: Tracing empirical developments and establishing conceptual direction." In GC Roberts (ed.), *Advances in motivation in sport and exercise* (pp. 183–234). Champaign, IL: Human Kinetics.

Hardy, L, Jones, G, and Gould, D. (1996). *Understanding psychological preparation in sport: Theory and practice for elite performers.* Chichester, England: Wiley.

Henderson, JM. (2003). "Human gaze control during real-world scene perception." *Trends in Cognitive Science,* 7(11), 498–504.

Jaakkola, T, and Digelidis, N. (2007). "Establishing a positive motivational climate in physical education." In J Liukkonen, YV Auweele, B Vereijken, D Alfermann, and Y Theodorakis (eds.). *Psychology for physical educators: Student in focus* (pp. 3–20). Champaign, IL: Human Kinetics.

James, W. (1890). *The principles of psychology.* New York: Holt.

Kahneman, D. (1973). *Attention and effort.* Englewood Cliffs, NJ: Prentice Hall.

Kane, T, Baltes, T, and Moss, M. (2001). "Causes and consequences of free-set goals: An investigation of athletic self-regulation." *Journal of Sport and Exercise Psychology,* 23, 55–75.

Kleininna, P, Jr., and Kleininna, A. (1981). "A categorized list of motivation definitions, with suggestions for a consensual definition." *Motivation and Emotion,* 5, 263–291.

Landin, D. (1994). "The role of verbal cues in learning. *Quest,* 46, 295–313.

Liukkonen, J, Auweele, YV, Vereijken, B, Alfermann, D, and Theodorakis, Y. (2007). *Psychology for physical educators: Student in focus.* Champaign, IL: Human Kinetics.

Locke, EA, and Latham, GP. (1990). *A theory of goal setting.* Englewood Cliff, NJ: Prentice-Hall.

Locke, EA, Shaw, KN, Saari, LM, and Latham, GP. (1981). "Goal setting and task performance." *Psychological Bulletin,* 90, 125–152.

Nideffer, RM. (1976a). *The inner athlete.* New York: King Features.

Nideffer, RM. (1976b). "Testing attentional and interpersonal style." *Journal of Personality and Social Psychology,* 34, 394–404.

Nideffer, RM. (1981). *The ethic and practice of applied sport psychology.* Ithaca, NY: Mouvement.

Nideffer, RM. (1993). "Attention control training." In RN Singer, M Murphy, and LK Tennant (eds.). *Handbook of research in sport psychology* (pp. 542–556). New York: Macmillan.

Nideffer, RM. (2007). "Reliability and validity of the attentional and interpersonal style (TAIS) inventory concentration scale." In D Smith and M Bar-Eli (eds.), *Essential readings in sport and exercise psychology* (pp. 265–277). Champaign, IL: Human Kinetics.

Nideffer, RM, and Segal, M. (2001). "Concentration and attention control training." In JM Williams (ed.), *Applied sport psychology: Personal growth to peak performance,* 4th ed. (pp. 312–332). Mountain View, CA: Mayfield.

Petri, HL. (2003). *Motivation: Theory, research, and applications,* 5th ed. Pacific Grove, CA: Brooks/Cole.

Shea, CH, Shebilske, WL, and Worchel, SW. (1993). *Motor learning and control.* Englewood Cliffs, NJ: Prentice-Hall.

Vickers, JN. (1996). "Visual control when aiming at a far target." *Journal of Experimental Psychology: Human Perception and Performance,* 22, 342–354.

Vickers, JN. (2004). "The quiet eye: It's the difference between a good putter and a poor one." *Golf Digest,* January, 96–101.

Vickers, JN. (2007). *Perception, cognition, and decision training: The quiet eye in action.* Champaign, IL: Human Kinetics.

Weinberg, RS, and Gould, D. (2007). *Foundations of sport and exercise psychology,* 4th ed. Champaign, IL: Human Kinetics.

Wilson, VE, Peper, E, and Schmid, A. (2001). "Strategies for training concentration." In J Williams (ed.), *Applied sport psychology,* 5th ed. (pp. 404–422). New York: McGraw-Hill.

Zelinsky, GJ, Rao, RPN, Hayhoe, MM, and Ballard, DH. (1997). "Eye movements reveal the spatial temporal dynamics of visual search." *Psychological Science,* 8(6), 445–453.

Answers to How Much Do You Know questions: (1) C, (2) D, (3) A, (4) C, (5) B, (6) D, (7) Empowerment, (8) Realistic, (9) Performance, (10) central-resource, (11) psychological refractory period, (12) selective.

CHAPTER 10

Instructions and Demonstrations

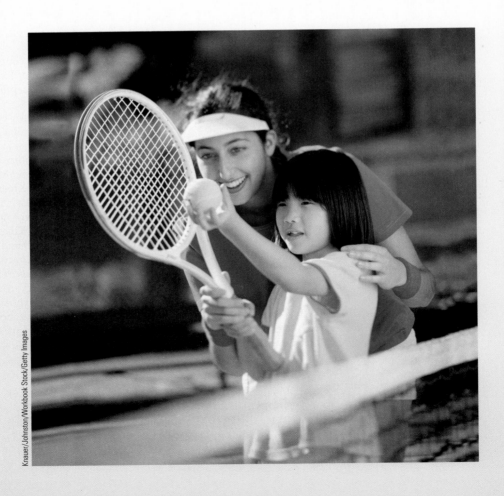

Knauer/Johnston/Workbook Stock/Getty Images

A mind without instruction can no more bear fruit than can a field, however fertile, without cultivation.
Cicero (c. 50 BC)

KEY QUESTIONS

- What types of pre-practice information are provided by verbal instructions and visual demonstrations?

- What are the most effective methods for providing verbal instructions?

- What is the difference between internal and external attentional focus when providing verbal instructions? Which is the most effective?

- What are the most effective methods for providing visual demonstrations?

- How do the characteristics of a model influence the quality and effectiveness of skill demonstrations?

- What are motor neurons? How might they explain the processes involved in learning?

CHAPTER OVERVIEW

If you needed surgery, would you be satisfied with a surgeon who had never been instructed concerning how to perform an operation? What if in the middle of a trans-Atlantic flight, you learned while cruising at 35,000 feet that the pilot flying the airplane you were on had never received flight training? Or what if on the first day with your new golf instructor, she informed you that she had never had a lesson in her life but had picked up all she needed to know simply by playing on her own? Would you ask for your money back and head to the clubhouse in search of a new instructor?

The problem in all of these scenarios, of course, is that we instantly recognize that people do not learn most skills adequately apart from the provision of formal instructions (and in the case of movement skills, demonstrations) provided by trained instructors. Even when a person may have acquired many hours of independent practice, we intuitively know that most motor skills are rarely, if ever, capable of being performed expertly apart from sufficient amounts of instructed practice.

Verbal instructions and visual demonstrations are critical to the effective acquisition of complex motor skills. They provide information necessary for successful practice that a learner would be incapable of discerning on his or her own. When delivered effectively, verbal instructions and visual demonstrations provide the learner optional practice experiences and the best opportunity for significant improvements in learning to occur. In this chapter, you will learn what is known about the provision of these two forms of practice guidance, and how instructions and demonstrations can be provided in ways offering learners the greatest opportunity for skill learning.

––––––––––––

When learning motor skills in formal instructional settings, information on how to perform the skills being practiced is typically provided in two different ways: verbal instructions and visual demonstrations. Both instructional methods convey to the learner information concerning the goals and proper mechanics of the task to be performed. Such information may be delivered before practice begins, as well as intermittently during a practice session. In either case, though, such information is task independent. That is, it conveys information concerning goals and techniques of skill performance based upon a learner's specific needs and stage of learning, but it does not address the results of any specific practice attempt. In this regard, verbal instructions and visual demonstrations are global in nature and address the general goals and requirements of skill development. Task-specific information about the consequences of particular practice attempts, which can be provided either during or after a practice attempt for purposes of either correcting performance errors or sustaining correct actions, is considered feedback and is the subject of Chapter 12.

Given the critical role they play in skill acquisition, it is pedagogically imperative that practitioners be capable of delivering instructions and demonstrations supported by sound theory and reliable empirical evidence. Far too frequently, however, techniques for providing these essential informational sources are based instead upon tradition, intuition, and emulation (Williams and Hodges, 2005). Considerable research supports the conclusion that practice based upon such subjective experiences is often ineffective and may actually hinder a learner's skill development (Hodges and Franks, 2005; Wulf, 2007; and Zemke, 1999). It is critical to good instructional practice that practitioners have a strong working acquaintance with current research findings addressing the important role played by pre-practice information (i.e., information provided prior to the performance of a trial or series of trials during a practice session), and knowledge of the most effective methods for providing instructions and demonstrations based upon such scientific evidence.

This chapter reviews the findings of empirical research on the role played by verbal instructions and visual demonstrations in the acquisition of motor skills, informing guidelines for their delivery based upon the best that current knowledge has to offer. How much do we currently know about providing instructions and demonstrations in the most effective manner? The answer to this question is that we understand a good deal, certainly enough to guide effective practice, but that a good deal also remains to be learned. Although other practice variables such as motivation, practice scheduling, and feedback

"Listen, watch, and learn" are frequent words of wisdom from parents, teachers, and coaches. The questioning learner might ask, "What should we listen to, what should we watch?" and the questioning teacher must equally decide what to tell and what to show.

—Nicola J. Hodges and Ian M. Franks (2004)

have received considerable attention from scholars and researchers over the years, the effects of various forms of instructions and demonstrations on skill acquisition have received relatively little attention. Though there is a strong indication that this lack of scholarly interest has begun to change, much work still remains to be done, and many questions remain unanswered or debated. Hodges and Franks (2002) have stated that "little scientific consensus exists about the role pre-practice information plays in the learning process, beyond the sometimes necessary role of relaying to the learner the goals of the task" (p. 794). Still, much that is valuable is known about how to increase the effectiveness of instructions and demonstrations, and the questions that remain have opened new and challenging avenues awaiting exploration (Shea et al., 2002). As new research is revealing, pre-practice instructions and demonstrations, properly combined with physical practice, can afford unique opportunities for learning.

VERBAL INSTRUCTIONS

Verbal instructions are a part of nearly every formal practice setting. They provide important information about both general and specific aspects of skill performance. Verbal instructions tell the learner what to think about and what to do. They help the learner acquire an appreciation and understanding of performance requirements and goals, direct actual practice performance, enhance learner confidence, promote skill learning, reinforce correct behaviors, and serve as a basis for the evaluation of learning goals. Provided correctly, they guide the learner's practice attempts toward optimal learning outcomes.

The provision of effective verbal instructions entails more than just "telling." To be effective, instructions need to be tailored to the learner and his or her specific needs and situation. This is really the initial key to providing good instructions. Movement skills instructors are typically highly skilled at the activities they instruct and may as a result fail to adequately appreciate the needs of beginners. What may seem obvious to the instructor can present a significant challenge for a beginner. Knowledgeable instructors recognize the needs of learners at various stages of skill development, including those of novice learners, and provide instructions that are developmentally appropriate. In doing so, instructors need to consider a number of features inherent in verbal instructions, including (1) the amount of information conveyed by instructional statements, (2) the precision of the information provided, (3) the critical features of the skill and environment, and (4) the skill outcomes on which learners should focus their attention.

Amount of Information

limited attentional capacity: The notion that individuals can only attend a limited amount of information at any one point in time, beyond which processing capabilities begin to be compromised.

As stated in the previous section, effective instructions begin with an empathetic consideration of the learner's developmental limitations and needs. Perhaps the first consideration along these lines is recognition of the limited capacity that learners have, especially when they are beginners, for attending to instructional information. We previously saw when discussing memory (Chapter 6) that humans have a **limited attentional capacity** for the amount of information that can be held and acted upon in short-term memory. That is,

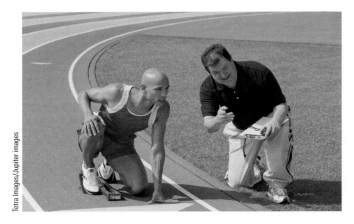

Tetra Images/Jupiter images

Verbal instructions help learners understand task requirements and goals.

a person can attend to only a limited amount of information at any one time; when too much information is presented within a single context, a person's ability to process it is overwhelmed. When practicing a new motor skill, in particular, a person is presented with numerous memory challenges at any single point during practice. Not only must the general goal of the skill be kept in the forefront of memory, but also: the patterning of muscular forces and timing, possibly over a system of multiple joints, must be coordinated; environmental features must be attended to and taken into account; balance and posture must be maintained; movements of others may have to be anticipated and responded to; and equipment may need be manipulated. Even simple motor skills may easily require responding to over a thousand items of information per second, and complex skills to many times that (Vanderbilt, 2009). Add to this the need on the part of the learner to divide attention between his or her actual performance and an instructor's directions about how to perform, and it is easy to see how the mental capacities of a learner can be easily overwhelmed. In fact, the principle cause of confusion on the part of those initially practicing new motor skills is typically the provision of too much information at any one time by well-intentioned but poorly informed instructors. As a general rule, instructions should be brief and to the point, focusing attention on a limited amount of information, perhaps only a single item or two at any one time. In the initial stages of learning, instructors should focus on providing the most elementary and basic information required, that which is most necessary to the execution of a new skill. As learners progress, instructions can become more detailed and be directed more toward the refinement of basic movement patterns.

Precision of Information

Learners can easily become confused by instructions that are nebulous and developmentally inappropriate. Telling a student in a softball class to "hug first-base more" may be the correct instruction for a given situation, but she may not understand what she is being asked to do. Instructions can also appear vague and cause confusion for relatively inexperienced learners when they are overly generalized. A patient learning to use crutches probably does not possess sufficient experience to respond correctly when instructed to "Contact the ground further out with the points of your crutches before starting your body swing," but probably can reliably interpret the instruction to "Place the point of your crutches one foot length in front of your toes." Descriptions that may seem clear to instructors because of their experience with a skill can be confusing to beginners who need more exact and precise movement descriptions.

When providing instructions to beginners, instructors should focus on providing descriptions that are quantitatively meaningful. "Step out one foot" rather than "Step out a little"; "Rotate your hips forty-five degrees" rather than "Rotate your hips more"; and "Keep no more than your body length from the base" rather than "Hug the base more" are examples. In each of these examples, the second way of stating the instruction could be interpreted in different ways by learners, but the first way of stating the instruction is precise and clearly conveys what the instructor intends.

Effectively communicating instructional goals can also be facilitated by using knowledge of skills that learners already possess. Many skills share similarities in movement patterns, for instance, and instructional communication can be greatly enhanced by drawing a learner's attention to those aspects shared by a skill currently being learned and one that is already possessed. For example, instructing a novice learner in the correct mechanics of the tennis serve might be accomplished with the instructions to "throw the head of the racquet at the ball." This instruction conveys considerable information to the learner because many mechanical aspects of the tennis serve are similar to the act of throwing a ball, a skill that most people possess to at least some degree of proficiency. The forward swing of the arm must be precisely coordinated with the rotation of the server's hips, for example, a difficult timing pattern for someone initially learning the skill. Transferring the movement patterns of ball throwing to the tennis swing, however, can greatly reduce the need for providing instructions on this aspect of the tennis serve. Instructors of motor skills should devote sufficient time and thought to developing a repertory of instructional procedures and images facilitating effective communication between themselves and learners (see Box 10.1).

BOX **10.1**   Good Verbal Instructions Are Precise

For the following instructions (and sports), think of two or three ways you could convey the same information in a more precise way.

- "Choke-up more on the bat." (baseball/softball)
- "Bring the club head back further." (golf)
- "Lift your arm higher." (lateral arm raises with a light weight for rehabilitation)

- "Turn sooner." (turning corners in a driver's education class)
- "Bring your knees in." (back-flip in gymnastics)
- "Do not release the ball so soon." (bowling)
- "Take bigger steps." (gait training for a Parkinson's patient)

The Use of Verbal Cues

verbal cue: A word or short phrase directing a learner's attention to a critical aspect of skill performance or of environmental factors influencing skill performance.

One way that practice information can be conveyed while limiting the attentional demands placed upon learners is through the use of verbal cues. **Verbal cues are words or short phrases that direct a learner's attention to some critical feature of skill performance.** Verbal cues can direct the learner's attention to a critical feature of the environment ("Watch the ball") or of a movement pattern ("Swing through the ball"). Well-conceived verbal cues provide effective instructional tools for both beginning and advanced learners. Research studies have demonstrated that well-developed and presented verbal cues have a significant impact on the amount and quality of learning that occurs during instructed skill practice (Rink, 2009). In designing verbal cues, instructors should consider four specific aspects of such instructions.

Verbal Cues Should Focus on Critical Features of Skill Performance

As already stated, motor skills instructors should strive to avoid overloading the limited attentional capacity of learners. One of the most important factors making verbal cues effective is that, when properly designed, they convey important instructional information in a brief and concise way. In limiting the amount of instructional information to which learners are exposed, instructors must focus verbal cues on those features of a skill that are the most critical to performance and learning. When designing verbal cues, instructors should begin by performing a critical and careful analysis of the skill to be instructed and of the most important features necessary to its proper performance. From such an analysis, critical features can be prioritized and the most important selected for initial instructional presentation. Even instructors who are well acquainted with a skill can often benefit from consulting authoritative sources such as textbooks, instructional videos, and experts in the skill area. However the information from which verbal cues are drawn is arrived at, it is of paramount importance that the most important features be correctly prioritized and that the information presented be accurate. Just as good verbal cues play a significant role in promoting good learning outcomes, inaccurate verbal cues can hinder learning. Accurately formed, verbal cues focus learners' attention on appropriate environmental and bodily features of performance, and significantly enhance learning.

Verbal Cues Should Be Stated Succinctly

Verbal cues should convey an immediately understandable and clear impression of the action required. To this end, verbal cues should consist of brief, succinct statements clearly directing the learner's attention to the action or environmental feature required without the need for unnecessary mental processing. Indeed, the meaning of a verbal cue should ideally be immediately discernible and easily grasped. Most experts suggest that no more than three or four words comprise verbal cues (Masser, 1993). To help learners grasp the intent of cues, words that convey a type of action are often useful (e.g., *snap, pull, hit, twist, punch, kick out, press*, etc.)

An exception to limiting the number of words included in a cue can occur when instructing skills having an internal rhythmic pattern. In such cases,

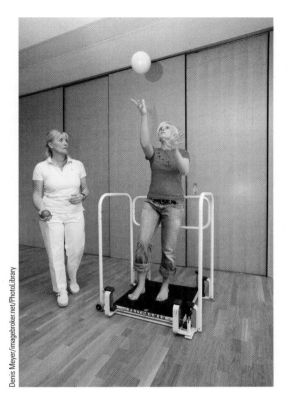

Denis Meyer/imagebroker.net/PhotoLibrary

Instructors should use verbal cues to direct learners' attention to critical features of the performance context.

longer sequences of words may be useful. The linkages between components of closed and serial skills often possess timing patterns that can be meaningfully expressed in rhythmic phases. Movement skills in aerobic and dance routines might, for example, be expressed by verbal cues something like "One-two-three-four-turn-slide-slide-hop." Such phases can be used by an instructor to guide an ongoing action, and can also be acquired by learners who can then use the cue as a method of "self-talk" to help remember and perform required actions.

Limit the Number of Verbal Cues Used to Those Most Needed at Any Point during Learning

Keeping in mind the need to limit demands placed upon learners' limited attentional resources, the number of specific cues used at any one point in the stages of learning should be limited to those most critical to a learner's progress. In the initial stage of learning, which we have previously seen as being labeled either the *cognitive stage* or *novice stage* (Chapter 7), two or three cues may be sufficient. Beyond that number, learners may begin to confuse the requirements of different cues, especially if more than a single cue pertains to the same action or environmental feature. Remember that one benefit of verbal cues is to keep learners' attention focused on those features of a skill most in need of their attention and practice at any particular time.

As learners progress into the middle stage of learning (i.e., associative or advanced), additional cues may be added in order to direct their attention toward new features of skill performance. Additional cues should only be added, however, as learners are able to respond to them appropriately without showing signs of hesitation or confusion. Although instructors need to be sensitive to the needs and attentional capabilities of individual learners, it is unlikely in most cases that the use of more than seven to nine verbal cues will prove beneficial in optimizing learning outcomes, and the elaboration of too many cues will eventually lead to confusion on the part of learners and detract from practice performance and its effectiveness for learning.

Repeat Verbal Cues Frequently

The repetition of the same verbal cues frequently during practice helps the learner form a strong association between the cue and the required action or environmental awareness. Especially in the initial stages of skill practice, frequent presentation of a verbal cue whenever the specific cue-relevant action is attempted can reinforce the connection between eliciting events or features and correct responses. As learners form stronger associations, instructors can gradually reduce the frequency of verbal cues in specific situations to encourage learners to recall and act upon the cues themselves.

To summarize, effective verbal cues should convey critical information that is developmentally appropriate and succinct, and should be limited in number and repeated frequently in the early stages of learning (see Boxes 10.2 and 10.3).

Attentional Focus

To what should learners pay attention when practicing a motor skill? The answer to this question may seem obvious at first: People should pay attention

---

BOX 10.2   Guidelines for Using Verbal Cues

- Cues should focus only on the most critical performance aspects of a skill or of environmental factors influencing skill performance.
- Cues should clearly direct the learner's attention to the critical aspects of performance.
- Generally, cues should contain no more than four words.
- Cues should contain action words indicating what the learner is to do.
- Cues should be precise and include quantitative information when appropriate (i.e., how many feet, how many degrees, "point to two o'clock," etc.).

- Meaningful images may also be used to guide action (i.e., "Make a 'T' with your body.," "Drop the apple in the basket," "Ring the bell," etc.).
- Limit the use of cues to no more than three or four in the early stages of learning; the number can be increased as learning progresses (though an upper limit of seven to nine is typically an optimal number of cues to actively use for instructional purposes).
- Encourage learners to repeat cues subverbally when they execute skills (i.e., "self-talk").
- Repeat cues frequently, especially in the early stages of learning.

to how they are performing the skill. That is, they should pay attention to how they move, to the bodily mechanics of a movement skill. If you are going to throw a ball, for instance, you must pay attention to how your limb movements are coordinated. What does your arm do? How much do you rotate your hips? Which comes first, hip rotation or arm action? Or are these movements timed together in some way? Given the perceived priority of such questions, it would appear apparent that a learner's attention should be focused on such aspects of movement. That is, learners should focus their attention on the actual movement patterns involved in producing a skilled action.

For a long time, this view predominated. In recent years, however, this prevailing view has been challenged and the premises upon which it is predicated brought into question (e.g., Byers, 2000; Hodges and Franks, 2004; Williams and Hodges, 2005; Wulf 2007; and Wulf and Prinz, 2001). To understand why this traditional view of the role of instructions has been challenged, we need to make a brief detour to consider the **problem of perception–action coupling** (review Chapter 2 for a discussion of this problem). In performing any skill, two distinct processes can be identified, which are labeled *perceptual processes* and *action processes*. First, the performer must perceive what is in the environment. This entails sensory information about external conditions. This information is transmitted over ascending pathways to cortical areas in the brain where it is organized, encoded, and brought to perceptional awareness (see Chapter 3). The second series of processes are action processes. Based upon perceptual information, a person decides upon, organizes, and initiates a motor response. Signals are conveyed over descending pathways to appropriate muscles to complete the responding action.

These two distinct processes result in two different kinds of mental information. Perceptual information forms what is known as an **event code**. The event code is shorthand for sensory information concerning the state of the environment. It is information that must be attended to and potentially acted upon. Information concerning the organization of an appropriate motor response forms an **action code**. The action code is formed by the mental operations involved in commanding a muscular response (in cognitive-based theories, action codes are motor programs). All voluntary motor behavior is, of course, a combination of event codes and action codes—that is, a combination

problem of perception–action coupling: The limitations of science in explaining how perceptual sensory information is turned into motor actions.

event code: Sensory information that has been encoded and brought to perception; information about a person's environment.

action code: Information encoded within the motor system related to the execution of some action.

BOX **10.3**   **Designing Verbal Cues**

For the following skills, suggest a verbal cue based upon the guidelines provided in this chapter for a beginner learning each skill. You may focus on a cue related to either the environment or movement pattern involved in each skill—or suggest a verbal cue for both!

- Free throw in basketball
- Performing CPR
- A social dance step with a partner
- Returning a tennis serve
- Handstand
- Downhill skiing

of perception and action. The problem of perception–action coupling comes in explaining how these two kinds of codes communicate with one another.

Traditionally, it was believed that event and action codes could not directly communicate. Like two individuals speaking different languages, direct communication was viewed as impossible. It was believed that a translator was required, just as with speakers of different languages. In this case, though, some transformation or translation of cognitive codes is required in order that perceptual events might be turned into motor actions. The exact nature of this translation has filled many volumes of neuroscience texts and need not concern us here. What is of concern is the conclusion that such a view leads to in terms of the proper role of instructions. In this view of perception–action coupling, an essential role of instructions is to promote the learning of mental operations responsible for translation. Individuals learn the rules of translation by becoming sensitive to what a proper response to a specific situation feels like, or, vice versa, by learning what happens when particular motor actions are produced. Given sufficient practice, learners can come to automatically match motor responses with desired perceptual outcomes. The focus of instructions in this view, therefore, is on learning to recognize the relationship between action and effect.

The theoretical bases for these conclusions were sharply challenged by a new view of perception–action coupling emerging in the 1990s, however (Hommel, 1996; Hommel and Elsner, 2000; and Prinz, 1992, 1997). In a seminal paper, Prinz (1997) proposed a new framework for understanding the functional relationship between perception and action. In this view, event codes and action codes are represented within a common cognitive domain. Prinz called this the **common coding approach** to perception and action. According to this approach, perceived events and planned actions share a common representational domain. That is, a cognitive translator is not required—action and effect are capable of direct communication. (This same premise is shared by Gibson's ecological theory discussed in Chapter 3, often considered one of the foundational assumptions of dynamical systems theory as applied to motor skills.)

An important premise of the common coding approach for the provision of motor skill instructions is that the execution of bodily movements (actions) are always coupled to representations of their effects. This idea actually goes back to the beginnings of psychology (Bliss, 1892–1893, and Boder, 1935). The **Bliss-Boder hypothesis**, an old principle in the psychology of learning, predicts a performance decrement when a performer thinks about body movement patterns or action plans during or immediately before the execution of a skill. Even Sigmund Freud (1922) recognized the ill effects of paying too close attention to how skills are performed, stating that "Many acts are most successfully carried out when they are not the object of particular concentrated attention . . . mistakes may occur just on those occasions when one is most eager to be accurate" (p. 23). Intuitively, many athletic coaches have for years cautioned their athletes about focusing too much attention on the actual movement patterns they use in executing skills. A commonly heard phrase in athletics expressing this caution is "Paralysis by analysis." In fact, this idea was the focus of a number of popular sports skill books marketed in the 1970s and 1980s concerning

common coding approach: The proposition that sensory and motor codes share a common domain and are capable of direct communication.

Bliss-Boder hypothesis: The idea that paying too much attention to one's movement patterns can disrupt efficient performance.

the "inner game" (i.e., mental game) of various skills. In one of the best sellers in this genre, Gallwey (1982) recommended that tennis players, when switching sides of the court, ask the opponent what he is doing to make his forehand so good that particular day, thus encouraging the opponent to think about his movements and thus disrupt his performance.

But if paying attention too closely to bodily movements when performing motor skills is detrimental, to what should performers pay attention? In answer to this question, Prinz (1997) suggested the **action effect hypothesis**. According to Prinz, because action and perception share a common domain and are directly linked, actions are best planned and controlled in relation to their perceptual consequences. Put most simply, actions should be planned in terms of their intended effect.

Based upon the implications of new theories of perception–action coupling such as Prinz's action effect hypothesis, motor skill researchers began to rethink the traditional approach to the provision of instructions which had emphasized the performer's actual movement pattern (see Hodges and Franks, 2005; and Wulf, 2007, for good reviews). In the first study to investigate the implications of such new conceptualizations for motor skills, Wulf, Hob, and Prinz (1998) studied the comparative effects of instructions directing learners' attention either to a movement itself, or to the effects of the movement. Instructions which focused learners' attention on the actual movement patterns involved in producing the skill were labeled as having an **internal focus of attention**, while instructions directing learners to the effects of their movements were labeled as having an **external focus of attention**.

In their study, Wulf and her colleagues had novice subjects learn a slalom-type movement on a ski simulator. The ski simulator device consisted of two bowed rails and a platform on wheels which could be moved across the rails, but which was continuously returned to the center by elastic bands (see Figure 10.1). The object of the task was for participants to move the platform sideways by exerting force on it in either direction, simulating slalom movements in skiing. The greater the amplitude of the subjects' movements (the greater distance back and forth from one side to the other) and the faster they could make them (the greater the frequency of side-to-side movements in a given time), the better the performance. Subjects were divided randomly into one of three different groups: an internal attentional focus group, an external attentional focus group, and a control group. The internal focus group was instructed to focus their attention on the force exerted by their outer foot in moving the platform. That is, when subjects wanted to move to the right, they concentrated on pushing with their right foot; and when they wanted to move to the left, they concentrated on the force produced by their left foot. The external focus group, in contrast, was instructed to concentrate on the force they exerted on the wheels of the platform directly under their feet, with force being placed on the right wheels when they wanted to move to the right, and on the left wheels when they wanted to move left. This may seem like a minor difference as the subjects' feet and the wheels of the platform were close to one another. The researchers hypothesized, however, that because the difference in instructions between the two groups was so minimal, any observed differences in learning would

---

action effect hypothesis: The concept that actions are best planned and controlled in relation to the desired effect of the action.

internal focus of attention: Attention directed toward the movement patterns used in generating a motor response.

external focus of attention: Attention directed toward the effects of a motor response within the environment.

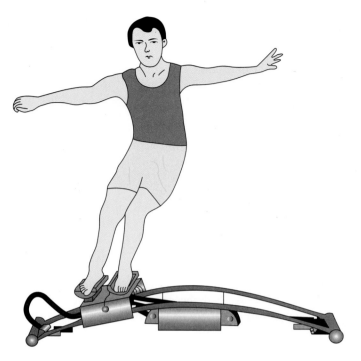

FIGURE **10.1** Ski Simulator Task Used by Wulf, Hob, and Prinz

Source: Adapted from Wulf, G, Hob, M, and Prinz, W (1998). "Instructions for motor learning: Differential effects of internal versus external focus of attention." *Journal of Motor Behavior, 30,* pp. 169–179.

strongly indicate that differences in attentional focus were the cause. A third group of subjects served as a control group and were provided with the same instructions as the two experimental groups concerning the goals of the task, but were not provided with instructions about where to focus their attention. This group was included so that the researchers could determine how effective, or perhaps ineffective, the internal and external focus groups were when compared to individuals left to their own devices and free to explore the performance environment.

All subjects in this experiment completed eight 90-second acquisition trials on each of two consecutive days. Appropriate instructions, either internal or external focus, were provided to participants before every other trial, beginning with the first trial (with the control group receiving no such instructions). One day after the acquisition trials were completed, a retention test was given. All subjects were tested on six 90-second trials. During these retention trials, however, none of the subjects were provided with instructions; instead, they were simply told to do their best.

Results of this study showed a clear advantage for the external focus group on both acquisition and retention trials (see Figure 10.2). All three

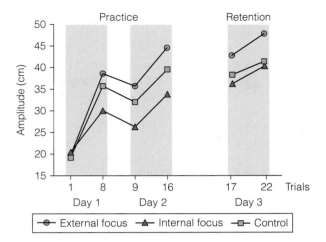

FIGURE **10.2** Results of Wulf, Hob, and Prinz Experiment

Source: Results of Wulf, Hob, and Prinz Experiment, *Journal of Motor Behavior* by Wulf, G, Hob, M, and Prinz. Copyright 1998 by Taylor & Francis Informa UK LTD - Journals. Reproduced with permission of Taylor & Francis Informa UK LTD - Journals in the format Textbook via Copyright Clearance Center.

groups performed similarly on the first trial of day one, producing amplitudes of approximately 20 cm (8 inches) to either side. (The maximum amplitude to either side, and therefore the maximum performance score obtainable, was 50 cm, or 20 inches.) Over the two days of acquisition trials, however, the external focus group demonstrated considerably greater improvements in performance than either of the other groups, obtaining a final average amplitude of 47 cm compared to 41 cm for the control group and 35 cm for the internal focus group. Interestingly, the group receiving internally focused instructions did not perform as well over practice sessions as did the control group receiving no instructions. Results of this original investigation of attentional focus effects was even more dramatic given the results of the retention test, however, because such results more accurately reveal the true measure of learning. The external focus group maintained its performance advantage averaging 47 cm on the final retention trial, compared to 41 cm for the control group and 40 cm for the internal group. Thus, the group provided instructions having an external attentional focus showed both better practice and learning outcomes than those receiving internally focused instructions, or no instructions at all. Perhaps as surprising, the internal focus group showed no better learning outcomes than did the group receiving no instructions. (Indeed, the results of this experiment were so contrary to prevailing beliefs of the time that the researchers were required to perform a second series of similar experiments to verify their results before their conclusions were accepted for publication.)

Since this original research was reported, many other studies have supported the conclusions reached. A number of sports skills have been investigated and similar findings reported; for instance, Maddox, Wulf, and Wright (1999) reported on the advantages of an external focus in learning the backhand stroke crosscourt in tennis. In their study, participants were instructed to either focus on the movement pattern of their swing (internal focus) or the trajectory of the ball and its landing point (external focus). Those following external focus instructions performed significantly better over both acquisition and retention trials. A transfer test also demonstrated that the external focus group was more proficient when performing the backhand to the opposite side of the court from the one they had practiced. Significantly, an analysis of the internal and external groups by expert raters also revealed that the external group's better performance was not obtained at the expense of technique, but that both groups rated similarly in the quality of their movements. In another study on the effects of practice instructions on learning a pitch shot in golf, Wulf, Lauterbach, and Toole (1999) instructed beginning golfers to either focus on the swing of their arms (internal focus), an instruction typical to golfing practice, or to focus on the pendulum-like motion of their club (external focus). Again, the external focus group performed significantly better than the internal focus group in both acquisition and retention trials. Other studies have reported similar advantages for an external attentional focus in basketball (Al-Abood et al., 2002), soccer (Wulf, Wachter, and Wortmann, 2003), football (Zachry, 2005), jumping (Wulf et al., 2006), balancing (Marchant, Greig, and Clough, 2005), and dart throwing (Marchant, Clough, and Crawshaw, in press, reported in Wulf, 2007). Examples of internal and external attentional focus are shown for a number of skills in Table 10.1. A perusal of this table should prove helpful in developing strategies for providing verbal instructions in specific skills.

Distance Effects

As we have observed, the benefits of focusing on the effects of one's movements rather than on the actual movement itself appears to be pronounced across a wide range of skills. There are, of course, many different movement effects to which learners could pay attention. One that has generated considerable interest is distance effects. Based upon early research studies, a number of researchers noted a tendency for the effects to which learners attend to be more or less beneficial as a function of their distance from the body. Specifically, the further an effect is from the bodily movements producing it, the more powerfully it appears to benefit learning. As one possible explanation for this observation, Wulf (2007) has speculated that "effects occurring in close spatial proximity to the body are less easily distinguishable from the body than are more remote effects" (p. 67).

To test this hypothesis, McNevin, Shea, and Wulf (2003) conducted a study in which they varied the distances of the effects to which subjects attended. The task they employed was a stabilometer task, basically a center-hung balance platform on which subjects stand while attempting to maintain the platform in a horizontal and level attitude. On the platform were two markers about three feet apart and each an equal distance from the center of the platform.

TABLE **10.1**
Internal and External Focus for Various Skills

Skill	Internal Focus	External Focus
Pitch shot in golf	Swing motion of arms	Pendulum-like motion of golf club
Throwing a ball	Arm movements	Path of the ball
Drive block in football	Explosive extension of body	Opponent driven back
Playing the piano	Accuracy of hand and finger movements	Quality of sound
One and a Half Gainer in springboard diving	Tuck knees close to body	Fast reverse rotation
Walking using crutches	Arm movements controlling action	Location where crutch tips are placed in front of body
Jump-and-reach	Force produced by legs	Target for finger touch
Dance routine	Individual steps	Path of dance steps
Turning corner while driving an automobile	Hand and arm movements controlling steering wheel	Motion and direction of car
Soccer kick	Kick ball with instep of foot	Kick ball with laces of shoe
Forearm pass in volleyball	Keep thumbs together and lock elbows	Pass ball low
Casting in fly fishing	Arm motion and wrist snap	Spot where fly is to land in water
Roller skating	Pressure exerted by feet	Pressure exerted by skate wheels on surface
Distance running	Mechanics of running	Environmental features (scenery along route)
Tennis serve	Coordinate arm movement with hip rotation	Visualize throwing racquet head at ball

All subjects were instructed to place their feet just behind these markers, which were called the *near markers*. Two other sets of markers were presented during the experiment. One set of markers was placed inside the near markers close to the center of the platform so that they almost touched; these were called the *far-inside markers*. Another set of markers was placed outside of the near markers at a distance of about 1.5 feet from each near marker; these were called the *far-outside markers* (see Figure 10.3).

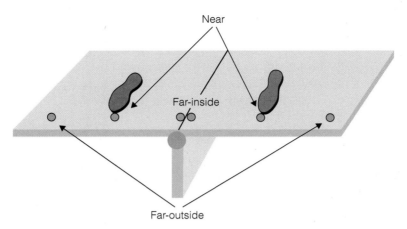

FIGURE **10.3** Marker Placement for Study
by McNevin, Shea, and Wulf (2003)

Source: Marker Placement for Study by McNevin, Shea, and Wulf (2003), *Journal of Motor Behavior*
by Wulf, G, Hob, M, and Prinz. Copyright 1998 by Taylor & Francis Informa UK LTD - Journals.
Reproduced with permission of Taylor & Francis Informa UK LTD - Journals in the format Textbook via
Copyright Clearance Center.

Subjects in this experiment were divided into three groups. All groups were
instructed to look forward toward a wall in front of them rather than to watch
the platform or any of the markers. All groups, however, were also instructed to
think about keeping one of the sets of markers horizontal to one another so that
the platform remained level and in balance. One group was instructed to keep
the near markers level to one another (near focus group), another to keep the
far-inside markers level (far-inside focus group), and the third group to keep
the far-outside markers level (far-outside focus group). The results supported
the original hypothesis in that both far groups (far-inside and far-outside) performed significantly better on both acquisition and retention trials than did the
near group. In fact, the two far groups performed approximately the same over
acquisition and retention trials. The researchers speculated, based upon these
findings, that the distance of the effect from the body is the critical factor in
enhancing the instructional benefits of an external focus, rather than the direction of the effect.

How far from the body an effect should be to maximize the benefits of an
external attentional focus remains a debated topic. Perhaps once the effect is
sufficiently distanced from the body to prevent any comparison with bodily
movements, the advantages of further distancing evaporate. What does seem
presently clear, however, is that practitioners should provide instructions focusing learners on external effects that are distinctly distinguishable from bodily
movements. Without more exact guidelines, practitioners will need to rely
upon their best professional intuition in forming such instructions. Hopefully,
further research will help to clarify this issue more exactly.

Directing Attentional Focus

Although the role played by promoting an external attentional focus through verbal instructions now appears well established, a number of important questions still remain. Possible differences in the effectiveness of an external focus are not well understood across various types of skills, for instance. There are also many different sources of information that could be used as focal points for internal and external instructions, and these have yet to be fully explored. Nor have the relationships among individual differences in learning styles, stage of learning, and psychological preferences been sufficiently investigated. There is some preliminary evidence, for instance, suggesting that those in the initial stages of learning may benefit most from a combination of internally and externally focused instructions (Perkins-Ceccato, Passmore, and Lee, 2003). Finally, the potential interaction between an external focus of attention and other instructional variables such as demonstrations, practice schedule, and feedback also remains to be explored.

Guidelines for providing externally focused instructions remain somewhat nebulous in several areas and await additional research for a more complete development of strategies that can be used by the practitioner. Until such strategies are more fully developed and supported through research, practitioners will need to exercise considered judgment in deciding how best to provide instructions focused on the effects of movement in their areas of instructional expertise (Box 10.4).

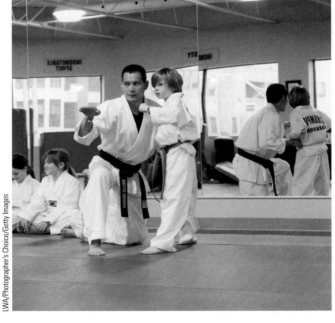

LWA/Photographer's Choice/Getty Images

Directing learners' attention to the external effects of their actions has been found to enhance learning in many instances, and may yet prove a general principle of learning.

VISUAL DEMONSTRATIONS

Although verbal instructions play a critical role in motor skill learning, visual demonstrations are the most frequently used method of conveying information to learners. It is easy to understand why this is so. Most motor skills, even relatively simple ones, require complex patterns of coordinated limb and body movements. Think about attempting to verbally describe to someone how to tie shoelaces, perform a dance routine, do a somersault, or hit a baseball. It is extremely difficult, if not impossible, to adequately convey how to perform these skills in words alone. Indeed, our natural tendency is to show someone how such skills are performed. The adage "A picture is worth a thousand words" reflects our natural human impulse to show rather than to tell.

Though demonstrations may be the most prevalent method for conveying practice information, they should not replace, but complement, verbal instructions. Verbal instructions may be limited in their capacity for conveying complex information about how to move when compared to demonstrations, but as we have seen, one advantage of verbal instructions is conveying to learners "what to pay attention to." An exclusive reliance on demonstrations, in fact, may focus learners' attention upon internal movement aspects of a skill, thus blocking attention directed to a movement's effects. In discussing the role of demonstrations, we must keep in mind that a combination of instructions and demonstrations is, in most cases, most effective for the presentation of practice information.

Keeping in mind the symbiotic relationship of instructions and demonstrations, demonstrations still play the primary role in helping learners grasp the basic movement patterns required when practicing new skills. An understanding of what constitutes effective demonstrations is therefore an essential link in the chain of instructional tools for effectively communicating skill practice information. And just as with verbal instructions, our understanding of what constitutes effective demonstrations has undergone significant revision in recent years. In the following section, we will explore some of these new perspectives as they inform methods for providing the most effective demonstrations for learners. Some brief background concerning the theory behind these recent methodological recommendations, however, is first necessary.

BOX 10.4 Directing Learners to an External Attentional Focus

For the following activities, think of how you could provide an instruction for each that would focus a learner's attention on an effect external to the movement itself.

- Kicking a football for an extra point
- Shooting an arrow at a target
- Ice skating
- Hammering a nail
- Learning to use a walker
- Bowling
- Parallel parking
- Walking using a walker
- Playing a guitar

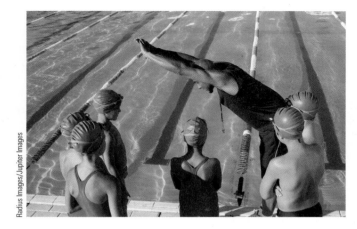

The ability to provide effective visual demonstrations is an essential skill for motor skill instructors.

Theoretical Considerations Supporting Research on Motor Skill Demonstrations

Visual demonstrations have long been viewed as an effective method for transmitting patterns of thought and behavior (Wesch, Law, and Hall, 2007). As early as 1896, the British psychologist C. Lloyd Morgan, based upon his observations of how animals learn, described imitation as an innate faculty of both animals and humans. Throughout the middle years of the last century, psychologists adhering to the behaviorist tradition, like Guthrie (1935), Hall (1943), Miller and Dollar (1941), and Skinner (1938, 1966), applied concepts of reinforcement to the study of imitative behavior, demonstrating that people not only learn through watching others, but that they also acquire attitudes motivating their acceptance or avoidance of those behaviors based upon the consequences such behaviors have for those performing them. In 1969, a cognitive psychologist named Albert Bandura proposed a new theory of how people learn through observation that eclipsed many of the premises and conclusions of previous theories. Recognizing that learning by observing others was a much more complex phenomenon than mere imitation shaped through reinforcement, Bandura preferred the term **observational learning** to describe the complex set of behaviors acquired through observing others. As he stated, "Learning would be exceedingly laborious, not to mention hazardous, if people had to rely solely on the effects of their own actions to inform them what to do. Fortunately, most human behavior is learned observationally through modeling: from observing others, one forms an idea of how new behaviors are performed, and on later occasions this coded information serves as a guide for action" (Bandura, 1977, p. 22).

Bandura's theory, which he originally called *social learning theory* but later revised to *social cognitive theory* (Bandura, 1986), has been the predominant theoretical foundation for most research relative to the demonstration of skills (motor and otherwise) since the theory's introduction. Over the years, Bandura

observational learning: The learning that occurs as a result of observing another perform a skill.

social cognitive theory: A theory advanced by Albert Bandura that all learning is observational by nature and occurs within a social context.

(1977, 1986, 1997) has refined and developed his theory. Since Bandura's social cognitive theory is, as its name suggests, a cognitively based theory, it has received challenges in the motor learning literature by those espousing a dynamical systems approach (see Scully and Newell, 1985, for a dynamical systems critique of social cognitive theory). Still, most research concerning the role of demonstrations in motor skill learning has been carried out under the auspices of social cognitive theory. We will therefore focus our discussion on Bandura's ideas as they have forged our current understanding of the role demonstrations play in the learning of motor skills. It should be noted that the empirical results of research on the effects of visual demonstrations conducted under assumptions of social cognitive theory are not challenged by dynamical systems theorists, who limit their critique to the underlying mechanisms responsible for those findings. Although important and interesting, these theoretical differences need not overly concern us in the search for practical guidelines for delivering effective demonstrations.

According to Bandura (1977), there are four distinct subprocesses that govern observational learning:

1. Attention
2. Retention
3. Reproduction
4. Motivation

The beginning of the observational learning process is attention. In order to learn, a person must first pay attention to a model engaged in a certain behavior. Bandura believed that attention is a selective mechanism. The information to which a learner attends is both externally and internally determined. Externally, the complexity of the modeled event (the number of parts in a skill, the coordination patterns involved, the speed with which it is modeled, the skill's distinctiveness, etc.) influences the learner's attention level. Attention is also influenced by internal determinants such as the learner's interest, awareness of salient factors to which attention should be directed (a primary role of practice instructions), previous knowledge, the functional value of the modeled task, and arousal level, among other factors. Bandura held that attentional level could be particularly enhanced by emphasizing the most important and relevant features of a skill to be learned, as well as by alternating good and bad performances of the skill. He also believed that various characteristics of a model, particularly the model's status relative to the observer, influenced attention level. See Box 10.5 for a consideration of factors influencing learner attention.

The second stage of the observational learning process is retention. Attending to modeled behavior would be ineffective if learners could not retain the information gained from their observations. For learning to occur, observed patterns of behavior must be transformed into representational form and stored in memory. Bandura believed that this process was the function of two subprocesses he called the *imaginal* and *verbal*. Imaginal processes refer to the abstraction of patterns and regularities from visual information. According to social cognitive theory, not all the elements of a skill need to be retained. Rather, an abstraction of relevant features is encoded and stored in memory. This is the same contention as postulated by schema theory (see Chapter 7). The cognitive processes that mediate behavior are believed to be verbal in nature. Bandura held that both visual demonstrations and verbal instructions were important for the formation of the memories underlying skilled behaviors.

Once retained, the observer must possess the capabilities to reproduce an action that is a copy of the observed behavior as represented in memory. Reproduction, the third stage of observational learning according to Bandura, refers to the active rehearsal of an observed skill. Because Bandura's primary interest was in the learning of social behaviors, he paid relatively little attention to this aspect of learning, although he did stress that practice helps to stabilize and strengthen an acquired response. In his later writings, Bandura (1986) did argue for an enhanced role of rehearsal for learning motor skills.

Finally, the fourth stage of observational learning is motivation. This final stage brings us back to the initial stage of attention. Bandura held that the degree to which someone is motivated to acquire a new behavior dramatically influences his or her level of attention. To encapsulate his ideas concerning motivation, he proposed the concept of self-efficacy (Bandura, 1997). **Self-efficacy**, simply stated, is a measure of one's confidence or belief concerning his or her ability of accomplishing an observed skill. The greater a person's self-efficacy, his or her belief that he or she possesses the ability to perform a modeled behavior, the more information he or she will be able to obtain and retain through observing a model. Demonstrations can play an important role in enhancing learners' level of self-efficacy, particularly when the model is assumed to have similar capabilities as those possessed by the observer. A summary of the four stages of observational learning is presented in Table 10.2.

self-efficacy: An individual's belief in his or her ability to master a task or skill.

Research on the Role of the Model in Observational Learning

Research into the effectiveness of modeling on motor skill learning has investigated a number of model characteristics predicted by Bandura's social cognitive theory to influence the effectiveness of demonstrations. Those characteristics receiving the most attention include the model's status, skill level, and similarity to the observer.

BOX **10.5**   **Attention-Grabbing Demonstrations**

Think about a time when you learned a motor skill from an instructor who taught you the skill using visual demonstrations. What was it about the way the instructor modeled the skill that attracted your attention? What was it about the way he or she modeled the skill that detracted from your attention? In other words, what worked and what

did not work about the instructor's demonstrations? Think of three things that were best about the skill demonstrations with which you were instructed and three things that were the least effective. Keep these features of your experience with skill demonstrations in mind as you continue reading this chapter.

TABLE **10.2**
Stages of Observational Learning

Bandura's theory of observational learning describes four stages in the learning of skills, with each stage influenced by the quality of visual demonstrations and modeling of skills, and all four stages necessary for the effective learning of motor skills.

1. **Attention**

Learner must observe and pay attention to a person engaged in the skill to be learned (i.e., a "model"). The learner's attention is influenced by his or her interest, motivation, previous experience, complexity of the skill being modeled, knowledge of the important skill features to which he or she should attend, arousal level, and model characteristics, among others. *Demonstrations should be developmentally appropriate to learners, focus attention on important skill features, and be accurate enough that they can be correctly imitated.*

2. **Retention**

Learners must be able to remember what the model has done. The model's movement patterns must be successfully encoded into memory and stored in a form readily retrievable. *Demonstrations, in connection with instructions such as verbal cues, should focus attention on the critical features of movement patterns such as transitional body positions and beginning and ending points of movement patterns. Accurate modeling of skills in the early stages of learning should be sufficient to convey correct images of movement patterns. The number of skill features modeled, and to which the learner's attention is verbally directed, should be limited in the early stages of learning so that attentional resources are not exceeded.*

3. **Reproduction**

The learner must be able to replicate the observed skill. Observed skills must be adequately rehearsed in order to stabilize and strengthen acquired responses. *Demonstrations can reinforce the correct reproduction of observed behaviors, demonstrate incorrect behaviors to be eliminated, and be expanded to include skill and performance context variations. Feedback plays an important role in this stage in conveying to learners how effectively they are reproducing observed behaviors.*

4. **Motivation**

The learner's degree of self-efficacy, his or her belief in being able to reproduce and acquire the observed skill, influences motivation which, in turn, enhances attention to subsequent observations (the four stages forming a continuous loop in the learning process). *The use of learning models can enhance a learner's belief that he or she can acquire the modeled skill, thus increasing feelings of self-efficacy and promoting further learning. Self-efficacy is also promoted by reinforcing and rewarding correct practice behaviors and patterns of skill performance.*

Status of Model

It has been known for some time that the social status of a model influences an observer's attention and likelihood of repeating the model's behavior. In an early study, Lefkowitz, Blake, and Mouton (1955) demonstrated that a jaywalking model dressed fashionably in business attire would induce significantly more passersby to jaywalk across a busy street than would a model dressed shabbily in soiled clothes. In developing social cognitive theory, Bandura (1986) hypothesized that characteristics of a model influence the attention phase of learning. He believed that a high-status model would elicit greater attention than a low-status model and therefore have a greater impact on learning. Although there have been few studies on the effect of model status in the literature, those that have been reported generally support slightly greater learning outcomes when observing a high-status as compared to low-status model.

In the first direct study on the influence of model status on motor learning, McCullagh (1986) had subjects learn a climbing task on the Bachman ladder, which consists of a 6-foot wooden ladder attached at the base to a pivot so that performers must maintain their balance while climbing. The number of rungs on the ladder that subjects can climb before losing their balance is taken as the measure of performance. Prior to practicing this climbing task, subjects first observed a model demonstrating how the task was to be performed. However, one group of subjects was told that the model demonstrating the task was especially highly skilled, while the other subject group, who watched the same model, was told that the model was not highly skilled and that they would be expected to do better. Because both groups observed exactly the same model performing the task, it was hypothesized that any differences between the two groups must be the result of attentional differences based upon perceived differences in model status. As predicted by McCullagh, the group of subjects who observed the model whom they perceived as having a high status did better on acquisition and retention tests than did those believing the model to have a low status, even though in fact both groups observed the same model.

Subsequent investigations have, however, failed to demonstrate a consistent pattern of superior learning when observing high-status models relative to the learning of motor skills (McCullagh and Weiss, 2001). Although the research reported does tend to support a slight benefit from observing high-status models, such differences do not now appear to play a major role in the effectiveness of modeling for motor skills.

Skill Level of Model

According to the predictions of social cognitive theory, expertly modeled skills are more beneficial to the encoding of memorial representations and therefore more effective in promoting learning. This conclusion resonates with considerable popular opinion. Indeed, many experts in the instruction of motor skills firmly believe that models should demonstrate skills correctly and as expertly performed as possible. Such beliefs are typically based upon the idea that learners encode and remember exact copies of the skills they observe. It would seem logical, therefore, to assume that the better a skill is performed, the better will be the representation of it formed in memory, thereby enhancing the learning of the skill. Observing skills poorly or even incorrectly performed, on the other hand, would logically seem to lead to the learning of bad habits. This line of reasoning underlies the popularity of the extensive commercial marketing of instructional videos by famous athletes and other experts. Indeed, many millions of dollars are spent every year on videos featuring various sports experts demonstrating how to perform the perfect golf swing, tennis serve, bowling motion, baseball pitch, dance routine, etc. Do such experts really make the most effective models, however?

So prevalent, and seemingly incontrovertibly logical, is the notion that modeled behaviors are best when they are correctly and expertly performed, that few learners or practitioners have stopped to question such wisdom, at least until fairly recently. Then in a 1986 review of a series of experiments, Jack Adams, a prominent motor learning theorist, proposed that observing models engaged in learning a skill might prove just as effective, if not even more so, than watching experts demonstrating a skill. Adams coined the terms **expert model** and **learning model** to differentiate between models who were highly skilled at a particular task and could demonstrate it correctly, if not perfectly, and those who were relatively unskilled but learning a motor task. In several experiments contrasting the benefits of expert and learning models that followed Adams' review in close succession, a number of researchers reported finding superior learning benefits from observing learning models when compared to expert models. In the first such study, McCullagh and Caird (1990), in an exploration of subjects learning a timing task, found that those subjects who first observed a learning model had better acquisition and retention performance than did those first observing an expert model demonstrating the task. Pollock and Lee (1992) compared two groups of subjects learning a computer tracking game, who observed either an expert or learning model prior to practicing the game, with a group of similar subjects not observing a model before practice. Their findings showed substantial observational learning for the two groups who observed a model compared to the no-model condition, but no differences between the groups observing the expert and learning models.

Given the contradictions between McCullagh and Caird's findings and those of Pollick and Lee's, Hebert and Landin (1994) suggested that the benefits of observing a learning model might be enhanced if subjects did not merely first observe the learning model performing a skill, but also heard corrective feedback provided to the model. To test this hypothesis, they had groups of female college students who were novice in tennis practice a tennis volley shot. Two groups of subjects observed a learning model prior to practice, with one group watching a learning model who received corrective feedback to which the subjects could attend, and a second group watching a learning model who received no feedback. A third group of subjects received feedback on their practice trials but did not observe a model. Results showed that both groups who observed the learning model performed better in both acquisition and retention tests than did the group receiving feedback on their own performance but without the benefit of observing a model. Of the two groups observing a learning model, the group who observed a model receiving feedback demonstrated both the best acquisition and retention measures.

expert model: A skilled model who demonstrates a skill correctly.

learning model: A person learning a skill who demonstrates both correct and incorrect aspects of performance relative to the model's stage of learning.

Results of these experiments demonstrated that the observation of a learning model could prove just as effective for purposes of learning as could observing an expert model, and that the learning model might, at least in some cases, prove better for learning. As to why learning models may be beneficial, it can be argued that motor learning is an essentially cognitive activity rather than one based upon mere imitation. Cognitive theories of motor learning, such as Schmidt's schema theory and Bandura's social cognitive theory, view skill acquisition as a problem-solving process. Especially important in this view is the role of feedback, which learners use to correct behaviors and develop their own error-correcting capabilities. As such, the observation of expertly modeled skills may block the problem-solving process because it fails to provide information concerning errors and how they might be corrected (Horn and Williams, 2004). When learners are observing a learning model, however, they are presented with the model's errors, which can serve as a source of cognitive problem solving on the observer's part. The benefits of observing a learning model without the provision of corrective feedback, therefore, are likely dependent upon the observer's knowledge and ability to detect errors and improvise corrective strategies on their own. The research literature clearly indicates, however, that the most critical factor in observing a learning model is that the observer receives the model's feedback. In contrasting expert and learning models, Darden (1997) has pointed out a number of important ways in which learning models present greater cognitive challenges, and therefore greater learning opportunities, compared to expert models for relatively unskilled observers. These are presented in Table 10.3.

TABLE **10.3**
Differences between Expert and Learning Model Demonstrations

Expert Model	Learning Model
The Model Should Represent	
• High status	• Similar status (peer)
• High-level performance	• Performance just above student's current level
• Repeated, continuous demonstrations	• Varied demonstrations
• Correct performance	• Correct performance + errors
• Verbal cues with demonstrations	• Verbal cues + instructor feedback with demonstrations
• Identification of model's correct technique	• Identification and correction of model's errors
• One correct technique	• Exploration of several task solutions
• Encouragement of mimicry and exact reproduction	• Encouragement of problem solving and thinking

Adapted from Darden, GF. (1997). "Demonstrating motor skills—Rethinking the expert demonstration." *Journal of Physical Education, Recreation and Dance*, 68(6), 31–35.

Similarity of Model

One model characteristic that may help explain the effectiveness of learning models is the similarity of a model to an observer. It has long been recognized that learners respond especially favorably to models they consider similar to themselves (McCullagh and Weiss, 2001; Rosenthal and Bandura, 1979). Presumably, those observing a model may believe themselves more capable of copying the model's behavior if they also see themselves as similar to the model in capability and stage of learning. Observing a similar model should, as suggested by Bandura, enhance an observer's feelings of self-efficacy and thereby increase motivational levels important for attending to and learning from modeled behaviors.

In a test of this hypothesis, Gould and Weiss (1981) had female college students perform a muscular endurance task (the leg extension) after watching one of two models. One group of women observed a nonathletic (similar) model demonstrating the task, whereas a second group observed an athletic (dissimilar) model demonstrate the task. Measures of both performance and self-efficacy were obtained. Results showed that those subjects who observed a similar model prior to practice scored higher on both performance and self-efficacy measures compared to those observing the dissimilar model. In a follow-up study, George, Feltz, and Chase (1992) replicated Gould and Weiss's study, but added the variable of sex by having both similar and dissimilar models of both sexes. Their results showed that both performance and self-efficacy were influenced by the similarity of a model's ability, but not by a model's sex. That is, the women who observed the similar (nonathletic) model, regardless of whether the model was male or female, performed better and gained more in self-efficacy than those women who observed the dissimilar (athletic) model of either sex. In a more recent study in which elementary school-age girls learned a scarf-juggling task, Griffin and Meaney (2000) have reported that same-sex models influenced the learning of performance strategies, although not actual retention or transfer of task skills.

The relatively limited research evidence available would seem to support the use of similar learning models, most likely because such models increase feelings of self-efficacy in learners, enhancing their motivational levels. Exactly which characteristics of a model are most relevant when similar to an observer's and how significant a role model's similarity is in the learning process, however, await further research.

Guidelines for Providing Effective Modeling of Skills

As our discussion has pointed out, research has brought into question a number of traditional beliefs and practices about the most effective methods of modeling motor skills for learners. Although additional research is needed to more fully explicate the complex and essential role of demonstrations in the learning process, a number of guidelines for providing effective demonstrations are well-supported by the scientific literature. A listing of some of the main findings and their implications for practice follows. Although not every guideline suggested can be followed in every learning situation, the assiduous use of these guidelines when providing demonstrations can frequently enhance learning outcomes.

The use of learning models for demonstrating skills can be just as effective, and in some cases more effective, than demonstrations performed by expert models. Growing and convincing evidence supports the conclusion that a novice who is learning a motor skill can be an effective model for demonstrations. Both cognitive and dynamical systems approaches to motor learning propose that a critical feature of the learning process is allowing learners to explore possible task solutions. From this perspective, an expert model may actually hinder the learning process. Learners should be encouraged to think about and find the best ways to move for themselves rather than merely mimic a model's behavior.

When using learning models, observers should be supplied with the model's feedback whenever possible. Learning models should be distinguished from those who are merely unskilled. To be the most effective, the observer should be privy to corrective feedback from an external source (teacher, coach, therapist, etc.) concerning a learning model's performance. A key to good learner modeling is that the observer be able to watch the model practice, receive feedback, and make corrections. Watching a model receive feedback and attempt task solutions encourages observers to engage in active problem-solving activities. Rather than observing movement patterns only, the observer perceives information about the strategies the model uses to correct errors, and can then decide whether it is best to apply the same or an alternative strategy during practice.

The use of models that observers view as similar to themselves, whether expert or learning models, is to be preferred. A number of studies have revealed that when learners observe models who share important similarities with them such as status, age, and sex, they perform and learn better than when observing a dissimilar model. Watching a model similar to oneself can make the modeled skill seem more within the reach of the observer's capabilities. It appears most likely that similar models promote better motivation on the part of observers by increasing observers' feelings of self-efficacy.

Use members of a group being instructed (i.e., class, team, etc.) as learning models. When demonstrating skills for a group, especially once a skill has been modeled several times correctly, ask individual members of the group to model the skill for the group, during which time feedback is provided. Having more than one group member model the skill will provide an opportunity to demonstrate critical features of the skill performed correctly while providing an opportunity to correct different errors. Be sure that the model demonstrating in front of the group is rewarded for those aspects of the skill he or she performs correctly, as well as for his or her contributions to the group.

To increase instructional effectiveness when teaching large groups, the use of peer models (a form of learning model) can be an effective method of providing demonstrations. When dealing with large numbers of learners, an effective method of implementing learning model demonstrations is to pair learners. Using this technique, one partner practices a skill for a number of trials while the other partner observes. After a certain number of practice trials, the pair alternates roles. One effective strategy is to provide the observer with a checklist of key aspects of the skill. The observer then looks for these key aspects and provides feedback to the performing partner. Under this scenario, the demonstrating partner benefits from the provision of corrective feedback, while the observing partner benefits from engaging in problem-solving activities while observing the partner's demonstrations. Small groups of learners may also be organized instead of learning pairs. Instructors can organize groups according to skill level, thereby enhancing the similarity of the learning model to observers. Feedback can then be provided either by an instructor or by alternating peer observers.

Mix demonstrations by expert and learning models for greatest effectiveness. Although learning models have important advantages when compared to expert models, the expert model is still the best way of demonstrating correct movement patterns. Creative instructors will gain the advantages of both model types by effectively mixing expert and learning model demonstrations. The expert model can be used to provide learners with an overall perspective of a skill, particularly in the initial stage of learning. Thereafter, the intermittent provision of expert modeling can be used to reinforce correct techniques, while the learning modeling is used to promote those cognitive processes important to learning.

Provide demonstrations before practice begins, and then space demonstrations throughout practice for the greatest benefit. For beginners, demonstrations provide the most effective means of conveying the general idea of how a skill is to be performed. Learning theory supports the importance of sufficient demonstration prior to actual practice so that learners comprehend the basic requirements of the movement patterns to be practiced. Once actual practice begins, demonstrations should continue to be provided as frequently as needed. Research has demonstrated that as learners progress through the stages of learning, they gain different kinds of information from observing models, and that in each stage of learning demonstrations play an important role in the learning process (Carroll and Bandura, 1990; Hand and Sidaway, 1993; Weeks and Anderson, 2000).

Arrange learners for the most effective viewing angles when observing demonstrations. How a model is positioned relative to an observer or observers when demonstrating is a consideration of practical concern, but one that has received little research attention in the literature (McCullagh and Weiss, 2001). One issue is whether models should face observers (called *mirror modeling*) or face away from them (thus making right and left orientations the same for model and observer). Traditionally, facing away modeling has been preferred because observers do not have to then rotate the mental image they observe before enacting movement. Models may also use a reverse mirror modeling technique to accomplish the same goal, facing observers but reversing right and left side movements so that both model and observer move in the same direction. Research has suggested, however, that the mental processes required in such image adjustments prior to overt practice may actually benefit learning by increasing the depth of cognitive processes involved in enacting the observed movement patterns (Ishikura and Inomata, 1995). When dealing with large groups of learners, whether facing away or mirror modeling is used, it is important to consider group arrangements that provide the best viewing angle for all learners (see Figure 10.4). It is also important to remember that learners need not only to clearly see demonstrations, but must also be able to clearly hear feedback and instructions provided during the demonstrations. Some formations, such as a circle pattern with the model in the center, are relatively

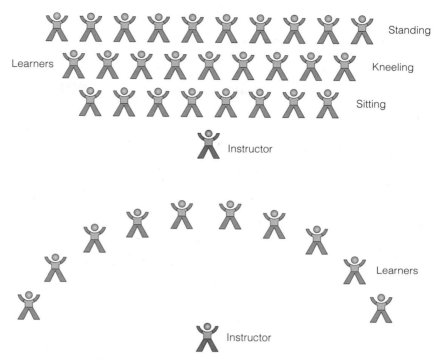

Standing

Learners

Kneeling

Sitting

Instructor

Learners

Instructor

FIGURE **10.4** Examples of Good Formations for Skill Demonstrations

Source: Adapted from Coker, CA (2004). *Motor learning and control,* 2e, pg. 170-172.
© 2009 Holcomb Hathaway Publishers.

ineffective because those learners positioned to the right or left of the model will have their view of some elements of the demonstration obscured. Another problem with a traditional circle formation is that learners will not see the demonstration from the same perspective, making the provision of feedback and instructions problematic. Good formations for providing demonstrations allow for all learners to clearly see the model from the same perspective and to be able to easily attend to salient aspects of the modeled skill.

Promising New Directions of Research on Observational Learning

As is the case with verbal instructions, scholarly attention on the role of visual demonstrations has fallen victim to greater interest in other areas of skill learning until fairly recently. Although the renewed interest in demonstrations and observational learning is encouraging and has already resulted in many new insights concerning the best ways of presenting demonstrations, further research is still needed to more adequately understand the role of visually modeled information when acquiring motor skills. This renewed focus on observational learning has received an unexpected boost in a recent discovery of potentially great importance to our developing understanding of how people acquire and control movement behaviors. This has been the discovery of the mirror neuron.

Mirror Neurons

One of the most exciting discoveries in neuroscience has been the recent identification of the brain's mirror neuron system. This discovery has been hailed as one of the most important findings in the history of neuroscience (Ramachandran, 2007). Offering new insights into many areas of human behavior, this discovery of **mirror neurons** has special significance for our understanding of the role demonstrations play in motor learning.

mirror neurons: Neurons that become activated when an animal or person is performing a particular action or watching another perform the same action.

The mirror neuron system was discovered quite by accident (a serendipitous and not uncommon happening in science). In 1992, an Italian research team at the University of Parma was conducting an experiment on monkeys designed to determine which areas of their brain were activated when grasping and moving objects. In their research laboratory, a monkey sat in a special chair, wires implanted in the region of its brain involved in planning and carrying out movements. Every time the monkey grasped and moved an object, specific cells in its brain would fire, activating a display of brain waves on a monitor and registering a "binging" sound. One day while the researchers were out, a graduate student entered the laboratory with an ice cream cone in his hand. The monkey stared at the graduate student. When the student raised the cone to his lips, an unexpected and amazing thing happened—the monitor sounded: "bing, bing, bing . . . ." Even though the monkey had not moved, the cells in its brain involved in planning and carrying out grasping and lifting movements became excited simply by observing the graduate student producing similar movements. Prompted by the graduate student's report, the researchers soon found that the same brain cells fired when the monkey watched humans or other monkeys bring peanuts to their mouth as when the monkey itself brought a peanut to its mouth (see Figure 10.5). In subsequent studies, the researchers found that cells fired when the monkey broke open a peanut or heard someone break open a peanut. The same thing happened with bananas, raisins, or any other object (see Rizzolatti and Sinigaglia, 2006, for a description of these experimental findings).

What the researchers had discovered, or at least stumbled upon, was a special class of neurons in the brain they soon labeled *mirror neurons*. Mirror neurons are neurons that fire both when an animal performs an action, and when it observes another animal performing the same action. These special neurons mirror the behavior of other animals, just as though the observing animal were performing the action itself. If the findings for monkeys were unexpected, however, the next discovery was even more unexpected. More recent research has revealed that humans also have mirror neurons, and that they are in fact far more flexible and highly evolved than those found in monkeys or any other animals so far studied. In fact, it is now known that the human brain has multiple systems of mirror neurons that are specialized for various activities including both motor and social behaviors (see Rizzolatti and Craighero, 2004, for a review).

In one of the first studies to identify mirror neurons in humans, researchers in England studied dancers from London's Royal Ballet and experts in capoeira, a martial arts dance form (Glaser, 2007). Both groups of dancers watched short videos of ballet and capoeira dance routines while lying

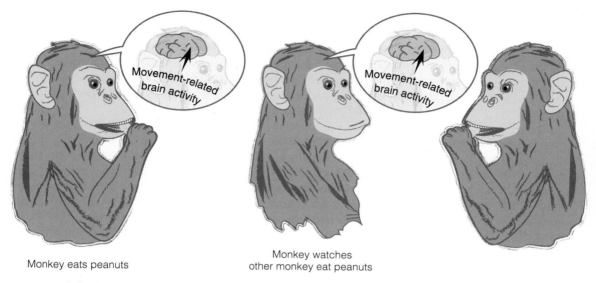

Monkey eats peanuts

Monkey watches
other monkey eat peanuts

FIGURE **10.5** The Mirror Neuron System: "Monkey See, Monkey Do"

perfectly still in an MRI brain scanner. A control group of nondancers also participated in the study. Two parts of the brain were monitored—the visual cortex, where visual signals of what we observe are processed, and the pre-motor cortex, the area of the brain involved in movement planning and execution (see Chapter 3). The same pattern of brain activity was observed in the visual cortex for all subjects. However, there was a distinct difference in pre-motor cortical activity among the groups. For the two groups of dancers, mirror neurons in the pre-motor cortex became excited when observing the dance form in which the subjects were expert, but not when observing the form in which they were not experienced. The control group of nondancers showed no increased activity of the mirror neuron system when watching either dance form. Even though the dancers were not moving, the part of their brains that controlled the dance movements in which they were expert acted the same as though they were actually dancing, although they were in reality only observing others.

It is now believed that mirror neurons are responsible for the planning and initiation of voluntary movements, though not the actual execution of movement (Rizzolatti and Craighero, 2004). That is, mirror neurons direct movement skills. Any skill that has been sufficiently practiced, even to only a minimum degree of proficiency, is encoded into the relevant mirror neuron system. It is the mirror neurons that activate the appropriate neural network to organize and activate muscular commands in order to accomplish a skill. And the system of mirror neurons is turned on when observing an action in another, whether one's own muscular system is initiated or not. We might think of mirror neurons as analogous to an engine in an automobile. The engine can be turned on whether or not the car is shifted into gear and actually moves. Similar to the transmission in an automobile, it now appears that a "neural gate" controls whether signals from the motor neuron system are sent to the musculature. The astonishing fact is, though, that once an individual has gained some experience, even minimally, with a specific skill, the mirror neurons controlling that skill are activated and strengthened (i.e., learning occurs) whether actually performing the skill or watching someone else perform it.

Even though the discovery of the mirror neuron system is still relatively recent and much remains to learn about it, it is now clear that the mirror neuron system plays an essential role in learning voluntary movement skills. The discovery of this system promises to focus new attention on the role of visual demonstrations in the learning of motor skills. Some recent studies have shown, for instance, that mirror neurons can be activated by observing only partial aspects of movements and that some parts of a movement are more essential than others in this process (Hamilton et al., 2007), the implication being that the demonstration of some features of skills may be more important than other features in promoting learning (Box 10.6). It has also been shown that mirror neurons are not only activated when a person sees an action (i.e., someone jump), but also when hearing the action (i.e., the sound of landing the jump) or even hearing the word describing the action (i.e., *jump*) (recall the earlier suggestion that instructions are more effective when action words are used).

The finding that the brain can simulate a learned skill simply through observation also has potential therapeutic relevance. Visual training protocols may, in the future, be developed to assist injured athletes retain skills during periods of recovery, as well as to better rehabilitate individuals whose motor skills have been damaged or impaired. The discovery of mirror neurons also promises an expanded role for visual training and psychological techniques involving imaging in the training of motor skills. The promise of the future is that as we learn more about mirror neurons, we will better understand the nature of motor learning and will be able to design methods that are more effective for providing demonstrations, mental training, and rehabilitative protocols.

BOX **10.6**   *Mirror Neurons Allow Us to Learn by Observing Others*

Somehow our brains must be able to learn from others. . . . To learn to make a spear, for instance, we have to convert the sight of someone else's manipulations into something very different—the nerve impulses required to move our own hands in similar fashion. Mirror neurons appear to have solved this difficult task: each time we see an action, they transform this sight into the motor commands necessary to replicate the action. While we watch an expert perform a series of action components, one after another, until a spear is made, our brain activates similar action components in the same order, composing the novel sequence of spear-making. . . .

—Christian Keysers (2009)

SUMMARY

Although physical practice is essential for the learning of motor skills, the provision of pre-practice information through verbal instructions and visual demonstrations can significantly influence the effectiveness of that practice. Correctly provided, they can reduce confusion, increase learner motivation, and significantly facilitate learning.

- When providing verbal instructions, motor skills instructors must take into consideration the limited attentional capacity of individual learners, keeping instructions brief, clear, and precise.
  - In the initial stage of learning, instructions should generally focus on the most elementary and basic information needed for practice performance.
- Research has recently highlighted the benefits of an external attentional focus when providing verbal instructions.
  - Although the benefits of an external attentional focus appear well established, many questions concerning its most effective use remain to be explored.
- Demonstrations can convey information concerning complex movement patterns that would be impossible to communicate verbally.
- Bandura's social cognitive theory has provided the theoretical framework for most research concerning observational learning and the presentation of demonstrations for motor skill learning.
  - According to social cognitive theory, four stages are essential for effective learning to occur as a result of observation; these are attention, retention, reproduction, and motivation.
- A number of model characteristics influence the effectiveness of demonstrations, including model status, skill level of model, and similarity of model to the learner.
- The recent discovery of the mirror neuron system has supported the effectiveness of observational learning and represents a promising avenue of research into the most effective methods of providing demonstrations as well as many other areas of skill learning.

LEARNING EXERCISES

1. For this exercise, you are to obtain permission to observe a professional (teacher, therapist, coach, trainer, etc.) instructing a motor skill in which both verbal instructions and visual demonstrations are used (typically involving learners in the initial or early stages of learning). During the actual observation of practice, position yourself where you can both see and hear the instructor clearly (you might need to work these arrangements out with the instructor prior to practice). You should observe at least 20 minutes of practice, taking notes on what you observe. Your task, once the observation is completed, is to prepare a

written report detailing your observations of the use of verbal instructions and visual demonstrations by the instructor during the practice session. Provide both your general impression as well as specific examples of the instructions and demonstrations you observed. Based on your observation and study of this chapter, what is your evaluation of the effectiveness of the instructions and demonstrations used during practice? What recommendations would you suggest for improving the quality of both?

2. For this exercise, you are to select a motor skill for which you are knowledgeable and which you can perform proficiently. Begin by analyzing the skill and developing a list of the most critical features necessary in performing the skill. (Be sure to include both movement and environmental features, and include the list as part of your written report.) From your list of critical skill features, develop 10 verbal cues that could be used when instructing someone in the skill. Keep your cues brief, succinct, and concise, and use action words where appropriate.

3. Select a motor skill of interest to you for this exercise (if you complete question 2 above, you may use either the same or a different skill.) Describe six different important movement components of the skill for which verbal instructions might be provided. For each of these movement components, provide an example of both an internally focused and externally focused instruction directing a learner's attention.

4. For a motor skill in which you consider yourself highly proficient, think about your experiences when originally learning the skill (select a different skill than that used to answer questions 2 and 3). Recalling your learning experiences, describe how your experience relates to each of the four stages of observational learning as described by social cognitive theory. That is, how do each of the four stages illustrate something different about your experiences learning the skill (be specific) that eventually resulted in your performance proficiency?

FOR FURTHER STUDY

HOW MUCH DO YOU KNOW?

For each of the following, select the letter that best answers the question.

1. Both research and experience support the conclusion that verbal instructions are
   a. superior to visual demonstrations in promoting learning.
   b. inferior to visual demonstrations in promoting learning.
   c. best when used in combination with visual demonstrations.
   d. not necessary if visual demonstrations are used sufficiently.

2. As a general guideline, verbal cues should contain no more than _____ words.
   a. one or two
   b. three or four
   c. six or seven
   d. ten

3. Concerning the use of instructions to focus a learner's attention, a significant body of recent research has demonstrated the benefits of promoting a(n) _____ attentional focus on the part of learners.

a. narrow
b. broad
c. internal
d. external

4. In providing instructions focusing a learner's attention on the effects of an action, research has generally supported the benefits of attending to those effects
   a. within the learner's body.
   b. occurring on the surface of the learner's body.
   c. external to but near the learner's body.
   d. at some distance from the learner's body.

5. Learning models have generally been found to be
   a. ineffective.
   b. less effective than expert models.
   c. as effective as expert models.
   d. vastly more effective than expert models.

6. _____ are brain cells that fire whether a person is initiating an overt action or merely watching someone else perform the same action.
   a. Mirror neurons
   b. Glial cells
   c. Action generators
   d. Excitatory neurons

Answer the following with the word or words that best complete each sentence.

7. When deciding how much information to provide to learners in the form of verbal instructions, it is essential that movement skills instructors keep in mind the limited _____ capacity of the learners.

8. A word or short phrase directing a learner's attention to some important feature related either to the execution of a skill or the environment in which the skill is performed, is labeled a _____.

9. The _____ is the notion that skills should be planned and executed in relation to their expected consequences.

10. Name the four stages of observational learning as proposed by social cognitive theory.

11. According to social cognitive theory, _____ is a measure of a person's belief in his or her ability to accomplish a goal or a task, such as learning a new motor skill.

12. The use of a learning model to demonstrate a motor skill has been shown to be most effective if, along with the demonstration, an observer also receives the learning model's _____.

Answers are provided at the end of this review section.

STUDY QUESTIONS

1. What roles do verbal instructions and visual demonstrations play in the acquisition of motor skills?
2. Why should verbal instructions generally be brief, concise, and limited?
3. In general, how much information should a movement instructor attempt to convey through a verbal instruction?
4. In what ways can verbal instructions be made more precise?
5. What are verbal cues and how should they most effectively be developed?
6. What guidelines concerning the number and frequency of verbal cues delivered during practice sessions should be followed?
7. Describe the perception–action coupling problem and explain the solution offered by the common coding approach.
8. Describe the difference between instructions having an internal and an external focus of attention.
9. What does research suggest about the relative benefits of internally and externally focused instructions?

10. How are distance effects related to the effectiveness of instructions having an external focus?
11. Describe the stages of observational learning as presented in social cognitive theory.
12. What characteristics of the model demonstrating a motor skill influence the effectiveness of the demonstration?
13. Define and contrast expert models and learning models.
14. What techniques can be used to increase the effectiveness of a learning model when providing skill demonstrations?
15. What are mirror neurons and how does the discovery of the mirror neuron system in humans support the importance of the role played by demonstrations in the learning of motor skills?

ADDITIONAL READING

Byers, BB. (2000). "Just do it—Commercial slogan or movement principle?" *Journal of Physical Education, Recreation and Dance*, 71(9), 16–19.

Darden, GF. (1997). "Demonstrating motor skills—Rethinking the expert demonstration." *Journal of Physical Education, Recreation and Dance*, 68(6), 31–35.

Hodges, JH, and Franks, IM. (2005). "Instructions, demonstrations and the learning process." In AM Williams and NJ Hodges (eds.), *Skill acquisition in sport: Research, theory and practice* (145–174), New York: Routledge.

Keysers, C. (2009). "Mirror neurons: Are we ethical by nature?" In M Brockman (ed.), *What's next: Dispatches on the future of science*, New York: Vintage Books.

Maddox, MD, Wulf, G, and Wright, DL. (1999). "The effect of an internal vs. external focus of attention on the learning of a tennis stroke." *Journal of Exercise Psychology*, 21, S78.

McCullagh, P, and Weiss, MR. (2001). "Modeling: Considerations for motor skill performance and psychological responses." In RN Singer, HA Hausenblas, and CM Janelle (eds.), *Handbook of sport psychology* (pp. 205–238), New York: John Wiley and Sons.

McNevin, NH, Wulf, G, and Carlson, C. (2000). "Effects of attentional focus, self-control, and dyad training on motor learning: Implications for physical rehabilitation." *Physical Therapy*, 80, 373–385.

Perkins-Ceccato, N, Passmore, SR, and Lee, TD. (2003). "Effects of focus of attention depend on golfers' skill." *Journal of Sports Sciences*, 21, 593–600.

Wesch, NN, Law, B, and Hall, CR. (2007). "The use of observational learning by athletes." *Journal of Sport Behavior*, 30(2), 219–231.

Williams, AM, and Hodges, JH. (2005). "Practice, instructions and skill acquisition in soccer: Challenging tradition." *Journal of Sport Sciences*, 23(6), 637–650.

Wulf, G, Lewthwaite, R, Landers, M, and Tollner, T (2009). The power of external focus instructions to enhance performance and learning. Physical Therapy, 89, 170–172.

REFERENCES

Adams, J. (1986). "Use of the model's knowledge of results to increase the observer's performance." *Journal of Human Movement Studies*, 12, 89–98.

Al-Abood, SA, Bennett, SJ, Hernandez, FM, Ashford, D, and Davids, K. (2002). "Effects of verbal instructions and image size on visual search strategies in basketball free throw shooting." *Journal of Sports Sciences*, 20, 271–278.

Bandura, A. (1969). *Principles of behavior modification*. New York: Rinehart-Winston.

Bandura, A. (1977). *Social learning theory*. Englewood Cliffs, NJ: Prentice-Hall.

Bandura, A. (1986). *Social foundations of thought and action: A social cognitive theory*. Englewood Cliffs, NJ: Prentice-Hall.

Bandura, A. (1997). *Self-efficacy: The exercise of control*. New York: Freeman.

Bliss, CB. (1892–1893). "Investigations in reaction time and attention." *Studies from the Yale Psychology Laboratory, 1,* 1–55.

Boder, DP. (1935). "The influence of concomitant activity and fatigue upon certain forms of reciprocal hand movements and its fundamental components." *Comparative Psychology Monographs, 11*(4).

Byers, BB. (2000). "Just do it—Commercial slogan or movement principle?" *Journal of Physical Education, Recreation and Dance, 71*(9), 16–19.

Carroll, WR, and Bandura, A. (1990). "Representational guidance of action production in observational learning: A causal analysis." *Journal of Motor Behavior, 22,* 85–97.

Darden, GF. (1997). "Demonstrating motor skills—Rethinking the expert demonstration." *Journal of Physical Education, Recreation and Dance, 68*(6), 31–35.

Freud, S. (1922). *Introductory lecture on psychoanalysis.* London: George Allen and Unwin.

Gallwey, WT. (1982). *The inner game of tennis.* New York: Bantam Books.

George, TR, Feltz, DL, and Chase, MA. (1992). "Effects of model similarity on self-efficacy and muscular endurance: A second look." *Journal of Sport & Exercise Psychology, 14,* 237–248.

Glaser, D. (2007). Nova ScienceNOW: Mirror neurons. Accessed at www.pbs.org/nova/sciencenow/3204/01-monkey.html.

Gould, D, and Weiss, M. (1981). "The effects of model similarity and model talk on self-efficacy and muscular endurance." *Journal of Sport Psychology, 3,* 17–29.

Guthrie, ER. (1935). *The psychology of learning.* New York: Harper.

Hall, C. (1943). *Principles of behavior.* New York: Appleton-Century-Crofts.

Hamilton, AF, Joyce, DW, Flanagan, JR, Frith, CD, and Wolpert, DM. (2007). "Kinematic cues in perceptual weight judgment and their origins in box lifting." *Psychological Research, 71*(1), 13.

Hand, J, and Sidaway, B. (1993). "Relative frequency of modeling effects on the performance and retention of a motor skill." *Research Quarterly for Exercise and Sport, 4,* 122–126.

Hebert, EP, and Landin, D. (1994). "Effects of learning model and augmented feedback on tennis skill acquisition." *Research Quarterly for Exercise and Sport, 65*(3), 250–257.

Hodges, JH, and Franks, IM. (2002). "Modelling coaching practice: The role of instruction and demonstration." *Journal of Sports Science, 20,* 793–811.

Hodges, JH, and Franks, IM. (2005). "Instructions, demonstrations and the learning process. In AM Williams and NJ Hodges (eds.), *Skill acquisition in sport: Research, theory and practice* (pp. 145–174). New York: Routledge.

Hommel, B. (1996). "Toward an action-concept model of stimulus-response compatibility." In B. Hommel and W. Prinz (eds.), *Theoretical issues of stimulus-response compatibility* (pp. 281–320). Amsterdam: North-Holland.

Hommel, B, and Elsner, B. (2000). "Action as stimulus control." In A Schick, M Meis and C Reckhardt (eds.), *Contributions to psychological acoustics* (pp. 403–424). Oldenburg, Germany: University of Oldenburg, BIS.

Horn, RR, and Williams, AM. (2004). "Observational learning: Is it time we took another look?" In AM Williams and NJ Hodges (eds.), *Skill acquisition in sport: Research, theory and practice* (pp. 175–206). New York: Routledge.

Ishikura, T, and Inomata, K. (1995). "Effect of angle of model demonstration on learning of a motor skill." *Perceptual and Motor Skills, 80,* 651–658.

Keysers, C. (2009). "Mirror neurons: Are we ethical by nature?" In M Brockman (ed.), *What's next: Dispatches on the future of science.* New York: Vintage Books.

Lefkowitz, M, Blake, RR, and Mouton, JS. (1955). "Status factors in pedestrian violation of traffic signals." *Journal of Abnormal and Social Psychology, 51,* 704–705.

Maddox, MD, Wulf, G, and Wright, DL. (1999). "The effect of an internal vs. external focus of attention on the learning of a tennis stroke." *Journal of Exercise Psychology, 21,* S78.

Marchant, D, Clough, PJ, and Crawshaw, M. (in press). "The effects of attentional focusing strategies on novice dart throwing performers and their experiences." *International Journal of Sport and Exercise Psychology.*

Marchant, D, Greig, M, and Clough, PJ. (2005). "Attentional focus as mediator of localized muscle fatigue in maintaining single legged balance." *Journal of Sports Sciences, 23*(11–12), 1258–1259.

Masser, LS. (1993). "Critical cues help first-grade students' achievement in handstands and forward rolls." *Journal of Teaching in Physical Education*, 12, 301–312.

McCullagh, P. (1986). "Modeling: Learning, developmental and social considerations." *Journal of Sport Psychology*, 8, 319–331.

McCullagh, P, and Caird, JK. (1990). "Correct and learning models and the use of model knowledge of results in the acquisition and retention of a motor skill." *Journal of Human Movement Studies*, 18, 107–116.

McCullagh, P, and Weiss, MR. (2001). "Modeling: Considerations for motor skill performance and psychological responses." In RN Singer, HA Hausenblas, and CM Janelie (eds.), *Handbook of sport psychology* (pp. 205–238). New York: John Wiley and Sons.

McNevin, NH, Shea, CH, and Wulf, G. (2003). "Increasing the distance of an external focus of attention enhances learning." *Psychological Research*, 67, 22–29.

McNevin, NH, Wulf, G, and Carlson, C. (2000). "Effects of attentional focus, self-control, and dyad training on motor learning: Implications for physical rehabilitation." *Physical Therapy*, 80, 373–385.

Miller, NE, and Dollard, J. (1941). *Social learning and imitation*. New Haven, CT: Yale University Press.

Morgan, CL. (1896). "On modification and variation." *Science*, 4, 733–743.

Perkins-Ceccato, N, Passmore, SR, and Lee, TD. (2003). "Effects of focus of attention depend on golfers' skill." *Journal of Sports Sciences*, 21, 593–600.

Pollock, BJ, and Lee, TD. (1992). "Effects of the model's skill level on observational motor learning." *Research Quarterly for Exercise and Sport*, 63, 25–29.

Prinz, W. (1992). "Why don't we perceive our brain states?" *European Journal of Cognitive Psychology*, 4, 1–20.

Prinz, W. (1997). "Perception and action planning." *European Journal of Cognitive Psychology*, 9(2), 129–154.

Ramachandran, VS. (2007). "Mirror neurons and imitation learning as a driving force in "the great leap forward" in human evolution. Online journal Edge, accessed at www.edge.org.

Rink, JE. (2009). *Teaching physical education for learning*, 6th ed. Boston: McGraw-Hill.

Rizzolatti, G, and Craighero, L. (2004). "The mirror-neuron system." *Annual Review of Neuroscience*, 27, pp. 169–192.

Rizzolatti, G, and Sinigaglia, C. (2006). *Mirrors in the brain: How our minds share actions and emotions*. New York: Oxford University Press.

Scully, DM, and Newell, KM. (1985). "The acquisition of motor skills: Toward a visual perception perspective." *Journal of Human Movement Studies*, 12, 169–187.

Shea, CH, Wright, DL, Wulf, G, and Whitacre, C. (2000). "Physical and observational practice afford unique learning opportunities." *Journal of Motor Behavior*, 32(1), 27–36.

Skinner, BF. (1938, 1966). *The behavior of organisms*. Englewood Cliffs, NJ: Prentice-Hall.

Vanderbilt, T. (2009). *Traffic: Why we drive the way we do (and what it says about us)*. New York: Vintage Books.

Weeks, DL, and Anderson, LP. (2000). "The interaction of observational learning with overt practice: Effects on motor skill learning." *Acta Psychologica*, 104, 259–271.

Wesch, NN, Law, B, and Hall, CR. (2007). "The use of observational learning by athletes." *Journal of Sport Behavior*, 30(2), 219–231.

Williams, AM, and Hodges, JH. (2005). "Practice, instructions and skill acquisition in soccer: Challenging tradition." *Journal of Sport Sciences*, 23(6), 637–650.

Wulf, G. (2007). *Attention and motor skill learning*. Champaign, IL: Human Kinetics.

Wulf, G, Hob, M, and Prinz, W. (1998). "Instructions for motor learning: Differential effects of internal versus external focus of attention." *Journal of Motor Behavior*, 30, 169–179.

Wulf, G, Lauterbach, B, and Toole, T. (1999). "Learning advantages of an external focus of attention in golf." *Research Quarterly for Exercise and Sport*, 70, 120–126.

Wulf, G, and Prinz, W. (2001). "Directing attention to movement effects enhances learning: A review." *Psychonomic Bulletin & Review*, 8, 648–660.

Wulf, G, Wachter, S, and Wortmann, S. (2003). "Attentional focus in motor skill learning: Do females benefit from an external focus?" *Women in Sport and Physical Activity Journal*, 12, 37–52.

Wulf, G, Zachry, T, Granados, C, and Dufek, JS. (2006). "Increases in jump-and-reach height through an external focus of attention." Manuscript submitted for publication.

Zachry, T. (2005). "Effects of attentional focus on kinematics and muscle activation patterns as a function of expertise." Master's Thesis, University of Nevada, Las Vegas.

Zemke, R. (1999). "Toward a science of training." *Training*, 36(7), 32–33.

Answers to How Much Do You Know questions: (1) C, (2) B, (3) D, (4) D, (5) C, (6) A, (7) attentional, (8) verbal cue, (9) action effect hypothesis, (10) attention, retention, reproduction, motivation, (11) self-efficacy, (12) feedback.

CHAPTER 11

Scheduling the Learning Experience

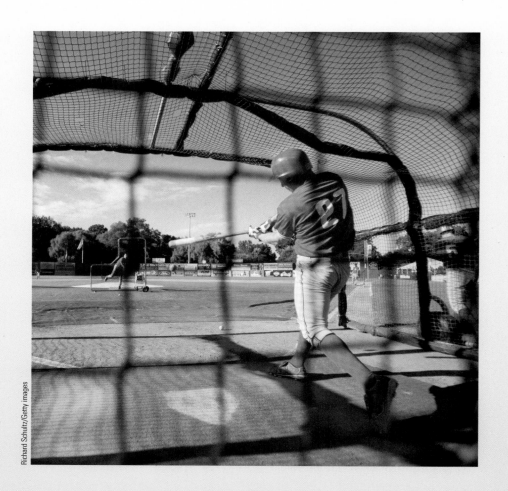

Richard Schultz/Getty images

Whatever you would make habitual, practice it.
Epictetus

KEY QUESTIONS

- Upon what basic principles of learning should practice be based?

- When practicing several different skills, what is the best way of ordering their presentation?

- When instructing a single skill that will be performed in one way only, is it ever best to practice it in different ways?

- How much rest between practice trials or between bouts of practice is best?

- How should individual practice sessions be distributed over time?

- How can skills be simplified during practice, and when is it a good idea to do so?

- Should practice be "perfect"?

CHAPTER OVERVIEW

There is an old joke that goes something like this. Two men meet on a busy street corner in New York City. The first man, a visitor to the city, asks the second man, a New Yorker, "Can you please tell me, sir, how can I get to Carnegie Hall?" The New York man, without missing a beat, replies, "Practice!"

This joke, of course, turns on the New York man's misconstruing the out-of-town visitor's question. But it also strikes an ironic chord of universal recognition. There is a truth, a recognized principle of learning, embedded within the humor of this story. Learning requires practice. Certainly if someone wants to acquire a skill well enough to perform in an elite venue like Carnegie Hall, practice is necessary. Although people may be born possessing innate capacities making learning a particular skill relatively easy practice is still necessary in order to optimize all but the simplest skills.

Practice is so central to learning that it can sometimes be easy to overlook the quality of practice experiences, as though the mere pursuit of practice, any type of practice, the repetitiveness of some skill over and over, is in itself all that learning requires. But all practice is not the same, and the quality of practice is as important as the time devoted to practice. Instructors of movement skills have access to a rich and broad inventory of practice methods from which to draw when designing practice experiences for individuals. The quality of those methods they select and how they are arranged play a major role in how well learners will acquire practiced skills. The same amount of time spent in practice can lead all the way from little or even no actual learning, to significant improvements in skill level, depending on how instructors design practice experiences. In this chapter we will explore issues related to the basic design of practice including those basic principles of sound design upon which learning is optimally promoted.

It is difficult to overstate the importance of practice. Practice and learning are so intertwined that it is tempting to use them synonymously. We do not think of practice apart from the learning we expect to occur as a result, or think about learning without reflecting on the practice that preceded it.

If, as is the consensus among both theorists and practitioners, practice is the single most important factor in the learning of motor skills, then it follows that the quality of that practice is essential for optimizing learning. Although almost any practice inevitably improves skilled performance, the way in which it is organized plays a significant role in the rate, stability, and amount of learning that will result. Instructors of motor skills must make important decisions concerning the organization of practice experiences, and their decisions play a critical role in the amount of learning individuals experience as a result of practice.

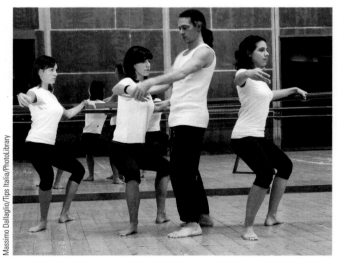

Massimo Dallaglio/Tips Italia/PhotoLibrary

Although practice is the most important factor influencing learning, the design of practice can enhance or detract significantly from the extent and quality of the learning that results.

In designing practice, instructors must answer many questions concerning the scheduling of practice experiences. These include questions concerning the order in which skills should be practiced, the amount of precision with which skills should be practiced, whether skills should be practiced in one way only or in a variety of different ways, how the amounts of rest and work should be balanced within practice sessions, the way in which individual practice sessions are distributed over time, and whether to practice new and complex skills in parts or as whole movements.

Although there is an abundance of research addressing each of these questions, answers to them are not always as clear as might be hoped. Though answers to many do appear clearly resolved and beyond dispute, others remain only partially solved. There is ample evidence, however, to clearly demonstrate that many common beliefs concerning the scheduling of practice experiences, those that are supported by tradition and that often also seem, at least initially, intuitively beyond question, are less than the most effective ways of instructing or learning motor skills. In this chapter, we will examine the research concerning what is known about scheduling practice experiences in the most effective manner, as well as those areas where debate still leaves issues unsettled.

SCHEDULING PRACTICE SESSIONS

One of the first questions motor skill instructors must answer when devising practice schedules concerns how many different skills to practice within a single practice session, as well as the order in which those skills should be presented. A related question concerns whether the skills should be practiced in one manner only, usually one promoting the best performance results, or in a variety of different ways. The answer to both of these questions depends to a large extent upon the answer to a more fundamental question concerning practice: Is it always desirable to promote optimal performance of a skill during practice?

Practice makes perfect. Correcting the overstatement of a maxim: Almost always, practice brings improvement, and more practice brings more improvement. We all expect improvement with practice to be ubiquitous, though obviously limits exist in scope and extent.

—A. Newell and P.S. Rosenbloom, 1981

An old saying about motor skills instruction addresses this question. The saying is "Practice makes perfect, but only if it is perfect practice," and it encapsulates a strongly held belief among many practitioners. This saying, and the belief that springs from it, are only partly true, however. The first part of the saying—"Practice makes perfect"—is true; all other things being equal, the more one practices a skill, the better will become one's performance of the skill, as the law of practice quantifiably stipulates (Chapter 5). It is the second part of the saying that can be misleading as a practice guideline.

The implication of stating that practice makes perfect "only if it is perfect practice" is that practice should result in learners performing skills in a way that optimizes their performance (that makes practice performance "perfect," or at least as close to perfect as possible given a person's capabilities and stage of learning). Instructors, following this formula for practice success, design practice experiences to promote the best (the "most perfect") performance of skills as an important practice principle. But this widely held belief, as we will see, often underlies poor practice decisions.

Scheduling Interskill Practice

The most common type of practice experience usually involves instruction for several different skills during a practice session. An individual practice session for tennis, for example, may involve practicing different shots including the forehand, backhand, and serve, as well as different return strategies. Patients in a clinical session may practice manipulating a variety of differently sized and shaped objects to help regain functional use of their hands and digits following an injury compromising manual control. Many other examples could easily be added.

interskill practice: The scheduling of different skills within a practice session or portion of practice session.

Whenever several different skills are to be practiced within a single practice session, a condition called **interskill practice** (i.e., "between skills"), one option is to arrange skills sequentially in some predetermined order and practice each skill for a requisite number of trials or amount of time, completing practice for each specific skill before moving on to practice the next skill, and so on. Such a practice schedule is termed **blocked practice** because individual skills are arranged in blocks to be practiced in isolation from other skills. By isolating the practice of a specific skill in this fashion, blocking out the effects of other skills, performance of the practiced skill is typically optimized. That is, the concentration on a single skill at one time allows individuals to devote their full attentional and memorial resources to performance of the skill and allows instructors to provide instructions and feedback maintaining high levels of performance. Thus, skills presented within a blocked schedule have the best chance of being practiced at optimal performance levels, so that practice becomes as "perfect" as possible.

blocked practice: A practice schedule in which the same skill is rehearsed in repetitive fashion.

But are blocked schedules always the most effective arrangement of interskill practice experiences? Are they always best for promoting learning (and recall here the distinction between performance and learning delineated in Chapter 5)? This is an old question, and the search for an answer goes back at least as far as a study by Pyle in 1919. In Pyle's study, subjects learning a card-sorting task, who alternated sorting cards into two different patterns of numbered sorting box compartments, performed better on a retention test (i.e., had better learning outcomes) than did subjects sorting cards into a single pattern (Pyle, 1919). The results of Pyle's research were largely forgotten, however, and both researchers and practitioners continued to echo the merits of blocked practice scheduling until two motor skills researchers reported results challenging this traditional view in a 1979 study that today is considered one of the most influential experiments in the literature on learning motor skills.

random practice: A practice schedule in which different skills are rehearsed in an unpredictable trial-to-trial order.

Based upon earlier research involving learning language skills (i.e., Battig, 1956, 1966), John Shea and Robyn Morgan designed an experiment to investigate whether arranging interskill practice schedules in a fashion making performance more challenging might actually benefit learning (Shea and Morgan, 1979). The experimental design of their study was discussed in Chapter 5, and we will not review it extensively here (although the reader interested in experimental arrangements can refer to the earlier description). In their experiment, Shea and Morgan compared subjects learning a novel task under either blocked or **random practice.** Unlike a blocked schedule where subjects complete a prescribed number of practice attempts for one skill before moving on to the next skill, random practice presents several skills within a single practice context in a randomized and unpredictable order. For example, if three skills labeled A, B, and C are presented during a practice period, a traditional blocked practice schedule would be illustrated as follows: A, A, A, A, A…, B, B, B, B, B…C, C, C, C, C…. Each skill would be practiced and the requisite number of trials completed prior to the presentation and practice of the subsequent skill. In random practice, the same number of practice trials for each skill may be completed, but the trials are presented in random fashion illustrated as follows: B, C, A, C, B, B, A, C, B, C, A, A…. Compared to blocked practice, random practice presents a greater immediate practice challenge to the learner.

The task that Shea and Morgan used to test their predictions consisted in having seated subjects grasp a tennis ball and knock down a series of barriers in front of them in a specified order as quickly as possible (see Figure 5.1 in Chapter 5). Three different patterns for knocking down the barriers were practiced. Depending on the color of the light initiating action, subjects would perform a series of movements knocking down the barriers in one of the three prescribed orders. All subjects performed the same number of total practice attempts (54) as well as the same number for each of the three patterns (18). However, half of the subjects completed their practice trials in a blocked fashion, whereas the other half of the subjects followed a random schedule.

Results of Shea and Morgan's study showed that subjects who practiced in the blocked schedule performed better than those practicing under a random schedule throughout acquisition, although the gap between groups did narrow toward the final acquisition attempts. Put into more general terms, blocked practice led to better performance during acquisition than did random practice. So far, the prediction about "perfect practice" making "perfect" seems safe. But as we have observed on other occasions, performance is not always the best predictor of learning, and the findings from this experiment highlighted another example of the learning–performance distinction. When subjects were tested on both retention and transfer tests, those who had acquired the three skill patterns under random practice conditions performed significantly better than did those practicing under blocked conditions. Based upon their results, Shea and Morgan concluded that blocked practice facilitated better acquisition performance than did random practice, but that random practice promoted better retention and transfer. Generalizing their conclusions, blocked practice enhances practice performance, but random practice results in better learning.

Contextual Interference Effects

contextual interference: The degree of interference created by the ordering of skills within a practice session; blocked practice results in low contextual interference, whereas random practice results in high amounts of contextual interference.

The practice variable that Shea and Morgan manipulated in their experiment is called **contextual interference**. Basically, contextual interference refers to the degree to which the arrangement of practice trials influences the amount of interference within memory experienced by a person during the practice of a skill. Blocked practice is believed to promote low contextual interference because the context in which skills are practiced remains constant from trial to trial, and so the memorial representation of any particular skill remains fairly stable over practice attempts. Random practice, on the other hand, is believed to promote high contextual interference because the context of practice

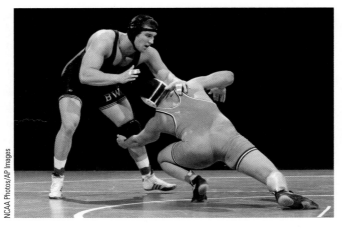

NCAA Photos/AP Images

Activities in which different skills must be performed in a rapid and unpredictable order, may especially benefit from employing random practice scheduling.

serial practice: A practice schedule resulting in moderate contextual interference in which several different skills are practiced in an alternating but predictable order.

constantly changes, leading to a constant shifting in memory states between practice trials. Contextual interference may also be specified as moderate, as is believed to be the case for **serial practice**, an arrangement of practice trials that are constantly changing but in a predictable order (e.g., A, B, C, A, B, C, A, B, C, … etc.).

Shea and Morgan's original study on the effects of contextual interference on motor learning led to an extensive and robust research agenda among scholars studying the effects of various practice variables on learning, with many issues still being investigated and debated (for reviews see Brady, 1998; Lee and Simon, 2004; and Magill and Hall, 1990). A conclusion emerging from the research literature is that low contextual interference (i.e., blocked practice) generally promotes better practice performance, but poorer learning of motor skills, than does high contextual interference (i.e., random practice), but that the benefits for learning of high-contextual interference are often masked by poorer practice performance during acquisition (see Box 11.1).

BOX **11.1**   Blocked Practice Can Mislead Instructors

Blocked practice can mislead motor skills instructors when they incorrectly judge the performance benefits of blocked practice as indicating better learning than is, in actuality, taking place. A prominent learning theorist, Robert Bjork, has stated the situation as follows: "The fact that blocked practice leads to better short-term performance but poor long-term learning has great potential to fool teachers, trainers and instructors…. It's natural to think that when we're making progress, we're learning, and when we're struggling and making errors, we're not learning as well. So people who are responsible for training can often be pushed toward training conditions that are far from optimal."

—Robert A. Bjork (1994)

Explaining Contextual Interference Effects

Observations about contextual interference effects may at first seem counterintuitive. Certainly, they are contrary to the old sayings concerning "perfect practice" with which we started our discussion. The more repetitions of a skill completed, and the more they are accomplished at or near a desired criterion of perfection, the better the skill should be learned, or so it would seem. After all, blocked practice promotes the most perfect practice possible at any given stage of learning. Why, then, the paradox of random practice, namely that deliberately compromising practice performance can lead to better learning?

Consider first that blocked practice has distinct advantages over random practice in promoting acquisition performance. Repetition of the same skill over a number of trials allows learners to make trial-to-trial adjustments within working memory. In essence, learners can fine-tune their performance over practice repetitions, a situation typically not available either in retention tests or real-life execution of skills. A number of temporary practice variables may also promote acquisition performance. The repetitiveness of blocked practices allows learners to search for and adjust their focus of attention on the most appropriate environmental cues, reach and maintain appropriate arousal levels, and may enhance motivation levels because of perceived elevated levels of success. All of these factors are temporary performance variables, however, whose benefits dissipate once practice is over.

If blocked practice facilitates practice performance due to temporary effects on performance, what is it about random practice, which has the effect of depressing practice performance, that promotes better learning outcomes? Two hypotheses have been advanced as explanations of contextual interference effects. These are the action plan reconstruction and elaboration hypotheses. Both hypotheses have been supported, but are believed to play different roles in promoting learning. The **action plan reconstruction hypothesis** is based upon the limited capacity of short-term memory (Lee and Magill, 1985). The argument is that when learners perform a particular skill (skill A), they must process incoming sensory information that is then coupled with retrieval of the long-term memory for the skill to produce an action plan (or motor program) guiding their performance of the skill. When they then shift to another skill (skill B), the action plan held in short-term memory for skill A is eliminated to make space within working memory available for retrieving and constructing the action plan for skill B. For this reason, this position is sometimes also referred to as the forgetting hypothesis—the plans for one skill are "forgotten" from short-term memory in order to make room for a different skill. The next time that skill A is performed, the action plan for it must be reconstructed within working memory.

Random practice leads to a continuous process of construction, forgetting, and reconstruction of the working memory (the action plan) for a skill. When performing a skill in blocked fashion, in contrast, once the action plan is retrieved and constructed in working memory, it can be held with little additional processing demand for each subsequent performance of the skill.

Blocked practice facilitates performance, but at the cost of limiting the cognitive effort associated with retrieving and constructing action plans that, in the long run, strengthen consolidation processes, thereby benefiting learning.

action plan reconstruction hypothesis: One explanation of the contextual interference effect holding that when people sequentially perform different skills during random practice, they continuously forget and must reconstruct the action plan for each skill each time that it is practiced, enhancing learning by leading to the development of a stronger memory representation.

The act of constantly retrieving and reconstructing the memory states for a skill, referred to as *retrieval practice* (Bjork, 1975), arguably results in a stronger memory of the skill that is manifested as greater learning when the skill is retrieved and performed at a later time.

elaboration hypothesis: One explanation of the contextual interference effect holding that random practice promotes a better appreciation of the distinctive features among skills, resulting in stronger memories and better learning.

A second explanation of the contextual interference effect is the **elaboration hypothesis.** In their original study, Shea and Morgan proposed that the advantages of random practice resulted because, when compared to blocked practice, random practice elaborated the memory representations of the skills or skill variations practiced. That is, random practice provided greater opportunities for individuals to distinguish both similarities and differences among the practiced skills. During random practice, learners continuously compare and contrast different skills and come to recognize both the similarities and differences among skills, making the memory for each skill more distinctive and meaningful. This greater distinctiveness or meaningfulness of memory not only enriches the memory of the skill but also provides important retrieval cues, making it easier to recall the skill from long-term memory at a later time.

Shea and Zimny (1983) conducted a study in which subjects performed the original barrier knockdown task conducted by Shea and Morgan, after which they were interviewed about their experiences. The investigators found that subjects who acquired the skill under random practice conditions possessed a much more rich and distinct memory of individual movement patterns associated with the tasks. The subjects had noticed relationships among the individual movements and were better at distinguishing both differences and similarities of the three separate skills. Those learning under a blocked practice condition, on the other hand, reported focusing their attention on the specific features of a single skill at a time and attempting to perform automatically. The performance of a single skill during a blocked series of attempts appears, in this view, to focus learners' attention on the rote production of a skill to the exclusion of cognitive processing that can otherwise enrich the mental representation of the skill. The result of such focused practice attention is to promote good practice performance, but to limit the development of memory and hinder learning.

Both the action plan reconstruction and elaboration hypotheses provide compelling explanations for the contextual interference effect, and it is likely that both are equally correct. The increased number of times motor commands must be structured as argued by the action plan reconstruction hypothesis, as well as the greater distinctiveness of those commands as the elaboration hypothesis suggests, are really two sides of the same coin. Perhaps the coin itself is forged in the crucible of greater attention and cognitive effort required of learners when practicing under random as compared to blocked conditions. Research has shown, for example, that during random practice learners take longer to prepare for each performance attempt, supposedly because of the additional time required by the increase in attention and cognitive effort required as tasks to be performed constantly vary (Li and Wright, 2000; and Smith, 1997). It is also interesting to note that learners practicing under blocked conditions are reported to overestimate the degree of their learning compared to those learning under random practice who often undervalue the degree of their learning, indicating that the performance advantages of blocked practice may lead to diminished attention and effort on the part of learners who perceive that their efforts are already successful (Simon and Bjork, 2001). However one weighs the various theoretical perspectives advanced as explanations of the contextual interference effect, that effect is one of the most strongly supported and significant findings in the motor skills learning literature. It is also a finding that has contributed significantly to the understanding of effective practice scheduling.

Practice Implications of the Contextual Interference Effect

The established benefits of high contextual interference during the acquisition of motor skills have strong implications for the design and implementation of practice schedules. Contrary to much common practice, research clearly supports the benefits of random practice in most motor skill–learning situations (Schmidt and Bjork, 1992). It would appear that virtually all populations of learners benefit from the increased attentional and cognitive demands placed upon them when employing random practice (Brady, 1998; and Lee and Simon, 2004). Beginning to advanced performers can benefit from randomly scheduled practice (Box 11.2). Even stroke patients (Hanlon, 1996), individuals with Alzheimer's disease (Dick et al., 2000), and children with Down's syndrome (Edwards, Elliot, and Lee, 1986) have been reported to benefit from early intervention employing random practice schedules.

As a general guideline, instructors of motor skills in educational, clinical, athletic, and occupational settings should strive to schedule practice sessions

---

BOX 11.2 **Random Practice Can Work for Advanced Performers Too**

The advantages of random practice have frequently been demonstrated for beginning and intermediate learners. To test the effects of random scheduling with advanced performers, Hall, Dominguez, and Cavazos (1994) investigated the effects of random practice on batting among collegiate baseball players. Thirty players were pre-tested and then divided into three equal ability groups. A random and blocked group received two additional practice sessions per week for six weeks, while a control group received no additional batting practice. The additional batting practice was comprised of 45 pitches consisting of 15 fastballs, 15 curveballs, and 15 change-up pitches. The random group received the pitches in a completely random order. The blocked group received the pitches in blocks of 15 counterbalanced across the players. All players continued to participate in normal team batting practice activities.

At the end of six weeks, all players received two post-tests of 45 pitches (15 of each type practiced), with pitches in one test presented in blocked order and randomly in the other. Results clearly favored the random practice group. The players receiving extra practice in random fashion performed significantly better than did the blocked practice group in both the random and blocked post-tests, whereas the blocked practice group performed better on both post-tests than the control group. (It was especially noteworthy to observe that the random group outperformed the blocked group even on the blocked post-test of pitches, on which the blocked group might have been expected to have some advantage.) In comparing pre-test to post-test scores, the random group clearly showed superior improvement, with an average improvement in score among the random group players of 56.7 percent compared to 24.8 percent for the blocked group and 6.2 percent for the control group.

Results of studies such as this one clearly point to the effectiveness of random practice scheduling for advanced performers as well as beginning learners.

employing random scheduling arrangements of skills early and often when presenting new skills. The advantages of random practice over blocked schedules of practice should outweigh concerns over the temporary depression in performance when learners practice under random practice conditions. Although the introduction of new skills may require some blocked presentation until learners acquire a basic grasp of the skill, transfer to random scheduling of practice experiences should proceed as soon as learners can produce rough approximations of the skills to be practiced (Shea, Kohl, and Indermill, 1990). The key question confronting instructors of motor skills is how soon to introduce random practice in a practice schedule. Should it be provided immediately or somewhat later in learning? The answer will depend upon several factors, including the age, experience, and ability level of the learner.

Although exact prescriptions are not possible, it is typical to initiate random practice once skills or skill variations have been presented and learners have a basic grasp of their mechanics and goals and are capable of producing approximations of correct movement patterns. The initial introduction to skills, however, typically entails a period of blocked presentation and practice so that learners might be provided sufficient practice attempts to enable them to produce approximations of correct mechanics. In many instances, this may require no more than a few practice attempts, and transfer to random practice will occur during the initial practice session in which skills are introduced. For more complex skills, introduction to several skills may occur over several practice periods before random practice is begun. Certainly, though, even for complex skills, random practice should typically be initiated before learners progress into the associative stage of learning. Research has indicated that blocked practice in the associative stage is significantly less effective compared to random practice and should be avoided.

Though instructors will typically strive to introduce random practice early, some factors can make a more delayed introduction advisable. Young learners may face greater challenges with both the cognitive and movement coordination patterns of motor skills and therefore require additional time to be sufficiently prepared for random practice (Wrisberg and Mead, 1983). Less skilled learners may also require additional time to master the basic skill fundamentals preparing them for random practice (Guadagnoll, Holcomb, and Weber, 1999). Of course, the number of skills introduced, as well as their complexity, may also necessitate a delay to the introduction of random practice.

When conditions such as age, learner capabilities, and task complexity delay its complete introduction, a gradual "fading in" of random practice can facilitate learners' ultimate readiness for it sooner than would otherwise be the case, as well as begin providing some of the benefits of practice variability associated with random practice. Serial practice schedules, in this regard, can provide gradual introductions of practice variability that help ease learners into random practice and promote better learning than does exclusive reliance on blocked practice (Al-Ameer and Toole, 1993; and Landin and Hebert, 1997). An example of various stages for gradually introducing random practice for the learning of four different skills is illustrated in Figure 11.1. Notice that three intermediate levels of serial practice between blocked and random schedules are illustrated. Depending on the complexity of the skills presented, as well

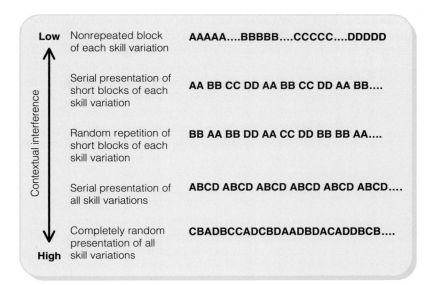

Low	Nonrepeated block of each skill variation	AAAAA....BBBBB....CCCCC....DDDDD
	Serial presentation of short blocks of each skill variation	AA BB CC DD AA BB CC DD AA BB....
	Random repetition of short blocks of each skill variation	BB AA BB DD AA CC DD BB BB AA....
	Serial presentation of all skill variations	ABCD ABCD ABCD ABCD ABCD ABCD....
High	Completely random presentation of all skill variations	CBADBCCADCBDAADBDACADDBCB....

Contextual interference (vertical axis label, arrow from Low to High)

FIGURE **11.1** Progression of Practice Schedule Designs Varying from Low to High Contextual Interference for Four Skills (A, B, C, D)

Source: Created by author.

as the needs of learners, only one or two intermediate levels of serially ordered trials may be sufficient (for simpler skills, or more experienced learners, transfer from blocked directly to random practice may be most appropriate). The number of practice trials within the serial blocks of skills can also be varied in length, with fewer trials within blocks of one skill increasing the amount of contextual interference within practice, and more trials of the same skill lessening the degree of contextual interference. By varying the order and number of practice attempts within blocks, movement skill instructors can vary the degree of contextual interference, and the concomitant challenges of practice presented to learners, in a variety of ways. The ability to effectively manipulate the degree of contextual interference in the practice schedule is one of the most important means instructors possess when designing practice experiences that will optimize learning (see Box 11.3).

BOX **11.3**   **Using Random Practice**

How could you design a schedule progressing from blocked to random practice for the following activities (include at least three intermediate steps, as well as completely blocked and random schedules)?

- Use of a manual wheelchair for daily activities

- Chest pass, set shoot, and rebound in basketball (practiced with other learners)
- Three tennis serves (flat, topspin, and slice)
- Basic throwing patterns taught to children (overhand, underarm, and sidearm)

When planning for the random scheduling of several skills during a practice session, instructors need not be overly concerned that only similar skills are presented. It is often the case that movement skill instructors feel that some coherence in similarity of skills must be maintained when using random practice. In fact, research indicates that random practice is most beneficial when skills are dissimilar (Magill and Hall, 1990). Instructors should plan for an arrangement of randomly practiced skills that facilitates ease of transition, allows for effective instruction, and keeps learners motivated; they need not worry about maintaining practice focus on a limited number of similar skills.

As can be gleaned from the previous discussion, the introduction of random practice into the design of practice schedules is both science and art. Although its benefits are solidly grounded in research, its most effective use entails informed application of principles as well as sensitivity to the needs of learners. Proper reliance on random practice in the design of practice experiences will, however, result in better learning outcomes for those under the instructor's guidance—though it may not make their practice *perfect*.

Scheduling Intraskill Practice

In the section just completed, we saw that increasing the practice variability among several skills (i.e., increasing the amount of contextual interference) enhances learning. Would increasing the amount of variability with which a single skill is practiced be as beneficial, however? Certainly, it might be argued, the practice of a specific skill should be attempted "perfectly," or at least in as perfect a fashion as possible. (Hopefully, the reader has come to question this argument by now.)

intraskill practice: The scheduling of a single skill or of variations of a single skill within a practice session or portion of practice session.

Questions concerning the scheduling of practice attempts for a single skill refer to **intraskill practice** (i.e., "within the same skill"). Whenever a single skill is practiced, whether over a number of repetitions in a blocked schedule, or intermittently in a random schedule, it can either be attempted the same way on each practice attempt or in a variety of different ways. When the skill is attempted in the same manner and under the same conditions each time it is practiced, the practice schedule is referred to as **constant practice**. When variations of the skill are attempted within practice, often varying from trial to trial, the schedule is referred to as **varied practice**. The skill variations in a varied practice schedule may refer to actually performing the skill in a different way (e.g., throwing a ball quickly on a flat trajectory or slowing its velocity to arch it over an object or opponent) or performing the skill in a different context (e.g., throwing to either a stationary or moving target). Analogous to the case with interskill practice, constant practice (like blocked practice) stabilizes behavior, benefits from the consistency of short-term memory, and results in relatively good performance during acquisition when compared to varied practice. But though it may seem obvious that trial-to-trial shifting of performance goals during varied practice scheduling will depress acquisition performance, we cannot jump to the conclusion that it will depress learning as well.

constant practice: A practice schedule in which the same skill is rehearsed in the same way, without variation, in a series of practice trials.

varied practice: A practice schedule in which the same skill is rehearsed in a variety of different ways.

What are the comparative results of constant and varied practice on the learning of motor skills? As with the comparisons of blocked and random practice, there has also been considerable research directed toward answering this question. The answer as to whether constant or varied practice is best is not quite as clear as the case for blocked and random practice, however, and depends on an analysis of the performance goals of practice. The essential question is whether the goal of practice is to acquire the ability to perform the practiced skill in a consistent manner and under consistent environmental circumstances or whether the goal is to acquire the capacity to perform the skill in a variety of ways and in differing environmental contexts.

For many skills, the goal of practice is to acquire the capacity to perform the skill under a variety of different circumstances. A person learning to shoot a basketball wants to be able to hit baskets from any distance and location on a basketball court; a physical therapy patient relearning to walk wants to be able to move about effectively in all of the possible locations with which he or she will daily be confronted; and someone learning to play the piano dreams of someday playing Mozart and Rachmaninov (or the Beatles and Bruce Springsteen), not just the beginning scales. In each of these instances, the goal of practice is to acquire the capacity to perform a specific skill in a new way, in a new environment, or under new conditions (or a combination of all three).

Whenever the goal of practice is to perform the practiced skill in a variety of different ways or under different conditions than those experienced during practice, an old idea in skill learning, known as the **specificity of practice principle**, applies. This principle, which has a long history in learning studies going back at least to the work of Thorndike and Woodworth at the beginning of the twentieth century, holds that the transfer between the conditions of practice and later performance in real-world settings depends upon the similarity between the elements of the practice and the real-world performance conditions. These ideas were embedded in the **theory of identical elements** (see Chapter 5). Put simply, the theory proposes that the greater the degree of similarity between the various elements of practice and those of the performance setting, the greater the degree of transfer between the two, which is an indication of learning. The notion that specificity of practice principles apply to motor skills is strongly grounded in the work of Franklin Henry (e.g., Henry, 1958; see also Barnett et al., 1973) and Jack Adams (Adams, 1971, 1987), who argued that the motor abilities underlying skilled performance are specific and change as the conditions or context of performing the skill change. Motor abilities, as we saw in Chapter 8, are considered the building blocks of motor skills (i.e., strength, speed, balance, endurance, coordination, reaction time, manual dexterity, etc.). Because motor abilities are specific to particular movement mechanics and environmental responses, any change from the practice condition will lead to a different collection of motor abilities underlying action. Skills practiced under constant conditions are consistently assembled through a specific set of motor abilities during acquisition, therefore leading to the skill being learned in a manner highly dependent upon those same motor abilities for any future performance. When the skill is performed differently or in response to a different set of environmental circumstances, a different set of motor abilities specific to the new situation must be assembled to produce the skill. To the degree that the motor abilities for the two conditions vary, transfer is weakened, resulting in poorer performance in the performance setting. The opposite is also true: The

specificity of practice principle: The notion that the best learning experiences are those that most closely approximate the movement components and environmental conditions of the target skill and target context.

theory of identical elements: The theory that the more similar the elements of two skills or two variations of the same skill are the greater will be the positive transfer between the two.

more similar the practice and performance situations, the more positive the transfer and the greater the learning. The similarity of elements between practice and later performance can refer to either the actual skill or to the context in which the skill is performed. In referring to the goals of practice, the manner in which a skill is meant to be performed as a result of practice is called the **target skill**, whereas the conditions in which the skill is expected to be performed are called the **target context**. The more faithful practice conditions are to mirroring the target skill and target context accurately, the greater will be the degree of positive transfer and the better the learning outcomes.

Practicing Skills Intended to Be Performed in a Variety of Ways

In real-world settings, many skills are performed in a variety of ways as well as in many diverse circumstances (this is especially the case with open skills). Successful acquisition of such skills depends, to a significant degree, upon the ability to perform the skills in many different ways and situations. That is, both the target skill and target context of practice are highly varied. Specificity of practice principles, in this case, dictate that a skill be practiced in a variety of ways and circumstances simulating the ways and circumstances in which it will be performed. Following a constant practice schedule would promote acquisition performance, but at the cost of more positive transfer to later performance conditions.

Consider, as a case in point, learning to throw a baseball or softball. A person learning to throw a ball under constant practice conditions might practice throwing to a stationary partner some moderate distance away on a series of attempts. A number of underlying motor abilities would be especially important in throwing under these practice conditions. We can further assume that such practice would lead to good practice performance.

But now assume that the target skill and target context are to throw runners out in game situations. The target skill may include throwing from various distances as well as from awkwardly contorted bodily positions assumed as a result of scooping up ground balls while on the run. The target context may now include throwing to a teammate who is also moving as he or she runs toward a base to tag an opponent out, as well as being able to decide which of two base-runners to attempt to throw out and then quickly responding with the correct throw. Though many of the motor abilities necessary to practice may also be necessary to the game situation, new ones may well take precedence. In our example, reaction time (quickly deciding on the correct throw to make), dynamic visual acuity (the ability to judge where to aim the ball to correspond to a teammate's movements), and gross body coordination (the ability to coordinate several movements simultaneously while the body is in motion) would all be required to a significant degree in throwing out the runner. Note that none of these specific motor abilities is required to perform well in the practice context, however. Constant practice would fail to adequately prepare our hypothetical player for throwing runners out in game situations, even though he or she might demonstrate considerable practice proficiency. In this case, the elements of practice and performance are too dissimilar, requiring an assemblage of different motor abilities to produce the same skill under the two differing conditions and leading to relatively poor learning outcomes.

target skill: The task a person wishes to be able to perform as a result of practice.

target context: The environmental context in which a person wants to be able to perform a skill as a result of practice.

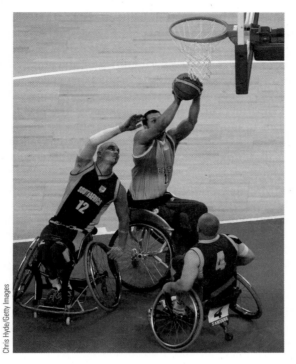

When a skill will be performed in a variety of different ways, varied practice methods should be employed during acquisition.

The implications for intraskill practice for the kinds of skills that will be performed under various transfer conditions are both theoretically and experientially straightforward. Varied practice is clearly indicated. The degree of practice variability will depend upon the extent to which the target skill and target context of practice vary. In our example, practice might reasonably include throwing from various distances (i.e., short, moderate, and long), both from a stationary position and while running, to both stationary and moving targets, and the practice of making rapid decisions and throwing quickly after fielding both fly and ground balls. This would result in practice entailing the broader range of abilities needed for the various kinds of throws and conditions confronted in game situations, resulting in better long-term learning.

As a general guideline, intraskill practice should entail the practice of a skill in a number of different ways and under a number of various conditions designed to represent the range of possibilities expected in the ultimate performance situation for which practice is designed to prepare learners. As was the case for interskill practice, it is also advisable to initially introduce a skill with little or no practice variability (i.e., constant practice) until learners have a grasp of it and can roughly approximate the correct movement patterns and situational responses. Once learners have demonstrated such a basic understanding, however, varied practice should be introduced. This introduction to varied practice conditions can be fairly quick or gradual depending upon the complexity of the skill and ability level of learners, as was also true when introducing random practice variability.

Instructors should be assured, though, that any brief periods of poorer practice performance will ultimately be replaced by superior learning and performance in real-world situations. Figure 11.2 presents a comparison of the typical performance curves for a skill learned under either constant or varied practice. Although the figure is admittedly hypothetical, it represents differences in performance curves as a function of practice variability consistent with the research literature. Note especially that though initial periods of practice are marked by depressed performance measures for varied practice, eventually varied practice results in superior performance compared to constant practice. The amount of time that it will take for such a crossover effect to become apparent in practice will depend upon a number of factors such as skill complexity and learner ability, and is a question in need of further research (Shoenfelt et al., 2002), though certainly such learning benefits of varied practice should become apparent by the associative stage of skill acquisition.

Practicing Skills Intended to Be Performed in the Same Way and under the Same Conditions as in Practice

A more challenging situation arises when designing intraskill learning experiences for skills designed to be performed in both a consistent manner and under nonvariable conditions (which is especially typical of closed skills). In other words, the target skill and target context are the same as the practice skill and context, respectively. Applying specificity of practice principles in this circumstance would lead to the conclusion that constant practice should result

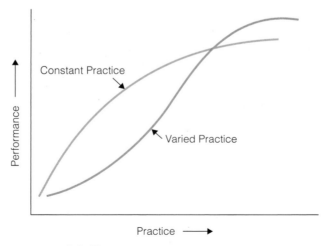

FIGURE **11.2** Hypothetical Comparison of Performance Curves for a Skill Acquired under Either a Constant or a Varied Practice Schedule

Source: Created by author.

not only in better practice performance, but also in better transfer and therefore better learning as well. After all, because the elements of practice and the intended performance setting are the same, the motor abilities underlying performance in both conditions are likewise the same. Logically, it can then be argued, transfer should be positive and learning maximized.

The validity of this reasoning, however, was challenged with the advent of schema theory (Schmidt, 1975). As we presented it in Chapter 4, schema theory is based on the notion that the memories underlying skills are constructed for entire classes of a skill rather than for each specific way in which a skill might be performed. That is, individual memories of skills across the variety of different ways and contexts in which they are practiced are not stored in memory. Rather, a single memory for all of the various ways a particular class of skill (i.e., throwing, jumping, walking, standing from a chair, using a fork, etc.) might be performed comprise a generalized memory of the skill that is then retrieved and "parameterized" for each specific way in which the skill is performed. Based upon the implications of schema theory, varied practice has been argued as being superior not merely for skills performed in a variety of different ways, but also for those skills in which performance conditions are consistent. This has led to the postulation of the **variability of practice principle**. This principle, contrary to specificity notions, proposes that practice consisting of skill variations is critical to the development of the memory for a skill and therefore results in better learning than does consistency of practice experiences. It is reasoned that because the memory for a skill, even one performed consistently, is generalized across all of the ways that it can be executed, varied practice leads to better development of the memory (i.e., the "motor program") underlying the skill (Christina and Alpenfels, 2002; Ghodsian, Bjork, and Benjamin, 1997; Schmidt and Bjork, 1992; and Shea and Kohl, 1990, 1991). Based largely upon the predictions of schema theory, varied practice has been recommended for consistently performed skills, a suggestion contradictory to specificity principles. (It can be noted that dynamical systems theory also supports the notion of practice variability, at least in the early stages of learning, as a way of promoting exploration of the constraint boundaries shaping motor control and learning.)

One of the first experiments to investigate the variability of practice hypothesis for consistently performed skills was conducted by Shea (a different Shea from the original co-investigator of random practice scheduling discussed earlier) and Kohl (1990, Experiment 2). These investigators had subjects learn a force production task under either constant or varied practice conditions. The task consisted of subjects lying supinely on a table and grasping a stationary handle positioned above their midline (see Figure 11.3). Subjects were to learn to produce a force of 175N by exerting a quick pushing action against the handle. A total of 289 practice trials were completed with a short rest between blocks of trials. Results were displayed on a monitor in view of the subjects at the completion of each attempt, providing an important source of feedback for learning the skill.

One-half of the subjects in the experiment were assigned to a constant practice group and completed all trials attempting the 175N criterion. The other half of the subjects comprised the varied practice condition. They performed the same number of practice trials, but their trials were equally divided

variability of practice principle: The notion that practicing skills or variations of the same skill in a variety of different ways and contexts has beneficial effects on learning; largely developed as a result of schema theory.

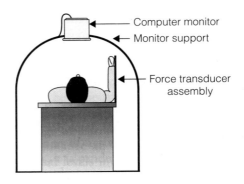

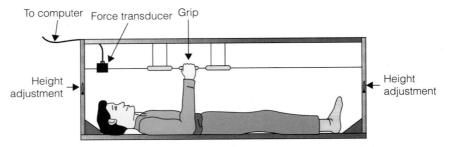

FIGURE **11.3** Shea and Kohl Experiment Comparing Constant
and Varied Practice for a Consistently Performed Skill

Source: Adapted from Shea, CH, and Kohl, RM (1990). Specificity and variability of practice.
Research Quarterly for Exercise and Sport, 61, 169–177.

among attempts to produce 125N, 150N, 200N, and 225N. The day after
completing the acquisition trials, all subjects completed a retention test of five
trials on the criterion task of 175N. Although both groups improved, the varied practice group demonstrated better learning on the retention test than did
the constant practice group. What is particularly noteworthy is that the varied group never practiced the criterion task (175N) during acquisition, yet they
were better able to perform it in the later recall test. These findings support the
predictions of schema theory that because memories for a skill are generalized,
varied practice will result in better learning. Such evidence lends credence to
the variability of practice principle.

Although such studies as Shea and Kohl's have supported recommending
varied practice for skills meant to be performed consistently, other studies have
resulted in findings that are more ambivalent. For example, two well-designed
studies testing the relative benefits of constant and varied practice in learning
a basketball free-throw skill demonstrated that both types of practice resulted
in good learning outcomes but that neither was clearly better than the other
(Landin, Hebert, and Fairweather, 1993; and Shoenfelt et al., 2002). So, though
there is strong support for variability of practice principles in the research

literature, results of other studies point out the need for more research to better understand exactly when and how varied practice might prove most effective. Until such answers are more clearly arrived at, however, the use of varied practice for skills that are performed with a high degree of movement consistency in stable environments will likely remain controversial and require keen discretion on the part of instructors.

The decision to employ varied practice scheduling for skills performed consistently requires careful analysis of the target performance and sensitivity to the needs of learners. Factors such as skill complexity, level of learner ability, age of learners, learners' needs for perceived success, and stage of learning can all play a role in deciding on the best scheduling of practice sessions. Even when the target skill of practice may remain highly consistent from practice to performance setting, the target context may change. In the basketball free-throw studies, where neither constant nor varied practice was clearly superior, it can be noted that the acquisition and retention phases of the investigations remained constant. In the real world, this skill is practiced in order to make free throws in the arenas of various opponents. The target context can change dramatically even when the performance of the target skill remains the same from practice to game. Coaches might use constant practice for the actual skill, but varied practice for the context conditions of practice. If free throws are to be made in the presence of an opposing team's home fans, who are notorious for booing opponents, for instance, practice might include free-throw attempts with the additional distraction of loud noises from a nearby music source (recall encoding specificity principles discussed in Chapter 6). They might also be practiced toward the end of a practice session when a player is fatigued. Practicing free throws when fresh and nondistracted may not optimize transfer to the game situation. In this case, even when the skill is practiced in a constant manner, the environment in which it is practiced is varied.

Varied practice may also lend interest to a practice situation, as well as require greater cognitive effort and attention on the part of learners, and these conditions may enhance learning quite apart from the actual variability of practice. So, the use of varied practice can play a role in the acquisition of consistently performed skills (see exercise in Box 11.4). Perhaps the best advice for

---

BOX 11.4 **Designing for Varied Practice of Closed Skills**

For the following list of closed skills designed to be performed in only one way, think about how and why you might design a varied practice schedule for each. How would you vary practice conditions? Do you believe that varied practice would be advisable for each of these skills? Why or why not?

- Getting out of bed (for a patient recovering from hip replacement surgery)

- Free throw
- Bowling (first ball of frame with 10 pins standing)
- Cartwheel in gymnastics
- Shooting an arrow at a stationary target
- Providing CPR
- Juggling three tennis balls

instructors of motor skills is to carefully observe what works during practice and to be willing to employ varied practice as part of an overall strategy to promote optimal learning.

THE DISTRIBUTION OF PRACTICE

distribution of practice:
The balancing of periods of rest and work within a practice schedule.

Once a decision concerning the ordering of skills in a practice schedule has been made, the next question will usually concern the spacing of practice. Instructors must decide how to space the time in which learners are actually engaged in practice. Should the practice within individual sessions be spread out over longer periods of time, with more time devoted to rest, or should it be packed together more closely in time? Should individual practice sessions be shorter but more frequent, or should there be fewer but longer sessions? Such questions concern the **distribution of practice.**

Research concerning the effects of practice distribution has a long history in the study of motor skills, with the period between 1930 and 1960 witnessing the greatest interest and number of studies (Adams, 1987). Since that time, however, partially because of shifting theoretical perspectives and the emergence of new topics of research interest (and also perhaps because many scholars thought little new was left to discover), few research studies have been directed toward further extending our understanding of practice distribution effects. There is, though, some evidence that this situation may be changing and a new era of research interest beginning (e.g., Dail and Christina, 2004; Shea et al., 2000; and Utley and Astill, 2008).

In studying the influence of practice distribution on motor skill learning, researchers have typically contrasted the effects of two types of practice schedules. These are *distributed practice* and *massed practice*. Unfortunately, a good deal of confusion has resulted from the fact that researchers have not always used these terms in the same way, leading to problems when comparing the results of various studies. Researchers frequently use these terms in a general way to indicate two extremes on a rest-to-work continuum, with **distributed practice** involving longer periods of rest and shorter periods of active practice (i.e., work), and **massed practice** involving less time in rest and longer periods in active practice (work). This way of defining the two terms is subjective and comparative in nature, and is typically used to contrast practice schedules across several practice sessions or within a single session when discrete skills are studied (because discrete skills are often completed quickly, therefore always necessitating relatively longer rest intervals between practice attempts than the actual time in practice). At other times, researchers also use a more objective method of defining both distribution schedules, particularly when distributive effects on continuous skills are contrasted within a single practice session. Under these circumstances, distributed practice may be defined as a practice session in which the amount of time in rest is equal to or greater than the amount of time in work, whereas massed practice is then defined as a practice schedule in which there is a greater amount of time in work than in rest.

distributed practice:
A practice schedule in which the amount of time in rest is relatively longer than the amount of time in actual practice.

massed practice: A practice schedule in which the amount of work or actual practice is relatively longer than the amount of time spent in rest.

Based upon the long history of research on practice distribution effects, strong consensus has emerged about the relative merits of distributed and massed practice schedules in some areas, whereas in other areas researchers remain divided (Dail and Christina, 2004; Lee and Genovese, 1988). Continuing controversies revolve mostly around the distributive influences vary for within and between practice sessions effects.

Within-Session Distribution Effects

In regard to the practice of motor skills within a single practice session, there is general consensus among researchers (echoed by practitioners) concerning the comparative effects of distributed and massed schedules on practice performance. Two major reviews of the literature support the conclusion that distributed practice promotes better acquisition performance than massed practice (Donovan and Radosevich, 1999; and Lee and Genovese, 1988). This may appear a somewhat obvious conclusion, because distributed practice, being more restful, leads to less fatigue and would therefore be expected to result in better acquisition performance than massed practice. The buildup of both physiological and psychological fatigue resulting from massed practice, imposing greater demands upon learners, can play a powerful role in depressing the ability to respond skillfully during practice. The critical question, though, is whether such effects on acquisition performance are only temporary or whether they are also mirrored in depressed measures of learning once the effects of fatigue have dissipated.

In their extensive review of the literature, Lee and Genovese concluded "that distributed practice is beneficial to both the performance and learning of motor skills, although the effect on performance is greater than the effect on learning" (p. 282). These reviewers also noted that almost all of the research reported contrasts the effects of distributed and massed practice on continuous skills. By their nature, continuous skills lend themselves more readily to experimental arrangements than do discrete skills because the amount of time devoted to actual work and rest can be more easily and objectively measured. In fact, in Lee and Genovese's review, they found that only one of 116 studies reported involved a discrete skill.

The exception to studies on continuous skills cited by Lee and Genovese was reported by Carron (1969). In Carron's study, subjects performed a peg-turning task. Beginning by grasping a key at the bottom of a board containing a number of pegs inserted into holes, the subjects' task was to release the key and move as quickly as possible to grasp a peg, turn it end to end, reinsert it in the hole, and move to re-grasp the key. Half of the subjects, who were assigned to the discrete condition, performed the task as quickly as possible with only a five-second rest after every 10th trial. The other half of the subjects, comprising the continuous condition, performed the same number of trials, but with a five-second rest between every practice attempt. All subjects were administered a retention test 48 hours later. Results showed no significant differences in performance during either acquisition or retention between the two groups, though in fact the massed group actually performed slightly better on the retention test. Lee and Genovese (1989) reported similar findings in a study of a discrete tapping task they carried out in an attempt to help clarify the discrepancy in findings between discrete and continuous skills. A more recent experiment by Dail and Christina (2004), employing a golf-putting task, found a slight benefit for both practice and learning as a result of distributed practice. In the absence of evidence to the contrary, most experts now believe that the massing of practice for discrete skills depresses practice performance, but not learning, when contrasted with distributed practice.

The few studies investigating distribution effects on discrete skills have initiated considerable debate concerning the relative effects of massed versus distributed practice for discrete skills. Although massing practice does depress practice performance, its effect on learning seems far less clear. The available evidence suggests that distributed practice is no more effective than is massed practice for the learning of discrete motor skills. Some studies have also reported superior benefits for massed practice compared to distributed practice as the time interval between acquisition and retention tests increases (Dail and Christina, 2004). Perhaps one reason this issue has remained unresolved, as well as under-investigated, is that no good theoretical explanation has been advanced to explain the differential distribution effects relative to continuous and discrete skills. Whatever the reasons, though, there exists little evidence on which to draw conclusions concerning the relative effects of massed and distributed practice on the learning of discrete motor skills, though what evidence does exist suggests no disadvantage for massed practice and may even point toward benefits in the long-term retention of discrete skills.

Practice Implications for Within-Session Distribution

The implications of research for the practice scheduling of continuous skills seems clear, which is to distribute practice to provide frequent rest periods while seeing that the total time in rest exceeds that in actual practice. The situation for the scheduling of discrete skills is not as readily clear, however, and requires careful analysis, observation, and a willingness on the part of instructors to make needed adjustments as practice results dictate.

In deciding upon the spacing of practice activities, instructors would be well advised to consider the pragmatic constraints of the time available for practice. Most practice situations, whether in schools, clinics, sports clubs, or on the job, are limited to predetermined amounts of time. A volleyball unit in a physical education class may be limited to twenty 30-minute sessions over a four-week period, and most physical therapy sessions are limited to a set time and number of appointments by insurance providers. In such cases, the urgency for scheduling sufficient practice experience within a limited time-frame must be weighed against the possible benefits of extending rest intervals within practice. Granting the ambivalent findings relative to massing practice, it is unequivocal that massing practice does allow for a greater amount of time in actual practice, and the amount of practice time is an essential ingredient for learning. In devising the practice recipe, instructors must weigh the relative benefits of practice time against the needs of learners for additional rest, as well as those factors that help learners gain from more massed practice. Individuals in good physical condition, who are highly motivated and who have acquired a good grasp of the skills being practiced, are most likely to benefit from additional massing of practice (Christina and Corcos, 1988).

Instructors might well keep in mind a conclusion drawn from the available research literature. If distributed practice benefits acquisition performance, its benefits for learning—if they exist—appear relatively slight. The imposition of time constraints on practice must be carefully considered, and the amount of actual practice time or number of practice trials deemed necessary to meet target goals balanced against the known beneficial distributive effects of practice.

Between-Session Distribution Effects

Besides making decisions regarding the spacing of practice within practice sessions, decisions concerning the distribution of practice over sequential sessions must also be made. Over what length of time should practice be distributed? Should practice sessions be scheduled daily, every other day, several days apart, or even further apart? Or, perhaps, would more than one daily practice session be most beneficial? Should sessions be short or long? Is it better to have shorter sessions frequently or longer sessions over a greater length of time? These questions concern between-session distribution effects.

Fortunately, the results of research concerning the distributive effects of practice are much more definitive regarding between-session effects than is the case for within-session effects. Though relatively few studies have been reported, the available evidence clearly supports the benefits of distributive practice (Schmidt and Lee, 2005).

The classic study supporting this conclusion was an investigation of postal workers learning to use a mail-sorting machine, reported by Baddeley and Longman (1978). This machine required workers to use a keyboard-like device to lift, address, and sort letters into appropriate routing lines for mail delivery. Workers, all of whom were inexperienced with the task, were divided into four different groups. All groups trained for a total of 60 hours, but using different distribution schedules. One group practiced one hour each day, five days a week, for a total of 12 weeks. A second group practiced in one-hour sessions twice a day, five days a week, completing 60 hours of practice in six weeks. A third group completed one 2-hour session each day, five days a week, also for a total of six weeks. Finally, a fourth group completed two 2-hour sessions a day, five days a week, for a total of three weeks. The groups varied on the amount of practice distribution experienced by the workers, with the first group representing the most distributed practice and the fourth group the most massed

BOX 11.5   Choosing a Massed or a Distributed Practice Schedule

For the following activities, decide whether emphasizing a more massed or distributed practice schedule within a practice session would be best advised. What is your reasoning for each choice?

- Square-dance routine
- Learning to play the keys on a piano

- Dribbling a basketball for a beginner
- Dribbling a basketball around moving defenders for an experienced learner
- Learning to use a walker
- Free-style stroke in swimming
- Golf putt

practice. Measurements of how long it took individual workers to learn the keyboard as well as to achieve a target goal of typing 80 correct keystrokes per minute were recorded and averaged over the four groups. The results are shown in Table 11.1.

As can be seen in Table 11.1, the workers in the most distributed practice group had the best learning outcomes, while learning was the worst for those workers in the most massed practice group. The number of hours it took workers to reach the target criterion of 80 correct keystrokes per minute was the measure of motor skill learning in this study. It took workers in the most distributed practice group 55 hours on average to reach this target, while after 80 hours of practice, the total hours available for training, the most massed practice group had failed to reach this target, averaging only 70 keystrokes per minute. Further retention tests were administered at three, six, and nine months after completion of the original training. On a keyboard speed test, the most distributed practice group performed the best, while the most massed group performed the worst. Interestingly, when workers were asked to rate the effectiveness of their training, the most massed group rated their practice experiences the best, while the most distributed group rated theirs as the worst, the exact opposite of the actual training outcomes.

Based upon the results of their study, Baddeley and Longman concluded that shorter practice sessions distributed over a longer time were more beneficial for learning than were longer practice sessions massed over a shorter time period. Similar results have been reported in the few other studies to investigate distributive practice effects for between-session scheduling (Annett and Piech, 1985; Bouzid and Crawshaw, 1987; and Shea et al., 2000). For between-session scheduling, the consensus of the research literature is that distributed practice benefits learning more than does massed practice. As a general guideline,

TABLE **11.1**
Results of Baddeley and Longman Study of Postal Workers

Practice Schedule	Hours to Learn Keyboard	Hours to Type 80 Keystrokes/Min.
1 hr. session, 1 session/day, 12 weeks	34.9	55
1 hr. session, 2 sessions/day, 6 weeks	43	75
2 hr. session, 1 session/day, 6 weeks	43	67
2 hr. session, 2 sessions/day, 3 weeks	49.7	80+*

*Achieved only 70 keystrokes/min. after 80 hours.

Source: "The influence of length and frequency of training sessions on the rate of learning to type", Baddeley, A.D., and Longman, D.J.A. *Ergonomics, 21,* 627–635. (1978). Reprinted by permission of the publisher (Taylor & Francis Group, http://www.informaworld.com)

shorter practice sessions, distributed over longer periods of time, are more beneficial for learning than are schedules where practice is massed in longer sessions and less time.

One possible explanation for the beneficial effects of practice distribution observed over practice sessions has to do with memory consolidation. Recall from our earlier discussion of memory in Chapter 6 that memories are consolidated (made permanent) through a series of biochemical processes. Those processes take time to be accomplished. When practice is distributed, there is simply more time for consolidation processes to be completed. Recall also serial order effects on learning. That is, those practice experiences occurring at the beginning and ending of practice sessions are the most easily consolidated into memory and therefore the best learned. Shorter and more frequent practice sessions also mean that more practice experiences occur in beginning and ending portions of practice than would be true for longer and fewer practice sessions, resulting in more practice experiences being effectively consolidated. Spacing out learning experiences also weakens the effects of interference on consolidation processes. Interestingly, evidence has begun to emerge in recent years that sleep may be essential for the consolidation of procedural memories, including those for motor skills (Kuriyama, Stickgold, and Walker, 2004; Walker et. al., 2003). One benefit of distributed practice may be that spreading practice out over more days results in more of the actual practice experiences being followed by periods of sleep, leading to more effective consolidation of those experiences in memory.

Another explanation for the relative benefits of distributed practice is the suggestion that massing practice may diminish the amount of cognitive effort exerted by learners after a certain point in practice is reached. Practice experiences may become so repetitive during massed practice that they become monotonous and boring to learners, who will then decrease the amount of cognitive effort they exert, which in turn will decrease the learning outcomes of practice.

However the causes underlying the benefits of distributed practice over massed practice are eventually sorted out, that distributed practice does promote better learning than massed practice is firmly established in the research literature. The question becomes one of how to translate this knowledge into effective practice designs.

Practice Implications for Between-Session Distribution

Based upon the available research evidence, the implications for scheduling of between-session practice are straightforward. Practice sessions that are shorter and distributed over a longer period (days/weeks, etc.) promote better learning than do practice sessions that are longer and massed over shorter periods of time. All other things being equal, instructors of motor skills are well advised to distribute practice experiences as much as possible.

Of course, a key phrase in this advice is "all other things being equal," which is seldom the case. For example, in referring to the study of postal workers discussed above, Schmidt and Lee (2005) have pointed out that although the most massed group (two-hour sessions twice a day for three weeks) had the poorest acquisition and retention performance, they completed their training in one-half the time used by two of the other groups, and in one-quarter the time used by the most distributed practice group (one-hour session daily for 12 weeks). Additional training for the most massed group would have resulted in additional learning, and in all likelihood they would have achieved the same level of learning as attained by the more distributed groups of workers in a shorter period of time.

Decisions concerning practice distribution and total time of training involve a trade-off. Distributed practice results in the most learning, but it also takes the most time. Massed practice results in less learning, but the learning is achieved in less time. Instructors must weigh the learning benefits of distributed practice against the time-saving benefits of massed practice, designing schedules that are most effective in balancing the length of time devoted to achieving target goals and the actual achievement of those goals (but see Box 11.6).

SIMPLIFYING SKILL PRESENTATION: THE USES OF PART PRACTICE

However it is scheduled, learning a new skill can be a daunting task. Learners can feel overwhelmed by the demands presented by new skills, and their inability to execute them correctly may even lead to frustration and withdrawal from further practice. Consequently, part practice is frequently employed as an

---

BOX **11.6**   **Three Caveats When Considering Massing Practice**

When considering massing practice within a single practice session, instructors must sometimes consider more than distribution effects on learning. Even when massing practice may benefit learning, other factors may dictate a more distributed schedule. The following three factors should be carefully evaluated whenever mass practice schedules are being considered.

Safety Massed practice can increase physiological and psychological fatigue, compromising both the learner's quality of movement and attentional focus. When practicing skills where safety issues are of concern, distributed practice, which is more restful, may be required in order to minimize the risk of injury.

Motivation The massing of practice does depress performance levels during acquisition, even when learning benefits remain present. Depressed performance levels, in addition to increased levels of fatigue, can affect a learner's motivation to continue practice. Especially with beginning learners, this factor requires due consideration. If adequate methods for encouraging and motivating learners are not sufficiently successful, greater distribution of practice may be indicated to reduce detrimental effects on learner motivation.

Kinematics If increased levels of fatigue associated with massing practice become sufficient to distort basic movement patterns, practice can quickly become ineffective. Both cognitive-based and dynamical systems theories of motor learning allow for beneficial effects of practice variability associated with fatigue, but both also recognize that when movement patterns exceed the kinematic boundaries inherent to a skill, practice is no longer effective. If the movement patterns of a skill become too greatly compromised due to a buildup of fatigue, rest periods should be increased until basic kinematic skill features are reestablished.

instructional strategy designed to reduce the demands on learners and provide them with early successes. Although part practice can greatly simplify the task confronted by learners early in practice, leading to experiences of success and progress, part practice does not in all cases lead to the best learning outcomes. **Part practice** refers to methods of presenting an otherwise complex skill in a more simplified form, usually involving separating the skill into component parts so that it can be more easily understood and executed by learners.

part practice: Any method of simplifying the performance of a skill, involving either the initial practice of component parts of the skill or the simplification of environmental features in which the skill is performed.

Methods of Part Practice

Three methods of part practice have traditionally been identified: segmentation, simplification, and fractionization (Wightman and Lintern, 1985).

Segmentation

segmentation: A part-practice method in which a skill is broken down into component parts and the parts practiced separately until some level of proficiency is obtained before practicing the skill in the whole.

progressive part method: A method of part practice in which the component parts of a skill are sequentially added to practice as each previous component is mastered.

Segmentation involves breaking a skill down into component parts or segments, which are then practiced separately until some level of proficiency is achieved. Once each part can be performed sufficiently, the individual parts are then reunited and the skill practiced as a whole. A variation of this method involves practicing the first part of a skill, then the second, then combining the two parts together. This method is continued by first practicing and then adding parts sequentially until the skill is completely reunited and being practiced in the whole. Similar to adding links to a chain, this method is also referred to as the **progressive part method,** or sometimes simply as *forward chaining.* In some instances, instructors will begin with the final part of a skill and then add parts in a backward direction, working toward the beginning of the skill, a method called *backward chaining.* An example of the progressive part method of segmentation practice is often seen in the teaching of dance and gymnastics floor routines, where learners are taught to correctly execute one of the many component parts of the skill at a time before additional parts are added.

Simplification

simplification: A method of part practice where a skill is practiced in the whole but in which the complexity of some feature of the skill or environment is reduced.

As the name suggests, **simplification** involves simplifying some aspect of practice. Technically, simplification is not a part method of practice because a skill is still performed in the whole. It is common, though, to classify it as a part-practice method because the goal is to simplify early practice experiences before adding the more difficult components of the skill, which is the same goal as for all part methods of practice. In simplification, various movement components of a skill or aspects of the environment in which the skill is performed are simplified. This may involve the simplification of movement patterns, as seen when ski instructors have beginners practice without the use of ski poles, thereby reducing the need to coordinate arm and leg actions. Simplification may also involve the use of equipment that reduces the perceptual demands on learners. An example is seen in teaching children to bat a stationary ball using a T-stand so that they can practice swinging without the need to coordinate their movements with the flight of an approaching ball. Another type of simplification occurs when providing auditory accompaniment for skills having a distinct rhythmic characteristic. For example, musical accompaniment can assist people with gait disorders while they practice walking.

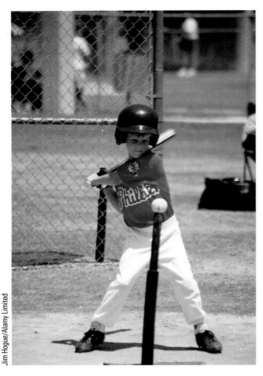

Jim Hogue/Alamy Limited

Simplification methods allow individuals to practice a skill in its entirety while reducing the perceptual and movement demands required in accomplishing the skill.

Fractionization

fractionization: A part method of practice involving the isolated practice of various skill components that would normally be performed simultaneously.

A third type of part practice, called **fractionization**, involves practicing in isolation the components of a skill that are normally performed simultaneously. For example, in learning the freestyle stroke in swimming, many beginners have initial difficulty coordinating the simultaneous actions of their legs and arms. A common solution to this problem is to have beginners practice leg and arm actions independently. This is usually accomplished by having beginners practice the kicking action of the stroke while facing and holding on to the side of the pool, and separately practicing arm strokes using a floatation device between the legs to eliminate the need for kicking while moving through the water. Although fractionization can dramatically reduce demands on learners and is a commonly employed method in many instructional settings, there is little support either theoretically or in the research literature for its use. The problem, as in the example of learning the freestyle stroke, is that the timing between limbs (in this case the arms and legs) is critical to performing the whole skill but is left out when the component parts are practiced separately. Of even greater concern, the separate practice of component parts may lead to learning them with entirely different timing characteristics than those necessary to successfully perform the skill as a whole.

Deciding When to Use Part and When to Use Whole Practice

As we have just seen in the case of fractionization, part practice may simplify practice and improve performance (at least of the skill elements performed separately) but may not always result in the most effective learning of skills. In fact, in some cases part practice hinders effective learning. An important question for practitioners is, When should part practice be used, and when should it be avoided? The answer to this question entails a careful consideration concerning the nature of the skills being instructed.

In a somewhat dated but still influential paper, Naylor and Briggs (1963) identified two aspects of a skill that determine whether part practice should be used. These two aspects are task complexity and task organization. Naylor and Briggs defined **task complexity** as referring to the number of parts or components of a skill and the level of attention demanded in performing the skill. A highly complex skill would have many components as well as require a high degree of attention. Examples of complex skills include shifting gears while driving an automobile, a wrestling takedown, performing a gymnastics routine, and relearning to walk up stairs following knee surgery. Low-complexity skills have few components and require relatively little attention. Bouncing a ball and lifting a glass are skills low in complexity. Another way to think about task complexity is in terms of the demands made upon a person's memory (Singer, 1980). How many things must a person think about during the execution of the skill? How much has to be remembered from previous experiences? How difficult does the person perceive the skill to be? Relative to the perceived difficulty of a task, an important distinction between complexity and difficulty should be kept in mind. Skills can be difficult and yet remain low in task complexity. Lifting a heavy barbell from the floor may be difficult, but it is relatively low in task complexity.

Task organization refers to the interdependence of the component parts of a skill. A skill is high in task organization when its parts are each related to a common spatial-temporal pattern inherent to the whole skill. Driving a golf ball, for example, requires coordinating the arm movements of the swing with the rotation of the hips and lower body, and the timing between these bodily segments must be precise if the skill is to be executed successfully. Dynamic forces arising from bodily movements may also act to link movement components together in a highly organized way. Hitting a baseball serves as an example of this. It would be easy to practice the backswing and forward-swing motions of hitting a baseball as separate parts, but consider the problem that would be encountered when reassembling them into the whole skill. Practicing the forward swing from a static beginning position looks like the same motion as when it is performed immediately after completing the backswing. Consider, however, that in the whole execution of the skill, there are elastic forces built up in the arm and shoulder muscles during the backswing phase that are then transferred to the forward-swing phase when the two components (backswing and forward swing) are joined together in a single quick motion, thereby contributing additional force to the forward swing that would not otherwise be present. For highly organized skills, the parts cannot be separated without destroying some essential coordinative feature of the task.

task complexity: The number of component parts of a skill.

task organization: The degree to which the component parts of a skill are interrelated and performance of the whole skill is dependent upon their integration.

Based upon analysis of the task complexity and task organization characteristics of skills, a useful guideline emerges for making decisions about the appropriate use of part and whole-practice methods. Skills that are high in task complexity are best suited to part method practice during initial phases of instruction, while skills low in task complexity are better served by the whole-practice method. On the other hand, skills high in task organization are best suited to **whole-practice** method, while skills low in task organization are better served by part method practice, during the initial phases of instruction. These guidelines, widely echoed in the research and professional literature concerning motor skills instruction, provide a sound basis for many, perhaps for most, instructional situations. Indeed, in most situations, an analysis of the task complexity and task organization characteristics of skills leads to an obvious conclusion. Skills high in task complexity and low in task organization can confidently be instructed using part methods of practice, at least until beginning learners have a sound grasp of the parts which can then be reassembled for practice in the whole. Conversely, for those skills low in task complexity and high in task organization, part-practice methods should be avoided and the skills practiced in the whole, and this is true even in the initial stages of learning.

> **whole practice:** Practice of a skill in its entirety as it is intended to be performed as a result of practice.

The decision to use part or whole practice can become much more difficult to make, however, as the differences between the criteria of task complexity and task organization blur. What about a skill that is fairly complex but also somewhat organized? What if a skill is both highly organized and highly complex? Although as a general guideline the analysis of task complexity and task organization can often lead to correct decisions regarding the use of part method practice, it may at other times prove too vague for useful application.

Some Additional Considerations

To help better clarify the situation of when to use part practice and when it should be avoided, several researchers have observed that the degree of task organization often corresponds to the type of skill being performed (Lee, Chamberlin, and Hodges, 2004; Schmidt and Lee, 2005). Serial skills, for example, often lend themselves to part-practice methods. In fact, because part practice may lead to the more difficult components of a skill being practiced with greater frequency than would result if the skill were practiced only in the whole, part practice can have significant benefits for learning many serial skills, producing transfer effects of greater than 100 percent. Although part practice for serial skills may be especially beneficial because of the additional practice of the more difficult parts of the skills, the mere repetition of the more difficult components apart from their progressive reassembly into whole practice (as in forward and backward chaining) does not appear to be beneficial. Of course, some serial skills do involve a high degree of organization among their component parts (e.g., playing the piano, shifting and clutching a standard-shift automobile), in which case part practice should be avoided. For continuous skills, in which the parts of a skill that can be isolated often occur simultaneously, part practice may not prove effective when those parts are highly coordinated in the target skill. If the task complexity of a continuous skill is especially high, however, some initial practice of the parts in isolation may be warranted, though expedient transfer to the skill as a whole should be a priority.

The least likely candidates for part practice are discrete skills, and especially discrete skills performed rapidly (e.g., hitting a baseball, returning a tennis serve, casting a fishing line). Schmidt and Wrisberg (2008) argue that because rapid discrete skills are believed to be controlled by a single motor program that is completely prestructured prior to the beginning of action (see Chapter 4), breaking such skills into constituent parts may involve the practice of new motor programs for each part that cannot then be effectively reassembled into the motor program for the whole skill. In an illustrative study by Klapp, Nelson, and Jagacinski (1998), participants were taught to tap a 3:2 bimanual polyrhythm (the right hand tapped three beats while the left hand tapped two beats in a 1,800 msec interval) in either a whole or part (right and left hand separately) method. Results showed that the whole group learned the task best. However, when asked to tap each hand rhythm separately, the whole group performed worse than the part group. Klapp, Nelson, and Jagacinski concluded that whole practice resulted in learning a motor program controlling the task as a whole rather than specifying actions for each hand independently. Practice of each hand in isolation, as Schmidt and Wrisberg contend, led to the learning of two separate motor programs distinct from the one used for accomplishing the skill as a whole. These recommendations based upon skill type, it should be noted, are really another way of focusing on the task organization of skills as originally recommended by Naylor and Briggs, but they offer another helpful guideline in deciding when part practice is appropriate. A summary of the uses of part- and whole-practice methods is presented in Figure 11.4.

A final caution should be kept in mind whenever the decision to use part practice is made, and that is that whenever learners practice in parts, it is critical that they understand the connections of those parts to the whole skill. Newell et al. (1989), for example, had subjects learn a computer game called Space Fortress developed by the United States Air Force as a training aid for pilots. The game required subjects to use both hands in controlling a joystick and buttons to execute a series of different actions designed to simulate aerial combat between two opposing forces, much like many popular video games. Two groups were taught the skills required for the game using part practice, but only one group was told how the individual parts related to the overall strategy of the game. Though both groups learned the parts equally well, the group instructed in the game's overall strategy was much more successful in transferring their newly acquired skills to performing well when playing the game. When employing part practice, then, helping learners understand how the individual components they are executing relate to the whole skill that represents the goal of practice is important in maximizing the benefits of part-practice methods.

Attentional Cueing

attentional cueing: A practice technique where an instructor directs a learner's attention to a specific aspect or component of a skill performed in the whole.

When part-practice methods are deemed inappropriate, some of their benefits may still be gained during whole practice by employing the technique of **attentional cueing**. Instructors use attentional cueing by focusing learners' attention on a single aspect or component of a skill being practiced in the whole. "Focus on your hips as you throw." "Concentrate on the position of your hand as you

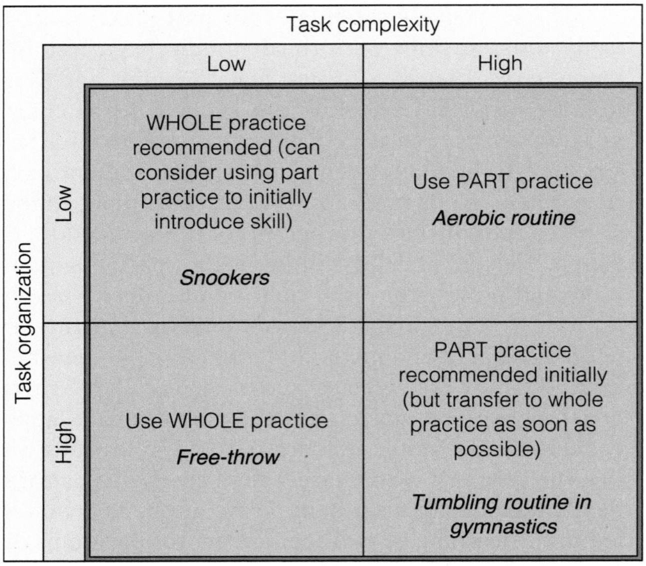

FIGURE **11.4** Weighing Task Complexity and Organization When Deciding on Using Part- or Whole-Practice Methods

Source: Created by author.

release the ball." "Think about keeping your elbows relaxed but locked as you position your crutches ahead of you." This strategy focuses learners' attention on one particular movement component (on one part of the skill) without disrupting the underlying spatial and temporal characteristics of the skill as a whole. Although little empirical research has yet confirmed the effectiveness of attentional cueing in facilitating the learning of specific task components (but see Gopher, Weil, and Siegel, 1989, for an example), it appears a promising area for further investigation.

BOX **11.7** **Deciding between Part and Whole Practice**

For the following activities, decide (a) whether each is high or low in both task complexity and task organization, and based upon your decision further decide (b) whether part or whole practice is most appropriate in the initial stages of learning.

- Typing a practice sentence
- Walking with a cane
- Parallel parking
- Heading a soccer ball
- Line dancing
- Using sign language
- Tying shoelaces
- Playing darts
- Performing CPR
- Pole vaulting

SEARCHING FOR GENERAL PRINCIPLES: COGNITIVE EFFORT AND THE CHALLENGE POINT MODEL

In this chapter, we have seen that a number of practice variables exhibit rather dramatic learning–performance distinctions. That is, methods that demonstrate good practice performance do not always promote good long-term learning. In the current chapter, we observed this in a number of instances when comparing the effects of blocked and random practice, constant and varied practice, massed and distributed practice, and part- and whole-practice methods. The same phenomenon is also evident when considering expert and learning models (Chapter 10) and frequency of feedback (Chapter 12), among other practice variables. Such pronounced differences in the effects on performance and learning of a number of practice variables present a challenge to motor skill instructors. Given these often counterintuitive aspects of practice manipulations, how can instructors select the best practice methods to optimize learning? Are there guidelines that can help in making practice decisions?

How can the motor skills instructor make sense of these seeming contradictions in patterns of performance and learning across many important practice methodologies? One particularly useful perspective aimed at helping practitioners make decisions regarding practice scheduling emerging in recent years has been advanced by Lee and his associates and focuses on the practice effects of **cognitive effort** (Guadagnoli and Lee, 2004; Lee, Swinnen, and Serrien, 1994; and Patterson and Lee, 2008). Cognitive effort is defined as "the mental work involved in making decisions" (Lee, Swinnen, and Serrien, 1994, p. 329). Some practice conditions require an intense use of cognitive resources, placing considerable processing demands on the performer. These entail instances of high cognitive effort. Other practice conditions, however, may lessen the cognitive demands placed upon performers, resulting in relatively little cognitive effort. Different practice arrangements may require different levels of cognitive effort. From an instructional viewpoint, practice provides opportunities for both promoting and impeding the amount of cognitive effort experienced when performing skilled movements. As is becoming more and more evident in recent years, the learning of motor skills is a highly cognitive process, so increasing levels of cognitive effort during the practice of skills (at least to a point) is generally beneficial for learning (Berthoz, 2000; Clark, 2008; and Rizzolatti and Sinigaglia, 2006).

As an illustration of the influence of cognitive effort on learning, Lee, Swinnen, and Serrien (1994) analyze its differential effects on learning when practicing under blocked and random practice conditions. Contextual interference, in this case, directly mirrors the degree of cognitive effort. The higher the degree of contextual interference within a practice schedule, the greater the amount of cognitive effort required, all other things being equal.

The reduced cognitive load required in blocked practice is obvious. Once the learner has processed information sufficiently to perform at an acceptable level given his or her stage of learning, maintenance of that performance level is simply a matter of holding the current movement solution in working memory—no further cognitive processing is required (or only minor adjustments are necessary). The ability afforded by blocked practice to fine-tune performance

cognitive effort: The amount of mental work involved in the retrieval, decision making, and planning leading to the execution of a skill.

Motor learning involves more than storing sensory and motor information that arises as a consequence of movement. Skill is highly cognitive, and the cognitive processes that subserve movement must be practiced as well.

—Lee, Swinnen, and Serrien, 1994

over several practice trials and then maintain motor commands within working memory keeps individuals performing around optimal levels of execution and, thus, maintaining high-acquisition performance. The story is different, however, for the effects on learning. By simplifying the cognitive processing requirements for performance, learners fail to maximize the full potential of practice by not including repetition of the cognitive elements of skill learning. Because random practice requires trial-to-trial retrieval and processing activities, it results in less stable execution of skills than is the case with blocked practice. The additional cognitive processing and decision-making activities required with random practice, though, do afford significantly greater opportunity for strengthening memory and other cognitive elements of skill supporting long-term retention. Increases in blocked practice performance are therefore realized because of reduced demands on cognitive effort, which in turn manifest themselves in less effective learning outcomes. Random practice suffers from higher comparative performance demands on cognition, resulting in relatively poor practice performance, but it is just that increased demand for additional cognitive processing that promotes greater retention of the practiced skills.

In using methods of practice that increase the cognitive demands placed upon learners, motor skill instructors are confronted with the challenge of increasing cognitive effort requirements to sufficient levels to promote optimal learning, but to refrain from presenting cognitive demands that are either too easy or too difficult for learners, both of which can compromise the benefits sought through the use of practice methods optimizing cognitive effort. A helpful way of assessing the proper point to which practice variables such as contextual interference might be varied to obtain the most appropriate levels of cognitive effort is captured in the **challenge point model** developed by Guadagnoli and Lee (2004).

challenge point model: A conceptual model relating the cognitive challenges inherent in practicing a skill to the learning potential available.

The challenge point model is illustrated in Figure 11.5. The base of the figure represents functional task difficulty. This term indicates the degree of difficulty for a particular individual considering his or her capabilities and stage of learning. Functional task difficulty pertains to an individual, not to a task itself. For a weekend golfer, a 130-yard drive to the green may be high in functional task difficulty; for a professional player on the PGA Tour, it is low. The solid line represents the learner's practice performance potential as levels of task difficulty are varied. If, for example, practice conditions are manipulated to reduce his or her task difficulty to a low level (e.g., by the use of blocked practice, part-practice methods, etc.), then practice performance will be optimized as shown by the solid line. As task difficulty is increased for the individual by making practice more difficult (e.g., by the use of completely random practice, whole practice, etc.), practice performance progressively decreases as the solid line shows. Reducing practice scheduling demands increases performance potential, while increasing cognitive demands reduces performance potential. There is a point, however, at which the two types of demands (practice scheduling and cognitive) balance one another, and the opportunity for learning is optimized, These learning opportunities are represented by the dashed line in the figure, with the optimal challenge point represented by the circle. It can be noted in the figure that practice performance increases as functional task difficulty is reduced (becomes lower) through the use of practice methods making fewer cognitive demands on learners. It can also be noted that the learning

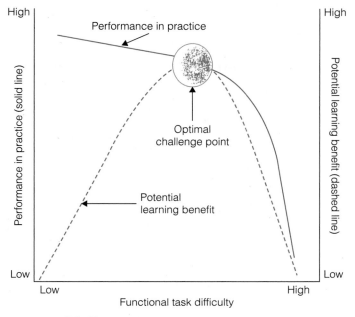

FIGURE **11.5** The Challenge Point Model

Source: Guadagnoli, MA and Lee, TD (2004). Challenge point: A framework for conceptualizing the effects of various practice conditions in motor learning. *Journal of Motor Behavior, 36*(2), 212–225. Copyright 2004 By Taylor & Francis Informa UK LTD - Journals. Reproduced With Permission of Taylor & Francis Informa UK LTD - Journals in the format Textbook via Copyright Clearance Center.

potential (the dashed line) is also reduced as functional task difficulty, along with cognitive effort, is reduced through the use of such methods.

One final point should be noted. The effects represented in Figure 11.5 are not static. As an individual becomes more proficient at a skill, his or her level of functional task difficulty also changes. This means that the optimal challenge point changes as well. The challenge for the motor skills instructor is gradually, but constantly, to monitor a learner's progress and increase the practice challenges through manipulating the many practice variables in the instructor's control in ways that will continually optimize learning.

SUMMARY

Practice is the single most critical factor in skill learning. Designing effective practice schedules requires a firm grasp of many practice principles. Though a great deal is known about effective practice scheduling, instructors of motor skills will also find that many trade-offs must be made in devising the most beneficial practice plans for those they instruct.

• Many practice variables manifest a learning–performance distinction. That is, one method of manipulating a specific practice variable results in optimal practice performance, while another method, often viewed as contradictory, results in optimal learning.

- When scheduling practice experiences, schedules that promote variability among practice trials may depress performance levels but often enhance long-term retention and the learning of skills.
  - In scheduling interskill practice sessions, blocked practice promotes better practice performance levels, although random practice often results in superior levels of learning.
  - In scheduling intraskill practice sessions, decisions regarding practice variability methods are not as clear, but certainly there are times when varied practice results in superior levels of learning, although at other times constant practice is preferred.
- The amount of actual work or practice within and between practice sessions is conceptualized as the distribution of practice and specified as being either massed or distributed.
  - Specific to within-session distribution effects, more distributed practice schedules promote both better performance and learning of continuous skills; for discrete skills, distributed practice promotes superior practice performance, but massed practice typically results in equal learning to distributed practice.
  - Specific to between-session distribution effects, more distributed practice schedules promote both better performance and learning for all skills, though there is a trade-off between the learning advantages of more distributed practice schedules and the additional amount of actual practice that can often be obtained through more massed practice designs.
- Part-practice methods may facilitate learning during the early stages of practice but should be used only after careful consideration of a number of factors, including task complexity and organization.
- The amount of cognitive effort required in the planning and execution of a motor skill is directly related to observed benefits in learning.

LEARNING EXERCISES

1. Conduct a survey of four or five people professionally engaged in teaching motor skills in a field of interest to you (teaching children, teaching adults, coaching, rehabilitation, training, dance instruction, instruction for a musical instrument, etc.). Ask each of the people in your survey to explain how they make decisions about scheduling practice experiences relative to (1) the ordering of skills, (2) the degree of variability with which specific skills are practiced, (3) practice distribution or spacing, and (4) the use of part-practice methods. Be prepared to ask questions and to probe for fairly complete descriptions in each of these areas. Also inquire about each instructor's belief concerning the degree to which maximizing practice performance should be a goal of practice. Select an appropriate method of recording answers to these questions from each of the people you interview (note taking, audio recordings, etc.). Remember that your task is simply to conduct a survey and collect answers,

not to judge or comment on an instructor's methods during an interview. After all of the interviews are completed, prepare a report of your findings. Describe the answers provided for each of the areas of practice concern. Based upon the information presented in this chapter, analyze the correctness or gaps in knowledge exhibited by your instructional sample. What conclusions can be drawn from the results of your survey?

2. Obtain your instructor's permission and prepare a 15-minute PowerPoint presentation addressing the question, Should practice be perfect? Present your presentation to your class or to another group on whom both you and your instructor agree. (As an alternative, prepare a 1,500-word paper of your position on this topic.)

3. Teach someone (a friend, family member, classmate, etc.) a skill with which you are familiar, using a part-practice method of instruction. You should instruct the person in the skill over a sufficient number of times (e.g., three or four) to observe progression toward whole performance of the skill (and perhaps full progression to whole practice). At the conclusion of the instructional sessions, prepare a written analysis of how well you believe the part-practice approach you used worked (be sure to consider the learner's observations on how he or she experienced the practice sessions). Describe why you chose the method that you did, your experience using it to teach the skill, and whether you believe it proved effective.

FOR FURTHER STUDY

HOW MUCH DO YOU KNOW?

For each of the following, select the letter that best answers the question.

1. A major theme developed in this chapter is that
   a. performance and learning are essentially the same thing.
   b. performance is always a good indicator of learning.
   c. optimal learning results from optimizing practice performance.
   d. optimal learning does not necessarily result from optimizing practice performance.

2. A random practice schedule results in _____ contextual interference.
   a. low
   b. moderate
   c. high
   d. varied

3. Introducing high levels of contextual interference into a practice schedule has generally been shown to
   a. depress both the performance and learning of motor skills.
   b. improve both the performance and learning of motor skills.
   c. depress the performance but improve the learning of motor skills.
   d. depress the learning but improve the performance of motor skills.

4. A practice schedule is defined as distributed if it
   a. maximizes performance measures.
   b. consists of a greater amount of rest than work.
   c. is experienced by the learner as restful.
   d. allows learners to rest whenever they become fatigued.

5. Part practice is recommended for motor skills that are
   a. high in task complexity and low in task organization.
   b. high in task complexity and high in task organization.

c. low in task complexity and low in task organization.

d. low in task complexity and high in task organization.

6. _____ skills are typically the best candidates for part practice.
   a. Serial
   b. Open
   c. Continuous
   d. Discrete

Answer the following with the word or words that best complete each sentence.

7. The _____ hypothesis suggests that learning is enhanced through random practice because it increases the meaningfulness and distinctiveness of skills making them more durable in long-term memory.

8. The task that a person wishes to be able to perform as a result of practice is called the _____ skill.

9. _____ is a type of part practice in which all component parts of a skill are practiced separately until each is mastered, and only then is the skill reassembled into a whole.

10. In the classic study by Baddeley and Longman in which the benefits of distributed practice were demonstrated for scheduling a series of practice sessions over an extended time, what was the skill that subjects in the experiment learned?

11. A practice technique in which an instructor tells a learner to focus his or her attention on a specific aspect of movement prior to executing a practice attempt is termed _____.

12. The mental work required when executing a motor skill is termed _____.

Answers are provided at the end of this review section.

STUDY QUESTIONS

1. Define and explain the differences between blocked and random practice schedules.
2. Define contextual interference, and describe how it is related to blocked, serial, and random practice.
3. When comparing the effects of blocked and random practice schedules, what are the differences, generally, between acquisition performance and long-term learning?
4. When and how should random practice be introduced into a practice schedule?
5. Compared to blocked practice, how effective is random practice across the stages of learning?
6. Define the action plan reconstruction and the elaboration hypotheses. How does each hypothesis account for contextual interference effects?
7. Define constant and varied practice. What factors should be considered when deciding whether to use constant or varied practice?

8. Define and contrast the implications of the specificity of practice and the variability of practice hypotheses.
9. Define massed and distributed practice. What factors should be considered when deciding on whether to use a massed or distributed practice schedule within a specific practice session?
10. What are the relative benefits of massed and distributed practice when considering the instruction of skills over a number of practice sessions? What is the trade-off that instructors typically should consider in deciding on the distribution of such schedules?
11. Describe the following methods of part practice: segmentation, progressive part, simplification, and fractionization.
12. What are task complexity and task organization, and how are they related to decisions about the use of part- and whole-practice methods?
13. How is cognitive effort related to the learning of motor skills? How does it help explain the learning–performance distinction?

ADDITIONAL READING

Brady, F. (1998). "A theoretical and empirical review of the contextual interference effect and the learning of motor skills." *Quest, 50,* 266–293.

Brady, F. (2008). "The contextual interference effect in sport skills." *Perceptual and Motor Skills, 106,* 461–467.

Chow, J-Y, Davids, K, Button, C, Shuttleworth, R, Renshaw, L, and Araujo, D (2006). "Nonlinear pedagogy: A constraints-led framework to understanding emergence of game play and skills." *Nonlinear Dynamics, Psychology and Life Science, 10,* 71-103.

Coker, CA. (2006). "To break it down or not break it down: That is the question." *Teaching Elementary Physical Education, 17,* 26–27.

Coker, CA, and Fischman, MG. (2010). Motor skill learning for effective coaching and performance. In JM Williams (ed.), *Applied Sport Psychology: Personal Growth to Peak Performance* (6th ed), (pp. 21–41). New York: McGraw-Hill.

Douvis, S. (2005). "Variable practice in learning the forehand drive in tennis." *Perceptual and Motor Skills, 101,* 531–545.

Jones, L, and French, KE. (2007). "Effects of contextual interference in acquisition and retention of three volleyball skills." *Perceptual and Motor Skills, 105,* 883–890.

Lee, TD, Chamberlin, CJ, and Hodges, NJ. (2001). "Practice." In RN Singer, HA Hausenblas, and CM Janelle (eds.), *Handbook of sport psychology* (pp. 115–143). New York: John Wiley and Sons.

Lee, TD, and Wishart, LR. (2005). "Motor learning conundrums (and possible solutions)." *Quest, 57,* 67–78.

Patterson, JT, and Lee, TD. (2008). Organizing practice: the interaction of repetition and cognitive effort for skilled performance. In D. Farrow, J Baker, and C MacMahon (eds.) *Developing sport expertise: Researchers and coaches put theory into practice* (pp. 119–134). London: Routledge.

Simon, DA, and Bjork, RA. (2001). "Metacognition in motor learning." *Journal of Experimental Psychology: Learning, Memory and Cognition, 27,* 907–912.

REFERENCES

Adams, JA. (1971). "A closed-loop theory of motor control." *Journal of Motor Behavior, 3,* 111–150.

Adams, JA. (1987). Historical review and appraisal of research on the learning, retention, and transfer of human motor skills. *Psychological Bulletin, 101,* 41–74.

Al-Ameer, H, and Toole, T. (1993). "Combinations of blocked and random practice orders: Benefits to acquisition and retention." *Journal of Human Movement Studies, 25,* 177–191.

Annett, J, and Piech, J. (1985). "The retention of a skill following distributed practice." *Programmed Learning and Educational Technology, 22,* 182–186.

Baddeley, AD, and Longman, DJA. (1978). "The influence of length and frequency of training sessions on the rate of learning to type." *Ergonomics, 21,* 627–635.

Barnett, ML, Ross, D, Schmidt, RA, and Todd, B. (1973). "Motor skills learning and the specificity of training principle." *Research Quarterly for Exercise and Sport, 44,* 440–447.

Battig, WF. (1956). "Transfer from verbal pretraining to motor performance as a function of motor task complexity." *Journal of Experimental Psychology, 51,* 371–378.

Battig, WF. (1966). "Facilitation and interference." In EA Bilodeau (ed.), *Acquisition of skill,* New York: Academic Press.

Berthoz, A. (2000). *The brain's sense of movement.* Boston: Harvard Press.

Bjork, RA. (1975). "Retrieval as a memory modifier." In R Solso (ed.), *Information processing and cognition: The Loyola Symposium* (pp. 123–144). Hillsdale, NJ: Lawrence Erlbaum.

Bjork, Robert A. (1994). "Memory and metamemory considerations in the training of human beings." In J Metcalfe and A Shimamura (eds.), *Metacognition: Knowing About Knowing,* Cambridge, MA: MIT Press.

Bouzid, N, and Crawshaw, CM. (1987). "Massed versus distributed word-processor training." *Applied Ergonomics, 18,* 220–222.

Brady, F. (1998). "A theoretical and empirical review of the contextual interference effect and the learning of motor skills." *Quest, 50,* 266–293.

Carron, AV. (1969). "Performance and learning in a discrete motor task under massed versus distributed practice." *Research Quarterly, 40,* 481–489.

Christina, RW, and Alpenfels, E. (2002). "Why does traditional training fail to optimize playing performance?" In E Thain (ed.), *Science and golf IV: Proceedings of the World Scientific Congress on Golf* (pp. 231–245). London: Routledge.

Christina, RW, and Corcos, DM. (1988). *Coaches guide to teaching sports skills.* Champaign, IL: Human Kinetics.

Clark, RC. (2008). *Building expertise: Cognitive methods for training and performance improvement.* San Francisco, CA: Pfeiffer.

Coker, CA. (2006). "To break it down or not break it down: That is the question." *Teaching Elementary Physical Education, 17,* 26–27.

Dail, T, and Christina, RW. (2004). "Distribution of practice and metacognition in the learning and long-term retention of a discrete motor task." *Research Quarterly for Exercise and Sport, 75,* 148–155.

Dick, MB, Hsich, S, Dick-Muehlke, C, Davis, DS, and Corman, CW. (2000). The variability of practice hypothesis in motor learning: Does it apply to Alzheimer's disease? *Brain and Cognition, 44,* 470–489.

Donovan, JJ, and Radosevich, DJ. (1999). "A meta-analytic review of the distribution of practice effect: Now you see it, now you don't." *Journal of Applied Psychology, 84,* 795–805.

Douvis, S. (2005). "Variable practice in learning the forehand drive in tennis." *Perceptual and Motor Skills, 101,* 531–545.

Edwards, JM, Elliott, D, and Lee, TD. (1986). "Contextual interference effects during skill acquisition and transfer in Down's Syndrome children." *Adapted Physical Activity Quarterly, 3,* 250–258.

Ghodsian, D, Bjork, RA, and Benjamin, AS. (1997). "Evaluating training during training: Obstacles and opportunities." In MA Quinoes and A Ehrenstein (eds.), *Training for a rapidly changing workplace* (pp. 63–88). Washington, DC: American Psychological Association.

Gopher, D, Weil, M, and Siegel, D. (1989). "Practice under changing priorities: An approach to training of complex skills." *Acta Psychologica, 71,* 147–177.

Guadagnoli, MA, Holcomb, WR, and Weber, TJ. (1999). "The relationship between contextual interference effects and performance expertise on the learning of a putting task." *Journal of Human Movement Studies, 37,* 19–36.

Guadagnoli, MA, and Lee, TD. (2004). "Challenge point: A framework for conceptualizing the effects of various practice conditions in motor learning." *Journal of Motor Behavior, 36*(2), 212–225.

Hall, KG, Dominguez, DA, and Cavazos, R. (1994). "Contextual interference effects with skilled baseball players." *Perceptual and Motor Skills, 78,* 835–841.

Hanlon, RE. (1996). "Motor learning following unilateral stroke." *Archives of Physical Medicine and Rehabilitation, 77,* 811–815.

Henry, FM. (1958). "Specificity vs. generality in learning motor skills." *Annual Proceedings of the Physical Education Association, 61,* 126–128.

Klapp, ST, Nelson, JM, and Jagacinski, RJ. (1998). "Can people tap concurrent bimanual rhythms independently?" *Journal of Motor Behavior, 30,* 301–322.

Landin, D, and Hebert, EP. (1997). "A comparison of three practice schedules along the contextual interference continuum." *Research Quarterly for Exercise and Sport, 68*(4), 357–361.

Landin, DK, Hebert, EP, and Fairweather, M. (1993). "The effects of variable practice on the performance of a basketball skill." *Research Quarterly for Exercise and Sport, 64,* 232–237.

Lee, TD, Chamberlin, CJ, and Hodges, NJ. (2001). Practice. In RN Singer, HA Hausenblas, and CM Janelle (eds.), *Handbook of sport psychology* (pp. 115–143). New York: John Wiley and Sons.

Lee, TD, and Genovese, ED. (1988). "Distribution of practice in motor skill acquisition: Learning and performance effects reconsidered." *Research Quarterly for Exercise and Sport, 59,* 277–287.

Lee, TD, and Genovese, ED. (1989). "Distribution of practice in motor skill acquisition: Different effects for discrete and continuous tasks." *Research Quarterly for Exercise and Sport, 60,* 59–65.

Lee, TD, and Magill, RA. (1985). "Can forgetting facilitate skill acquisition?" In D Goodman, RB Wilberg, and IM Franks (eds.), *Differing perspectives in motor learning, memory and control* (pp. 3–22). Amsterdam: North-Holland.

Lee, TD, and Simon, DA. (2004). Contextual interference. In AM Williams and NJ Hodges (eds.), *Skill acquisition in sport: Research, theory, and practice* (pp. 29–44). London: Routledge.

Lee, TD, Swinnen, SP, and Serrien, DJ. (1994). "Cognitive effort and motor learning." *Quest, 46,* 328–344.

Li, Y, and Wright, DL. (2000). An assessment of attention demands during random and blocked practice. *Quarterly Journal of Experimental Psychology, 53A,* 591–606.

Magill, RA, and Hall, KG. (1990). "A review of the contextual interference effect in motor skill acquisition." *Human Movement Science, 9,* 241–289.

Naylor, J, and Briggs, G. (1963). "Effects of task complexity and task organization on the relative efficiency of part and whole training methods." *Journal of Experimental Psychology, 65,* 217–244.

Newell, A, and Rosenbloom, PS. (1981). "Mechanisms of skill acquisition and the law of practice." In JR Anderson (ed.), *Cognitive skills and their acquisition* (pp. 1–56). Hillsdale, NJ: Lawrence Erlbaum.

Newell, KM, Carlton, MJ, Fisher, AT, and Rutter, BG. (1989). "Whole-part training strategies for learning the response dynamics of microprocessor driven simulators." *Acta Psychologica, 71,* 197–210.

Patterson, JT, and Lee, TD. (2008). "Organizing practice: The interaction of repetition and cognitive effort for skilled performance." In D Farrow et al. (eds.), *Developing sport expertise* (pp. 119–134). London: Routledge.

Pyle, WH. (1919). Transfer and interference in card-distributing. *Journal of Educational Psychology,* 10, 107–110.

Rizzolatti, G, and Sinigaglia, C. (2006*). Mirrors in the brain: How our minds shape actions and emotions.* New York: Oxford Press.

Schmidt, RA. (1975). "A schema theory of discrete motor skill learning." *Psychological Review, 82,* 225–260.

Schmidt, RA, and Bjork, RA. (1992). "New conceptualizations of practice: Common principles in three paradigms suggest new concepts of training." *Psychological Science, 3,* 207–217.

Schmidt, RA, and Lee, TD. (2005). *Motor control and learning: A behavioral emphasis,* 4th ed. Champaign, IL: Human Kinetics.

Schmidt, RA, and Wrisberg, CA. (2008). *Motor learning and performance: A problem-based learning approach,* 3rd ed. Champaign, IL: Human Kinetics.

Shea, CH, and Kohl, RM. (1990). "Specificity and variability of practice." *Research Quarterly for Exercise and Sport, 61,* 169–177.

Shea, CH, and Kohl, RM. (1991). "Composition of practice: Influence on the retention of motor skills." *Research Quarterly for Exercise and Sport,* 62(2), 187–195.

Shea, CH, Kohl, R, and Indermill, C. (1990). "Contextual interference: Contributions of practice." *Acta Psychologica, 73,* 154–157.

Shea, CH, Lai, Q, Black, C, and Park, J. (2000). "Spacing practice sessions across days benefits the learning of motor skills." *Human Movement Science, 19,* 737–760.

Shea, JB, and Morgan, RL. (1979). "Contextual interference effects on the acquisition, retention, and transfer of a motor skill." *Journal of Experimental Psychology: Human Learning and Memory, 5,* 179–189.

Shea, JB, and Zimny, ST. (1983). "Context effects in memory and learning in movement information." In RA Magill (ed.), *Memory and control of action* (pp. 345–366). Amsterdam: North-Holland.

Shoenfelt, EL, Snyder, LA, Maue, AE, McDowell, CP, and Woolard, CD. (2002). "Comparison of constant and variable practice conditions on free-throw shooting." *Perceptual and Motor Skills, 94,* 1113–1123.

Simon, DA, and Bjork, RA. (2001). "Metacognition in motor learning." *Journal of Experimental Psychology: Learning, Memory and Cognition, 27,* 907–912.

Singer, RN. (1980). *Motor learning and human performance: An application to motor skills and movement behaviors,* 3rd ed. New York: Macmillan.

Smith, PJ. (1997). "Attention and the contextual interference effect for a continuous task." *Perceptual Motor Skills,* 84(1), 83–92.

Snoddy, GS. (1926). "Learning and stability: A psychophysical analysis of a case of motor learning with clinical applications." *Journal of Applied Psychology, 10,* 1–36.

Utley, A, and Astill, S. (2008). *Motor control, learning and development.* New York: Taylor & Francis.

Wightman, DC, and Lintern, G. (1985). "Part-task training strategies for tracking and manual control." *Human Factors, 27,* 267–283.

Wrisberg, CA, and Mead, BJ. (1983). "Developing coincident-timing skill in children: A comparison of training methods." *Research Quarterly for Exercise and Sport, 54,* 67–74.

Answers to How Much Do You Know questions: (1) D, (2) C, (3) C, (4) B, (5) A, (6) A, (7) elaboration, (8) target, (9) segmentation, (10) letter sorting, (11) attentional cueing, (12) cognitive effort.

Providing Feedback

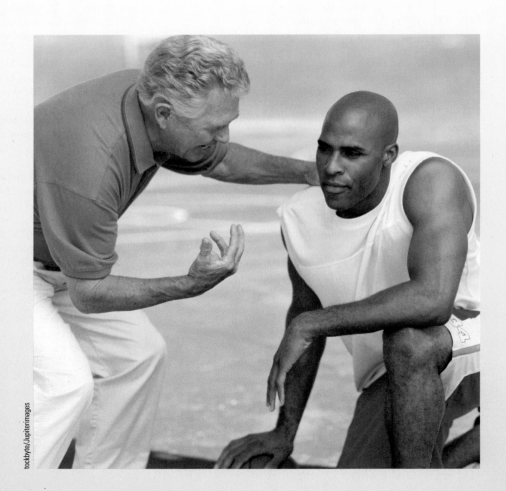

Advise not what is most pleasant, but what is most useful.
Solon (c. 500 BC)

KEY QUESTIONS

- What is feedback?

- How is feedback classified?

- Why is feedback important when learning motor skills?

- What are the best methods for providing feedback?

- What information should feedback convey to learners?

- When might it be beneficial not to provide feedback?

CHAPTER OVERVIEW

Think about a time when you were first learning a new skill. It might be when you learned how to drive an automobile or solve a quadratic equation or serve a tennis ball, or even how to tie your shoelaces, if your memory goes back that far. What do your recollections of each of these things have in common? Probably, whatever else your memories of learning each skill share, you will remember the uncertainty and confusion that accompanied your initial practice attempts for each skill. You may even remember becoming frustrated, perhaps even to the point of wanting to give up altogether at times.

Hopefully, though, you were lucky enough to have someone who knew how to perform the skill help you when you were first learning each of them—perhaps the driver's ed teacher at school, your 10th-grade math teacher, a recreation department tennis instructor, or your parents or an older sibling who understood and unlocked the mysteries of tying shoelaces. In each of these cases, your uncertainty about what to do and how to do it was lessened by the feedback provided as you tentatively practiced each new step along the path to ultimately mastering the skill. "Let out gradually on the clutch as you press down on the gas peddle." "Solve the expression under the square root sign before calculating the value of the numerator." "Pretend you are throwing the racquet head like a ball." "Loop the two ends of the laces around one another like this." Such feedback reduced your uncertainty, instructed you on what to do next, and encouraged you to continue practicing in the belief that, as long as feedback continued, you would ultimately master the skill.

Feedback is essential to effective learning. In fact, after the amount of time spent in practice, it is probably the most important factor in how well a person initially learns a new skill. In this chapter, we will examine the role feedback plays in learning, the types of feedback that can be provided, and methods for providing the most effective feedback to learners.

In both of the major theoretical approaches to the study of motor skills discussed in this book, feedback holds a central place among those factors responsible for learning. Cognitive-based theories, both closed-loop and open-loop approaches, view the development of motor programs as the codification within memory of response-produced information derived through various feedback sources. In dynamical systems theory, the learning of motor skills is viewed as a transformative adaptive process of mapping motor output to sensory consequences, a process facilitated by the provision of instructional feedback (Cheng and Sakes, 2006).

Very few people understand their talents and potential to the level which they exist. Feedback is a catalytic mechanism; it produces a desired result in a predictable way.

—Robert A. Laffreda

Whichever theoretical approach is adopted as the best explanation for motor skill learning, feedback remains a central concern. Indeed, many experts in the field of motor skill learning have argued that the effective delivery of feedback is the most crucial factor, apart from amount of practice, involved in learning and that any instructional situation will be significantly less effective if feedback is not provided correctly (Adams, 1987; Bilodeau, 1966; Chen, 2001; Christina and Corcos, 1988; Fischman and Oxendine, 2001; Salmoni, Schmidt, and Walter, 1984; and Wrisberg et al., 1995). We will begin our inquiry into feedback by first developing a working vocabulary for the many roles feedback can play in the learning process.

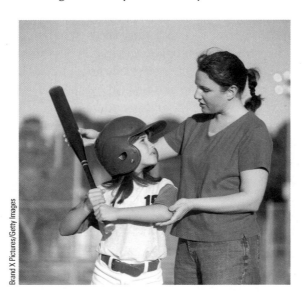

Brand X Pictures/Getty Images

The learning of motor skills is significantly enhanced through the effective provision of feedback.

FEEDBACK CAN BE CLASSIFIED IN A NUMBER OF WAYS

feedback: All sources of information available to a performer regarding the consequences of a practice attempt, including both sensory information and information provided through external sources.

Feedback is defined as any response-related information received either during or after the production of a movement skill. There are two broad categories of feedback. These are called *sensory feedback* and *augmented feedback*. The first, sensory feedback, is always present to individuals through their various sensory modalities. The second, augmented feedback, is only available when provided by an external source and plays a key role in the learning process.

Sensory Feedback

sensory feedback: Information available to a performer concerning the consequences of a practice attempt that is provided directly through the performer's various sensory systems.

Sensory feedback is information received directly by the performer through his or her various sensory systems. This can include what the performer feels, sees, hears, smells, or tastes (only the first three are typically important in motor skill learning). This category of feedback is also termed *intrinsic feedback*, because it is inherent in the performer's own movements.

Sensory feedback can further be divided into proprioceptive feedback and exteroceptive feedback. **Proprioceptive feedback** includes all sensory information concerning the performer's body (i.e., the "feel" of a movement informed by proprioceptors including muscle spindles, joint receptors, golgi tendon organs, and the vestibular apparatuses). **Exteroceptive feedback** includes all information about the external environment provided by the performer's visual, auditory, and tactile sensory systems (i.e., what can be seen, heard, and perceived by touch). Unless some sensory deficit is present, sensory feedback is always present to an individual.

proprioceptive feedback: Sensory feedback concerning the visual, auditory, and tactile consequences of a practice attempt.

exteroceptive feedback: Sensory feedback concerning features of the environment in which a skill is performed.

Augmented Feedback

augmented feedback: Information about the performance of a skill that is supplied by a source external to the performer and that supplements or adds to the performer's sensory feedback.

The second broad category into which feedback is classified is information about an action provided by a source external to the performer. This can include information supplied by an observer (e.g., instructor, coach, trainer, therapist, etc.), a video replay of the performance, a graph or computer-generated display of some aspect of the performance (often used in research situations), or biofeedback, as the most common types of external feedback. This category of feedback is called **augmented feedback**, because it comes from sources outside of the performer and it augments (i.e., complements or adds to) sources of sensory feedback. Augmented feedback is also referred to as *extrinsic feedback* because it is supplied by a source external to the receiver.

verbal augmented feedback: Augmented feedback that is either delivered verbally or that is capable of being verbalized even when provided in a nonverbal form.

Augmented feedback can further be classified as being either verbal or nonverbal. Although the distinction between verbal and nonverbal feedback would seem obvious, it is not quite as clear as seems the case at first blush. **Verbal augmented feedback** refers to all information delivered verbally by another person (e.g., a coach telling an athlete his or her time after a 100-yard dash), but also to information that is capable of being verbalized but may be delivered in another fashion (e.g., the same coach showing the athlete his or her time for the dash on the stopwatch used in timing the run).

Nonverbal augmented feedback is not only delivered in a form other than spoken, but is also not capable of accurate verbalization, usually because of the amount, complexity, or abstract nature of the information provided (e.g., videotape replays, performance graphs, computer-generated graphic displays, biofeedback, etc.).

Of the various forms feedback may take, verbal augmented feedback has received the majority of research attention, in part because it is the most frequently used type of feedback in a wide range of motor skill settings including clinical, educational, athletic, artistic, and job training. There is good reason that this form of feedback is so pervasive across instructional settings. It provides the learner with information concerning both the causes and outcomes of a performance in terms that are readily comprehended. It informs the learner how well he or she accomplished the goal of a skill and something about the correctness (or incorrectness) of his or her movements in performing the skill. It is also easily deliverable and does not require the use of any equipment or special devices.

Augmented feedback is further classified on the basis of whether it provides information concerning the outcome of an action or of the movements produced in accomplishing the action. The first of these two ways of classifying augmented feedback is called **knowledge of results (KR)**. KR can be defined as any response-related information provided by an external source concerning the outcome of an action in terms of the goal of the action. Said in another way, KR is augmented feedback concerning the degree to which a performer achieves his or her performance goal. Here are the major questions answered by KR: What happened? What was the outcome? How successful was the attempt? In these examples, it should be noted that no information concerning the possible causes of the outcome are conveyed, or is information provided concerning how to correct future movements in order to perform the skill better. Only information about the outcome in terms of the goal of a skill is available to the learner by KR.

In reference to KR, it should also be noted that it is often redundant with sensory feedback, a phenomenon referred to as KR redundancy. That is, KR statements may convey information about the results of an action that merely duplicates sensory sources of information the person performing receives him- or herself. Telling someone attempting a free throw in basketball that he or she made the basket adds nothing to the information already available through visual feedback. In such cases, KR is of little value in promoting movement correction and learning. At other times, though, KR may be valuable in supplying information learners cannot extract from the performance experience themselves, even when sensory information is available. This is often the case when movement outcomes are judged on form or quality of movement, such as is the case in gymnastics, diving, modern dance, and playing a musical instrument. Even when sufficient proprioceptive information is available for evaluating the correctness of performance, those in the initial stages of learning usually lack the requisite capabilities necessary for evaluating their own sensory sources of feedback. At other times, KR may supply useful performance information not available through a learner's sensory systems (words typed per minute, time in the mile run, timing of a bat swing for children learning nonsighted softball).

The second type of augmented feedback is **knowledge of performance (KP)**. KP is defined as any information provided by an external source concerning the mechanics of a movement in terms of its effectiveness in meeting an action goal. Said in another way, KP is augmented feedback concerning the cause(s) of a performance response relative to the performance goal. Major questions answered by KP include: Was the movement correct? What caused an outcome error? How can the error be corrected? How should the movement be changed? Examples of verbal KP statements include the following: "Bend your elbow a little more on the next attempt." "You didn't follow through on your swing that time." "Keep your wrist straight." "Watch your opponent—not the ball." "Think about contracting your hip muscles on each step that you take." Note that in all of these examples of KP, information is provided to a learner about why his or her actions were either correct or incorrect (why they resulted in a particular outcome), and when incorrect, either explicitly or implicitly how to correct the errors on future attempts.

Our discussion of feedback in the remainder of this chapter shall be limited to augmented feedback, both KR and KP, because it is this form of feedback that is under the direct control of an instructor and for which techniques of delivery can be structured to affect—often dramatically—the learning of motor skills. The classification of feedback as presented here is illustrated in Figure 12.1.

Before leaving our discussion of basic terms used to describe feedback, two additional categories for describing augmented feedback are useful. First, the delivery of KR and KP can be described as being either concurrent or terminal. **Concurrent feedback** is that provided during the production of a motor skill; **terminal feedback,** on the other hand, is provided after an action is completed (and is sometimes further classified as being either immediate or delayed, though this distinction is somewhat subjective). A second method of describing augmented feedback is to distinguish between distinct and accumulated

concurrent feedback: Augmented feedback delivered during the execution of the motor skill for which it is provided.

terminal feedback: Augmented feedback delivered after the completion of the motor skill for which it is provided (can be either immediate or delayed).

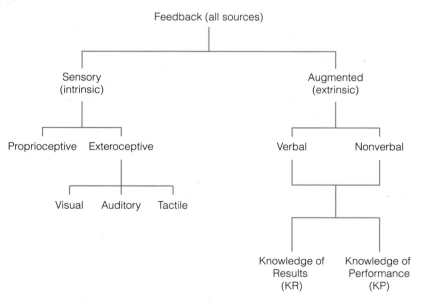

FIGURE **12.1** The Classification of Feedback

Source: Created by author.

distinct feedback:
Augmented feedback
provided for a single
motor response.

accumulated feedback:
Augmented feedback
provided for a series
of motor responses at
the completion of the
responses in the series.

sources of feedback. **Distinct feedback** is provided after a specific performance attempt and represents only that particular performance. **Accumulated feedback** represents information on a series of performance attempts (minimally at least two attempts, though the number can be considerably greater).

Finally, because KP provides direct information concerning the causes of performance errors, as well as information concerning corrective actions, it typically plays a greater role in facilitating learning than does KR, though both types of feedback have important places in the augmentation of sensory feedback for learners. Because augmented feedback plays such a critical role in the learning of motor skills and is under the control and instructional manipulation of the motor skills instructor (unlike sensory feedback), it is typical for movement scientists concerned with the learning of motor skills to refer to augmented feedback somewhat generically simply as feedback, while referring to sensory feedback specifically when distinctions are to be noted. We will follow this consensus of usage in this chapter. As a test of your ability to distinguish between KR and KP statements, see Box 12.1.

Having mastered the terms for describing feedback, we will next turn to the roles it plays in learning.

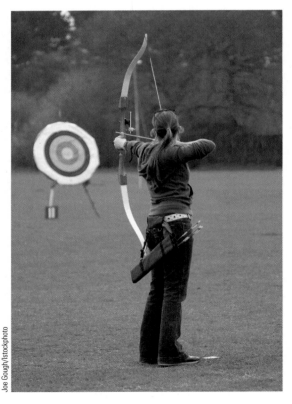

Joe Gough/Istockphoto

For many motor skills, KR (knowledge of results) is redundant with the performer's sources of intrinsic feedback.

THE FUNCTIONS OF AUGMENTED FEEDBACK

As we have already noted, feedback plays a critical role in the acquisition of motor skills. An initial question of interest to the student of motor learning, therefore, might reasonably concern what functions feedback plays in learning. Why is it so critical? What are the functions of feedback that account for its significant influence on learning? Understanding how feedback functions to promote the learning of motor skills is prerequisite to understanding how to provide it effectively in instructional settings.

In the long and extensive literature on the role of augmented feedback, four critical functions that it plays in the learning of motor skills have been identified (see, for example, Adams, 1968, 1987; Annett, 1969; Bilodeau, 1966; Coker, 2009; Hull, 1943; Lavery, 1962; Rose and Christina, 2006; Salmoni, Schmidt, and Walter, 1984; Silverman, Tyson, and Krampitz, 1992; and Thorndike, 1931). These are informational, motivational, reinforcement, and guidance functions. We will examine each of them in turn.

The Informational Function of Feedback

When performing a motor skill, and especially a new and relatively unpracticed one, learners often experience considerable difficulty interpreting the flood of response-produced sensory feedback resulting from their actions. What happened? Were there performance errors? What caused the errors? Learners require sufficient information to answer these questions, but may be too inexperienced to accurately interpret their sources of sensory feedback for such answers. The most obvious function of augmented feedback is that it provides learners with a source of interpretable information concerning the results (KR) and causes (KP) of their actions. Such feedback allows learners to assess performance outcomes and, when required, correct errors on subsequent practice attempts.

The informational content of feedback can function to inform learners of both correct and incorrect action outcomes and movement patterns. Providing information on the correct features of a performance may lead to learners repeating the same performance patterns on future attempts, thereby stabilizing their performances around correct behaviors. If information is provided on

---

BOX 12.1   Is It KR or KP?

Can you correctly classify each of the following feedback statements as being either KR or KP?

1. Release the bowstring sooner next time.
2. You missed the bull's-eye by 6 inches to the left.
3. You are not keeping your wrist fixed all the way through the racquet swing.
4. Good effort! You achieved 5 degrees greater knee flexion today compared to last week.
5. Next time, keep your eye on the headpin as you release the ball.
6. Did you feel your toes clip the last hurdle as you went over it?
7. You typed the sentence without making any errors, and that was your best time yet. Well done!
8. That was perfect. Do it exactly the same way next time.

incorrect features of skill attempts, on the other hand, it can be used as a source of error information to help generate corrective actions.

The question of whether augmented feedback should convey information related to the correct features of a skill attempt or to errors in need of correction has received considerable research inquiry. Although information concerning both the correct and incorrect aspects of a skill attempt is valuable to learners, a consistent finding of the research literature supports the greater effectiveness of information concerning errors (Coker, 2009; Fischman and Oxendine, 2001; Lintern and Roscoe, 1980; and Williams and Briggs, 1962). From a cognitive-based perspective such as schema theory, this finding makes perfectly good sense. Information on errors provides a greater range of information on the parameters of a skill that should benefit the processes involved with abstracting relative timing and force associations required of generalized motor programs. Dynamical systems theory argues that learning is, in part, a result of coming to identify a greater range of affordances, and again the identification of errors would provide a greater range of individual and environmental information from which affordances are constructed. Whatever the theoretical explanations, however, the conclusion can be strongly supported that feedback fulfills a critical function in learning by supplying learners a much needed source of usable information, with information on movement errors being especially valuable in promoting learning.

The Motivational Function of Feedback

Besides leading to the identification and correction of movement errors, feedback has an important role in motivating learners. As we have seen in Chapter 9, being properly motivated is important in preparing individuals for optimal learning.

The feedback a movement instructor provides can strongly motivate learners. It has an energizing effect, keeping learners alert, maintaining their interest, prompting them to set higher performance goals, and generally making practice more enjoyable (Schmidt and Lee, 2005). Learners use instructional feedback to compare their completed performance to established practice goals. Based upon such feedback, they decide whether to correct previous actions (which we have seen as the informational function of feedback). When such corrective actions lead to improvements in performance, learners perceive their practice attempts as being effective and are encouraged to continue exerting efforts toward further improvement (Fredenberg, Lee, and Solmon, 2001; and Silverman, Woods, and Subramaniam, 1998). If feedback conveys a message of nonimprovement to learners, however, it can have the opposite effect, resulting in their becoming discouraged, and even ceasing further participation. In either case, changes in learner motivation can have a significant effect on learning.

Some researchers have pointed out that because enhanced levels of learner motivation do not directly lead to the correction of specific errors, but only to continued effort and participation on the part of learners, motivation should be considered a performance variable rather than a learning variable. That is, motivation may energize learners so that they perform better, but it provides no information on how errors might be corrected and so does not have a direct effect on learning processes. While this is technically true, Schmidt and Lee

(2005) have argued convincingly that though not a direct learning variable, motivation functions as a strong indirect learning variable (see also McMorris, 2004, on this point). These authors point out that motivated learners are more likely to engage in a kind of deliberate practice that is more intense, longer, and in which greater amounts of effort are exerted than would otherwise be the case. Such highly motivated behaviors are all associated with enhanced learning outcomes (Ericsson, 1996), supporting the observation that motivation plays a strong role in the learning process.

Finally, although most research has examined the effects of feedback in enhancing motivation relative to skill development, some research has also pointed to the beneficial effects of augmented feedback in the development of physiological measures of fitness (Annesi, 1998; Dishman, 1993). Just as in skill learning, feedback motivates individuals' efforts and adherence to training in exercise and rehabilitation settings, and can play a significant role in increasing the effectiveness of such training.

The Reinforcing Function of Feedback

reinforcement: Any change in an organism's surroundings that occurs regularly when the organism behaves in a certain way (i.e., the change is contingent on the response).

A major instructional goal of practice for motor skills is to get learners to continue doing the things they are doing correctly and to change the things they are doing incorrectly. The role of **reinforcement** in learning has been recognized since the early part of the last century and is one of the most widely accepted and applied principles in learning theory. Basically, the function of reinforcement is to increase the probability that desired (correct) behaviors will be repeated in practice situations, and that undesired (incorrect) ones will be diminished and ultimately eliminated. Feedback plays an important role in this goal by reinforcing desirable actions and discouraging the continuance of undesirable ones.

law of effect: Law first formulated by Thorndike stating that an organism will tend to repeat behaviors resulting in desirable consequences and avoid behaviors resulting in undesirable consequences.

The prominent American psychologist E. L. Thorndike (1874–1949) was perhaps the first to offer a satisfying explanation for the role of feedback in learning. His observations concerning reinforcement are best summed up in his influential **law of effect**. In formulating the law of effect, Thorndike (1927) stated, "An action elicited by a stimulus and followed by pleasant, or rewarding, consequences tends to be repeated when that stimulus appears again; an action followed by unpleasant, or punishing, consequences tends not to be repeated." (Anyone who has trained a puppy knows how to apply this law already. Little Fido's misadventures in the house are met with unpleasant shouts of "No!" from you, and his desired behaviors greeted with lavish petting and rewarding praise for being a "good boy!")

According to Thorndike, learning consists of trial-and-error behavior and a gradual "stamping in" of some behaviors (those leading to satisfaction) and "stamping out" of other behaviors (those leading to discomfort). In other words, rewarded behaviors are experienced pleasantly and are more likely to be repeated, which over time leads to learning. Behaviors not rewarded, or even punished, tend not to be repeated and are eventually discontinued. Over time, behaviors that are rewarded are increased, and those that are not rewarded (or even punished) are decreased, shaping the learner's behavior toward the desired goal.

Three types of reinforcement are important to consider in instructional situations; these are positive reinforcement, punishment, and negative reinforcement.

positive reinforcement: Occurs when a response is followed by a desired consequence and increases the likelihood that the response will be repeated in similar situations in the future.

punishment: Occurs when a response is followed by undesirable consequences and decreases the likelihood that the response will be repeated in similar situations in the future.

negative reinforcement: Occurs when a response is followed by the removal of undesirable consequences previously associated with the response and increases the likelihood that the response will be repeated in similar situations in the future.

sandwich technique: A method of providing augmented feedback in which a negative or punishing reinforcing statement is immediately preceded and followed by a positively reinforcing statement.

Positive reinforcement is defined as a pleasantly experienced reward presented after a response. Positive reinforcement may point out what a learner is doing correctly ("You turned your body in the right direction that time—good work!" "That was a good follow-through." "Your time was five seconds faster than before.") or provide a more global statement concerning a movement's general correctness ("Good work—keep it up." "Much better that time.")

Punishment is reinforcement designed to decrease the likelihood that learners will continue practicing in an inappropriate or incorrect way. Punishment tells a person what not to do rather than what to do. Again, punishment can be either specific ("Don't step out so far next time." "You didn't bring your hips around." "You were much slower that time.") or can be provided as a more generalized evaluation of performance ("That was not as good as before." "You're not following through")

Negative reinforcement consists of the removal of punishment. A common misconception is that negative reinforcement and punishment are the same things—both experienced unpleasantly by the learner. On the contrary, however, learners experience negative reinforcement in a pleasant way. When an instructor has been punishing undesirable motor behaviors for a series of practice trials through the delivery of unpleasantly experienced feedback statements and then withdraws such punishment on a subsequent trial (i.e., provides no feedback), the learner interprets this absence of correction in a rewarding way (i.e., the practice attempt must have been correct—or at least better—than previous attempts that were punished).

A well-established principle in learning theory is that positive reinforcement promotes the greatest improvement in learning, followed by negative reinforcement and then punishment. Although the application of all three types of reinforcement is necessary in motor learning situations, a goal of motor skill instructors should be to supply a majority of augmented feedback as positive reinforcement.

The astute reader may well be asking here, "How can the majority of feedback be positive if learners make so many errors initially?" Of course, the reader is right, and corrective feedback is necessary for effective learning. Still, the balancing of corrective feedback with positive reinforcement should be the goal of motor skill instructors, as should be the provision of corrective information in positively experienced ways by learners. An interesting application of positive reinforcement is illustrated by what is known as the **sandwich technique** of providing feedback. Suppose, for example, that an individual who is learning a drive shot in golf is continually keeping his or her arm too straight, thereby leading to poor performance. An instructor could provide feedback after each attempt such as "You still need to relax your elbow more!" Although it is important to convey this information to the learner in order to promote a change in behavior (in this case from a rigid to a more relaxed elbow), such unpleasantly experienced feedback provided over a period of time can lead to frustration and a decrease in motivation, especially when the learner is not experiencing obvious success. In this case, the sandwich technique could be used by an instructor, which allows for the provision of positive reinforcement along with the corrective punishing reinforcement. In the sandwich technique, an instructor provides a punishment statement (the "meat") between two positive reinforcement statements (the "bread"). In our example, this technique might result in a feedback statement something like: "Much better that time—your mechanics are improving ("bread"). You still need to relax your elbow more, though ("meat"). Good effort, though—keep it up! ("bread")." Such a statement provides corrective information (the need to relax the elbow) while at the same time telling the learner that he or she is doing some things correctly (better mechanics and good effort) and is showing improvement (see Box 12.2 for a further consideration of these principles).

Before leaving our discussion of the role of feedback in reinforcing correct movement behaviors, one final point is important to note. Another well-established principle of learning is that **intermittent reinforcement** through the occasional provision of feedback is more beneficial in promoting learning than is feedback provided frequently, especially if it is provided after every practice attempt. Apparently, the withholding of feedback on some practice attempts that might otherwise be punished or positively reinforced is beneficial in strengthening the reinforcement of desired behaviors. This well-established observation supports the use of faded schedules of feedback delivery, an important pedagogical principle discussed later in this chapter.

intermittent reinforcement: Reinforcement of a response after some but not all instances in which a contingency for reinforcement is present; often more powerful in shaping behavior than reinforcement provided in every contingent situation.

The Guidance Function of Feedback

A final function of feedback is to act in such a way as to guide learners to correct actions. In much the same way as physical guidance—manually moving a person's limbs to produce the correct kinematics of a skill—keeps a learner on

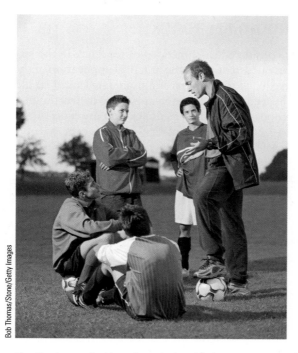

Bob Thomas/Stone/Getty Images

Feedback supplied by a knowledgeable instructor can reinforce correct skill behaviors, while distinguishing incorrect behaviors.

task, so feedback also keeps learners performing within a prescribed range of performance. When people perform skills and receive instructional feedback about errors, they will typically change their behavior on subsequent attempts in order to correct those errors (i.e., a reshaping of behavior due to reinforcement). For example, a student driver learning to make left-hand turns may time the beginning of turning the automobile's steering wheel either too soon or too late. If on each practiced left-hand turn the driving instructor informs the student that the turn was begun too late, the student will make corrections by beginning the next turn earlier, until he or she is starting turns at the correct time. The feedback provided will guide the student driver toward the correct approximation of when to begin a left-hand turn. Once performing correctly and with some consistency (or at least correctly enough to make left-hand turns without his or her car ending up on the sidewalk), other learning processes may take over and help the student develop good driving skills.

Although this guidance function played by feedback may seem at first to be beneficial to learning, considerable research has challenged this conclusion. Indeed, the prevailing opinion among experts is that guidance has more of an adverse effect on learning than it does a beneficial one. For now, though, we will leave further consideration of the guidance properties of augmented feedback, and of the reasoning behind viewing it as detrimental to learning, for discussion later in this chapter. A summary of the four functions of augmented feedback is shown in Box 12.3.

GUIDELINES FOR PROVIDING FEEDBACK

Having considered the functions of feedback in the learning of motor skills, we now turn our attention to the practical application of those functions in the delivery of feedback to learners. What guidelines can be gleaned from the functions played by feedback that, when applied to instructional settings, will inform effective methods of providing feedback that are most likely to optimize learning?

Three concerns are particularly relevant when formulating methods of providing feedback. First, how precise should feedback be? Should it contain

---

BOX 12.2   The Role of Reinforcement in Providing Feedback

A new high school girls' volleyball coach, who was an outstanding college player known for being a perfectionist both on the court and in practice, believes strongly that to help her players reach their greatest potential, she must keep them from becoming complacent by constantly challenging them and pointing out ways in which they can improve. Even a well-executed spike is likely to be met with "You are fortunate that worked. The ball should have been hit down at a greater angle and more to the left." The coach's philosophy is that players should never become satisfied with their current levels of performance and that her role as the coach is to continually point out errors, even minor ones, challenging players to improve. She believes that praise, on the other hand, leads to complacency and to a lack of one's best efforts.

How would you evaluate this coach's philosophy? Based upon a consideration of the law of effect, why are the coach's instructional principles either effective guides or relatively ineffective guides for providing feedback?

information of a general nature concerning errors, or should it be detailed and specific? Second, when should feedback be provided? Is feedback most effective when provided immediately after a practice attempt, or should it be delayed for some period of time? What about feedback given while a performance is ongoing? Third, how frequently should feedback be provided? Should feedback be given on all, or at least on most, practice attempts? Or should it perhaps be provided on relatively few attempts? If only for a few, how many?

These three concerns involve the precision, timing, and frequency with which feedback is delivered. Each is equally important. Together, they form the guidelines for providing effective feedback to learners of motor skills, and a sound grasp of their principles is essential for motor skill instructors.

Precision of Feedback

It should be noted initially that most research concerning the effects of feedback precision has investigated the effects of KR, and typically verbal KR. The reason for this is that KR has distinct advantages when designing research studies. For one thing, KR is easily manipulated (it is present or not), whereas KP may be represented by a broad range of behaviors. Even though most research involves KR, the assumption is that findings from KR studies also apply to other forms of feedback such as KP and nonverbal feedback, which has generally held true when such other forms are used as the research variable investigated.

It is typical, as well as pedagogically relevant, when conducting research relative to precision to vary the precision of feedback around two broad categories referred to as *qualitative* and *quantitative* feedback. **Qualitative feedback** statements contain information about the direction of an error, without reference to the magnitude of the error. Examples of qualitative feedback statements include: "That was too far." "Bend your elbow more." "That was faster than last time." "That was better." Note that in each case the feedback statement indicates a needed direction of change (more/less, faster/slower, etc.), but not how much of a change should be made. Adding information to a feedback statement

qualitative feedback: Augmented feedback that supplies information about the direction of an error (e.g., too much, too little; too fast, too slow) without reference to the magnitude of the error.

BOX **12.3**   **The Functions of Feedback**

Whenever movement instructors provide feedback to learners, it functions in at least four different ways. Although the instructor's purpose for providing feedback may focus on only one of these functions, it should be kept in mind that all four function to some degree every time feedback is given.
Feedback is a source of

1. **Information**   Informs learners about the outcomes of their actions as well as the correctness or incorrectness of their movement patterns.

2. **Motivation**   Energizes learners and encourages them to continue exerting efforts to accomplish learning goals.

3. **Reinforcement**   Promotes correct behaviors and discourages continuance of incorrect behaviors.

4. **Guidance**   Acts to guide learners toward correct actions (which can create dependency on feedback as a source of information).

about how much change is needed increases the precision of feedback. In our examples this could be accomplished by adding modifiers such as: "That was a little too far." "Bend your elbow just a little bit more." "That was a lot faster that time." "That was much better." Using word descriptions, the precision of feedback can be increased only to a point, however.

Although qualitative feedback statements contain useful information, they still lack the informational properties most useful for initiating corrections. The problem is really one of communication. For example, if an instructor tells a learner, "Bend your elbow a little more," how is the learner to interpret that statement? Does the instructor mean 5 degrees more, 10 degrees more, or even perhaps 15 degrees more? To the instructor "a little more" may mean 5 degrees, but the learner may interpret "a little more" to mean 10 degrees. The statement does serve to elicit change in the correct direction, but the amount of change required is not clearly specified.

The precision of feedback is significantly increased by providing information not only concerning the direction of an error, but also about the magnitude of the error. **Quantitative feedback** provides information about both the direction of an error and its magnitude in numerical terms. That is, quantitative feedback tells the learner how to change and also how much to change in a quantitatively precise way. Examples of quantitative feedback statements include these: "That was six inches too far." "Bend your elbow to a 45-degree angle." "Your time was 11.2 seconds." "Your flexion has improved by five degrees." Note that these statements contain more precise information about needed corrections than do qualitative feedback statements. Not only is the information in such statements more precise, both the instructor and learner are more likely to interpret it in the same way. Though "a little more" is ambiguous, "six inches more" means the same thing to both instructor and learner, so communication is significantly improved between them.

There is a point, however, where too much quantitative information can be provided in a feedback statement. Consider the following: "Bend your elbow to 12.5 degrees." Such a statement, although precise (and we will assume correct), would most likely lead to confusion on the part of the learner. Additionally, the learner would also more than likely engage in too much cognitive effort attempting to duplicate the precise angle specified. In this case, such a high degree of feedback precision could prove detrimental to the learning process. A learner could easily become frustrated by his or her inability to make such precise corrections and might also become disenchanted with the instructor providing such confusing feedback, which in turn could lead to disregarding further feedback altogether.

As a general guideline, we can say that feedback should be provided with as much precision as a learner can meaningfully interpret, and that this typically implies using quantitative feedback as preferable to qualitative feedback. There is a point, however, beyond which quantitative feedback can become too precise and can lead to poor learning outcomes. Figure 12.2 illustrates the relationship between feedback precision and learning (this is referred to as a curvilinear relationship). A general finding of research on the relationship between the precision of feedback and learning is that learning is enhanced as

quantitative feedback: Augmented feedback that supplies information about both the direction and magnitude (in numerical terms) of an error; is considered more precise than qualitative feedback.

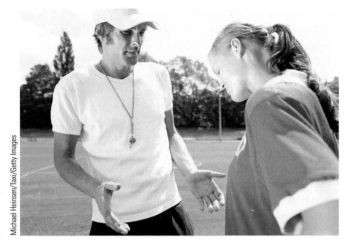

Good feedback statements are precise enough (quantitative) to be meaningfully interpreted by the performer, though too much precision can lead to confusion and ineffectiveness.

the precision of feedback becomes greater, but only up to a point (McMorris, 2004; Rogers, 1974; and Smoll, 1972). After that point, continued increases in precision become less useful to learners, who are unable to effectively respond to the more precise corrective information, which leads to diminished performance and learning.

Descriptive and Prescriptive Feedback

As we have just seen, in most instructional situations KP is to be preferred over KR because it provides for greater precision in conveying information. Where KR supplies information only about the outcome of a performance attempt,

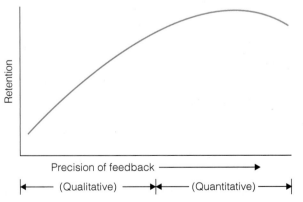

FIGURE **12.2** Precision of Augmented Feedback

Source: Created by author.

descriptive feedback:
Knowledge of performance describing errors a learner makes, but not the causes of the errors or suggested corrections.

prescriptive feedback:
Knowledge of performance concerning both an error made by a performer and suggestion for correcting the error.

KP supplies relevant information upon which specific errors can be identified and corrections made. The precision of KP in facilitating error correction responses can be specified as being either descriptive or prescriptive. **Descriptive feedback** simply describes the error a learner has made, without any suggestion about how the error might be corrected. A basketball coach would be providing descriptive feedback if she told one of her players during a practice session: "You reacted too slowly to your opponent's cutback. That is why she faked you out and got to the basket!" In this example, the player's error is clear (she reacted too slowly), but there is no information concerning the possible causes for her slow response or how she might correct it.

Prescriptive feedback supplies learners with useful information on how they can correct their errors. It not only describes an error, but also what can be done to correct the error (Newell and McGinnis, 1985). In our example of the basketball player, her coach would have been supplying prescriptive feedback if, instead of merely describing the player's error, she had offered the following statement suggesting a course for correcting the error in subsequent performance: "You reacted too slowly to your opponent's cutback because you were watching the ball. Focus your attention on her number next time, not where the ball is. Your reactions will be much quicker that way."

Prescriptive feedback is more useful for beginners because it guides them into corrective actions they would not likely determine on their own. Once individuals have acquired sufficient knowledge concerning how to correct specific errors, descriptive feedback becomes useful. In the early stages of practice, movement instructors should focus on providing prescriptive feedback. Once learners have the skill and knowledge to determine corrective actions on their own when a specific error is identified, descriptive feedback can be provided as well as prescriptive feedback (To assess your ability to provide prescriptive and descriptive feedback see Box 12.4).

A Caveat Regarding Feedback Precision

Although in general greater feedback precision is typically beneficial, there are, however, times when less precision may be more appropriate. Magill and Wood

BOX 12.4 Providing Descriptive and Prescriptive Feedback

Feedback can be either descriptive or prescriptive in content. Of these two types of feedback, research shows that prescriptive feedback is more beneficial to learners in the early stages of learning. Once learners acquire sufficient skill and knowledge, including the knowledge of how to correct specific errors, descriptive feedback can be used effectively. Effective motor skills instructors need to be able to provide feedback in both ways and to understand when learners are sufficiently capable of benefiting from descriptive feedback.

For the following activities, suggest an example of both a descriptive and a prescriptive feedback statement.

- Putting in golf
- Kicking a soccer ball
- Shifting when driving an automobile
- Painting a room
- Hammering a nail
- Learning to walk on crutches
- Swimming using the freestyle stroke

(1986) reported the results of an experiment that suggests some caution in applying the principle of feedback precision too exclusively. Their study has served as an influential reminder to those suggesting all-encompassing learning principles regarding the provision of feedback. Few research findings are universal and exceptions to general findings may appear and must be taken into account when searching for the most effective instructional practices. Factors such as stage of learning and the nature of the task, for example, may play a role in determining the proper amount of precision required for maximizing skill acquisition.

In their study, Magill and Wood had two groups of subjects practice a timed movement task in one of two KR conditions. To perform the task, subjects were seated before a flat response board consisting of four padded, wooden, and hinged barriers. The goal of the task was to learn to make a series of six quick, discrete hand and arm movements striking the barriers in a prescribed order and in a specified movement time. The six movements varied in distance between 28.5 and 43 cm, and in time between 300 and 900 ms. Subjects performed 100 trials of the task on two consecutive days with KR, and each practice session was completed with an additional 10 retention trials with no KR. At the completion of each trial, subjects received KR on a computer monitor for each of the six movement segments. One-half of the subjects received qualitative KR. For each of the six movement segments the subjects' performance was reported as being "too fast," "too slow," or "correct" (with correct considered as being $+/-10$ ms from the criterion time). The other half of the subjects were provided with quantitative KR. That is, both the direction and the amount of error were reported for each of the six movement segments (e.g., $+50$ ms, -120 ms, etc.).

Results of Magill and Wood's study revealed an interesting, and somewhat unexpected, finding. Contrary to expectations, both groups, those receiving qualitative and quantitative KR, performed similarly in early practice trials. As illustrated in Figure 12.3, both groups of subjects experienced roughly the same amount of error during their initial practice trials (i.e., the first 60 trials represented by blocks 1–6). In the later trials (blocks 7–10 representing the final 40 acquisition trials), however, the subjects receiving the more precise quantitative KR consistently outperformed the subjects receiving qualitative KR. Differences in the effects of KR were especially evident in the two retention tests (blocks 11 and 12), where the quantitative KR group clearly showed a learning advantage over the group receiving the less precise qualitative KR.

Based upon the results of their experiment, Magill and Wood concluded that providing more precise feedback early in the learning of a motor skill does not always lead to better performance and learning. Indeed, they suggested that the more precise delivery of feedback could wait until learners are experienced enough to benefit from the additional information available through greater feedback precision. In the early stages of learning, it may at times be more appropriate to provide general (qualitative as opposed to quantitative) information about errors.

In making decisions regarding the precision of the feedback to provide learners during the initial stages of learning a new skill, instructors would be

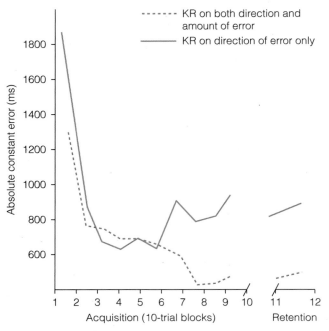

FIGURE **12.3** Effect of KR Precision on Initial Acquisition Pattern of a Motor Skill

Source: Adapted from Magill, RA and Wood, CA (1986). Knowledge of results precision as a learning variable in motor skill acquisition. *Research Quarterly for Exercise and Sport, 57,* 170–171.

well advised to consider the complexity of a task relative to the usefulness of information provided by feedback. When a learner can easily translate the information provided by feedback into the execution of accurate movement responses (i.e., place your hand four inches closer to the handle, bend your arm to 45 degrees), then the greater precision provided by quantitative forms of KR are appropriate. However, in the case where information cannot be effectively translated into accurate movement responses because of the relative inexperience of learners (such as was the case with the sequenced timing patterns in Magill and Wood's study), more general information about the direction of error (more or less, faster or slower, etc.) is warranted and probably of greater value to learners. Such considerations point to the need of motor skill instructors not only to understand learning principles based upon research, but also to be sensitive to the individual needs of learners when applying such principles.

How Many Errors Should a Feedback Statement Identify?

Another factor to consider relative to feedback precision pertains to how many errors should be identified in a feedback statement. In this case, greater precision is measured by increasing the number of errors corrected (or reinforced) by feedback. Consider the following example of a feedback statement: "Bend your elbow more next time. Step out further. Rotate your hips more. Don't choke up on the racquet as much. Watch the angle of the ball coming off the wall. Got it?"

Obviously the above feedback statement contains too much information for learners to internalize and effectively respond. Instructors are often anxious to over-correct learners' behaviors, however, because they themselves see so much in need of correction. Learners, though, especially ones in the early stages of learning, are not capable of internalizing so many corrections at a time, and attempting to get them to will only lead to confusion, frustration, and poor performance and learning outcomes. As a general rule, knowledgeable movement skill instructors provide feedback statements concerning a single needed correction (or the reinforcement of a correct action) at a time. Because learners can also become overwhelmed when too many different corrections are indicated in a single practice session, skills instructors should also focus their feedback around the two or three most crucially needed corrections in any single practice session rather than attempt to over-correct too many errors during a single practice (see Box 12.5) (Chen, 2001; Knudson and Morrison, 1997).

The Effects of Imprecision: The Case of Erroneous Feedback

The influence of feedback precision on learning is dramatically illustrated when we consider its opposite—feedback that is imprecise to the point of being incorrect. What happens when learners are provided **erroneous feedback** that is not only incorrect, but that clearly contradicts their sources of sensory feedback? It would seem logical to assume that learners would simply disregard the erroneous information in favor of what they could clearly see and feel. Buekers and colleagues studied the effects of erroneous feedback in several studies (Buekers, Magill, and Hall, 1992; Buekers, Magill, and Sneyers, 1994; and Buekers and Magill, 1995) involving subjects learning an anticipation timing task (i.e., observing a light target moving down a runway and depressing a button coincidently with their prediction of when the light would reach the end of the runway). The subjects could clearly see the light travel and reach the

erroneous feedback: Augmented feedback provided in an intentionally incorrect and misleading fashion.

BOX **12.5**   **When Is Precise Too Precise?**

A young man interested in learning golf goes to the driving range with his boss, who is an avid golfer with a 10 handicap. The man's boss suggests they start by learning to hit using a driver. During the course of practice, the boss is heard providing the following feedback after one practice swing: "Remember to keep your heels shoulder-width apart and to shift your body weight to your left foot as you swing. Do not look up; keep your head still as you swing. Remember what I said about keeping your left elbow in and rotating your hips; let the club come around like a pendulum. Your belt buckle should be pointing toward the target when you complete your swing, not off to the side like it was. And remember to stay relaxed throughout your swing."

Can you explain why the boss's feedback was probably ineffective, as well as how it could have been improved?

end of the runway, as well as perceive when they depressed the response button. Although the subjects might not be able to accurately judge how precise their responses were in quantitative terms, they were clearly able to perceive whether they were early or late depressing the response button. When provided with KR regarding their response error, however, the subjects were given false information indicating an error in the opposite direction (early or late) from their true performance. For example, a subject responding 50 ms early might be provided KR indicating an error of 100 ms late. What is interesting is that even when such KR contradicted their sensory feedback, subjects made corrections based upon the erroneous KR. That is, they conformed their subsequent actions to the incorrect KR while negating their own sensory feedback, even though they could perceive a conflict between these two informational sources. The effect of the erroneous KR on learning was so great, in fact, that when later tested in no-KR retention tests, the subjects duplicated their incorrect timing responses from acquisition—they had learned incorrect movement patterns (see Ryan and Roby, 2002, for similar findings).

One interpretation of these results is that individuals in the early stages of learning can be so uncertain about the meaning of their own sensory feedback and of their ability to accurately interpret it that they will rely upon external sources of information even when that information seems clearly contradictory to what they perceive. The results of such studies on the effects of erroneous feedback highlight the powerful effect that instructional feedback has on learners and should encourage those responsible for providing feedback to individuals learning motor skills to exercise due care and studied thoughtfulness in order to deliver feedback that is accurately and appropriately precise.

The Timing of Feedback

Another aspect of feedback that movement skill instructors must consider involves the timing of feedback delivery. How soon after a practice attempt should feedback be given? Once learners are provided with feedback, how soon should they practice the next attempt?

An answer to these questions frequently heard among some practitioners is that feedback should be given immediately upon the completion of a practice attempt and that learners should then quickly practice the next attempt. The reasoning behind both of these notions is that learners are subject to a limited attention span. Therefore, feedback should be provided immediately because learners begin to forget elements of their practice attempts as soon as each is completed. The same reasoning follows for how soon after the provision of feedback learners should engage in subsequent practice attempts. By this reasoning, learners also begin to lose focus on the provided feedback almost immediately or may become distracted by other thoughts or activities, and so should attend to corrective actions quickly. It might on initial reflection seem reasonable to mitigate these detrimental effects associated with time delays by reducing them as much as possible. But is such a conclusion warranted? Much research has been directed toward answering this (Adams, 1968; Bilodeau and Bilodeau, 1969; Magill, 2001; Swinnen, 1996; and Swinnen et al., 1990).

KR-delay interval: The period of time between the completion of a practice attempt and the presentation of augmented feedback.

post KR-delay interval: The period of time between the presentation of augmented feedback and the beginning of the next practice attempt of the skill for which it was provided.

interresponse interval: The total time between the completion of a practice attempt for which KR is provided and the beginning of the next practice attempt.

Before discussing the results of research in this area, however, some description of the temporal sequences involved in the provision of feedback needs to be addressed. Between completing one practice attempt for which feedback is provided and the beginning of the following practice attempt, three temporal intervals can be identified. The first of these is called the **KR-delay interval** and refers to the time between the completion of the reinforced response and the delivery of KR (note that though KR is specified in this terminology, the same sequences follow whether KR or KP is the type of feedback considered). The second temporal interval is the **post KR-delay interval** and refers to the time from the delivery of KR until the beginning of the next response (which is presumed to benefit from the KR). Finally, the total time between the two responses is referred to as the **interresponse interval**. These three intervals are illustrated in Figure 12.4.

Let us first consider the KR-delay interval. Should feedback be provided immediately? Or should it be given after a few seconds delay? Or does the length of time really even matter?

Research and a little thought support the conclusion that at least a few seconds delay between an action attempt and the provision of feedback maximizes learning (though not necessarily performance). Consider the mental processes occurring in learners between completion of a response and delivery of feedback. The completion of a response is attended by the generation of sensory feedback, both what performers felt in completing the response and what they saw and heard as a result. The internalization of this sensory information requires some amount of time for processing (at least from a cognitive-based theoretical perspective). Generally, learners need from three to five seconds, depending upon the complexity of a task, for attending to this response-produced sensory feedback. The learners' next task is to compare their sensory feedback with that feedback provided by an external source (the instructor) and determine needed corrections (or reinforce correct actions). Again, once feedback is delivered, another few seconds (approximately 3–5) are needed for learners to engage in cognitive activities associated with comparing their sensory-produced feedback with the instructional feedback provided, thus either stabilizing or correcting the reinforced response.

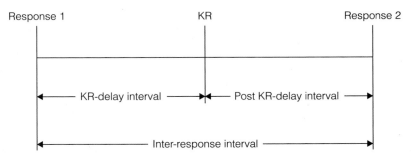

FIGURE **12.4** Timing Intervals of Augmented Feedback

Source: Created by author.

In an influential study on the effects of the temporal positioning of feedback, Swinnen et al. (1990) compared three groups of subjects learning a timing task who received KR either instantaneously upon completion of each practice attempt, three seconds after each attempt, or eight seconds after each attempt. In comparing results for the three groups, those subjects who received instantaneous KR performed significantly worse in acquisition than did the two groups receiving delayed KR. Further, retention tests revealed that the subjects experiencing the longest KR-delay interval (8 seconds) learned the task best. Additional research has supported the benefits of delaying the delivery of feedback for several seconds after the completion of a practice attempt, and it even appears that longer delays are not detrimental to learning (but see Box 12.6 for another view).

The effects of extending the post KR-delay interval are somewhat similar. Again, studies have consistently found delays of several seconds from the delivery of feedback to the execution of the subsequent action attempt to result in superior retention compared to instantaneous or very short delays in performance. In fact, even performance delays of several days have not been found to dampen the beneficial effects of feedback on subsequent practice attempts. There are, of course, good reasons not to delay further practice attempts for too long once feedback has been provided. First, even though learning may not be affected by the delay, performance often is. Once learners complete the cognitive processes involved in comparing their response-produced sensory feedback to externally delivered feedback, they will tend to quickly lose immediate access to their short-term memories of these processes as other activities intervene, which in turn will degrade subsequent performance. Decreases in performance can then threaten motivational levels and, therefore, adversely impact learning. More practically, however, increasing the delay interval between practice attempts decreases the number of practice trials that can be attempted in any given practice period—and the number of practice trials is strongly related to learning outcomes. Still, instructors need not be overly concerned when there is good reason to delay practice attempts after feedback is administered, as long as a sufficient amount of practice is still provided.

The Frequency of Feedback

One final guideline needs to be developed concerning the effective presentation of feedback, and that entails how frequently feedback should be provided to be of most benefit for learners. Should feedback be provided after every practice attempt to be of greatest benefit? Would some other schedule of feedback prove more beneficial—every other attempt, every third attempt, or even every tenth attempt, for example? The answer to this question is one of the most intriguing—and strongly supported—in the research literature concerning feedback.

Well into the last century, it was believed that feedback should be provided on every practice attempt. This conclusion was based on Thorndike's law of effect and the principles of operant conditioning. If feedback were essential in strengthening stimulus–response connections, it was argued, then it seemed obvious that the more frequently feedback was delivered, the more reinforced the correct response would become. This conclusion, which seems intuitively appealing at first, is still held by many of those responsible for motor skill instruction today. One reason that this conclusion continues to exert an influence on instructional thinking is that frequent feedback does promote practice performance, a fact that becomes obvious to anyone who provides feedback to learners of motor skills for any period of time.

Beginning in the mid 1960s and continuing into the 1970s, however, researchers began to observe laboratory results that contradicted the accepted wisdom that the greater the frequency of feedback, the greater the degree of learning that would occur. In perhaps the first study to challenge such conventional wisdom, Bilodeau and Bilodeau (1969) demonstrated that reduced frequencies of feedback proved more beneficial than higher frequencies in promoting learning outcomes.

To discuss the findings of Bilodeau and Bilodeau, we must first define two terms used in the research literature. The frequency of feedback can be defined in terms of both its *absolute frequency* and its *relative frequency*. The **absolute frequency of feedback** refers to the total number of practice attempts in a series of attempts in which feedback is delivered. If feedback is provided for every practice attempt in a series of 10 attempts, then the absolute frequency of feedback is 10. If in the same series of 10 practice attempts, feedback were provided for only a single attempt, then the absolute frequency of feedback is one. Absolute frequency refers to the total number of reinforced trials in a series of practice trials, regardless of the total number of practice trials in the series.

absolute frequency of feedback: The total number of practice attempts for which KR is provided during a specific practice period.

| BOX **12.6** | **Is Concurrent Feedback Beneficial?** |

Although feedback is typically provided at the conclusion of a practice attempt, there are times when it may be provided during the actual performance. This is the case for many continuous skills such as dancing, driving an automobile, cycling, typing, sawing wood, and tracking on a rotary pursuit device in a laboratory setting. When feedback is provided during the ongoing execution of a skill, it is termed *concurrent feedback*.

There has been considerable research concerning the benefits of concurrent feedback, but the findings have led to a good deal of ambivalence and uncertainty about when, or if, it is advisable to deliver feedback concurrently with actual skill performance. The evidence suggests, however, that there are distinct differences in the ways that visual and auditory sources of concurrent feedback work. Providing auditory feedback during a performance, such as keeping pace with audio cues when learning a rowing pattern or dance routine, appears

to enhance both the performance and learning of skills (though learning appears to be as effective when terminal feedback is supplied). When visual sources of feedback are supplied concurrently with performance, however, such as the use of mirrors in dance practice, performance during practice is enhanced, but learning appears to be significantly hindered when compared to the delivery of post-performance feedback.

The reasons for these differences are not well understood, though evidence suggests that visual information captures too much of a learner's attention, which in turn may block other important processing activities associated with learning. Until further research is available, the effectiveness of concurrent feedback will remain debated, although it can be pointed out that no evidence exists suggesting it as being superior to post-response feedback, especially when the feedback may be provided visually.

relative frequency of feedback: The proportion of practice attempts in a series of attempts for which KR is provided (equal to the percentage of attempts on which KR is given).

The **relative frequency of feedback** refers to the percentage of trials in a series of practice trials in which feedback is provided. If 10 trials in a series of 10 practice trials each receive feedback, then the relative frequency is 100 percent (10/10 × 100 = 100%). If only one trial in the series of 10 practice trials receives feedback, the relative frequency is 10 percent (1/10 × 100 = 10%). The relative frequency of feedback is the proportion of practice attempts for which feedback is provided; it is equal to the absolute frequency of feedback divided by the total number of practice attempts and then multiplied by 100 to give a percentage figure.

Returning to the research of Bilodeau and Bilodeau, they investigated the effects of manipulating feedback frequency on learning. In a series of studies, they were the first to observe that reducing the relative frequency of feedback enhanced learning outcomes when compared to higher relative frequencies of feedback. They also reported that this effect was observed only for retention measures (i.e., learning), and not for performance (which appeared to benefit as the relative frequency of feedback increased). Bilodeau and Bilodeau's findings helped establish the existence of a curvilinear relationship between learning and the relative frequency of feedback. That is, in their studies Bilodeau and Bilodeau found that high relative frequencies of feedback actually depressed optimal learning, whereas reducing relative frequencies of feedback improved learning outcomes. At some point, however, reducing the relative frequency of feedback further begins to impede further learning and, in fact, actually begins to depress learning. A generalized curve illustrating these findings is shown in Figure 12.5 (see also Box 12.7).

The 1970s witnessed an abundance of research on the benefits of reducing the relative frequency of feedback, with many studies confirming Bilodeau and Bilodeau's original observations. The beneficial effects of reduced relative frequencies of feedback on learning (and the relatively less useful

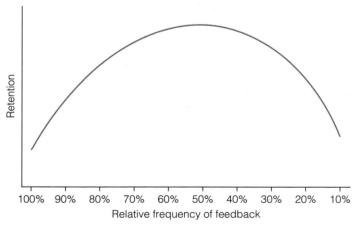

FIGURE **12.5** Retention and Relative Frequency of Feedback

Source: Created by author.

effects of high relative frequencies of feedback—with 100% relative frequency almost always proving less than optimal for learning) became accepted among experts in the field. What was also gleaned from this spate of research activity was that a number of variables seemed to shift the benefits of reduced feedback frequencies, with stage of learning and skill complexity having the most pronounced effects. It became apparent that although Bilodeau and Bilodeau's original findings held up in nearly every context, the benefits of reducing feedback frequency were more pronounced in some circumstances than they were in others. One such factor strongly influencing the benefits of reduced feedback frequency was the learners' previous experience

---

BOX 12.7 Reducing the Frequency of Feedback Can Promote Better Learning Outcomes

Effects of various relative frequencies of feedback on learning were demonstrated by Vander Linden, Cauraugh, and Greene (1993) in a therapeutic setting. Subjects in the experiment were patients relearning to perform basic movement patterns after shoulder surgery. The task performed entailed learning to produce an isometric contraction and relaxation pattern of the upper arm similar to patterns required for elbow extension. Subjects were seated with their dominant arm positioned in a semirigid forearm splint at 90-degrees flexion at the elbow. A load cell was attached to the splint that was capable of exerting from 0 to 50 pounds of force pulling downward on a subject's forearm (i.e., exerting an extension force). The subjects' task

was to learn to duplicate a five-second isometric contraction mirroring a force pattern represented by a power-curve graph displayed on the screen of an oscilloscope visible directly in front of them (see figure below). All subjects completed 100 acquisition trials and 30 trials in a 48-hour retention test.

Subjects were provided KR by viewing their results on the screen showing their movement pattern curve displayed over the criterion pattern they were attempting to duplicate. Three groups of subject were used: One group received 100 percent KR, a second group received 50 percent KR, and a third group received concurrent KR on every trial (100% KR). Results of the study showed that during acquisition, the concurrent KR group performed significantly better

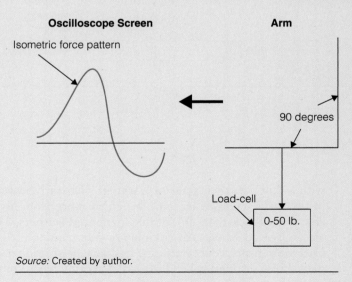

Source: Created by author.

BOX **12.7** *(Continued)*

than did either of the terminal KR groups, and the 100 percent KR subjects performed significantly better than those receiving 50 percent KR. On the retention test, however, the results were quite different. Both terminal KR conditions proved significantly better for retention than did concurrent KR, and of the two terminal KR conditions, subjects receiving the less frequent KR (50%) showed superior learning in comparison to the 100 percent KR group subjects (see figure below). The researchers concluded that more frequent KR, and especially KR provided concurrently, exerts a strong influence on performance, but that reducing the frequency of KR and making it less immediately available enhances learning outcomes.

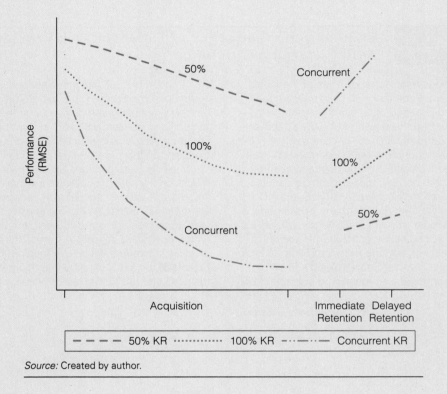

Source: Created by author.

with a skill (i.e., their stage of learning). Generally, it was observed that those in the early stages of learning benefited more from higher relative frequencies of feedback than did more experienced learners. This same pattern was also observed when task complexity was manipulated. Simpler skills benefited more from reduced relative frequencies of feedback than did more complex skills (see Figure 12.6). As skills became more complex, and as learners

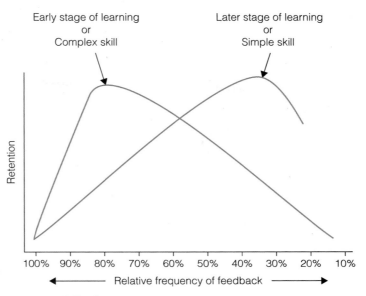

Early stage of learning
or
Complex skill

Later stage of learning
or
Simple skill

Retention

100% 90% 80% 70% 60% 50% 40% 30% 20% 10%

◄——— Relative frequency of feedback ———►

FIGURE **12.6** Interaction of Relative Frequency of Feedback with Stage of Learning and Task Complexity

Source: Created by author.

progressed through the stages of learning a skill, the beneficial contributions of high relative frequencies of feedback decreased, and reduced relative frequencies became more beneficial in promoting continued skill development. These findings soon became axiomatic in the literature of skill learning. By the early 1980s, it had become a well-accepted principle in motor learning that reducing the relative frequency of feedback proved beneficial to learning, at least up to some point (Adams, 1987; Salmoni, Schmidt, and Walter, 1984). Research continues, up to the present, to investigate the effects of frequency manipulations of feedback in a number of areas of theoretical and practical interest. Of particular interest has been the question of how much feedback may be needed by beginners learning complex skills. There is evidence, for instance, suggesting that high relative frequencies of feedback, even as high as 100 percent, may be beneficial for individuals in the initial stages of learning particularly complex and challenging skills (e.g., Wulf, Shea, and Matschiner, 1998).

EXPLAINING RELATIVE FREQUENCY EFFECTS

The beneficial effects on learning from reducing the relative frequency of feedback were strongly supported by early research investigations, as we have just seen. It remained, however, for an adequate theoretical explanation of these effects to be advanced. A widely accepted explanation came in 1984 in the

guidance hypothesis:
The notion that high relative frequencies of augmented feedback can lead to a learner's overreliance on the guidance properties of feedback to the detriment of optimal learning outcomes.

form of the guidance hypothesis (Salmoni, Schmidt, and Walter, 1984; see also Winstein and Schmidt, 1990). The **guidance hypothesis** provided a theoretical foundation for the observed effects of reduced KR frequency on learning and performance as well as being intuitively compelling.

Recall that earlier in this chapter we discussed four functions played by feedback: information, motivation, reinforcement, and guidance. Of these four, we stated that the first three were beneficial to learning, but that the fourth—guidance—was problematic. That is, feedback provides a source of information that guides a learner's performance during practice much in the way that physical guidance does, thus keeping performance close to the desired goal of the skill. When feedback is removed, however, subsequent performance suffers. The guidance role of feedback maintains a high degree of performance but leads to poorer levels of retention. Reducing the relative frequency of feedback is beneficial because it lessens the temporary and negative effect of guidance.

In explaining the relatively detrimental effects of high relative frequencies of feedback, the guidance hypothesis posited three reasons why it typically proves less beneficial to learning than does a reduced schedule of relative feedback frequency. These three reasons are that high relative frequencies of feedback (1) become part of the task to be learned so that learners do not learn independently of feedback, (2) lead to maladaptive short-term corrections, and (3) block other important processing functions like the development of error-correction capabilities. We will look more closely at each of these in turn.

Feedback Becomes a Part of the Task

If feedback is provided frequently when initially learning a skill, then it may become part of the task itself in much the same way as any other sensory stimulus or cue that is present during acquisition. Learners, as a result, build in sources of instructional feedback along with the set of other stimuli forming the memory of the skill. Feedback then functions like any other stimulus associated with performing the skill—proprioceptive feedback, environmental information, etc. Learners do not practice performing independently of feedback, so when it is withdrawn (as in a retention test), they cannot produce an effective performance apart from it (any more than they could if any other sensory cue were removed).

Maladaptive Short-Term Corrections

A second problem associated with frequent feedback is that it encourages learners to make too many corrections during practice, so they fail to produce stable and consistent behaviors. Since the time of Thorndike, it has been recognized that feedback elicits a change in behavior (whereas the absence of feedback tends to stabilize current behaviors). The problem with too much feedback is that changes in behavior take place on too many practice attempts, thus preventing the establishment of stable processes in movement production. On the other hand, when feedback is withheld, at least on some practice attempts, the practiced behaviors tend to stabilize. By withholding feedback, especially on a learner's better performances, the processes leading to those better performance outcomes become more consistent (whereas feedback provided on the worse performance outcomes discourages the repetition of the cognitive processes leading to them). These conclusions reflect perfectly the reasoning of Thorndike's law of effect. As Thorndike's law teaches, providing too much feedback causes learners to make continuous short-term corrections, which in turn fails to adequately reinforce correct behaviors. (It can be noted that an alternative to the guidance hypothesis, called the *consistency hypothesis*, focuses attention more or less exclusively on this **maladaptive short-term correction** aspect of high relative frequencies of feedback.)

maladaptive short-term correction: Inappropriate corrections in the production of a motor skill resulting when relatively minor movement errors are corrected through the provision of augmented feedback.

error detection capability: The capacity of individuals to detect and correct their own errors as a result of sensory sources of feedback.

Blocking Other Processing Activities

A third reason suggested by the guidance hypothesis for the detrimental effect of frequent feedback is that it may, because it attracts so much attention, interfere with or block other important processing activities that are important to learning. This is especially true for the important learning role played by the processing of response-produced sensory feedback in the learner's development of an **error detection capability**. That is, the learner pays too much attention to processing instructional feedback, and insufficient attention to attending to and processing sensory sources of feedback information. This, in turn, inhibits the development of internal mechanisms of error identification and correction essential for effective learning.

SCHEDULES FOR FADING FEEDBACK

When providing for reduced relative frequencies of feedback, several methods are available. Although some of these methods were originally developed for use in research studies, their use as field methods has become more common among practitioners as they focus on methods of fading feedback over practice attempts. That is, if reduced feedback has the advantages suggested by the guidance hypothesis, then it makes sense to find appropriate methods for gradually reducing—fading—the frequency of feedback over practice attempts in order to promote better learning outcomes.

feedback fading: An augmented feedback schedule in which feedback is provided most frequently early in practice and then gradually reduced in frequency as practice continues.

Feedback fading works much in the same way as teaching a child to ride a bicycle. Initially, the child begins by using training wheels and having a parent run alongside holding onto the bicycle's handlebars. In other words, a high degree of guidance is provided. If the provision of this level of guidance continued, the child would perform well, but obviously would not learn to ride a bicycle (because once the training wheels and adult support were removed, the child could not perform well independently, having come to rely upon such guidance). Over time, though, the parent gradually removes more and more guidance, forcing the child to take on more and more responsibility for the task of bicycle riding (i.e., learning to ride). First, the training wheels come off; next, parental control of the handlebars is loosened; soon the parent releases the handlebars altogether, though a hand may still support the bicycle seat. Finally, even this last support on the seat is removed, and the child is left to control the bicycle relying only on his or her own sensory sources of feedback—he or she has become an independent learner.

In an analogous fashion, the gradual fading of feedback over practice trials promotes learning. Practitioners use several methods for scheduling the relative frequency of feedback, each of which can also lead to schedules of fading feedback over practice attempts. We will look at four of the more commonly used methods: summary feedback, bandwidth feedback, and average feedback, as well as an extension of these methods used in practice we will call *intuitive feedback*. Finally, we will mention a method of providing feedback called *learner-requested feedback*, where, as the name suggests, learners establish their own schedules.

Summary Feedback

summary feedback: The provision of augmented feedback for each practice attempt in a series of attempts, but only after the series is completed.

Summary feedback is defined as the provision of feedback after a predetermined number of practice attempts in a series of attempts in which feedback (usually in the form of KR) is provided for each of the attempts in that series. If, for example, a summary length of 10 were determined as the criterion in a series of practice attempts, feedback would be provided for the first 10 attempts *after* the 10th attempt was completed. For the second block of

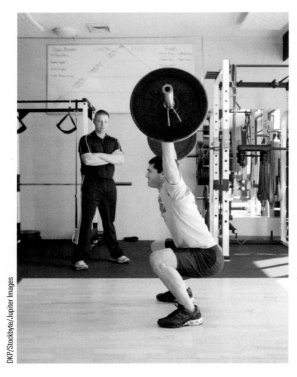

DKP/Stockbyte/Jupiter Images

Effective instructors use a variety of methods to fade feedback over practice so that learners come to increasingly rely upon their own sources of intrinsic feedback and perform independently of the instructor's augmented feedback.

10 practice attempts—trials 11 to 20—feedback would again be provided for each and every attempt at the completion of the 20th trial. The completion of trial 30 would be attended by feedback for each of the practice trials 21 to 30, and so on, until the series of practice attempts was completed. In a summary feedback schedule, every practice attempt receives feedback, but only at the completion of a predetermined number of attempts in the series.

Summary feedback is widely used as a method for manipulating feedback frequency in research studies. Most of the original research studies exploring frequency effects of feedback on performance and learning, such as those by Bilodeau and Bilodeau, used summary KR schedules to manipulate the relative frequency of feedback.

As an example of summary feedback, consider training for a patient with balance impairment. For such training, kinetic or force feedback about postural alignment and weight-bearing by the legs and feet is often used (Shumway-Cook and Woollacott, 2007). One technique involves having a patient repeatedly step on and off of a forceplate that registers the amount of weight-bearing for each foot, with the goal of achieving correct body alignment by equally distributing the force exerted between the patient's left and right feet. The patient performs repeated trials with a two to three second pause on each trial while attempting to achieve correct vertical body alignment.

In this example, the instructor has decided to employ a summary length of 10. The instructor records the best balance score achieved on each trial. Scores are recorded as the percentage of weight-bearing greater on one foot than on the other, with either left or right indicating on which foot the greater force was exerted. A score of "0" indicates that the patient distributed weight evenly on both feet. After the patient's tenth practice trial, the instructor shows the patient a graph of the individual trial scores. An example of this graph is shown in Figure 12.7. Note that the learner receives information about every practice attempt, but not until completing the prescribed number of practice trials. Also note, in this case, that observing the summary information readily conveys the patient's bias for exerting greater force on the right foot than on the left, something that might not be as apparent if feedback were received on every trial.

How many attempts should practitioners include in such summary schedules? Evidence suggests that there is an optimal number and that anything over or under detracts from learning (Schmidt, Lange, and Young, 1990). For simple tasks, or for learners having gained a good grasp of a skill, 15 or 20 trials may be appropriate as a summary length. On the other hand, when a task is complex, fewer practice attempts are indicated—perhaps 5 or 10. When a complex task is coupled with an inexperienced learner in the early stages of learning, 2 or 3 practice attempts may be best as a summary length. For extremely complex tasks practiced by novice learners, the optimal summary length may even be 1, at least until learners master the essential movement elements. Over the course of practice, instructors can fade feedback by progressively lengthening the summary length, thereby promoting learning.

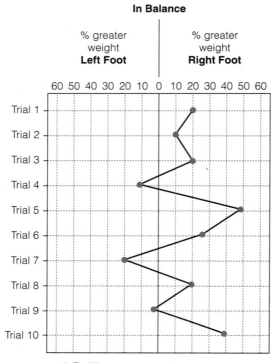

FIGURE **12.7** Summary Feedback

Source: Created by author.

Bandwidth Feedback

bandwidth feedback:
Augmented feedback
that is provided only
when performance
error falls outside of a
predetermined criterion
of correctness.

A second way of fading the frequency of feedback is by the method of
bandwidth feedback First introduced by Sherwood (1988), in this method
the instructor only provides feedback when a learner's performance falls outside of some predetermined and acceptable level of correctness, or bandwidth.
When providing beginning learners feedback for free-throw attempts in basketball, for example, the basket, net, and backboard could constitute the bandwidth within which feedback is withheld. As long as the basketball initially
strikes the basket, net, or backboard, no feedback is delivered. Anything outside of this criterion, however, will result in the provision of corrective feedback. As other examples, a bandwidth when practicing the tennis serve might
include any serve that passed legally over the net and landed safely within
bounds. The bandwidth for bowling might be any ball that remained on the
alley and hit the pins without going into the gutter. As individuals improve
their performance capabilities, these criteria could be narrowed. For the basketball example, once learners were performing fairly consistently within the
original bandwidth, an instructor could set a new criterion in which feedback would be withheld only for those attempts where the basket or net were

initially contacted. Outside of these limits, now including the backboard, feedback would be provided.

The bandwidth feedback method has several advantages. First, it fades the amount of feedback in a natural way as learners become more skilled. In this way, learners themselves actually determine the frequency of feedback by their own performances. In the early stage of learning, individuals will naturally make more mistakes, leading to more practice attempts outside of the bandwidth criterion and therefore a higher relative frequency of feedback. As learners become more skilled, their performances will more frequently fall within the bandwidth criterion of correctness, thereby fading the amount of feedback they receive. Second, because only the worse attempts fall outside of the bandwidth criterion and receive feedback, only the worse mistakes (relatively) will receive feedback, whereas the best attempts (relatively) will not receive feedback. That is, learners receive feedback encouraging changes in behavior only for their worse mistakes. For their better practice attempts, they do not receive feedback (a form of negative reinforcement), thus stabilizing behaviors around correct actions. Finally, the absence of feedback on some attempts acts to focus learners' attention on intrinsically produced feedback rather than extrinsic forms of feedback, thus promoting the development of self-reliance and error-correction capabilities.

Average Feedback

average feedback: Augmented feedback provided at the completion of a series of practice attempts regarding the average performance of the attempts (often as a numerical average).

A third method of scheduling feedback is **average feedback**. In this method, a predetermined number of practice attempts are completed before feedback is provided, as is the case also in summary feedback. Unlike summary feedback, however, the average of error scores for all practice attempts is provided rather than individual error scores. In the tennis example cited for summary feedback, the instruction might have used average feedback by stating something like, "Your serves were, on average, about one meter short of the service line." (Note, though, that when used as a laboratory research variable the average error is typically provided as a quantitatively precise measurement.)

Average feedback probably functions in much the same way as summary feedback but is easier for practitioners to give in most situations. Rather than recording (or remembering) error scores on every practice attempt, the instructor need only provide a single error estimate (or score). Moreover, average feedback is more likely to provide learners with a general sense of their movement errors, more clearly indicating what aspects of movement they need to change on the next series of practice attempts.

Intuitive Feedback

intuitive feedback: The intentional fading of augmented feedback to a learner based on an instructor's perception of the learner's needs and capabilities.

A technique of combining all three of the methods of feedback scheduling discussed here is **intuitive feedback**. This is not so much a formal method of feedback scheduling as it is a description of what practitioners typically do in actual practice.

In the field, practitioners are frequently faced with numerous instructional challenges that make the provision of formal schedules of feedback difficult, if not impractical. An instructor with 30 students, each at a different skill level, and a limited time in which to provide instruction is not able to watch each learner on every practice attempt or to devote the attention or time necessary to schedule a formal method of fading scheduling (though when practical, this is always preferable).

Good instructors use their intuition, experience, and understanding of feedback frequency effects to provide effective feedback to learners. This may entail some general notion of how many practice attempts each individual learner should be provided free of feedback relative to their stage of learning (summary feedback), some criterion of performance beyond which corrective information will be provided and within which it will not (bandwidth feedback), and feedback provided in general terms concerning a series of practice attempts rather than specific information on single attempts (average feedback). Providing feedback based on the practitioner's intuition informed by a knowledge of the principles of feedback fading, a knowledge of the skills being instructed, and a sensitivity to individual differences and levels of learning is one of the most important skills (if not the most important one) effective motor skill instructors can process.

Learner-Requested Feedback

learner-requested feedback: A technique for providing feedback only when a learner requests it.

Although not formally designed as a method for fading feedback, the technique of **learner-requested feedback** (also called self-controlled, self-requested, and self-regulated feedback) typically results in effective patterns of feedback fading as a natural outcome of learner perceived needs. Applying this technique, learners receive feedback only when they request it.

While not a great deal of research has been focused on this technique as yet, two particularly interesting findings have consistently emerged from reported studies. The first is that learners request feedback on a small percentage of their practice experiences, with reports of as few as 7 and 11 percent of practice trials for which feedback was requested (Janelle, Kim, and Singer, 1995; Janelle et al., 1997). A second major finding reported in the research literature is that learners who could request feedback when they desired it were significantly more likely to request feedback on the practice attempts they perceived as correct (or "good") than they were for those attempts they experienced as incorrect (or "bad") (see Chiviakowsky and Wulf, 2002; and Chiviakowsky and Wulf, 2005).

The reasons for the observed patterns of learner-requested feedback remain somewhat unclear and remain debated. From theoretical perspectives of both cognitive-based and dynamical systems theories, however, there are considerable reasons to support the practice. From a cognitive-based perspective, it can be pointed out that this method may well involve greater attention and problem-solving strategies on the part of the learner, both conditions facilitating effective encoding of information into long-term memory. From a dynamical systems perspective, the technique can be viewed as increasing exploration of the movement environment as well as self-discovery on the part of the learner, who more actively engages in seeking problem-solving strategies to achieve action goals. For a review of the various methods of fading feedback, consider the examples shown in Box 12.8.

| BOX **12.8** | **How Many Ways Can You Fade Feedback?** |

One of the most important things a movement skills instructor can do to enhance learning opportunities for those he or she instructs is to design meaningful ways of fading feedback over the course of skill practice. Formal methods of doing this include the use of summary, bandwidth, and average fading schedules. Suggest specific methods you could use to apply each of these techniques when instructing someone learning the following skills:

- Target shooting on a rifle range
- 20-foot golf putt on a practice green
- Pilot practicing landings in a flight simulator
- Performing a back handstand
- Patient moving from a sitting to a standing position
- Tennis serve
- Moving a handgrip 50 cm in exactly 500 ms on a linear movement device in an experiment

SUMMARY

- Feedback refers to any response-related information concerning a motor skill provided either during or subsequent to production of the skill. Feedback can be either sensory or augmented.
  - Sensory feedback is response-produced information from the performer's own sensory sources.
  - Augmented feedback is supplied by a source external to the performer.
- Augmented feedback can be further classified as being of two types:
  - Knowledge of results (KR) is information concerning the outcome of a response.
  - Knowledge of performance (KP) is information concerning the causes of a response outcome.
- Augmented feedback plays an essential role in the acquisition of motor skills; it is believed to have four important functions in skill acquisition:
  - It provides information necessary to correct errors.
  - It reinforces behaviors.
  - It acts to motivate learners.
  - It guides practice experiences before learners have developed internal templates of reference.
- Three especially important principles in providing effective augmented feedback concern the precision, timing, and frequency with which feedback is delivered.
  - Generally, quantitative feedback statements are more effective than are qualitative feedback statements, although an inverted-U relationship

exists such that overly precise quantitative statements become increasingly ineffective.

- Post-response feedback is more effective than is concurrent feedback, and a minimum post-response period of two to three seconds should elapse before the delivery of feedback.
- High relative frequencies of feedback are generally less effective than are reduced relative frequencies, and this becomes increasingly true as learners acquire motor skills.

- Effective motor skills instructors use various methods to fade the relative frequency of feedback over time. These might include summary, average, bandwidth, intuitive, or learner-requested methods of feedback fading.

LEARNING EXERCISES

1. Identify a motor skill in which you have an interest and for which you have a good working knowledge concerning its correct performance. Next, identify five key performance errors that a beginner learning the skill might typically be expected to make. For each of these key errors, write a hypothetical feedback statement representing qualitative KR, quantitative KR, qualitative KP, quantitative KP, descriptive feedback, and prescriptive feedback. Examining your feedback statements, do you believe that one of the types of feedback would prove more beneficial than the others to a beginner learning the skill? Explain your answer.

2. Select a skill in which you are interested (choose a different skill than you used for question 1), and design for it a bandwidth feedback fading schedule. Identify a population for whom you will develop the schedule, and consider feedback criteria that can be used to progress learners from an initial novice stage of learning to a skilled autonomous or expert learning stage. Specify the bandwidth criteria that you will use as learners progress through the various stages of learning, as well as the criteria you will set for transitioning learners from one bandwidth to the next.

3. For this exercise, observe an instructor providing feedback in a skill practice setting. Instructions can be provided either for an individual or for a group. The learner or learners should be in the initial or early stage of learning the skill. Position yourself where you can clearly observe the practice activities and can hear feedback as it is provided. You should be able to complete at least 20 minutes of observations in this fashion.

   Your task is to observe and take notes on the type of feedback and the manner of delivery used by the instructor. After completing the field portion of this exercise, prepare a written report on the quality of feedback you observed. Comment both on what you felt the instructor did well and on those things you believe could have been done more effectively. What specific suggestions would you make for improving the quality of feedback that you observed? Your paper should reflect your understanding of the principles and methods presented in this chapter.

FOR FURTHER STUDY

HOW MUCH DO YOU KNOW?

For each of the following, select the letter that best answers the question.

1. Which of the following is *not* a primary function of augmented feedback?
   a. Guidance function
   b. Motivation function
   c. Reinforcement function
   d. Comparative function

2. The observation that rewarded behaviors tend to be repeated and that punished behaviors tend to be changed is formalized by the
   a. guidance hypothesis.
   b. law of effect.
   c. relative frequency rate.
   d. specificity hypothesis.

3. As what type of feedback would you *best* classify the following statement: "The reason that the ball popped up like that is that you're holding your racquet too loosely and your grip is too high."
   a. Qualitative KR
   b. Quantitative KR
   c. Qualitative KP
   d. Quantitative KP

4. As a general rule, providing feedback to a learner after every practice attempt
   a. depresses performance but improves learning.
   b. improves performance but depresses learning.
   c. improves both performance and learning.
   d. depresses both performance and learning.

5. For feedback to be most effective, it should typically be provided—
   a. 3 to 5 seconds after a response.
   b. 20 to 30 seconds after a response.
   c. immediately after a response.
   d. during a response.

6. When beginners are provided with erroneous feedback that clearly contradicts their sources of sensory feedback, they are most likely to
   a. disregard the erroneous feedback in favor of their sensory sources of feedback.
   b. disregard both the erroneous feedback and their own sensory feedback.
   c. disregard their sensory sources of feedback and rely instead on the erroneous feedback.
   d. compromise between the two sources of feedback information.

Answer the following with the word or words that best complete each sentence.

7. If a person performs 30 trials of a particular skill during a practice session, and he or she receives feedback on 6 of those trials, then the relative frequency of feedback is ____(a)____ and the absolute frequency of feedback is ____(b)____, respectively.

8. During a physical therapy session, a patient attempts a set of three elbow extension exercises. Upon completion of the three exercises, her therapist provides her with feedback concerning the numerical angle of elbow extension achieved on each of the three exercises. What type of feedback did the therapist provide?

9. What kind of reinforcement is being provided when an instructor corrects five practice attempts in a row and then withholds feedback on a sixth attempt in which there is improvement?

10. KP is an abbreviation for _____.

11. A gradual reduction in the relative frequency of feedback designed to promote learning is termed feedback _____.

12. The period of time between the delivery of feedback and the person who receives the feedback attempting his or her next response is referred to as the _____ interval.

Answers are provided at the end of this review section.

STUDY QUESTIONS

1. Define feedback. Into what two basic categories is feedback classified?
2. In what different ways can augmented feedback be classified? Define each of these ways.
3. What four functions, as described in this chapter, does feedback play in the learning of motor skills? Describe what is meant by each of these functions.
4. Define the law of effect. Define and provide an example of each of the following types of feedback reinforcement: positive, negative, and punishment. What are the relative effects of each type of reinforcement on learning?
5. What advice, based upon research in motor learning, would you offer a movement instructor concerning the precision with which feedback should be provided?
6. How soon should feedback be provided after an action is completed? What is the effectiveness of delivering feedback concurrently? Explain your reasoning in both cases.
7. What general principles apply to the frequency with which feedback should be provided?
8. How should skill complexity and learner experience influence decisions concerning feedback frequency?
9. What is the guidance hypothesis and what reasons does it advance as explanations for reduced relative frequency effects on the performance and learning of motor skills?
10. Define and provide examples for each of the following methods for fading feedback: summary, bandwidth, average, intuitive, and learner-requested.

ADDITIONAL READING

Aruin, AS, Hanke, TA, and Sharma, A. (2003). "Base of support feedback in gait rehabilitation." *Journal of Rehabilitation Research, 26,* 309–312.

Chambers, KL, and Vickers, JN. (2006). "Effects of bandwidth feedback and questioning on the performance of competitive swimmers." *The Sport Psychologist, 20,* 184–197.

Chen, DD. (2001). "Trends in augmented feedback research and tips for the practitioner." *Journal of Physical Education, Recreation and Dance, 72*(1), 32–36.

Chiviakowsky, S, and Wulf, G. (2007). "Feedback after good trials enhances learning." *Research Quarterly for Exercise and Sport, 78*(1), 40–47.

Cronin, JB, Bressel, E, and Finn, L. (2008). Augmented feedback reduces ground reaction forces in the landing phase of the volleyball spike jump, *Journal of Sport Rehabilitation, 17,* 148–159.

McNevin, CJ, and Liogas, V. (2001). "Type and frequency of feedback used by physical therapists: Effects on patient performance." *Physical Therapy, 81*(5), 81.

Mouratidis, A, Vansteenkiste, M, Lens, W, and Sideridis, G. (2008). The motivation role of positive feedback in sport and physical education: Evidence for a motivational model. *Journal of Sport and Exercise Psychology, 30,* 240–268.

Peterson, AP. (1981). "Using feedback to develop tennis skills." *Journal of Physical Education, Recreation, and Dance, 52*(7), 54, 57.

Swinnen, SP. (1996). "Information feedback in motor skill learning: A review." In HN Zelaznik (ed.), *Advances in Motor Learning and Control* (pp. 37–66). Champaign, IL: Human Kinetics.

Winchester, JB, Porter, JM, and McBride, JM. (2009). Change in bar path kinematics and kinetics through use of summary feedback in power snatch training. *Journal of Strength and Conditioning, 23,* 444–454.

Wulf, G, and Shea, CH. (2004). "Understanding the role of augmented feedback: The good, the bad and the ugly." In AM Williams and NJ Hodges, *Skill Acquisition in Sport: Research, Theory and Practice.* London: Routledge.

REFERENCES

Adams, JA. (1968). "Response feedback and learning." *Psychological Bulletin, 70*, 486–504.

Adams, JA. (1987). "Historical review and appraisal of research on the learning, retention, and transfer of human motor skills." *Psychological Bulletin, 101*, 41–74.

Annett, J. (1969). *Feedback and human behavior.* Middlesex, England: Penguin.

Aruin, AS, Hanke, TA, and Sharma, A. (2003). "Base of support feedback in gait rehabilitation." *Journal of Rehabilitation Research, 26*, 309–312.

Bilodeau, IM. (1966). "Information feedback." In EA Bilodeau (ed.), *Acquisition of skill* (pp. 255–296). New York: Academic Press.

Bilodeau, IM, and Bilodeau, EA. (1969). *Principles of skill acquisition.* New York: Academic Press.

Buekers, MJ, and Magill, RA. (1995). "The role of task experience and prior knowledge for detecting invalid augmented feedback while learning a motor skill." *Quarterly Journal of Experimental Psychology, 48A*, 84–97.

Buekers, MJ, Magill, RA, and Hall, KG. (1992). "The effect of erroneous knowledge of results on skill acquisition when augmented information is redundant." *Quarterly Journal of Experimental Psychology, 44A*, 105–117.

Buekers, MJ, Magill, RA, and Sneyers, KM. (1994). "Resolving a conflict between sensory feedback and knowledge of results, while learning a motor skill." *Journal of Motor Behavior, 26*, 27–35.

Chambers, KL, and Vickers, JN. (2006). "Effects of bandwidth feedback and questioning on the performance of competitive swimmers." *The Sport Psychologist, 20*, 184–197.

Chen, DD. (2001). "Trends in augmented feedback research and tips for the practitioner." *Journal of Physical Education, Recreation and Dance, 72*(1), 32–36.

Cheng, S, and Sakes, PN. (2006). "Modeling sensorimotor learning with dynamical systems." *Neural Computation, 18*(4), 760–792.

Chiviakowsky, S, and Wulf, G. (2002). "Self-controlled feedback: Does it enhance learning because performers get feedback when they need it?" *Research Quarterly for Exercise and Sport, 73*(4), 408–414.

Chiviakowsky, S, and Wulf, G. (2005). "Self-controlled feedback is effective if it is based on the learner's performance." *Research Quarterly for Exercise and Sport, 76*(1), 42–48.

Chiviakowsky, S, and Wulf, G. (2007). "Feedback after good trials enhances learning." *Research Quarterly for Exercise and Sport, 78*(1), 40–47.

Christina, RW, and Corcos, DM. (1988). *Coaches' guide to teaching sports skills.* Champaign, IL: Human Kinetics.

Coker, CA. (2009). *Motor learning and control for practitioners.* Scottsdale, AZ: Holcomb Hathaway.

Dishman, RK. (1993). "Exercise adherence." In RN Singer, M Murphey, and LK Tennant (eds.), *Handbook on sport psychology* (pp. 779–798). New York: Macmillan.

Ericsson, KA. (1996). *The road to excellence: The acquisition of expert performance in the arts and sciences, sports, and games.* Mahwah, NJ: Lawrence Erlbaum.

Fischman, MG, and Oxendine, JB. (2001). "Motor learning for effective coaching and performance." In JM Williams (ed.), *Applied sport psychology: Personal growth to peak performance* (pp. 13–28). Mountain View, CA: Mayfield.

Fishman, S, and Tobey, C. (1978). "Augmented feedback." In W Anderson and G Barrette (eds.), *What's going on in the gym: Descriptive studies of physical education classes* (pp. 51–62), *Motor skills: Theory into practice,* Monograph 1.

Fredenberg, KB, Lee, AM, and Solmon, ML. (2001). "The effect of augmented feedback on students' perception and performance." *Research Quarterly for Exercise and Sport, 72*, 232–242.

Hull, CL. (1943). *Principles of behavior.* New York: Appleton-Century-Crofts.

Janelle, CM, Barba, DA, Frehlich, SG, Tenant, LK, and Cauraugh, JH. (1997). "Maximizing performance feedback effectiveness through videotape replay and a self-controlled learning environment." *Research Quarterly for Exercise and Sport, 68*, 269–279.

Janelle, CM, Kim, J, and Singer, RN. (1995). "Subject-controlled performance feedback and learning of a closed motor skill." *Perceptual and Motor Skills, 81*, 627–634.

Lavery, JJ. (1962). "Retention of simple motor skills as a function of type of knowledge of results." *Canadian Journal of Psychology, 16*, 300–311.

Lintern, G, and Roscoe, SN. (1980). "Visual cue augmentation in contact flight simulation." In SN Roscoe (ed.), *Aviation Psychology* (pp. 227–238). Ames, IA: Iowa State University Press.

Magill, RA. (2001). "Augmented feedback and skill acquisition." In RN Singer, HA Hausenblaus, and C Janelle (eds.), *Handbook on Research in Sport Psychology*, 2nd ed. (pp. 86–114). New York: Wiley.

Magill, RA, and Wood, CA. (1986). "Knowledge of results precision as a learning variable in motor skill acquisition." *Research Quarterly for Exercise and Sport, 57*, 170–173.

McMorris, T. (2004). *Acquisition and performance of sports skills.* Chichester, England: Wiley.

McNevin, CJ, and Liogas, V. (2001). "Type and frequency of feedback used by physical therapists: Effects on patient performance." *Physical Therapy, 81*(5), 81.

Newell, KM, and McGinnis, PM. (1985). "Kinematic information feedback for skilled performance." *Human Learning, 4*, 39–56.

Peterson, AP. (1981). "Using feedback to develop tennis skills." *Journal of Physical Education, Recreation, and Dance, 52*(7), 54, 57.

Rogers, CA. (1974). "Feedback precision and postfeedback interval duration." *Journal of Experimental Psychology, 102*, 604–608.

Rose, DJ, and Christina, RW. (2006). *A multilevel approach to the study of motor control and learning*, 2nd ed. San Francisco: Benjamin Cummings.

Ryan, LJ, and Roby, TB. (2002). "Learning and performance effects of accurate and erroneous knowledge of results on time perception." *Acta Psychologica, 111*, 83–100.

Salmoni, AW, Schmidt, RA, and Walter, CB. (1984). "Knowledge of results in motor learning: A review and reappraisal." *Psychological Bulletin, 95*, 355–386.

Schmidt, RA, and Lee, TD. (2005). *Motor control and learning: A behavioral emphasis,* 4th ed. Champaign, IL: Human Kinetics.

Schmidt, RA, Young, DE, and Lange, C. (1990). "Optimizing summary knowledge of results for skill learning." *Human Movement Science, 9*, 325–348.

Sherwood, DE. (1988). "Effect of bandwidth knowledge of results on movement consistency." *Perceptual and Motor Skills, 66*, 535–542.

Shumway-Cook, A, and Woollacott, M. (2007). Motor control: Translating research into clinical practice. Philadelphia: Lippicott, Williams, & Walkins.

Silverman, S, Tyson, LA, and Krampitz, J. (1991). "Teacher feedback and achievement in physical education: Interaction with student practice." Paper presented at the American Education Research Association, Chicago, IL.

Silverman, S, Woods, AM, and Subramaniam, PR. (1999). "Feedback and practice in physical education: Interrelationships with task structures and student skill level." *Journal of Human Movement Studies, 36*, 203–224.

Smoll, FL. (1972). "Effects of precision of information feedback upon acquisition of a motor skill." *Research Quarterly, 43*, 489–493.

Swinnen, SP. (1996). "Information feedback in motor skill learning: A review." In HN Zelaznik (ed.), *Advances in Motor Learning and Control* (pp. 37–66). Champaign, IL: Human Kinetics.

Swinnen, SP, Schmidt, RA, Nicholson, DE, and Shapiro, DC. (1990). "Information feedback for skill acquisition: Instantaneous knowledge of results degrades learning." *Journal of Experimental Psychology: Learning, Memory, and Cognition, 16*, 706–716.

Thorndike, EL. (1927). "The law of effect." *American Journal of Psychology, 39*, 212–222.

Thorndike, EL. (1931). *Human learning.* New York: Century.

Vander Linden, DW, Cauraugh, JH, and Greene, TA. (1993). "The effect of frequency of kinetic feedback on learning an isometric force production task in nondisabled subjects." *Physical Therapy, 73*, 79–87.

Williams, AC, and Briggs, GE. (1962). "On-target versus off-target information and the acquisition of tracking skill." *Journal of Experimental Psychology, 64*, 519–525.

Winstein, CJ, and Schmidt, RA. (1990). "Reduced frequency of knowledge of results enhances motor skill learning." *Journal of Experimental Psychology: Learning Memory, and Cognition, 16*, 677–691.

Wrisberg, CA, Dale, GA, Liu, Z, and Reed, A. (1995). "The effects of augmented information on motor learning: A multidimensional assessment." *Research Quarterly for Exercise and Sport, 66*, 9–16.

Wulf, G, Shea, CH, and Matschiner, S. (1998). "Frequent feedback enhances complex motor-skill learning." *Journal of Motor Behavior*, *30*, 180–192.

Wulf, G, and Shea, CH. (2004). "Understanding the role of augmented feedback: The good, the bad and the ugly." In AM Williams and NJ Hodges, *Skill Acquisition in Sport: Research, Theory and Practice*. London: Routledge.

Answers to How Much Do You Know questions: (1) D, (2) B, (3) C, (4) B, (5) A, (6) C, (7) 20%, 6, (8) summary feedback, (9) negative reinforcement, (10) knowledge of performance, (11) fading, (12) post-KR delay.

Measuring Performance: Time and Magnitude

In assessing an individual's or a group's performance in meeting the goals of a task, a number of trials or performance measurements are evaluated. A single trial or other performance measurement is seldom an accurate representation of performance capability, so a number of individual performance measurements are averaged in order to provide a more stable and accurate picture of an individual's (or group's) generalized performance capabilities.

In assessing performance in motor learning, three types of measurements are typically collected and evaluated. These include measurements of time, magnitude, and error. The first two of these, time and magnitude, refer to the kind of task outcomes that are the criteria of performance; these measures are discussed here. The third, error measurements, refers to the assessment of accuracy and are presented in Appendix B.

Measurements of time and magnitude are readily applicable to motor skill learning where time (how fast) and magnitude (how much, how far) are frequently the criteria most indicative of performance success. That is, success in many motor skills depends primarily on how well an individual meets the environmental goals of a task in terms of time (i.e., speed) or some measure of magnitude (i.e., distance, force, or weight).

Measurements of Time

Two measurements of time are used extensively in motor learning research: reaction time (abbreviated RT) and movement time (abbreviated MT).

Reaction time is a measurement of how long it takes a person to perceive, process, and initiate a movement in response to a stimulus. As can be seen in the figure below, RT is the time between the presentation of a stimulus signal and the beginning of movement in response to that signal. It is important to note that RT does not include any movement component, but is the time prior to initiation of movement in response to the initiating stimulus.

In laboratory settings, the stimulus signal can take the form of a light, a sound, or even a slight electric shock, so that RT can be measured in response to any sensory modality. The response to the initiating sensory signal may be as simple as lifting one's finger from a telegraph key or as difficult as the completion of a complex movement sequence, so that RT is a measurement of the time needed to prepare and initiate movement responses ranging from the very simple to the very complex. Reaction time may also be measured as the time required for responding to a single stimulus, called simple RT, or from among different stimuli requiring alternative response choices, called choice RT. An example of choice RT in a laboratory setting could include the presentation of lights of different colors, with each colored light requiring a different response such as depressing a particular key from among a series of different keys. Finally, it is typical in most laboratory measurements of RT to include a short warning period (usually between one-half and five seconds) prior to the presentation of the stimulus signal.

Movement time is the time between the beginning of movement in response to the stimulus signal and the completion of that response. Thus, MT begins where RT ends; it represents a carrying out of the response that was planned and initiated during the RT period. Movement time can last anywhere from a fraction of a second for a ballistic discrete skill such as batting a pitched ball, to hours for a continuous skill like running a marathon race. In laboratory settings, movements requiring no more than a few seconds at most are typical.

The combination of RT and MT is called response time (i.e., RT + MT = Response Time). Though it might seem that those individuals possessing quick reaction times would also demonstrate quick movement times, and therefore also quick response times, research has revealed a low correlation between RT and MT. The processes underlying RT and MT are relatively independent of one another, so performance on one does not predict performance on the other. An individual demonstrating very quick RT may well prove, upon measurement of MT, to be

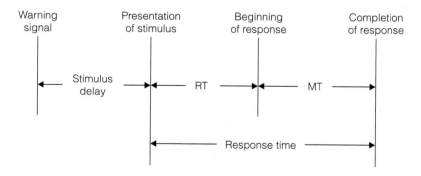

relatively slow. Thus researchers need to separate response time into RT and MT in order to understand the contribution of each to overall response time.

Measurements of Response Magnitude

The second basic method of assessing the performance of motor skills is the measurement of response magnitude. These measurements involve the magnitude (i.e., the "amount") of the performance. For example, measurements of magnitude include the distance a javelin is thrown, the amount of weight lifted in an overhead press, the angle of flexion obtained at the knee joint by a patient in therapy, and the distance for a long jump. Such measurements are often the determinants of competitive success in sports and so might seem valid performance measures, especially in applied sports-related studies. Surprisingly, though, they are little used in motor learning research (at least they are not used much in laboratory research, though research conducted in field settings is more likely to employ measurement of magnitude as the dependent variable). One reason that such measurements are little used is no doubt attributable to researchers' inclination toward the use of performance tasks that can be carefully controlled and measured, such as those pertaining to the measurement of time and speed. Not only are tasks in which performance is recorded through various measurements of magnitude more difficult to control and measure accurately, but subjects in such studies are more likely to bring transferable skills and experiences to the experimental task conditions (i.e., measurement of the distance a research subject can throw a ball may be more a factor of previous learning experiences in ball throwing than of experimental manipulations).

Another reason magnitude measurements may play a small role in laboratory research is that skills in which some magnitude measurement is significantly related to performance are typically gross motor skills in which fatigue builds up over trials. The problem with using such skills experimentally is that it is difficult to isolate changes in performance that are due to learning or skill enhancement from those caused by fatigue, at least in the relatively short time periods typical of laboratory protocols. It is also problematic that subjects in an experiment employing gross skills, and resulting in fatigue, may become less motivated in their efforts as the experiment proceeds. Fatigue, then, acts as a confounding variable, weakening experimental control and interacting with treatment variables so that it is difficult to disentangle the effects of one from the other. Simply stated, it is difficult to tell which changes in observed magnitude measurements are due to experimental manipulations and which are due to temporary fatigue conditions that build up in subjects.

Noteworthy exceptions do exist to this general lack in the use of magnitude measurements in laboratory research. Both the Bachman Ladder and Stability Platform have a long history in motor learning research, and a number of important recent investigations have employed the Ski Simulator (see Chapter 10); all of these are experimental tasks in which measurements of magnitude represent the criteria of performance. Gross motor tasks like these have the advantage of closely duplicating the requirements of most sports skills, thereby increasing the external validity of experimental findings.

Measuring Accuracy

Three methods for averaging individual performance measures are used when assessing an individual's (or group's) accuracy in meeting task goals. Each of these provides different information concerning performance; taken together, they provide a comprehensive analysis of performance. These three methods for assessing accuracy include absolute error (AE), constant error (CE), and variable error (VE).

Absolute Error (AE)

AE represents the average deviation from the performance criterion or goal, disregarding the direction of error. That is, mathematically the deviation from the performance criterion or goal is deduced for each performance trial, disregarding plus or minus sign; summed; and then averaged. The value of AE represents the average error committed during a series of performance attempts evaluated without reference to the direction of error (for example, whether errors were, on average, too long or too short). The formula for AE is as follows:

$$AE = \Sigma|X-C|/k$$

In the formula, X represents individual performance trials, C is the criterion or performance goal, and k the number of trials being averaged. As an example, consider an individual performing five golfing putts, whose individual trials are 8 feet short, 4 feet short, 3 feet long, 7 feet long, and 12 feet long. In this case, there are five X scores of -8, -4, 3, 7, and 12; and because there are five trials, k = 5. The criterion, C, is 0 because a successful putt is neither short nor long, but meets the goal of the task. Substituting these data into the equation for AE yields the following:

$$AE = |-8-0|^* + |-4-0| + |3-0| + |7-0| + |12-0|/ \ 5$$
$$= (8)+(4)+(3)+(7)+(12) \ / \ 5$$
$$= 34/5$$
$$= 6.8$$

*[The straight brackets (||) mean disregard the sign of the individual scores.]

An AE of 6.8 means that, on average, an individual deviates 6.8 units (in whatever units of measurement are being used) from achieving the criterion performance goal when measured for a series of performance attempts. In our example, the performer missed the target of sinking a putt by an average of 6.8 feet, though AE provides us with no information on whether the putts were more likely to be short or long, or evenly distributed among both short and long putts. AE is very useful, however, as an easily calculated overall measurement of average performance error.

Constant Error (CE)

Like AE, CE provides information concerning average error, but unlike AE, CE also provides information concerning the direction of that error. It is calculated the same way as AE, with the exception that the direction of an error (the + and − signs) is taken into account. CE provides an average measure of both the direction and distance from the criterion or performance goal on a series of performance trials. The formula for CE follows, with X, C, and k maintaining their previous meanings:

$$CE = \Sigma(X-C)/k$$

Using the same example as for AE above, and substituting the data into the equation yields the following:

$$CE = (-8-0) + (-4-0) + (3-0) + (7-0) + (12-0)/ \ 5$$
$$= (-8) + (-4) + (3) + (7) + (12) \ / \ 5$$
$$= 10/5$$
$$= 2.0$$

A CE score of 2.0 is interpreted as meaning that a performer's average deviation from the criterion or performance goal is 2.0 units in the positive direction of measurement. CE is a measurement of performer bias, indicating the average amount and direction of error during performance trials. In our example, a CE of 2.0 indicates that on average the performer's putting attempts were 2.0 feet too long, indicating a slight tendency toward overshooting the performance target (i.e., the hole). Note that CE provides a measurement of average bias, but not average error. Following our putting example, three putts of 1 foot, 2 feet, and 3 feet long would yield a CE of 2; but so would three putts of 10 feet short, 2 feet long, and 14 feet long. The second series of three putts represents significantly greater average error per putt than does the first series, though both result in the same amount of bias. To be interpreted most meaningfully, then, CE is typically coupled with VE indicating the range of error scores.

Variable Error (VE)

VE provides information concerning the variability of performance trials. A relatively low VE score indicates consistency of performance, with less performance consistency indicated as VE progressively increases. VE is a measurement of how consistently, or inconsistently, an individual performs over a series of performance trials. It is important to recognize that VE is a measurement of variability, rather than accuracy. An individual could produce the same very large error on every performance attempt, and have a VE score of 0 because trial-to-trial performance is consistent (even though highly inaccurate). VE does not depend upon how closely an individual comes to achieving a performance goal, but indicates the spread or dispersion of performance trials about the individual's own average performance (i.e., CE score). The formula for VE is shown here:

$$VE = \sqrt{[\Sigma(X - C)^2/k] - CE^2}$$

Continuing with our same example yields the following calculations:

$$VE = \sqrt{[(-8)^2 + (-4)^2 + (3)^2 + (7)^2 + (12)^2/5] - (2.0)^2}$$

$$= \sqrt{[(64 + 16 + 9 + 49 + 144)/5] - 4}$$

$$= \sqrt{(282/5) - 4}$$

$$= \sqrt{56.4 - 4}$$

$$= \sqrt{52.4}$$

$$= 7.2$$

A VE of 7.2 means that approximately 68 percent of an individual's performance scores varied 7.2 units of measurement from the individual's CE score (the 68% figure is related to the standard deviation of scores in a normally distributed data array, which need not be of concern here). What is important is that a high VE score indicates inconsistency of performance, and a low VE score indicates consistent performance in a series of performance trials. The exact interpretation of what constitutes high and low consistency will depend upon the relation of the units being measured to the task requirements and accuracy criteria established in any given situation. In our putting example, a VE of 7.2 is interpreted as meaning that a majority of the performer's putting attempts varied by an average of 7.2 feet.

Using AE, CE, and VE Scores

As we have seen, AE provides a general indication of accuracy for a series of performance measurements and can be valuable as a single general index of accuracy that is easily and quickly calculated. AE masks two important features of any array of scores, however, these being the bias and consistency associated with the scores. For this reason it is important to use both CE and VE scores when evaluating any set of performance data (and, in fact, these are often the only two scores that are reported). VE indicates the relative consistency or inconsistency of performance trials, while CE provides a measurement of bias or general direction of error without reference to the variability of performance scores. The differences in the information provided by CE and VE error scores can better be seen in the figure below for the sample data we have been discussing. The figure illustrates a fairly even dispersion of the five performance scores, but also makes clear that there is a slight tendency for the scores to represent long rather than short putts (i.e., there are three "long" scores compared to two "short" scores, and the longest of these is a full 4 feet further from the hole than is the shortest error score). The VE represents the amount of consistency, or sameness, of the individual scores. Observing the dispersion of the five putts about the CE score in the figure, they are fairly evenly spread out and range from 8 feet short to 12 feet long, indicating less consistency in achieving the performance goal than the CE score of 2 feet might suggest.

This illustration highlights the problem with using a single error measurement. The performance scores in our example tend toward a perfect putting score of 0. When CE is calculated, the relatively large scores (e.g., −8 and 12 feet) partially cancel each other out, so that the resulting CE score is much closer to zero (i.e., 2) than is the actual case when considering the spread of scores for all putts. The CE score by itself, then, is misleading. It is still extremely useful in telling us about performance bias and the tendency of scores toward a particular value, but without the balancing measure of VE indicating how consistent or inconsistent the individual scores are relative to the performance criterion, we could be easily led to drawing false conclusions concerning the meaning of these performance data.

Preparing Laboratory Reports

Laboratory research has been the main vehicle for the advancement of knowledge in motor learning and motor control. Conducting laboratory research and preparing laboratory reports is an important part of the learning experience for students enrolled in introductory motor learning and control courses. The preparation of laboratory reports has several purposes and advantages. First, it requires the processing and analysis of new ideas and information that help to reinforce material presented in class lectures and readings, often leading to a deeper and richer understanding of course concepts. Second, it helps illuminate the methods by which ideas are tested, practices evaluated and either supported or discarded, and new theories developed. Third, laboratory research promotes an appreciation for the role that the scientific method plays in advancing our understanding of how people acquire, control, and rehabilitate motor skills. The completion of laboratory research and preparation of a comprehensive report of such research, then, is one of the most important learning experiences in promoting critical thinking abilities concerning the practice of motor skills.

A laboratory report is similar in many ways to an essay you might write for a non-science class. It adheres to all of the standard rules of grammar and of sentence and paragraph structure. The same rules for good composition followed in essay writing also apply to scientific writing. It is, in fact, especially important that ideas be expressed clearly and unambiguously in scientific writing. The clarity of written laboratory reports corresponds directly to the clarity of the findings, interpretations, and conclusions reached in scientific reports. The major differences between the typical essay and the laboratory report are that information in laboratory reports is presented more concisely and with greater precision; objectivity is emphasized and subjective interpretation scrupulously avoided; and laboratory reports are organized in a particular format.

Sections of the Laboratory Report

Reports of laboratory research follow a fairly fixed structure of well-agreed-upon sections. This structure is designed to emphasize accuracy and objectivity in reporting, as well as to standardize the reporting of scientific findings. Because of this standard format for scientific reporting, readers can quickly and easily assess only those parts of a report that may be of interest to them. Readers may, for example, be interested only in the methods used for conducting a research investigation and may only decide whether to read additional sections depending upon the methods that were employed for the study.

This appendix discusses the common sections of a laboratory report, which are listed below:

Introduction

Methods

Results

Discussion

This basic format, sometimes labeled "IMRAD" (Introduction, Methods, Results, And Discussion), is standard in all scientific disciplines, although it may be found in slightly different shades depending on the discipline and nature of the particular research inquiry. Some reports may include an abstract of the study, or a separate section for hypotheses or methods of statistical analysis, or may label the methods section as Experimental Design or Procedures, or the discussion section as Conclusions. Regardless of the specific disciplinary or reporting particulars, the same components are found in all scientific reporting. In this appendix, we will focus on the basic elements of all laboratory reports, leaving more advanced considerations for discussion as warranted within students' specific courses. We will also leave out of our presentation methods of statistical analysis; information on various methods of statistical analysis is readily available from many sources, should it be included as part of the laboratory experience for a particular course.

Introduction

The introduction identifies the general aims and purpose of the study. It informs the reader of the need for the study and the specific objectives of the research. It also places the study in a theoretical context and enables the reader to understand and appreciate the purpose of the research. The introduction should answer three questions:

1. *Why was the study conducted?* What is the need for the study? What problem exists that the research is designed to address? How will the

results of the study potentially be beneficial and help to address the problem identified?

2. *What knowledge already exists about the particular subject?* This question entails a review of the literature specifically related to the study. What has previous research reported regarding the subject? What gaps in knowledge exist? What do we know, and what is unknown or contended? If you think of scientific research as a conversation, then a single research report continues the conversation of previous researchers. It is your way of advancing the ongoing conversation concerning the specific subject of your study. Science is built through a series of small exchanges among scientists working in a particular area of specialization. A research report is a way of joining that chorus. Your review of literature need not be exhaustive or complete, but should show how your research builds upon previous research. Assume that the reader has a broad knowledge of the field, but not of the specifics related to your research question. One purpose of the introduction is to demonstrate the logical continuity between previous research and your study.

3. *What is the specific purpose of your research?* Your research should be designed to answer one specific question. Beginning researchers typically make the mistake of attempting to answer too many questions or to answer a single question too broadly, rather than focusing on a more delimited question that can be investigated and answered precisely and well. What is the specific question that you hope to answer through your laboratory investigation? This question is often posed as a separate section within the laboratory or scientific report called "The Purpose of the Study."

Based upon the review of previous literature, you may be able to make an educated guess concerning what answer you might derive relative to the purpose of the study. Such an educated guess, in scientific terms, is a hypothesis. It is really the hypothesis that is tested in experimental research, which states the expected relationship between two variables (i.e., what is the relationship between practice time and skill level, or between the frequency of feedback one receives and learning?). The hypothesis is a declarative sentence stating the expected relationship between two variables that are measured in the research study, and may be included as a separate section within the introduction labeled "Hypothesis" (or "Hypotheses" if there are more than one).

It should be noted that hypotheses are evaluated through statistical analyses. In laboratory reports completed within a class setting, the purpose of the study and hypothesis are often collapsed into a single research question, which may also be included as a section within the introduction. Data from the research are then used to evaluate and draw conclusions concerning this research question, though without the greater certainty possible through statistical analysis (this is allowed for educational purposes but would not be acceptable for broader scientific dissemination such as journal articles or scientific meetings).

Methods

The methods section, as the name implies, tells the reader how the research was conducted. The objective of this section is to supply sufficient detail so that another researcher could use some or all of the methods in another study or judge the scientific merits of your approach. The methods used in the study should be described clearly and extensively enough so that your research investigation could be duplicated and the same results obtained, but should not be so detailed as to overwhelm the reader. The methods section includes descriptions of the sample, task, and procedures for conducting the study and gathering data. Each of these is a separate subsection within the methods section, and they may each be additionally divided into further subsections if needed.

Sample. Describe the subjects used in the study with sufficient detail that the population represented is clear. A description of how the sample was formed (especially if different groups are formed) is necessary. When possible, groups should be formed through random methods of assignment, though this is not always possible when a sample is drawn from an intact laboratory class. In such cases, the researcher must take special care to describe subjects and groups so that readers can assess the potential for any sampling bias.

Task. This section includes a description of the task or tasks that subjects performed. The nature of the task, equipment used, and the performance criteria or goal of the task are described.

Procedures. In this section the design of the study, including the arrangement of acquisition trials and retention and transfer tests used, is described. Any instructions given to subjects are also described. It is here also that the methods for collecting data are delineated. As previously stated, the description should be detailed enough for the reader to replicate the essential elements of the study.

Results

The purpose of this section is to present and illustrate the findings of the study. This section is an objective report of results and does not include any interpretation or conclusions (which come in the following section).

If necessary, start this section with a description of any complications arising during the investigation, such as subject misinterpretation or violations of instructions; missing data or equipment, or recording problems; or data anomalies such as outliers.

The data are presented in summary form such as averages. Do not report results for individuals within groups, or complete results for every trial on which data were collected. If hypotheses have been tested, report on their acceptance or rejection based upon your results.

Your data may be organized into tables or graphs for summary purposes, but data shown in a table should not be duplicated in another form such as a graph or figure. All tables and graphs should have descriptive titles and should include a legend explaining any symbols or abbreviations. Tables and graphs should be numbered and should be referred to by number in the text. Tables and graphs should also be self-explanatory; that is, the reader should be able to understand them without needing to refer to the text.

The results section should focus on general trends and on the differences between or among groups, and not upon minor details within the data. The section should, though, provide sufficient details to support the interpretation and conclusions reached, which are reported in the discussion section.

Discussion

The purpose of this section is to provide an interpretation of your results and to draw conclusions that seem warranted based upon those results. Begin the section with a brief, concise summary of the results attained in the study. From this, explain how the results should be interpreted and how they answer your research question or hypothesis. The objective is to use evidence from your results, as well as generally accepted knowledge if appropriate, to support the conclusions you reach regarding your findings. When connections are obvious, relate your findings to the literature in the field that was discussed in the introductory section of the report, or to broader theoretical issues if applicable. The significance or importance of your findings, including their relevance to applied practice, should be clearly described.

Title and References Cited

Besides the four major sections described above, two other important elements are included in the laboratory report: the title of the report and a section for references of works cited.

The title of your research report should be short (generally 15 or fewer words) and descriptive, clearly indicating what the study is about. If in doubt, try specifying the relationship investigated in the study. What did you manipulate or change in the study, and what did you expect to observe as a result? If you can clearly identify a cause (what you changed, called the "independent variable") and effect (what you observed or were expecting to observe called the "dependent variable"), then these should both be part of the title. For example: "The Use of Whole and Part Methods of Practice [the cause] and the Acquisition of a Novel Discrete Motor Task [the effect]." That is, you manipulated the practice conditions (whole or part practice) to investigate the effect on the acquisition of a specific kind of task.

Finally, all references mentioned in the report should be listed in the reference section of the report. Your class instructor may require a specific referencing style, such as APA, for purposes of citation.

Guidelines for Preparing the Laboratory Report

Specific course requirements for the submission of laboratory reports will always supercede instructions presented in these general guidelines:

- Use 12-point standard font such as Times, Times New Roman, CG Times, Courier, Bookman, Helvetica, or Lucida Sans.
- Text is double-spaced on 8½-inch by 11-inch white paper with 1-inch margins all around.

- All pages are single-sided.
- Number all pages consecutively starting with the title page. A header, which is a shortened three- to four-word version of the paper's title, and the page number appear in the upper right-hand corner of pages.
- Tables, graphs, and figures must be shown entirely on a single page; do not break or split these between pages.
- Tables, graphs, and figures requiring more than one-half of a page should be shown on a separate page following their first textual mention.
- Present your points in logical order and stay focused on the research question.
- Scientific writing is parsimonious; make your points clearly and concisely, avoiding superfluous and flowery wording.
- Use the present tense when reporting well-established and accepted facts: "Average reaction time for adult males is 210 ms."
- Use the past tense to describe information or results specific to the study: "The average reaction time of subjects was 210 ms." Remember that your research and the results that you obtained occurred in the past when you are writing your report.
- Refer to information reported by other authors in the past tense.
- Avoid using the first person (I or we) in writing. Scientific writing is objective, so keep your writing impersonal and write in the third person using the passive voice. The passive voice is used in scientific reporting to convey that the researcher was impartial and objective in carrying out and interpreting the results of the research. Instead of saying "We told subjects to keep their eyes on the target," say "Subjects were instructed to watch the target."
- When drawing conclusions, interpreting results, or making recommendations, be careful to distinguish data generated by your study from information gathered from other sources.
- Avoid offering personal opinion; your interpretations must be based on fact and supported by the results of your research.

Example of Laboratory Report Pages

On the following pages are displayed several examples of laboratory report pages. These are intended to illustrate features presented in this appendix.

CONSTANT AND VARIED PRACTICE   1

> Page numbers begin on the title page

Constant and Varied Practice in the Acquisition
of an Arm-Positioning Task

John C. Student
Normal University

> Complete title repeated on the first page of the report

CONSTANT AND VARIED PRACTICE   2

Constant and Varied Practice in the Acquisition
of an Arm-Positioning Task

Traditionally, practice for discrete skills performed in closed environments is completed using constant practice. Constant practice consists in the repetitive sequencing of multiple practice attempts in exactly the same way and under the same conditions. Practice trials are typically performed in conditions as closely to those of the anticipated performance as possible. Motor skills such as the free throw in basketball, drive in golf, serve in tennis, or performance of a specific dance routine do not change, at least significantly, from one time they are performed to the next. The goal of practice, then, is to learn to perform such skills in a specific and constant way.

> 1" margins on all sides

Short title included on every page

Methods

Sample

Subjects in the study included 16 male (n=8) and female (n=8) students enrolled in an undergraduate motor learning course at a four-year university. None of the subjects had previous experience with the task used in the experimental procedures. Participation in the laboratory exercise was part of the regularly assigned class activities and was required for

Task

The task

a kinesthesiometer (

Instrument Company

to swivel about its ba

their forearm with th

post between the sub

extraneous movemen

extension of the fore

fied angle measured

the subject's arm is p

ment is measured as

After a 10-minute retention interval, all subjects in both groups A and B performed a five-trial retention test of 40 degrees. No feedback was provided on these retention trials. One minute after completion of the retention test, all subjects performed a transfer test of five trials attempting a forearm movement of 60 degrees. Again, no feedback was provided for the transfer trials. In summary, the experimental conditions are shown below in Table 1.

Table 1

Experimental Design

	Practice Group	
	Group A	Group B
Testing Phase	Constant Practice	Varied Practice
Acquisition	3 blocks of 15 trials,	3 blocks of 15 trials, alternating in series of 30, 40, and 50 degrees
		40 degrees
Retention	5 trials, 40 degrees	5 trials, 40 degrees
Transfer	5 trials, 60 degrees	5 trials, 60 degrees

Tables, figures, or graphs shown immediately after paragraph in which first mentioned

CONSTANT AND VARIED PRACTICE   8

Discussion

The purpose of this study was to investigate the benefits of varied practice in learning a discrete motor skill performed in a closed environment. For the purposes of this study, an arm-positioning task using a kinesthesiometer was used. Subjects practiced under either a constant or a varied practice schedule to learn a target skill of a 40-degree movement on the kinesthesiometer. After 45 acquisition trials performed under their group's practice condition, all subjects performed a five-trial retention test of the criterion 40-degree movement goal, and a five-trial transfer test of 60 degrees.

Results of the study showed that the group learning under a constant practice schedule performed better during acquisition than did the varied practic

group was 5.1 compa

tionally, the constant

rion target of 40 degr

(CE = 9.9), and also

scores (VE = 11.0 fo

for the varied practic

proved an advantage.

> Double-spacing throughout paper

> Only works cited in text included in references

CONSTANT AND VARIED PRACTICE   11

References

Davids, K, Button, C, and Bennett, S. (2008). *Dynamics of skill acquisition: A constraints-led approach.* Champaign, IL: Human Kinetics.

Landin, D, Hebert, EP, and Fairweather, M. (1993). "The effects of variable practice on the performance of a basketball skill." *Research Quarterly for Exercise and Sport.* 64, 232–237.

Lee. TD, Chamberlin, CJ, and Hodges, NJ. (2001). Practice. In RN Singer, HA Hausenbles, and CM Janelle (eds.). Handbook of sport psychology, pp. 115–143, New York: Wiley.

Schmidt, RA. (1975). "A schema theory of discrete motor skill learning." *Psychological Review*, 82. 225–260.

Shea, CH, and Kihl, RM. (1990). "Specificity and variability of practice." *Research Quarterly for Exercise and Sport*, 61, 169–177.

Utley, A, and Astill, S. (2008). *BIOS instant notes: Motor control, learning and development.* New York: Taylor and Francis.

10-year rule A rule derived from observation across several skill domains that it generally requires a minimum of 10 years of deliberate practice to attain expertise in a skill.

ability A genetically endowed trait underlying the performance of motor skills.

absolute frequency of feedback The total number of practice attempts for which KR is provided during a specific practice period.

accumulated feedback Augmented feedback provided for a series of motor responses at the completion of the responses in the series.

acetylcholine A neurotransmitter released by motor neurons.

acquisition Those practice experiences of a skill designed to influence the learning of the skill.

action A term used synonymously with motor skill.

action code Information encoded within the motor system related to the execution of some action.

action effect hypothesis The concept that actions are best planned and controlled in relation to the desired effect of the action.

action plan reconstruction hypothesis One explanation of the contextual interference effect holding that when people sequentially perform different skills during random practice, they continuously forget and must reconstruct the action plan for each skill each time that it is practiced, enhancing learning by leading to the development of a stronger memory representation.

action potential A temporary electrical signal that propagates along the axon of a neuron and at the presynaptic terminal triggers the release of a neurotransmitter to target neurons.

activation The persistence and energy level of behavior indicating motivation.

advanced stage of learning The intermediate stage of learning in Vereijken's dynamical systems model of the stages of learning.

afferent pathway The path of a neural signal traveling toward the CNS (also referred to as the *ascending pathway*).

affordance The properties of an object or of the environment that offer opportunities for action.

all-around athlete Description of an individual who appears to excel at most motor activities he or she attempts.

all-or-none law Law stating that all of the muscle fibers of a motor unit will contract maximally when the motor neuron propagates sufficient stimulation, or none of the muscle fibers will contract in the absence of a sufficient action potential.

alpha motor neuron A motor neuron that innervates skeletal muscle (also called a *motoneuron*).

ambient visual system Nonconscious visual system specialized for movement control.

anxiety Feelings of threat or apprehension in a given situation, accompanied by an increasing state of arousal.

arousal General physiological and psychological activation of an individual; varies from a state of sleep to extreme excitement.

ART measures An acronym for the acquisition, retention, and transfer measurements used in assessing learning in an experiment.

associative stage of learning The intermediate stage of learning in Fitts and Posner's three-stage model of learning.

asymptote Theoretical upper limit to learning that is progressively approached with practice but that is never reached.

attention The direction of conscious mental resources toward specific sensory stimuli.

attentional cueing A practice technique where an instructor directs a learner's attention to a specific aspect or component of a skill performed in the whole.

attentional focus The allocation of attentional resources along dimensions of width of focus (broad to narrow) and direction of focus (external or internal).

attractor A preferred pattern of stability toward which a system tends.

augmented feedback Information about the performance of a skill that is supplied by a source external to the performer and that supplements or adds to the performer's sensory feedback.

automaticity The capacity of individuals to access and operate on procedural memory without the need for conscious attentional resources when executing well-learned skills.

autonomous stage of learning The third and final stage of learning in Fitts and Posner's three-stage model of learning.

average feedback Augmented feedback provided at the completion of a series of practice attempts regarding the average performance of the attempts (often as a numerical average).

axon A long fiber extending from the cell body of a neuron and ending in presynaptic terminals that send signals to other neurons.

bandwidth feedback Augmented feedback that is provided only when performance error falls outside of a predetermined criterion of correctness.

basal ganglia A group of four brain structures lying within the central region of the brain that help regulate motor activity.

Bliss-Boder hypothesis The idea that paying too much attention to one's movement patterns can disrupt efficient performance.

blocked practice A practice schedule in which the same skill is rehearsed in repetitive fashion.

bottleneck theories The perspective that attention is limited to the processing of only one or two chunks of information at a time, which must be completed before additional sensory information can be processed.

brain The organ that mediates all mental functions and all behaviors.

brain stem Part of the brain just above the spinal column housing the medulla, pons, and reticular formation.

cell body (soma) The metabolic center of a neuron containing the nucleus and other organelles.

central nervous system All of the nerve cells within or originating within the brain or spine.

central-resource theories The perspective that attention consists of a limited resources pool from which one must decide how much attention to allocate among competing needs.

cerebellum One of the major parts of the brain involved in motor control; involved in motor coordination, muscle tone, balance, and the learning of motor skills.

cerebral cortex Outer layer of the cerebrum composed of gray matter, and the major site of higher brain functions such as abstraction, reasoning, decision making, and voluntary motor control.

cerebrum Composed of two large hemispheres comprising the majority of the brain, it functions as the center for learning, emotional control, memory, and voluntary movement.

challenge point model A conceptual model relating the cognitive challenges inherent in practicing a skill to the learning potential available.

chunk A singularly coherent and meaningful unit of information within short-term memory.

chunking The process of grouping skill elements into meaningful units for purposes of instruction.

clasp-knife reflex A protective reflex initiated by Golgi tendon organs, resulting in the relaxation of a muscle stretched beyond a familiar load.

closed control system A system in which the mechanisms of control are internal and closed to influences outside of the system itself.

closed motor skill A skill in which action occurs in a stable and predictable environment.

closed-loop control A system of control in which feedback is compared to a reference of correctness during the course of action and errors corrected when necessary.

cognitive effort The amount of mental work involved in the retrieval, decision making, and planning leading to the execution of a skill.

cognitive skill A skill for which success is primarily determined by an individual's knowledge and cognitive capabilities.

cognitive stage of learning The initial stage of learning in Fitts and Posner's three-stage model of learning.

common coding approach The proposition that sensory and motor codes share a common domain and are capable of direct communication.

complexity A characteristic of systems that are comprised of diverse elements that are connected and interdependent, and capable of adaptation.

concurrent feedback Augmented feedback delivered during the execution of the motor skill for which it is provided.

cones Visual receptors specialized for discerning detail and color in objects and subserving focal vision.

consolidation The process by which a new memory trace is gradually transferred to long-term memory.

constant practice A practice schedule in which the same skill is rehearsed in the same way, without variation, in a series of practice trials.

constraint Boundaries that limit the possible values or patterns that a system can assume that are imposed by the organism, physical environment, and task itself.

contextual interference The degree of interference created by the ordering of skills within a practice session; blocked practice results in low contextual interference, whereas random practice results in high amounts of contextual interference.

continuous motor skill A motor skill in which the beginning and ending of action are arbitrary.

convergence center A theory that memories are stored in parts across the brain and only brought together through retrieval processes near the sites where they were initially perceived.

corpus callosum The thick band of neurons connecting the two cerebral hemispheres and acting as a communications bridge between them.

correlation The degree of association between two things, or the percentage of component parts the two things have in common; the strength of a correlation is mathematically expressed as a number ranging from -1.00 to $+1.00$.

cutaneous receptors Receptors located in the dermis and epidermis throughout the body and specialized to monitor one of several types of sensory stimulation, including pressure, heat, cold, pain, and chemical stimuli.

decision-making stage The second stage of information processing in which decisions are made concerning what actions, if any, should be carried out.

declarative memory A memory system specialized for holding and operating on information concerning objective facts and events.

degrees of freedom The number of dimensions in which a system can independently vary.

degrees of freedom problem How the many degrees of freedom available in the human motor system are controlled to produce a particular movement.

deliberate practice Practice that is effortful, highly structured and organized, and directed toward extrinsic goals and rewards.

dendrites Branching fibers extending from the cell body of neurons that receive signals from other neurons.

depolarization A change in the membrane potential of a cell, reducing its negativity and making it more excitable and likely to generate an action potential.

descriptive feedback Knowledge of performance describing errors a learner makes, but not the causes of the errors or suggested corrections.

diencephalon The part of the cerebrum containing the hypothalamus and thalamus.

directionality The specific behaviors indicating a person's level of motivation.

discovery learning Practice based upon the theory that learners learn best when they discover through exploratory methods the most effective ways of accomplishing motor skills.

discrete motor skill A motor skill in which the beginning and ending points are clearly defined.

distinct feedback Augmented feedback provided for a single motor response.

distributed practice A practice schedule in which the amount of time in rest is relatively longer than the amount of time in actual practice.

distribution of practice The balancing of periods of rest and work within a practice schedule.

dynamical system Any system that is in motion or exhibits change over time.

dynamical systems theory A theory of motor control and learning having as a major assumption that the human motor system interacts with the larger environment surrounding it and reacts to organize movement patterns establishing internal system stability.

ecological psychology A branch of psychology emphasizing the role of the environment in human behavior, especially the interface between perception and action.

efferent pathway The path of a neural signal traveling away from the CNS (also referred to as the descending pathway).

elaboration hypothesis One explanation of the contextual interference effect holding that random practice promotes a better appreciation of the distinctive features among skills, resulting in stronger memories and better learning.

emergence The spontaneous creation of a new state or pattern resulting from the self-organization of the elements of a complex system.

empowerment The degree to which a person feels in control of his or her own learning.

encoding condition The context in which a skill is practiced and learned.

encoding specificity principle The principle that skills executed in situations similar to those in which they are learned will be better remembered and performed.

encoding The processes involved in transferring sensory information into various memory systems in such a way that it can be retained and acted upon.

environmental constraint Features of the physical environment such as gravity, temperature, and light that act to constrain movement patterns; also includes social features such as cultural norms that constrain movement behavior.

episodic memory A memory system specialized for holding and operating on information of a personal nature and specifying the time and place that events occurred.

erroneous feedback Augmented feedback provided in an intentionally incorrect and misleading fashion.

error-correction capability The capacity of individuals to detect and correct their own errors as a result of sensory sources of feedback.

event code Sensory information that has been encoded and brought to perception; information about a person's environment.

excitation The depolarization of a cell, increasing the likelihood that an action potential will be propagated.

expert model A skilled model who demonstrates a skill correctly.

expert stage of learning The third and final stage of learning in Vereijken's dynamical systems model of the stages of learning.

expert-induced amnesia A term used to describe the tendency for highly skilled performers to exclude episodic monitoring during the execution of skills.

expertise Refers to a stage of learning indicating the attainment of superior levels of performance and knowledge related to a specific skill, and attained only by those experts at the very highest levels of achievement.

explicit memory Memory that is open to intentional retrieval (synonymous with declarative memory).

exploiting the degrees of freedom Using passive and reactive forces inherent in bodily systems and in the environment to assist in producing bodily movements.

external focus of attention Attention directed toward the effects of a motor response within the environment.

exteroception Perception of information in the environment external to the body.

exteroceptive feedback Sensory feedback concerning features of the environment in which a skill is performed.

extrafusal muscle fiber Skeletal muscle attached to bones and capable of generating significant contractile forces; responsible for purposeful movements and under voluntary control.

faded feedback An augmented feedback schedule in which feedback is provided most frequently early in practice and then gradually reduced in frequency as practice continues.

fallacy of observed correlation The tendency to draw conclusions based only upon relationships that can be readily observed.

fast-twitch muscle fibers Muscle fibers capable of producing quick, high contractile force responses.

feedback All sources of information available to a performer regarding the consequences of a practice attempt, including both sensory information and information provided through external sources.

feedforward Sensory information related to the production of an action prior to the initiation of the action.

fine motor skill A motor skill in which the precision of movement is the primary requisite for performance success.

Fitts's law Law expressing the mathematical relationship between speed of movement and accuracy for discrete aiming tasks.

Fleishman's taxonomy of motor abilities A widely used classification of motor abilities identifying 21 separate abilities.

focal visual system Conscious visual system specialized for object identification.

forgetting The loss of, or failure to retrieve, information from memory.

fovea Central area of the retina comprised entirely of cones and responsible for both focal and color vision.

fractionization A part method of practice involving the isolated practice of various skill components that would normally be performed simultaneously.

freeing the degrees of freedom Releasing frozen limbs and joints to move freely.

freezing the degrees of freedom Limiting the movement of limbs and joints.

gamma motor neuron A motor neuron that innervates the fibers of a muscle spindle.

general cognitive abilities A generalized ability broadly encompassing such cognitive traits as reasoning, problem solving, and verbal abilities.

generalized motor abilities hypothesis (GMA) The notion that motor abilities are positively correlated, and that a person's percentile rank in one motor ability is fairly similar to his or her comparative ranking in all other motor abilities.

generalized motor program (GMP) The concept of a motor program as proposed by schema theory; an abstract representation of rules generalized to control an entire class of actions.

glia Supportive cells of the central nervous system.

global motor ability The notion that a single global factor is responsible for the relative strength of all motor abilities.

goal setting The process of establishing targets for skill improvement as a result of practice.

Golgi tendon organ Mechanoreceptor located in the muscle-tendon junction of all skeletal muscles providing information about tension.

gross motor skill A motor skill in which the contributions of muscular force are the primary requisite for performance success.

guidance hypothesis The notion that high relative frequencies of augmented feedback can lead to a learner's overreliance on the guidance properties of feedback to the detriment of optimal learning outcomes.

hippocampus Part of the limbic system especially responsible for the formation of long-term memories.

homunculus A bodily representation indicating size of body regions as proportional to area devoted to them by either the somatosensory cortex or motor cortex.

hypothalamus The brain structure just below the thalamus that is responsible for regulating body temperature and energy use.

identical elements theory The theory that transfer is positively related to the number of elements that two skills share in common.

implicit memory Retrieval of information from long-term memory through performance rather than conscious recall; nondeclarative memory.

incentive motivation The idea that people have greater incentive to behave situationally in ways that have previously been rewarded.

information processing A model of cognitive processes occurring in the central nervous system underlying the production of motor skills; three stages are identified, including the perceptual, decision-making, and programming stages.

interference A theory of forgetting in which memories encoded into long-term storage may fail to be retrieved into short-term memory because other memories stored in the long-term system block retrieval processes.

intermittent reinforcement Reinforcement of a response after some but not all instances in which a contingency for reinforcement is present; often more powerful in shaping behavior than reinforcement provided in every contingent situation.

internal focus of attention Attention directed toward the movement patterns used in generating a motor response.

interneuron One of three major types of neurons; they connect and convey signals between sensory and motor neurons.

interresponse interval The total time between the completion of a practice attempt for which KR is provided and the beginning of the next practice attempt.

interskill practice The scheduling of different skills within a practice session or portion of practice session.

intrafusal muscle fiber Muscle fiber making up part of the muscle spindle, the deformation of which initiates afferent signal stimulation.

intraskill practice The scheduling of a single skill or of variations of a single skill within a practice session or portion of practice session.

intuitive feedback The intentional fading of augmented feedback to a learner based on an instructor's perception of the learner's needs and capabilities.

invariant features The components of a movement that remain the same, or constant, regardless of the timing, force, muscles used, or other features of a movement. Three invariant features are recognized in schema theory, including muscle sequencing, relative timing, and relative force.

inverted-U theory A psychological theory that increases in the state of a person's arousal are beneficial to performance up until a point when they then begin to detract from performance.

joint receptor Mechanoreceptor located in the capsules of all synovial joints and which provide information on joint angle.

kinesthesis Sense of position and movement of the body and limbs and of external forces acting on the body.

kinesthetic system The system composed of muscle spindles, Golgi tendon organs, joint receptors, and the vestibular apparatus, which together provide the sense of kinesthesis.

knowledge of performance (KP) Augmented feedback concerning the causes of a movement outcome; typically provided in terms of bodily mechanics.

knowledge of results (KR) Augmented feedback concerning the results or outcome of a movement response.

KR-delay interval The period of time between the completion of a practice attempt and the presentation of augmented feedback.

law of effect Law first formulated by Thorndike stating that an organism will tend to repeat behaviors resulting in desirable consequences and avoid behaviors resulting in undesirable consequences.

law of practice Improvement in performance continues as long as practice continues, but the rate at which it occurs gradually and predictably diminishes over time or number of practice trials; it can be expressed mathematically as a power function.

learner-requested feedback A technique for providing feedback only when a learner requests it.

learning A relatively stable change in performance resulting from practice or experience.

learning model A person learning a skill who demonstrates both correct and incorrect aspects of performance relative to the model's stage of learning.

learning-performance distinction Refers to the well-established finding that performance measures during acquisition may mask the true degree of learning that has occurred.

limbic system Composed of a number of structures deep within the cerebrum, this system plays a critical role in motivation, emotions, value judgments, and the control of movements.

limited attentional capacity The notion that individuals can only attend a limited amount of information at any one point in time, beyond which processing capabilities begin to be compromised.

linear performance curve A performance curve in which equal amounts of time or number of trials during practice correspond to equal increases in performance measures.

location-suppression hypothesis The notion that fixation of one's visual gaze on a specific location before and during the execution of a skill enhances performance by stabilizing processing activities.

long-term memory A memory system that permanently stores all information encoded from short-term memory; responsible for learning.

magic number 7+/–2 The number of chucks, or bits, of information that short-term memory is capable of holding and operating on at any one time.

maladaptive short-term corrections Inappropriate corrections in the production of a motor skill resulting when relatively minor movement errors are corrected through the provision of augmented feedback.

massed practice A practice schedule in which the amount of work or actual practice is relatively longer than the amount of time spent in rest.

mastery level A predetermined performance level established as the goal of practice.

medulla Part of the brain stem responsible for regulation of respiration, blood pressure, and heart rate.

memory The processes enabling humans to retain information over time.

memory trace A network of neuronal brain cells encoded to store a specific memory.

mirror neurons Neurons that become activated when an animal or person is performing a particular action or watching another perform the same action.

monotonic benefits assumption The notion that learning occurs at the same rate as long as practice continues, though its manifestation in performance decreases at a predictable rate.

motivation An internal state or condition directing and energizing behavior.

motivational climate The curricular and instructional factors influencing performers' motivation in structured performance environments.

motor ability A trait that specifically supports the performance of motor skills.

motor consistency The capacity to achieve the goals of motor skills consistently; the capacity of the human motor system to learn.

motor control The discipline concerned with the underlying mechanisms responsible for human movement and stability.

motor cortex Area of the cerebral cortex where afferent signals directly controlling each of the body's skeletal muscles originate.

motor educability The concept that a single factor underlies all motor skills and that an individual possesses the same performance potential in all skills.

motor equivalence The capacity to produce many different movement patterns to accomplish the same action goal.

motor learning The discipline concerned with the processes underlying the acquisition and performance of motor skills.

motor modifiability The capacity to alter a movement pattern to achieve a new action goal.

motor neuron One of three major types of neurons; they form synapses with muscle cells conveying information from the CNS and converting it into movement.

motor program A procedural memory comprised of the rules commanding muscular activity for producing specific skills.

motor skill A learned, goal-directed activity accomplished primarily through muscular contributions to action.

motor unit An alpha motor neuron and all of the muscle fibers that it innervates.

motor unit pool All of the motor units controlling a specific muscle.

motor variability No two movement patterns, even of the same skill, are ever produced in exactly the same way.

movement A change in the position of limbs or body segments; the behavioral components used to assemble motor skills.

movement class All of the possible movements controlled by a single generalized motor program, typically sharing common coordination patterns.

muscle spindle A proprioceptor found in all skeletal muscles that supplies information concerning stretch and changes in the length of muscle.

near transfer Positive transfer between similar skills.

negative correlation A correlation between two things such that increases in the value of the first are accompanied by decreases in the value of the second.

negative reinforcement Occurs when a response is followed by the removal of undesirable consequences previously associated with the response and increases the likelihood that the response will be repeated in similar situations in the future.

negative transfer When learning one skill negatively influences the learning of another skill or of the same skill in a new context.

negatively accelerating performance curve A performance curve exhibiting diminished improvements in performance measures as a function of time or trials of practice.

neuron The basic cell for communication within the central nervous system.

neurotransmitter A chemical substance that is released from one neuron and binds with receptors in another neuron to either convey or inhibit transmission of a signal.

nonverbal feedback Augmented feedback that is not capable of being verbalized because its content is too complex or abstract and which therefore must be presented in another fashion.

normal distribution The tendency for individuals within a population to cluster about the average value on any given measurement of trait strength, and for progressively fewer individuals to exhibit measurements of either high or low trait strength as distance increases from the norm.

novelty problem A deficiency of simple motor program theory based on the notion that individuals should be unable to effectively produce unpracticed variations of learned movements because they have not developed specific motor programs for them.

novice stage of learning The initial stage of learning in Vereijken's dynamical systems model of the stages of learning.

observational learning The learning that occurs as a result of observing another perform a skill.

open control system A system that interacts with the environment outside of itself and responds to external influences in its mechanisms of control.

open motor skill A skill for which the object acted upon or the context in which action occurs varies from one performance to the next.

open-loop control A system of control in which movement commands are prestructured and executed without corrective intervention from feedback.

optic flow The patterning of light rays moving across the retina that supplies information concerning the speed and direction of the movement of objects in the environment.

organismic constraint Characteristics of an individual that act as constraints on movement, including structural characteristics such as height, weight, and body shape, as well as functional characteristics such as intelligence, motivation, and psychological states.

original learning The amount of practice required to attain a specified level of mastery.

outcome goals Targets for skill improvement focusing on the results of performance and often involving comparison to others.

overlearning The concept that practice of a newly acquired skill beyond the point of mastery benefits long-term retention of the skill.

parameters Features of a skill that must be added to the invariant features of a generalized motor program to meet the specific demands of a situation. Parameters include overall duration, overall force, and muscle selection.

part practice Any method of simplifying the performance of a skill, involving either the initial practice of component parts of the skill or the simplification of environmental features in which the skill is performed.

peer-referenced judgments Evaluation of skill performance in comparison to the performance of others.

percentile rank A ranking indicating a person's position relative to trait strength among the general population of people and being equal to the percentage of persons below him or her in strength of the trait.

perception The process by which sensations arising from within or outside of the body are brought to conscious awareness.

perceptual skill A skill for which the ability to discern and discriminate among sensory stimuli is of primary concern in successfully accomplishing the skill.

perceptual speed ability The ability to assess environmental stimuli and respond quickly.

perceptual stage The first stage of information processing in which sensory information is detected and identified.

perceptual-motor integration problem The intellectual problems arising when attempting to explain how perception is coupled with human movement to produce motor skills.

performance Qualitative or quantitative assessment of what can be observed during the execution of a skill.

performance curve A two-dimensional graph of the changes in performance measures over time as a result of practice.

performance goals Targets for skill improvements in comparison to a person's previous skill level.

performance variable A variable influencing performance measures during acquisition, but which has little or no influence on learning.

peripheral nervous system All of the nerve cells originating or contained entirely outside of the central nervous system.

phase shift In a dynamical system, the spontaneous transition from one organizational pattern to another as a result of self-organization.

play Activity that is spontaneous, intrinsically motivated, enjoyable and imaginative, and not pursued for any external rewards or goals.

polarization A change in the membrane potential of a cell increasing its negativity and making it less excitable and less likely to generate an action potential.

pons Portion of brain stem responsible for integrating sensory signals and routing them forward to higher brain centers.

positive correlation A correlation between two things such that increases in the value of the first are accompanied by increases in the value of the second.

positive reinforcement Occurs when a response is followed by a desired consequence and increases the likelihood that the response will be repeated in similar situations in the future.

positive transfer When learning one skill positively influences the learning of another skill or of the same skill in a new context.

positively accelerating performance curve A performance curve exhibiting increasing improvements in performance measures as a function of time or trials of practice.

post KR-delay interval The period of time between the presentation of augmented feedback and the beginning of the next practice attempt of the skill for which it was provided.

prescriptive feedback Knowledge of performance concerning both an error made by a performer and suggestion for correcting the error.

primacy-recency effect The phenomenon that information presented at the beginning and ending of a practice session is more readily learned, all other factors being equal, than is information presented in the middle of practice.

priming The brief introduction of new information prior to the time when it is actually practiced; increases the likelihood that the information will be learned when it is later practiced.

proactive inhibition The interference of older memories with the learning and retrieval of newer memories.

problem of perception–action coupling The limitations of science in explaining how perceptual sensory information is turned into motor actions.

problem of the homunculus A criticism of cognitive-based theories that the brain alone is incapable of controlling all aspects of an action.

procedural memory A memory system specialized for holding and operating on information pertaining to the execution of skilled behaviors and functioning at a nonconscious level.

process goals Targets for skill improvement that emphasize the quality of a movement.

programming stage The third stage of information processing in which the motor program is prepared and action initiated.

progressive part method A method of part practice in which the component parts of a skill are sequentially added to practice as each previous component is mastered.

proprioceptive feedback Sensory feedback concerning the visual, auditory, and tactile consequences of a practice attempt.

proprioceptors Sensory receptors located in the body that supply information about forces within muscles, joint and limb position, movement, and general body orientation.

psychological refractory period Delay in responding to the second of two stimuli occurring closely in time.

punishment Occurs when a response is followed by undesirable consequences and decreases the likelihood that the response will be repeated in similar situations in the future.

qualitative feedback Augmented feedback that supplies information about the direction of an error (e.g., too much, too little; too fast, too slow) without reference to the magnitude of the error.

quantitative feedback Augmented feedback that supplies information about both the direction and magnitude (in numerical terms) of an error; is considered more precise than qualitative feedback.

quiet eye The fixation of one's visual gaze prior to and during the execution of an action.

random practice A practice schedule in which different skills are rehearsed in an unpredictable trial-to-trial order.

rate modulation The frequency with which action potentials are propagated between a motor unit and its associated muscle fibers, affecting force produced by the muscle fibers.

reactive motor skill A commonly used term denoting an open motor skill.

recall condition The context in which a skill is performed as a result of practice.

refresher practice A form of overlearning in which continued practice of a skill is carried out beyond the attainment of the original performance goal in incrementally spaced practice intervals as a method of maintaining achieved performance levels.

regression toward the mean The intergenerational tendency for individuals, regardless of their parents' trait characteristics, to move toward the 50th percentile rank on specific motor abilities.

regulatory conditions Features of the performance environment that determine how a skill must be performed in order to be successful.

reinforcement Any change in an organism's surroundings that occurs regularly when the organism behaves in a certain way (i.e., the change is contingent on the response).

relative frequency of feedback The proportion of practice attempts in a series of attempts for which KR is provided (equal to the percentage of attempts on which KR is given).

response A term used synonymously with motor skill, especially by those favoring a cognitive perspective of motor behavior.

retention The persistence of improvement in the performance of a skill over a period of no practice; it is interpreted as a measure of learning.

retention interval The time elapsed between the completion of acquisition trials and a retention test in a learning experiment.

retention test A measurement of performance conducted subsequent to acquisition trials and after sufficient time has elapsed to allow any effects of performance variables to dissipate.

reticular activating system A grouping of cells within the reticular formation responsible for general alertness and arousal levels.

reticular formation Area of the brain stem that acts to filter out irrelevant sensory input from further processing activities.

retrieval Processes involved in accessing information from long-term memory into working short-term memory.

retroactive inhibition The interference of newer memories with retrieval of older memories.

rods Visual receptors specialized for detecting movement and subserving ambient vision.

S-shaped performance curve A performance curve exhibiting relatively slow rates of improvement both early and late during acquisition, but accelerated rates of learning during the middle phase of acquisition.

sandwich technique A method of providing augmented feedback in which a negative or punishing reinforcing statement is immediately proceeded and followed by a positively reinforcing statement.

schema A set of rules relating the various outcomes of an individual's actions (e.g., short distance of a throw) to the parameter values the individual chooses in order to produce those outcomes (e.g., small amount of force).

schema theory A theory of motor programs first proposed by Schmidt in 1975 that assumes that motor programs are made up of an abstract set of rules that can begeneralized to control an entire class of actions.

segmentation A part practice method in which a skill is broken down into component parts and the parts practiced separately until some level of proficiency is obtained before practicing the skill in the whole.

selective attention The human capacity for choosing among the many sources of sensory information to which one's attention could be directed.

self-efficacy An individual's belief in his or her ability to master a task or skill.

self-organization The tendency for elements within a complex system to synergistically adapt so that new states or patterns emerge.

self-paced motor skill A commonly used term denoting a closed motor skill.

self-referenced judgments Evaluation of skill performance in comparison to one's previous performance levels.

semantic memory A memory system specialized for holding and operating on information of a generalized factual nature.

sensation Sensory information that reaches the cortex and is capable of being perceived and acted upon.

sensory feedback Information available to a performer concerning the consequences of a practice attempt that is provided directly through the performer's various sensory systems.

sensory memory A memory system specialized for encoding all incoming sensory signals and transferring relevant information to short-term memory for attention and possible action.

sensory neuron One of three major types of neurons, it conveys information about the environment from sensory receptors to the CNS.

serial motor skill A motor skill composed of a series of discrete skills such that the integration of each discrete component into a continuous movement pattern is crucial to performance success.

serial practice A practice schedule resulting in moderate contextual interference in which several different skills are practiced in an alternating but predictable order.

serial-order problem The problem arising in attempting to provide an adequate explanation for how the order and timing of movement elements forming motor skills are organized and controlled.

short-term memory A memory system that holds and operates on information transferred from sensory memory or retrieved from long-term memory; it is under conscious control and capable of operating on only a limited amount of information at a single point in time.

simplification A method of part practice where a skill is practiced in the whole but in which the complexity of some feature of the skill or environment is reduced.

size principle Mechanism for motor unit recruitment where motor units with smallest axons are recruited first and those with largest axons recruited last; the order is reversed in deactivation.

skill A learned, goal-directed activity entailing a broad range of human behaviors.

skill acquisition problem An intellectual or research problem arising in attempting to explain how motor skills are learned.

skill domain A categorical classification of skills possessing similarities specific to cognitive, perceptual, and motor characteristics.

slow-twitch muscle fibers Muscle fibers that produce low contractile forces and that are relatively slow in responding, but capable of maintaining sustained workloads.

social cognitive theory A theory advanced by Albert Bandura that all learning is observational by nature and occurs within a social context.

somatosensory cortex Band of neurons on cerebral cortex where sensory information is organized and brought to perception.

specificity of motor abilities hypothesis (SMA) The notion that motor abilities are not significantly correlated and that a person's percentile rank in one motor ability does not predict his or her ranking for any other motor ability.

specificity of practice hypothesis The notion that the best learning experiences are those that most closely approximate the movement components and environmental conditions of the target skill and target context.

speed–accuracy trade-off The observation that in the performance of many skills an increase in the speed with which the skill is performed is accompanied by a decrease in performance accuracy, and vice versa.

stage of learning Phase in the learning process exhibiting distinct behavioral characteristics; Fitts and Posner have identified three such stages: the cognitive, associative, and autonomous.

state space All of the possible patterns or states that a system is capable of assuming.

storage Retaining information in memory in a nonactive form for later use.

storage problem A deficiency of simple motor program theory based on the notion that a vast memory capacity would be needed to store all of the separate programs for controlling the nearly countless movement skills people are able to produce.

summary feedback The provision of augmented feedback for each practice attempt in a series of attempts, but only after the series is completed.

synapse The site of communication between two neurons consisting of a presynaptic terminal, postsynaptic cell, and synaptic cleft.

synergy A grouping of joints, muscles, and cells that temporarily cooperate in acting together as a single collective action unit; can be assembled and unassembled as the need arises; also called a *coordinative structure.*

system A collection of interacting parts that functions as a single entity.

target context The environmental context in which a person wants to be able to perform a skill as a result of practice.

target skill The task a person wishes to be able to perform as a result of practice.

task complexity The number of component parts of a skill.

task constraint Constraints on human movement imposed by the task performed, including task goals, equipment used, and mandated rules and procedures.

task organization The degree to which the component parts of a skill are interrelated and performance of the whole skill dependent upon their integration.

temporal summation The summation of several postsynaptic action potentials on the contraction of an extrafusal muscle fiber because of the rapid successive firing of a single presynaptic alpha motor neuron.

terminal feedback Augmented feedback delivered after the completion of the motor skill for which it is provided (can be either immediate or delayed).

tetany The maximal contractile force that can be produced by a muscle and that results from rapid frequency of stimulation from presynaptic motor neurons.

thalamus Brain structure just above the hypothalamus responsible for relaying sensory inputs to sensory areas of the cerebral cortex.

theory A coherent statement or set of statements relating a large number of observations into a logical and testable framework; a theory must be open to empirical verification and prediction of future observations within its conceptual area of phenomena.

theory of identical elements The theory that the more similar the elements of two skills of two variations of the same skill are, the greater will be the positive transfer between the two.

trace decay A theory of forgetting that the memory trace fades over time and reverts to its original state; an explanation of forgetting from sensory memory and short-term memory.

trait-centered view of motivation The theory that a person's motivational proclivities and tendencies are the result of genetic factors.

traits Inherited factors that are stable and enduring and that underlie and support activity across the entire spectrum of human behaviors.

transfer The influence of practicing one skill on the learning of another skill or of the same skill in a new context.

transfer test A type of retention test in which the object is to measure the amount of learning that can be transferred to a similar but different skill, or to the original skill in a new context.

transfer-appropriate processing theory The theory that transfer between skills is positively related to similarities in required mental operations shared by the skills.

unit of action A specified component of movement that can be used repeatedly in various actions, producing essentially the same results.

variability of practice hypothesis The notion that the best learning experiences are those that vary the movement components and environmental conditions of the target skill and target context.

variability of practice principle The notion that practicing skills or variations of the same skill in a variety of different ways and contexts has beneficial effects on learning; largely developed as a result of schema theory.

variant feature The aspects of a motor program that change from one

performance attempt to another, including bodily states, environmental factors, and task goals.

varied practice A practice schedule in which the same skill is rehearsed in a variety of different ways.

verbal cue A word or short phrase directing a learner's attention to a critical aspect of skill performance or of environmental factors influencing skill performance.

verbal feedback Augmented feedback that is either delivered verbally or that is capable of being verbalized even when provided in a nonverbal form.

vestibular apparatus Region of the inner ear that provides sense of equilibrium and controls head movements, as well as coordinates head and eye movements; it consists of the utricle, saccula, and semicircular canals.

vestibulo-ocular reflex A reflex initiated by the vestibular system in which head and eye movements cooperate in compensatory actions designed to maintain visual focus on moving targets.

visual dominance The tendency for vision to dominate in the processing of sensory information during the initial stage of learning.

von Restorft effect An exception to the primacy-recency effect in that information presented during the middle of a practice session in a particularly meaningful or dramatic fashion increases the likelihood that it will be learned.

whole practice Practice of a skill in its entirety as it is intended to be performed as a result of practice.

working memory A temporary work space within short-term memory combining incoming perceptions with information from long-term memory.

zero correlation A complete lack of association between two things, such that changes in the value of the first are not accompanied by any predictable changes in the value of the second.

zero transfer When the learning of one skill has no influence on the learning of another skill or of the same skill in a new context.

INDEX

Note: Figures and tables are indicated by *f* or *t*, respectively, following page numbers.